Recent Advances in Neuroscience

Recent Advances in Neuroscience

Edited by Conelth Dickerson

hayle medical

New York

Hayle Medical,
750 Third Avenue, 9ᵗʰ Floor,
New York, NY 10017, USA

Visit us on the World Wide Web at:
www.haylemedical.com

ISBN: 978-1-63241-667-4

Cataloging-in-Publication Data

Recent advances in neuroscience / edited by Conelth Dickerson.
    p. cm.
Includes bibliographical references and index.
ISBN 978-1-63241-667-4
1. Neurosciences. 2. Neurology. 3. Nervous system. 4. Nervous system--Diseases.
I. Dickerson, Conelth.
RC341 .R43 2019
612.8--dc23

Table of Contents

Preface

This book aims to highlight the current researches and provides a platform to further the scope of innovations in this area. This book is a product of the combined efforts of many researchers and scientists, after going through thorough studies and analysis from different parts of the world. The objective of this book is to provide the readers with the latest information of the field.

Neuroscience studies the nervous system to understand the biological basis of memory, perception, learning, behavior and consciousness. Specific areas of the cerebral cortex codes for specific psychological functions. Nearly 20,000-25,000 genes of the human genome find expression in the brain. Also, owing to the plasticity of the brain, the synaptic structures and their functions change throughout life. These aspects present a complex challenge to the understanding of the brain. Recent advances in neuroscience have been brought about by a progress in the fields of electrophysiology, molecular biology and computational neuroscience. This allows better understanding of the structure of the nervous system, along with the way it works, malfunctions, develops and changes. This book is a valuable compilation of topics, ranging from the basic to the most complex advancements in the field of neuroscience. Different approaches, evaluations, methodologies and advanced studies on neuroscience have been included in this book. It will prove to be immensely beneficial to students and researchers in this field.

I would like to express my sincere thanks to the authors for their dedicated efforts in the completion of this book. I acknowledge the efforts of the publisher for providing constant support. Lastly, I would like to thank my family for their support in all academic endeavors.

Editor

Delayed and repeated intranasal delivery of bone marrow stromal cells increases regeneration and functional recovery after ischemic stroke in mice

Monica J. Chau[1], Todd C. Deveau[1], Xiaohuan Gu[1], Yo Sup Kim[1], Yun Xu[3], Shan Ping Yu[1,4] and Ling Wei[1,2,5*] (iD)

Abstract

Background: Stroke is a leading cause of death and disability worldwide, yet there are limited treatments available. Intranasal administration is a novel non-invasive strategy to deliver cell therapy into the brain. Cells delivered via the intranasal route can migrate from the nasal mucosa to the ischemic infarct and show acute neuroprotection as well as functional benefits. However, there is little information about the regenerative effects of this transplantation method in the delayed phase of stroke. We hypothesized that repeated intranasal deliveries of bone marrow stromal cells (BMSCs) would be feasible and could enhance delayed neurovascular repair and functional recovery after ischemic stroke.

Results: Reverse transcription polymerase chain reaction and immunocytochemistry were performed to analyze the expression of regenerative factors including SDF-1α, CXCR4, VEGF and FAK in BMSCs. Ischemic stroke targeting the somatosensory cortex was induced in adult C57BL/6 mice by permanently occluding the right middle cerebral artery and temporarily occluding both common carotid arteries. Hypoxic preconditioned (HP) BMSCs (HP-BMSCs) with increased expression of surviving factors HIF-1α and Bcl-xl (1×10^6 cells/100 µl per mouse) or cell media were administered intranasally at 3, 4, 5, and 6 days after stroke. Mice received daily BrdU (50 mg/kg) injections until sacrifice. BMSCs were prelabeled with Hoechst 33342 and detected within the peri-infarct area 6 and 24 h after transplantation. In immunohistochemical staining, significant increases in NeuN/BrdU and Glut-1/BrdU double positive cells were seen in stroke mice received HP-BMSCs compared to those received regular BMSCs. HP-BMSC transplantation significantly increased local cerebral blood flow and improved performance in the adhesive removal test.

Conclusions: This study suggests that delayed and repeated intranasal deliveries of HP-treated BMSCs is an effective treatment to encourage regeneration after stroke.

Keywords: Ischemic stroke, BMSC, Intranasal, Hypoxic preconditioning, Trophic factors

Background

Stroke is a leading cause of death and disability worldwide with only one FDA-approved drug treatment, tissue plasminogen activator (tPA), in the U.S. [1]. tPA is a thrombolytic agent that may show therapeutic effect acutely after stroke; delayed administration of tPA after its therapeutic window of 4.5 h has increased risk of hemorrhagic conversion [2]. Additionally, a set of exclusion criteria precludes many patients from receiving the tPA treatment regardless of the time window. These may include uncontrolled hypertension, indication of intracranial hemorrhage, seizure at the onset of stroke, and a history of arteriovenous malformation or aneurysm. As another impedance, patients that were asleep during the onset of stroke cannot accurately pinpoint the time of

*Correspondence: lwei7@emory.edu
[5] Woodruff Memorial Research Building, Suite 617, Emory University School of Medicine, 101 Woodruff Circle, Atlanta, GA 30322, USA
Full list of author information is available at the end of the article

occurrence. Thus, it appears necessary and important to develop delayed treatments several hours or even several days after stroke.

Transplantation of cells such as bone marrow stromal and bone marrow stem cells (BMSC) has been explored as a regenerative avenue for stroke therapy [3–5]. The regenerative phase is thought to have a wide therapeutic window. Cells can be transplanted in the delayed phase of stroke, from days to a month after stroke [6, 7]. BMSCs are already clinically used for therapy in autologous and allogeneic transplantation for diseases such as leukemia and sickle cell anemia [8, 9]. Similar to other types of stem and progenitor cells, BMSCs produce trophic factors that are beneficial for the recovery of brain damage. For example, BMSC-conditioned media enhances neurite outgrowth and neurite length in Ntera-2 neurons, demonstrating the paracrine effects of BMSCs in vitro [10]. Adaptive factors released by mesenchymal stem cells include cytoprotective factors (endothelin-1), angiogenic factors (VEGF, Smad4, and Smad7), and pro-migration factors (LRP-1, LRP-6) [11]. Previous studies showed that trophic factors secreted by transplanted BMSCs contributed to tissue repair, ultimately leading to improved functional recovery [12, 13]. An intravenous infusion of BMSC- and BMSC-conditioned media led to neurogenesis and an attenuation of macrophage/microglia invasion in the brains of ischemic stroke mice [14]. Although the exact mechanism remains to be further identified, it is suggested that transplanted BMSCs can serve as vehicles for regenerative and anti-apoptotic factor delivery through their paracrine actions after administration [11].

Endogenous regeneration occurs in the adult mammalian brain through processes such as neurogenesis in which neural progenitor cells are continuously generated in regenerative niches such as the subventricular zone (SVZ). Following ischemic injury, neuroblasts are diverted from the rostral migratory stream toward the ischemic region by chemoattractive factors specifically the stromal cell-derived factor-1 α (SDF-1α) [15–17]. This response appears to be an attempt at self-repair after a CNS injury. However, it is estimated that as many as 80% of SVZ-derived new neurons at the ischemic site die 6 weeks post-ischemia, possibly due to the detrimental cytotoxic effects of the injured environment [18]. Treatments aimed at bolstering this endogenous repair may prove to be a promising strategy for stroke therapy.

There are currently several methods of stem cell delivery for brain disorders: intravenous/intra-arterial infusion, intracerebral injection, and more recently, intranasal administration. Previous studies with BMSC transplantation focused on intracerebral and intravascular routes [19–21]. Even though these studies demonstrate the therapeutic potential of BMSCs after stroke, these delivery methods are either invasive or inefficient. For example, intracranial administration requires a craniotomy surgery and cell injection with a needle or a pipette that can damage brain tissue. Cells delivered systemically have low homing rates to the brain; the majority of cells are found in peripheral organs primarily in the lungs, liver, and spleen following delivery [22, 23].

As a way to bolster transplantation efficacy, our group has reported that hypoxic preconditioning (HP) of BMSCs and neural progenitor cells conveys several benefits [3, 24, 25]. HP increases the survival of transplanted cells in the ischemic heart and brain [3, 25], enhances BMSC homing capacities to the brain infarct region through increased expression of the SDF-1 ligand CXCR4 [3]. Intranasally delivered BMSCs in the acute phase of stroke reduced the volume of the ischemic infarct, decreased the number of TUNEL-positive cells in the peri-infarct region, and improved sensorimotor functional recovery of after stroke [3]. In the present investigation, we aimed to demonstrate that the time window for intranasal administration of BMSCs can be extended past 24 h after stroke. Taken the advantage of the noninvasive nature of the nasal route, we demonstrated that delayed and repeated administrations of BMSCs could be applied for enhancing endogenous regenerative activities and sustainable functional recovery after stroke.

Methods

The experimental timeline is summarized in Fig. 1.

BMSC cell culture

BMSCs were isolated and cultured as previously described [3, 24]. Briefly, GFP-expressing BMSCs were dissected from the tibias of postnatal day 21 transgenic Wistar rats (Charles River Laboratories, Wilmington, MA). Cells were cultured and maintained in DMEM media with 15% BMSC Fetal Bovine Serum (FBS) and 1% Penicillin–Streptomycin to prevent contamination of cell culture. Cells were trypsinized with 0.25% trypsin–EDTA and then deactivated with 15% FBS media before being plated into dishes. After 24 h, non-adherent cells were removed and fresh medium was added to adherent cells. Upon isolation, the BMSC population was characterized via fluorescence-activated cell sorting using cell surface markers CD34, CD45, CD73, CD90, and CD105 (eBioscience, San Diego, CA or BD Pharmingen, Rockville, MD). All cells used in this study were freshly isolated, used at low passages (within 4 passages) when they were 80-90% confluent, and maintained at normoxic oxygen until hypoxic preconditioning.

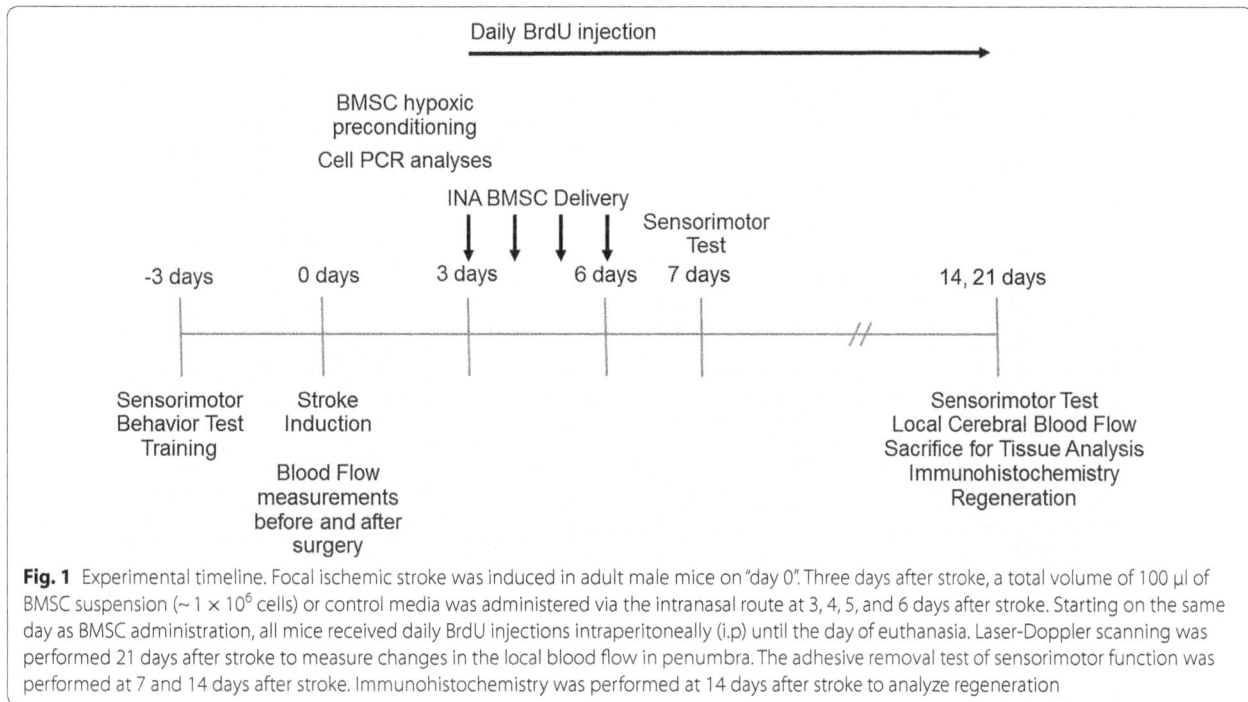

Fig. 1 Experimental timeline. Focal ischemic stroke was induced in adult male mice on "day 0". Three days after stroke, a total volume of 100 µl of BMSC suspension (~ 1 × 10^6 cells) or control media was administered via the intranasal route at 3, 4, 5, and 6 days after stroke. Starting on the same day as BMSC administration, all mice received daily BrdU injections intraperitoneally (i.p) until the day of euthanasia. Laser-Doppler scanning was performed 21 days after stroke to measure changes in the local blood flow in penumbra. The adhesive removal test of sensorimotor function was performed at 7 and 14 days after stroke. Immunohistochemistry was performed at 14 days after stroke to analyze regeneration

Immunocytochemistry

Cells in 3.5 cm tissue culture dishes were fixed with 4% paraformaldehyde for 10 min. The dishes of cells were washed with 1× phosphate buffered saline (PBS) 3 times for 5 min per wash. Ethanol:acetic acid (2:1) was applied for 10 min and washed with PBS. 0.2% Triton-X 100 was applied for 10 min for cell permeabilization and washed out with PBS (3 times, 5 min each). The cells were blocked with 1% cold fish gelatin (Sigma, St. Louis, MO) for 1 h and primary antibodies were applied at a concentration of 1:100 overnight at 4 °C for SDF-1α (MAB350, R&D Systems, Minneapolis, MN), CXCR4 (R&D Systems), VEGF (Millipore, Billerica, MA) and FAK (c-20; Santa Cruz Biotechnology). A secondary antibody (Jackon ImmunoResearch, West Grove, PA) corresponding to the host animal of the primary antibody was applied and incubated at room temperature for 1 h then washed with PBS. Hoechst 33342 was applied at a concentration of 1:25,000 for 5 min and washed with PBS. Dishes were cover-slipped with Vectashield mounting media (Vector labs, Burlingame, CA). Photographs were taken with a fluorescent microscope (BX51, Olympus, Tokyo, Japan).

Hypoxic preconditioning of BMSCs

BMSCs (70–90% confluent) were incubated for 24 h in the ProOx-C-chamber system (Biospherix, Redfield, NY) at 0.1–0.3% oxygen. After 24 h, the cells were returned to normoxic, culture conditions for 1 h of reoxygenation.

Following reoxygenation, cells were either harvested for PCR analysis, fixed for immunohistochemistry, or harvested for intranasal delivery (Fig. 1). Only HP-treated BMSCs were used for transplantation in this investigation; comparisons between HP-BMSCs and non-HP BMSCs have been established where HP benefits were great enough for us to continue the use of HP on BMSC as standard protocol [3].

PCR analysis

mRNA was harvested from the control BMSC and HP-BMSC culture dishes using Trizol reagent (Invitrogen Life Technologies, Grand Island, New York). 250 µl of Trizol was used per 3.5 cm dish of BMSC. The cells were scraped in Trizol and collected, vortexed, and briefly incubated for 5 min to allow for the full dissociation of nucleoprotein complexes. Fifty µl of choloroform was added to the mixture to separate RNA into a colorless phase from the mixture. This colorless aqueous phase was separated into a new tube. One hundred and twenty five µl of isopropyl alcohol was used to precipitate the RNA. The RNA was centrifuged down into a pellet and washed with 75% ethanol two times. The alcohol was discarded and the RNA pellet was dried and resuspended in molecular grade water. RNA concentration was measured (Take3, BioTek Instruments, Winooski, VT).

RNA was converted to cDNA using the High Capacity RNA-to-cDNA kit™ (Life Technologies). Reverse transcription PCR was performed on 1 µg of total cDNA from each sample for control and HP-BMSCs. Each PCR reaction was performed with a mixture of Taq polymerase (New England Biolabs, Ipswich, MA) and its corresponding 10x Taq buffer (New England Biolabs), forward and reverse primers, 10 mM dNTP, water, and cDNA. In particular, we used primers probing for anti-apoptotic and trophic factors. PCR samples were run out on a 1.8% agarose gel with ethidium bromide and visualized under UV light. A list of the factors that we probed for and their primer pairs are listed below alphabetically. All lane intensities were normalized against the corresponding 18S control. PCR gels were captured with a gel imaging system and levels of intensity were quantified with ImageJ.

Primer pairs (5′->3′):

18S (NCBI Accession: NR_003278):
GACTCAACACGGGAAACCTC (forward), ATGCCAGAGTCTCGTTCGTT (reverse)

Bcl-xL (NCBI Accession: L35049):
GCTGGGACACTTTTGTGGAT (forward), CAGTGTCTGGTCACTTCCGA (reverse)

CXCR4 (NCBI Accession: NM_022205):
GCCATGGCTGACTGGTACTT (forward), CACCCACATAGACGGCCTTT (reverse)

FAK (NCBI Accession: JN971016.1):
CAGGGTCCGACTGGAAACC (forward), GTTACTTCCTCGCTGCTGGT (reverse)

HIF-1α (NCBI Accession: AF057308.1):
TGGTCAGCTGTGGAATCCA (forward), GCAGCAGGAATTG (reverse)

SDF-1α (NCBI Accession: BC006640):
GCTCTGCATCAGTGACGGTA (forward), CCAGGTACTCTTGGATCCAC (reverse)

VEGF (NCBI Accession: NM_001287056.1):
CTCACCAAAGCCAGCACATA (forward), AAATGCTTTCTCCGCTCTGA (reverse).

Focal ischemia stroke model of the adult mouse

All animal experiments and surgical procedures were approved by the Emory University Animal Research Committee and met NIH standards. The animal protocol (2001290-021015BN) specifies the housing location of animals in the temperature and huminity controlled rooms in the Emory University animal facility. The justification of using the mouse stroke model and the number of animals were provided in the protocol. The sterile method, surgery proceudres, pre-surgery and post-surgery procedures are specified. The animal monitoring methods for anesthesia, during surgery, after surgery, the sign of pain and infection are specified in the protocol. The post-surgery care including food and water supplies and prevention of pain and infection using antibiotics and analgesic drugs are described. At the endpoint of

experiments, animals will be euthanized using overdose isoflorune.

The sensorimotor cortex ischemic stroke was induced based on previous reports [26, 27]. 8–10 week-old adult male C57BL/6 mice from Jackson Laboratories weighing 26–30 g were used in this investigation. The ischemic surgery procedure was performed following our published method [27]. Briefly, anesthesia was induced using 3.5% isoflurane followed by the maintenance dose of 1.5% isoflurane. Both the tail and paws of the animal were pinch-tested for anesthetic depth. The right middle cerebral artery (MCA) was permanently ligated using a 10-0 suture (Surgical Specialties Co., Reading, PA), accompanied by a bilateral common carotid artery (CCA) ligation for 10 min. This ischemic procedure was suitable and sufficient for the induction of focal ischemia in the mouse brain, resulting in specific infarct formation in the right sensorimotor cortex [27]. Body temperature remained at 37 °C using a heating pad and a temperature-controlled incubator. Three days after stroke, all mice received 50 mg/kg daily BrdU injection i.p. until they were euthanized Fig. 1).

Intranasal administration of BMSCs

BMSCs were treated with HP as described above. Prior to transplantation, HP-BMSCs were incubated in Hoechst 33342 (1:10,000) for 1 h during reoxygenation. The cells were rinsed with PBS and dissociated from the dish with 0.25% Trypsin–EDTA. 15% FBS growth medium was added to inactivate the trypsin and the cell suspension was collected and centrifuged at $1000 \times g$ for 3 min, the media was removed, and cells were resuspended at approximately 1×10^6 cells/100 μl. Three, 4, 5, and 6 days after stroke and 30 min prior to BMSC administration, each mouse received a total of 10 μl (10 mg/ml) hyaluronidase (Sigma, St. Louis, MO; dissolved in sterile PBS) delivered into the nasal cavity (5 μl in each nostril). Hyaluronidase increases tissue permeability of the nasopharyngeal mucosa that facilitates stem cell invasion into the brain [28]. One set of animals was randomly designated as the control group receiving cell culture media (100 μl total/animal) and the other set was given BMSCs (approximately 1×10^6 cells/100 μl). Rat cells were used in this experiment due to the greater yield of cells from rats compared to mice. Five drops containing control media or cell suspension were pipetted in each nostril, alternating each nostril with 1-min intervals.

Tracking BMSCs after transplantation

Six and 24 h after intranasal administration of BMSC, mice were anesthetized with 4% chloral hydrate (10 ml/kg, i.p.) and euthanized once deemed non-responsive. Their brains were dissected out, flattened for tissue sectioning tangential to the surface of the cortex, and mounted in Optimal Cutting Temperature (OCT) compound (Sakura Finetek USA Inc., Torrence, CA, USA) on dry ice. Tissues were sectioned at 10 μm thickness and counterstained with propidium iodide (PI) for nuclear label. Co-labeling of Hoescht 33342 dye positive cells with PI counterstain verified true nuclear labeling of BMSCs in the brain. The peri-infarct area of the cortex was examined for transplanted BMSCs.

Immunohistochemistry and quantification

Immunohistochemistry was performed to analyze neurogenesis and angiogenesis in vivo. Design-based stereology was used when sectioning fresh frozen brains coronally at 10 μm thickness on a cryostat (CM 1950, Leica Biosystems, Buffalo Grove, IL). Every tenth section was collected such that two adjacent tissues were at least 100 μm apart to avoid counting the same cell twice during analysis. Tissues were collected to include the peri-infarct and infarct areas 1 mm anterior and 1 mm posterior to bregma.

Brain sections were dehydrated on a slide warmer for 15 min and fixed with 10% buffered formalin for 10 min. The sections were washed with PBS (1×, pH 7.4) three times and fixed with methanol twice for 7 min each. Slides were air-dried for several seconds then rehydrated in PBS. Sections were incubated in 2 N HCl for 1 h at 37 °C and then washed in borate buffer for 10 min. Tissue sections were permeabilized with 0.2% Triton X-100 for 45 min and washed in PBS three times. Brain sections were blocked with 1% cold fish gelatin (Sigma) and incubated overnight at 4 °C with the following primary antibodies: Ms anti-NeuN (1:200; MAB377, Millipore, Billerica, MA), Rat anti-BrdU (1:400; AbD Serotec, Hercules, CA), and Rabbit anti-Glut-1 (Chemicon Millipore). Slides were then incubated for 1 h at room temperature with the following secondary antibodies: BrdU: Cy3 anti-rat (1:300, Jackon ImmunoResearch); NeuN: anti-Mouse (1:100, Alexa Fluor 488, Life Technologies, Grand Island, NY); and Glut-1 Cy5 anti-Rabbit. Slides were mounted with Vectashield mounting media and cover-slipped and stored at − 20 °C.

Brain sections were imaged under fluorescent microscopy. Six fields per section were photographed at 40x magnification of both sides of the peri-infarct area in the cortex. Six tissue sections of per animal were photographed. The numbers of BrdU/NeuN co-labeled cells and BrdU/Glut-1 co-labeled cells were quantified using the Image J software (NIH). The reported number for each animal is the sum number of NeuN/BrdU and Glut-1/BrdU co-labeled cells in the image sampling.

Local cerebral flood flow (LCBF) measurement

Animals were anesthetized with 4% chloral hydrate (10 ml/kg, i.p.). The skin was incised to expose the skull over the peri-infarct area for blood flow measurement. Laser scanning imaging was performed by Laser Doppler flowmetry [29] (PeriFlux System 5000-PF5010 LDPM unit, Perimed, Stockholm, Sweden) and used to estimate the LCBF. The laser was placed to scan above the right MCA and blood flow was measured by the LDPI program. Blood flow was recorded at the same location at the stroke penumbra before stroke, during, and 21 days after stroke. Values were averaged from 6 repeated readings from each time point for both BMSC and control mice. Quantification of the post-stroke mean intensity values were normalized to pre-stroke mean values to measure the change in blood flow over time.

Adhesive removal functional behavior test

The adhesive removal test was used to evaluate the animal's sensorimotor impairment after an ischemic stroke as previously described [30]. The stroke affects the forepaws somatosensory cortex thus affecting forepaw sensation in this focal ischemia model. Briefly, an adhesive sticker (Tough-Spots 3/8″ diameter, Diversified BioTech, Dedham, MA) was cut into quarters and placed on one paw of the animal. The time required for the animal to remove the adhesive sticker was recorded in seconds. All mice were trained for 3 days before stroke with one trial run per day to ensure that animals were able to remove the adhesive sticker. Animals were then tested 3 days before, 7, and 14 days after ischemia. The time was averaged from 4 trials per animal. Stereotypically, theunimpaired right paw (contralateral to the unimpaired cortex) has a quicker detection and removal time compared to an impaired left paw (contralateral to the impaired cortex).

Statistical analysis

Data was graphed and statistically analyzed using GraphPad Prism, version 4 (GraphPad Software, Inc., San Diego, CA). Data analysis was performed using a student's two-tailed t test for the comparison of the two experimental groups (hypoxic preconditioning PCR, angiogenesis, and neurogenesis data) and two-way ANOVA for multiple comparisons with Bonferroni post hoc tests (Laser Doppler blood flow and adhesive removal test). Changes were identified as significant if p was less than 0.05.

Results

Regenerative factors expressed in BMSCs

Immunocytochemical staining (Fig. 2A–E) and reverse transcriptase PCR analysis (Fig. 2F) revealed that rat

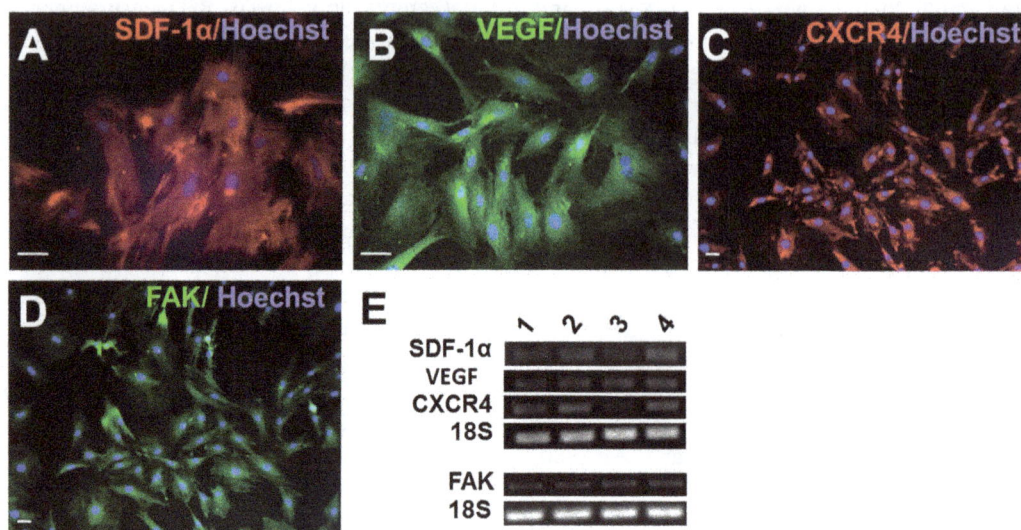

Fig. 2 Regenerative factors expressed in BMSCs. Immunocytochemistry was performed in cultured BSMCs for the expression of several regenerative factors. **A–D** Expressions of SDF-1α, VEGF, CXCR4, and FAK were detected in BMSCs. Scale bars represents 20 μm. **E** Reverse transcription PCR analysis confirms the expression of SDF-1α, VEGF, CXCR4, and FAK in four different batch of BMSCs

BMSCs in cultures expressed several regenerative and migration factors such as SDF-1α, VEGF, CXCR4 and FAK.

Hypoxic-preconditioning increases survival factors in BMSCs

To enhance the survival and regenerative potential of BMSCs, cultured BMSCs were subjected to 24-h hypoxic preconditioning (HP) treatment in a hypoxic chamber of 0.1–0.3% oxygen. To verify that BMSCs were responsive to hypoxia, RT-PCR showed that the HIF-1α expression was drastically higher after HP (Fig. 3a). Bcl-xl is a prominent downstream factor of HIF-1α [31]. The Bcl-xl level was also significantly increased in BMSCs treated with HP compared to control (Fig. 3b).

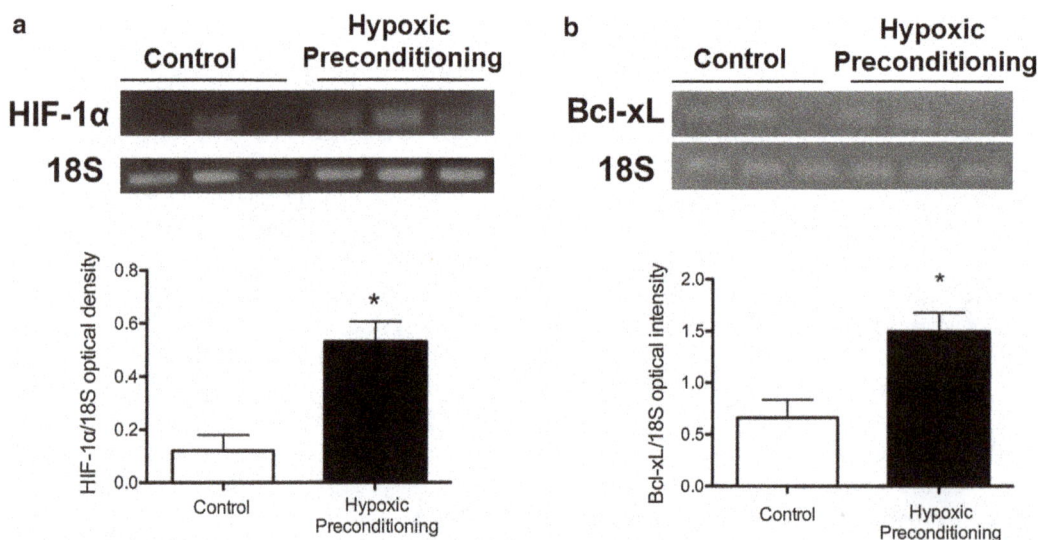

Fig. 3 Hypoxic-preconditioning increases survival factors in BMSCs. BMSCs were subjected to 24 h hypoxic preconditioning (0.1–0.3% oxygen) and 1 h of reoxygenation. RT-PCR analysis was used to detect the mRNA level of two key genes for cell survival, HIF-1α and Bcl-xL. **a** HIF-1α in HP-BMSCs was increased compared to control BMSCs. N = 3, p = 0.013; student's t test. **b** Increased Bcl-xL after HP treatment compared to control BMSCs. N = 3, *p < 0.05, student's t test

Intranasally delivered BMSCs migrated to the peri-infarct region of the ischemic brain

In a mouse model of focal ischemic stroke targeting the right sensorimotor cortex, HP treated rat BMSCs (HP-BMSCs; 1×10^6 cells/100 µl) were intranasally administered at 3, 4, 5, and 6 days after stroke. Transplanted BMSCs were pre-labeled with Hoechst 33342 for in vivo tracking. Due to the well-established and overwhelming benefits of HP, we opted to only use preconditioned cells in this investigation [3]. BMSCs labeled with Hoechst 33342 were detected in the peri-infarct region 6 and 24 h after single BMSC administrations (Fig. 4).

Intranasally delivered BMSC increased neurogenesis and angiogenesis in the ischemic brain

To assess neurovascular regeneration, we quantified NeuN/BrdU and Glut-1/BrdU co-labeled cells in the peri-infarct area of each animal (Fig. 5). In the peri-infarct cortex 21 days after stroke (18 days after the first delivery of BMSCs), there was a significant increase in NeuN/BrdU co-labeled cells (Fig. 5C, D) and Glut-1/ BrdU co-labeled cells (Fig. 5E, F) compared to vehicle-treated stroke controls.

BMSC transplantation increased local cerebral blood flow (LCBF)

The laser Doppler scanning method was used to survey the LCBF at the stroke peri-infarct region before, during, and 21 days after focal stroke [29]. The measurement was taking at the same location over the right somatosensory cortex bordering the ischemic core (Fig. 6a). The mean post-stroke blood flow value was normalized to the mean pre-stroke value. There was a significant increase in LCBF in the BMSC treatment group compared to vehicle controls (Fig. 6b).

BMSC transplantation increased functional recovery after stroke

The adhesive removal test was used to assess sensorimotor deficits in mice 7 and 14 days after stroke induction. In the focal stroke model with damaged right somatosensory cortex, the left paw of the animal is affected. We tested both left and right paws for comparisons. The data

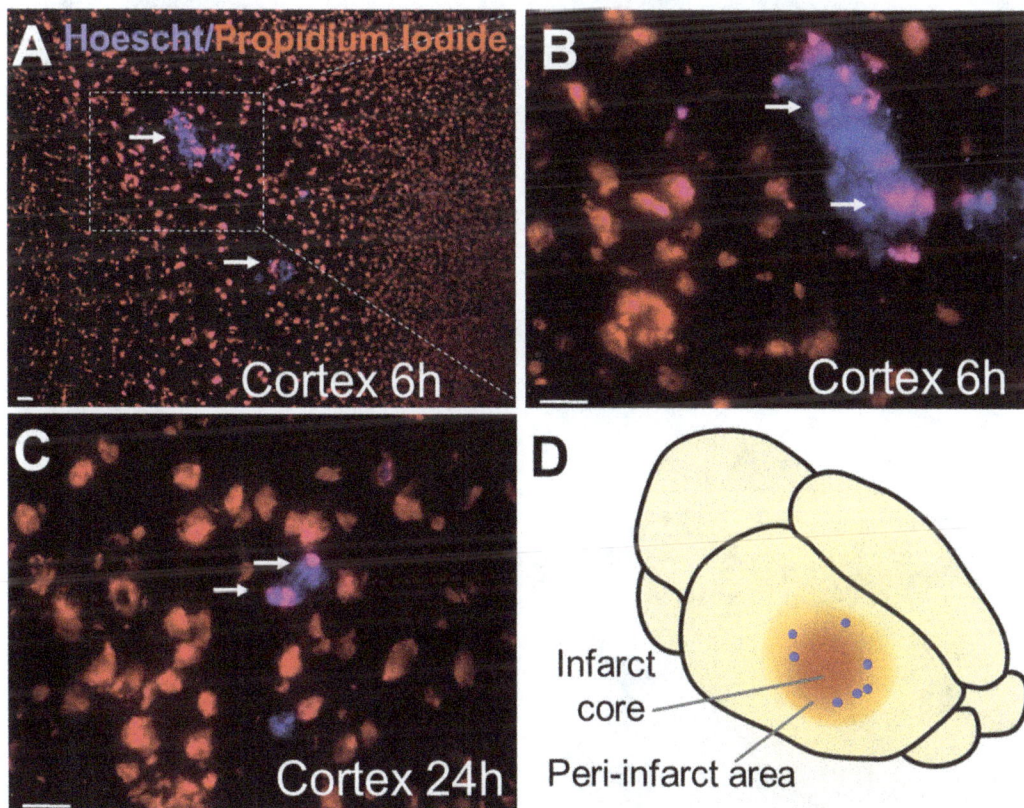

Fig. 4 Intranasally delivered BMSCs migrated to the peri-infarct region of the ischemic brain. **A–C** Brain sections at the stroke penumbra region were collected and analyzed to examine cell presence of BMSCs delivered intranasally. Hoechst-positive BMSCs (blue) counterstained with Propidium Iodide (PI, red) were detected in the peri-infarct area of the cortex at 6 and 24 h after BMSC delivery at 3 days after stroke. Scale bars = 20 µm. **D** An illustration of the mouse ischemic brain where the cells were found in the cortex

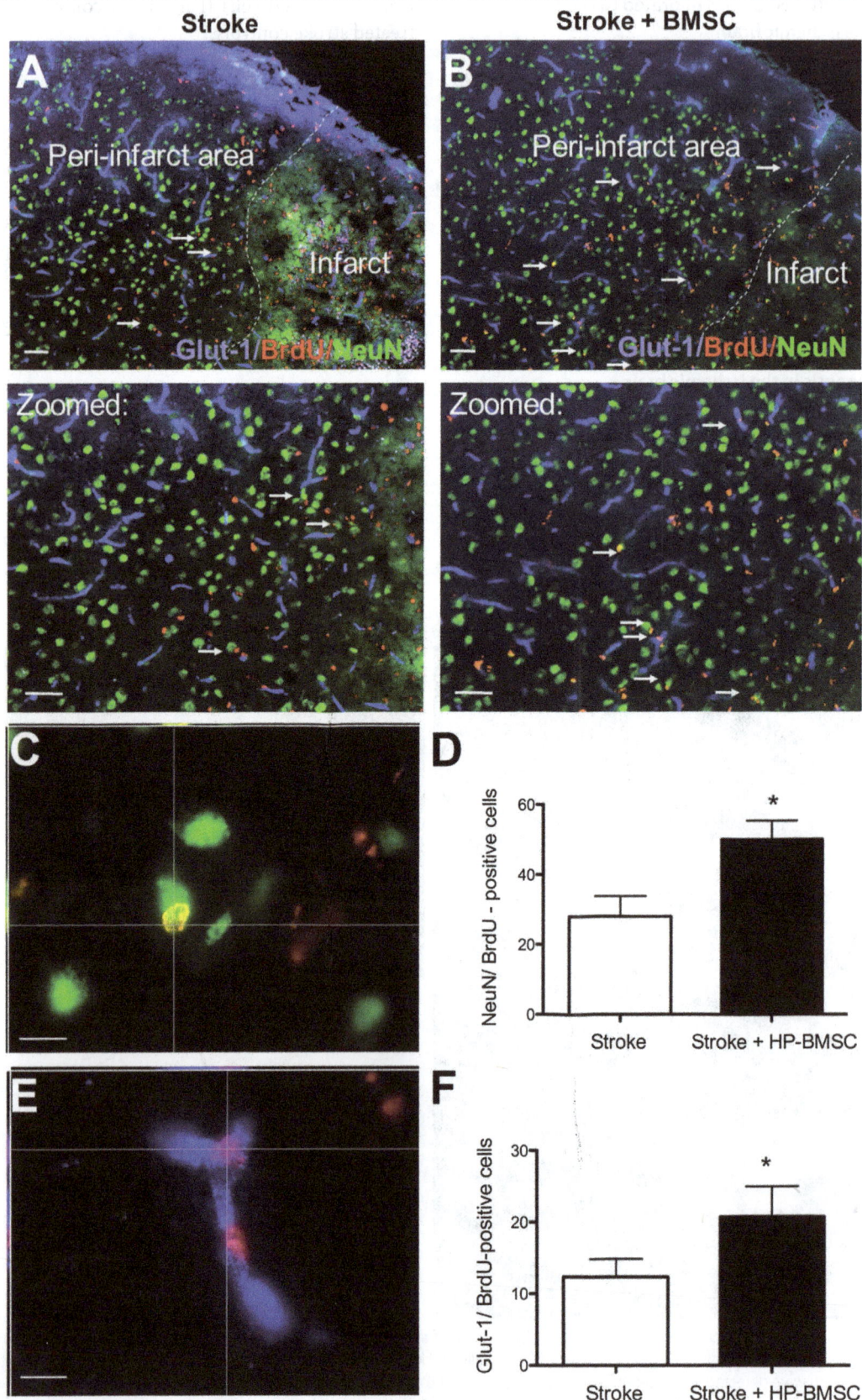

(See figure on previous page)

Fig. 5 Intranasally delivered BMSC increased neurogenesis and angiogenesis in the ischemic Brain. **A, B** Animals were euthanized 14 days after stroke with and without BMSC treatment. Immunohistochemistry stained for BrdU (red), NeuN (green), Glut-1 (blue). Arrows point to the presence of co-labeled cells in the peri-infarct region 14 days post stroke. BrdU/NeuN co-labeled cells indicate the presence of proliferating neuronal cells. BrdU/Glut-1 co-labeled cells indicate the presence of proliferating blood vessel cells. Scale bars $= 40$ μm. **C, D** Enlarged image to show a colabeled NeuN and BrdU cell and the counting result of these cells is shown in the bar graph. There was a significant increase in the total number of NeuN/BrdU co-labeled cells in the BMSC treatment group compared to control. N $= 5$–6, p $= 0.024$; student's t test. Scale bar $= 10$ μm. **E, F** Enlarged image shows Glut-1 and BrdU double positive endothelia cells. There was an increase in Glut-1/BrdU co-labeled cells in the HP-BMSC treatment compared to control. N $= 5$–6, *p < 0.05, student's t test. Scale bar $= 10$ μm

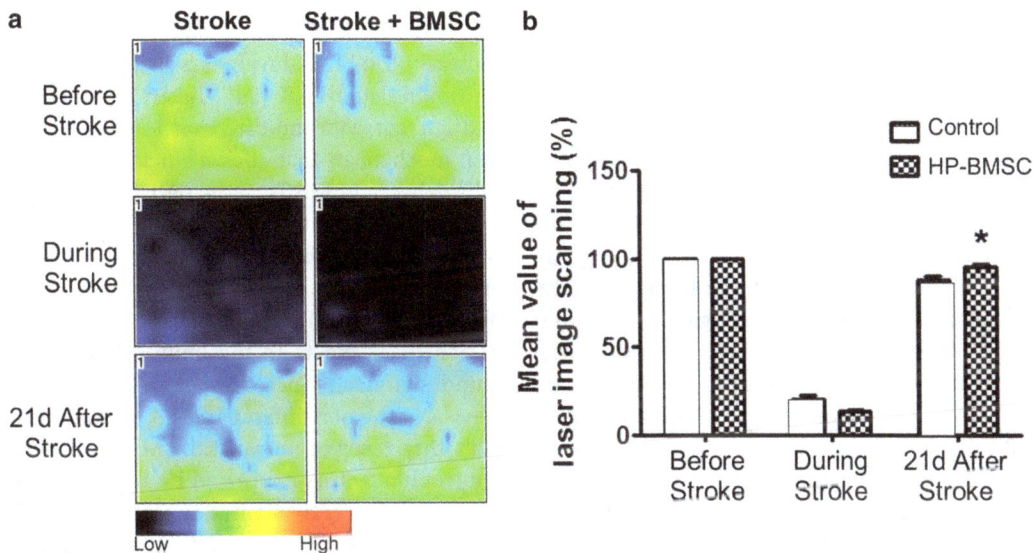

Fig. 6 BMSC transplantation increased local cerebral blood flow. Laser-Doppler blood perfusion monitor (PeriFlux System 5000-PF5010 LDPM unit, Perimed, Stockholm, Sweden) was used to measure changes of local cerebral blood flow in the penumbra. **a** Laser scanned images of the stroke penumbra before, during and 21 days after cerebral ischemia in control and BMSC treatment groups. **b** Quantified data of flow measurement 21 days after stroke show similar flow reduction during the ischemic surgery but better restoration of the local cerebral blood flow in BMSC treatment animals compared to controls. N $= 5$–10, *p < 0.05, two-way ANOVA

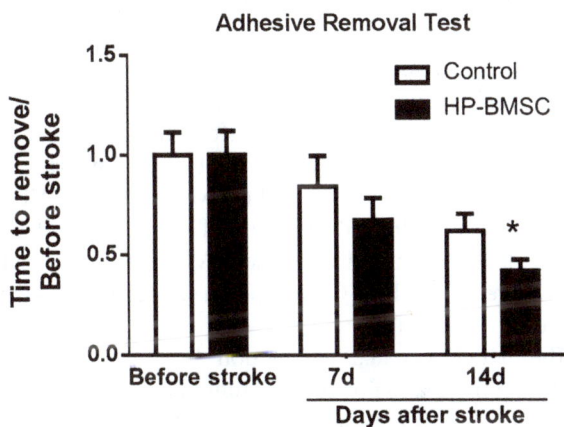

Fig. 7 BMSC transplantation increased functional recovery after stroke. The adhesive removal test was used to assess the sensorimotor impairment after ischemic stroke. The test on both control and treatment groups was performed at 3 days before stroke, and 7 and 14 days after stroke. The BMSC treatment group at 14 days displayed significant improvement (shorter time) to remove the sticky dot compared to control mice. N $= 8$, *p $= 0.0503$, two-way ANOVA

was then normalized to the pre-stroke baseline of each individual mouse to account for the natural variation of their removal times before injury. The BMSC treatment group showed significant reduction in removal time of the left paw at 14 days compared with vehicle-treated mice (Fig. 7).

Discussion

In the present investigation, we demonstrated that delayed multiple intranasal deliveries of BMSCs showed improved vascular and neural regeneration and functional recovery in a focal ischemic stroke model of adult mouse. We confirmed previous findings that BMSCs express several trophic and migratory factors including SDF-1α, CXCR4, VEGF and FAK [24]. These factors play prominent roles in cellular migration, neurogenesis, and angiogenesis [15, 24, 32, 33]. It is predicted that the BMSCs acted as carriers to deliver these factors to the ischemic brain for recovery. As a strategy to enhance the endogenous repair potential of these cells, hypoxic preconditioning was applied as a routine pre-treatment of transplanted cells [3, 34]. Our present study further confirms that HP treatment effectively increases the expression of several pro-survival and pro-regenerative factors in BMSCs, which prime them for greater therapeutic benefits after transplantation.

To be successful in a regenerative therapy, several obstacles must be overcome. One of the major issues of stem cell transplantation after stroke is cell survival after engraftment. Previous studies report that the survival rate of transplanted cells is low, most cells die within 3 days of engraftment likely due to the cytotoxicity from the ischemic environment [35–37]. The timing of stem cell administration may impact graft survival. To maximize transplant efficacy, delayed administration of BMSCs until after levels of inflammatory cytokines have significantly subsided is a feasible approach [38]. To increase the tolerate of transplanted cells to the harsh ischemic environment of the post-stroke brain, we have shown before and in the current investigation that preconditioning BMSCs with hypoxia before transplantation is an effective strategy to increase the expression of specific gene transcripts that are adaptive to low oxygen conditions [39, 40].

The intranasal route can be used to non-invasively deliver neuropeptides and drugs to the brain, but is relatively a new method for cell treatment of stroke [41–43]. It was necessary to demonstrate the feasibility and efficacy of delayed and repeated administration of BMSCs. Intranasally delivered cells can bypass the BBB at the nasal mucosa, pass through the nasal epithelium, and enter the brain via olfactory sensory nerves, such as the trigeminal nerve [28, 42]. It is also possible that intranasally delivered cells can gain access to the CSF and perivascular spaces, further facilitating their transport into deeper brain regions. In the present study, intranasally delivered BMSCs reached the peri-infarct region as early as 6 h after delivery. This is consistent with our previous report showing the ability for the cells to quickly migrate to the brain parenchyma within 1.5 h after intranasal delivery [3].

The homing mechanisms of the SDF-1α/CXCR4 axis and FAK pathways are known to contribute to the migration of HP-BMSCs [3, 44]. SDF-1α is endogenously upregulated in the brain after ischemic injury, forming a chemoattractive gradient that is strongest in the core starting at 7 days after stroke [17]. HP of BMSCs increases CXCR4 expression, suggesting an important role of the SDF-1α/CXCR4 axis in HP-mediated homing of HP-BMSCs to the stroke region [3, 26]. We demonstrate that CXCR4 is expressed in BMSCs, thus these cells can respond to SDF-1α signaling for directed migration toward the lesion site. A previous study of BMSCs

injected into the retro-orbital venous sinus of stroke animals revealed that BMSCs migrated to ischemic region closely associating with reactive astrocytes and vessels expressing SDF-1α [44].

FAK is an essential downstream signaling partner in the CXCR4 signaling cascade. FAK phosphorylation can increase cellular migration. We demonstrated before that HP increased BMSC homing to the stroke site was mediated by the mechanism involving FAK and CXCR4 upregulation [3]. FAK is a crucial protein kinase integrating extracellular signaling and cellular migration [45]. HP increases total FAK levels as well as the activated form of phosphorylated FAK [24]. Taken together, our previous and current data indicate that HP promotes the migration mechanism that allows efficient homing of intranasally delivered BMSCs to the peri-infarct region.

Our goal was to test whether or not delayed and repeated administration of BMSCs could increase regenerative activities after stroke. In the current study, we observed that BMSC transplantation exhibits a number of beneficial effects to the injured brain [3, 46, 47]. We found significant increases in neurogenesis and angiogenesis in the peri-infarct area 14 days after stroke in animals that received intranasal BMSCs. It is thought that the trophic factors expressed by BMSCs played a role in neurogenesis. Transplantation of BMSCs with SDF-1α released into this area may attract more endogenous neural progenitors to the peri-infarct area. VEGF is a major trophic factor for the stimulation of angiogenesis. For example, VEGF increased tubule formation and vessel growth of human endothelial cells (HUVEC) in vitro [48]. In stem cell transplantation, neural stem cells that secrete VEGF increased the neovascularization and overall blood vessel density in the peri-infarct area [49]. Further, neural stem cell transplantation enhances angiogenic pathways with increased levels of VEGF and its ligands [49]. VEGF can be neuroprotective and neurogenic. For example, VEGF was shown to promote neurogenesis in the SVZ and SGZ and endogenous migration of neural progenitors from the SVZ [50]. Mice over-expressing VEGF had fewer neurological deficits and smaller infarct volumes after a stroke [51]. Release of VEGF by intranasally administered HP-BMSCs may play a similar role in facilitating angiogenesis.

The neural-vascular interaction in the neurovascular niche plays a major role for functional recovery after stroke [52]. New neurons must interact with the vasculature for the remodeling process and ultimately for animal functional recovery. We tested the effect of intranasally delivered BMSC on blood flow recovery by measuring cerebral blood flow in the peri-infarct area. Mice that received BMSCs had increased local cerebral blood flow 21 days after stroke indicative of vascular improvement.

This is consistent with the increased angiogenic activity in BMSC-treated mice at 14 days after stroke.

Our stroke model creates an infarct in the forepaw somatosensory area, thus forepaw somatosensation deficits can be evaluated with the adhesive removal behavioral assay. By measuring the animals' time to remove the adhesive from the paw contralateral to the ischemic cortex, we assessed functional improvements after the intranasal BMSC therapy. Animals received BMSCs had quicker removal times of the adhesive dot compared to controls. These behavioral data are consistent with the observed increase in neurogenesis, angiogenesis, and local cerebral blood flow. It is postulated that both neurogenesis and angiogenesis worked synergistically to rebuild the neurovascular unit to allow for sustained improvements in somatosensory function.

Conclusions

We demonstrate the success of repeated administrations of BMSCs, which could increase the number of stem cells delivered to the target site. The time for the regenerative treatment can be delayed beyond 24 h after stroke, which is a clinically relevant therapeutic window for most stroke patients.

Abbreviations

BDNF: brain-derived neurotrophic factor; BMSCs: bone marrow stromal cells; BrdU: bromodeoxyuridine (5-bromo-2'-deoxyuridine); CCA: common carotid artery; CNS: central nerves system; CXCR4: C-X-C chemokine receptor type 4; FAK: focal adhesion kinase; Glut-1: glucose transporter 1; HP: hypoxic preconditioning; HIF-1α: hypoxia induced factor-α; LCBF: local cerebral blood flow; MCA: middle cerebral artery; OCT: optimal cutting temperature; PBS: phosphate buffered saline; RT-PCR: reverse transcription polymerase chain reaction; SDF-1α: stromal cell-derived factor-1α; SVZ: subventricular zone; tPA: tissue plasminogen activator; VEGF: vascular endothelial growth factor.

Authors' contributions

MC performed most experiments, data analysis and wrote the first draft of the paper. She also participated in revision of the manuscript. TCD helped in the experimental design and initiation of the project. XG performed ischemic surgery in mice, YSK participated in cell culture and animal experiments including behavioral tests. YX helped with concept development and data analysis, SPY contributed to data analysis, wrote and revised the manuscript, LW developed the concept, in charge of experimental design and data analysis. She provided financial support to this project. All authors read and approved the final manuscript.

Author details

¹ Department of Anesthesiology, Emory University School of Medicine, Atlanta, GA 30322, USA. ² Department of Neurology, Emory University School of Medicine, Atlanta, GA 30322, USA. ³ Department of Neurology, Nanjing University School of Medicine, Nanjing, China. ⁴ Center for Visual and Neurocognitive Rehabilitation, Veteran's Affair Medical Center, Atlanta, GA, USA. ⁵ Woodruff Memorial Research Building, Suite 617, Emory University School of Medicine, 101 Woodruff Circle, Atlanta, GA 30322, USA.

Acknowledgements

We appreciate the comments and final editing of this manuscript by Myles R. McCrary.

Competing interests

The authors declare that they have no competing interests.

Funding

This study was supported by NIH grants NS075378 (SPY), NS085568 (LW/SPY), NS091585 (LW), AHA Established Investigator Award (LW) and AHA Predoctoral Fellowship Award (MC). This work was also supported by the NIH grant C06 RR015455 from the Extramural Research Facilities Program of the National Center for Research Resources.

References

1. Go AS, Mozaffarian D, Roger VL, Benjamin EJ, Berry JD, Borden WB, Bravata DM, Dai S, Ford ES, Fox CS, et al. Heart disease and stroke statistics—2013 update: a report from the American Heart Association. Circulation. 2013;127(1):e6–245.
2. Zoppo D. Expansion of the time window for treatment of acute ischemic stroke with intravenous tissue plasminogen activator: a science advisory from the American Heart Association/American Stroke Association (vol 40, pg 2945, 2009). Stroke. 2010;41(9):E562.
3. Wei N, Yu SP, Gu X, Taylor TM, Song D, Liu XF, Wei L. Delayed intranasal delivery of hypoxic-preconditioned bone marrow mesenchymal stem cells enhanced cell homing and therapeutic benefits after ischemic stroke in mice. Cell Transplant 2013;22(6):977–91.
4. van Velthoven CT, Kavelaars A, van Bel F, Heijnen CJ. Nasal administration of stem cells: a promising novel route to treat neonatal ischemic brain damage. Pediatr Res. 2010;68(5):419–22.
5. van Velthoven CT, Sheldon RA, Kavelaars A, Derugin N, Vexler ZS, Willemen HL, Maas M, Heijnen CJ, Ferriero DM. Mesenchymal stem cell transplantation attenuates brain injury after neonatal stroke. Stroke. 2013;44(5):1426–32.
6. Shen LH, Li Y, Chen J, Zacharek A, Gao Q, Kapke A, Lu M, Raginski K, Vanguri P, Smith A, et al. Therapeutic benefit of bone marrow stromal cells administered 1 month after stroke. J Cereb Blood Flow Metab. 2007;27(1):6–13.
7. Komatsu K, Honmou O, Suzuki J, Houkin K, Hamada H, Kocsis JD. Therapeutic time window of mesenchymal stem cells derived from bone marrow after cerebral ischemia. Brain Res. 2010;1334:84–92.
8. Walters MC, Storb R, Patience M, Leisenring W, Taylor T, Sanders JE, Buchanan GE, Rogers ZR, Dinndorf P, Davies SC, et al. Impact of bone marrow transplantation for symptomatic sickle cell disease: an interim report. Multicenter investigation of bone marrow transplantation for sickle cell disease. Blood. 2000;95(6):1918–24.
9. Butturini A, Gale RP. Allogeneic bone marrow transplantation for leukemia. Curr Opin Hematol. 1994;1(6):402–5.
10. Oh JS, Liu ML, Jin HL, An SS, Kim KN, Yoon DH. Effect of bone marrow derived mesenchymal stem cell conditioned media for neurite outgrowth in human ntera-2 neurons. Tissue Eng Regen Med. 2009;6(4):562–7.
11. Nguyen BK, Maltais S, Perrault LP, Tanguay JF, Tardif JC, Stevens LM, Borie M, Harel F, Mansour S, Noiseux N. Improved function and myocardial repair of infarcted heart by intracoronary injection of mesenchymal stem cell-derived growth factors. J Cardiovasc Transl Res. 2010;3(5):547–58.
12. An SS, Jin HL, Kim KN, Kim DS, Cho J, Liu ML, Oh JS, Yoon do H, Lee MH, Ha Y. Neuroprotective effect of combined hypoxia-induced VEGF and bone marrow-derived mesenchymal stem cell treatment. Childs Nerv Syst. 2010;26(3):323–31.
13. Chen J, Zhang C, Jiang H, Li Y, Zhang L, Robin A, Katakowski M, Lu M, Chopp M. Atorvastatin induction of VEGF and BDNF promotes brain plasticity after stroke in mice. J Cereb Blood Flow Metab. 2005;25(2):281–90.
14. Tsai MJ, Tsai SK, Hu BR, Liou DY, Huang SL, Huang MC, Huang WC, Cheng H, Huang SS. Recovery of neurological function of ischemic stroke by application of conditioned medium of bone marrow mesenchymal stem cells derived from normal and cerebral ischemia rats. J Biomed Sci. 2014;21:5.
15. Robin AM, Zhang ZG, Wang L, Zhang RL, Katakowski M, Zhang L, Wang Y, Zhang C, Chopp M. Stromal cell-derived factor 1alpha mediates neural progenitor cell motility after focal cerebral ischemia. J Cereb Blood Flow Metab. 2006;26(1):125–34.
16. Kokaia Z, Thored P, Arvidsson A, Lindvall O. Regulation of stroke-induced neurogenesis in adult brain—recent scientific progress. Cereb Cortex. 2006;16(Suppl 1):i162–7.
17. Miller JT, Bartley JH, Wimborne HJ, Walker AL, Hess DC, Hill WD, Carroll

JE. The neuroblast and angioblast chemotaxic factor SDF-1 (CXCL12) expression is briefly up regulated by reactive astrocytes in brain following neonatal hypoxic-ischemic injury. BMC Neurosci. 2005;6:63.

18. Arvidsson A, Collin T, Kirik D, Kokaia Z, Lindvall O. Neuronal replacement from endogenous precursors in the adult brain after stroke. Nat Med. 2002;8(9):963–70.

19. Onda T, Honmou O, Harada K, Houkin K, Hamada H, Kocsis JD. Therapeutic benefits by human mesenchymal stem cells (hMSCs) and Ang-1 gene-modified hMSCs after cerebral ischemia. J Cereb Blood Flow Metab. 2008;28(2):329–40.

20. Shen LH, Li Y, Chen J, Zhang J, Vanguri P, Borneman J, Chopp M. Intracarotid transplantation of bone marrow stromal cells increases axon-myelin remodeling after stroke. Neuroscience. 2006;137(2):393–9.

21. Cui X, Chopp M, Zacharek A, Roberts C, Lu M, Savant-Bhonsale S, Chen J. Chemokine, vascular and therapeutic effects of combination Simvastatin and BMSC treatment of stroke. Neurobiol Dis. 2009;36(1):35–41.

22. Fischer UM, Harting MT, Jimenez F, Monzon-Posadas WO, Xue H, Savitz SI, Laine GA, Cox CS Jr. Pulmonary passage is a major obstacle for intravenous stem cell delivery: the pulmonary first-pass effect. Stem Cells Dev. 2009;18(5):683–92.

23. Detante O, Moisan A, Dimastromatteo J, Richard MJ, Riou L, Grillon E, Barbier E, Desruet MD, De Fraipont F, Segebarth C, et al. Intravenous administration of 99mTc-HMPAO-labeled human mesenchymal stem cells after stroke: in vivo imaging and biodistribution. Cell Transplant. 2009;18(12):1369–79.

24. Hu X, Wei L, Taylor TM, Wei J, Zhou X, Wang JA, Yu SP. Hypoxic preconditioning enhances bone marrow mesenchymal stem cell migration via Kv2.1 channel and FAK activation. Am J Physiol Cell Physiol. 2011;301(2):C362–72.

25. Hu X, Yu SP, Fraser JL, Lu Z, Ogle ME, Wang JA, Wei L. Transplantation of hypoxia-preconditioned mesenchymal stem cells improves infarcted heart function via enhanced survival of implanted cells and angiogenesis. J Thorac Cardiovasc Surg. 2008;135(4):799–808.

26. Li WL, Yu SP, Ogle ME, Ding XS, Wei L. Enhanced neurogenesis and cell migration following focal ischemia and peripheral stimulation in mice. Dev Neurobiol. 2008;68(13):1474–86.

27. Jiang MQ, Zhao YY, Cao W, Wei ZZ, Gu X, Wei L, Yu SP. Long-term survival and regeneration of neuronal and vasculature cells inside the core region after ischemic stroke in adult mice. Brain Pathol. 2017;27(4):480–98.

28. Danielyan L, Schafer R, von Ameln-Mayerhofer A, Buadze M, Geisler J, Klopfer T, Burkhardt U, Proksch B, Verleysdonk S, Ayturan M, et al. Intranasal delivery of cells to the brain. Eur J Cell Biol. 2009;88(6):315–24.

29. Stern MD, Lappe DL, Bowen PD, Chimosky JE, Holloway GA Jr, Keiser HR, Bowman RL. Continuous measurement of tissue blood flow by laser-Doppler spectroscopy. Am J Physiol. 1977;232(4):H441–8.

30. Bouet V, Boulouard M, Toutain J, Divoux D, Bernaudin M, Schumann-Bard P, Freret T. The adhesive removal test: a sensitive method to assess sensorimotor deficits in mice. Nat Protoc. 2009;4(10):1560–4.

31. Chen N, Chen X, Huang R, Zeng H, Gong J, Meng W, Lu Y, Zhao F, Wang L, Zhou Q. BCL-xL is a target gene regulated by hypoxia-inducible factor-1{alpha}. J Biol Chem. 2009;284(15):10004–12.

32. Thored P, Wood J, Arvidsson A, Cammenga J, Kokaia Z, Lindvall O. Long-term neuroblast migration along blood vessels in an area with transient angiogenesis and increased vascularization after stroke. Stroke. 2007;38(11):3032–9.

33. Wang L, Chopp M, Gregg SR, Zhang RL, Teng H, Jiang A, Feng Y, Zhang ZG. Neural progenitor cells treated with EPO induce angiogenesis through the production of VEGF. J Cereb Blood Flow Metab. 2008;28(7):1361–8.

34. Wei ZZ, Zhu YB, Zhang JY, McCrary MR, Wang S, Zhang YB, Yu SP, Wei L. Priming of the cells: hypoxic preconditioning for stem cell therapy. Chin Med J (Engl). 2017;130(19):2361–74.

35. Ishibashi S, Sakaguchi M, Kuroiwa T, Yamasaki M, Kanemura Y, Shizuko I, Shimazaki T, Onodera M, Okano H, Mizusawa H. Human neural stem/progenitor cells, expanded in long-term neurosphere culture, promote functional recovery after focal ischemia in Mongolian gerbils. J Neurosci Res. 2004;78(2):215–23.

36. Park KI. Transplantation of neural stem cells: cellular & gene therapy for hypoxic-ischemic brain injury. Yonsei Med J. 2000;41(6):825–35.

37. Kelly S, Bliss TM, Shah AK, Sun GH, Ma M, Foo WC, Masel J, Yenari MA, Weissman IL, Uchida N, et al. Transplanted human fetal neural stem cells survive, migrate, and differentiate in ischemic rat cerebral cortex. Proc Natl Acad Sci USA. 2004;101(32):11839–44.

38. Wei L, Wei ZZ, Jiang MQ, Mohamad O, Yu SP. Stem cell transplantation therapy for multifaceted therapeutic benefits after stroke. Prog Neurobiol. 2017;157:49–78.

39. Huang LE, Pete EA, Schau M, Milligan J, Gu J. Leu-574 of HIF-1alpha is essential for the von Hippel-Lindau (VHL)-mediated degradation pathway. J Biol Chem. 2002;277(44):41750–5.

40. Ogle ME, Gu X, Espinera AR, Wei L. Inhibition of prolyl hydroxylases by dimethyloxaloylglycine after stroke reduces ischemic brain injury and requires hypoxia inducible factor-1alpha. Neurobiol Dis. 2012;45(2):733–42.

41. Danielyan L, Schafer R, von Ameln-Mayerhofer A, Bernhard F, Verleysdonk S, Buadze M, Lourhmati A, Klopfer T, Schaumann F, Schmid B, et al. Therapeutic efficacy of intranasally delivered mesenchymal stem cells in a rat model of parkinson disease. Rejuvenation Res. 2011;14(1):3–16.

42. Lochhead JJ, Thorne RG. Intranasal delivery of biologics to the central nervous system. Adv Drug Deliv Rev. 2012;64(7):614–28.

43. Hanson LR, Frey WH 2nd. Intranasal delivery bypasses the blood-brain barrier to target therapeutic agents to the central nervous system and treat neurodegenerative disease. BMC Neurosci. 2008;9(Suppl 3):S5.

44. Hill WD, Hess DC, Martin-Studdard A, Carothers JJ, Zheng J, Hale D, Maeda M, Fagan SC, Carroll JE, Conway SJ. SDF-1 (CXCL12) is upregulated in the ischemic penumbra following stroke: association with bone marrow cell homing to injury. J Neuropathol Exp Neurol. 2004;63(1):84–96.

45. Mitra SK, Hanson DA, Schlaepfer DD. Focal adhesion kinase: in command and control of cell motility. Nat Rev Mol Cell Biol. 2005;6(1):56–68.

46. Theus MH, Wei L, Cui L, Francis K, Hu X, Keogh C, Yu SP. In vitro hypoxic preconditioning of embryonic stem cells as a strategy of promoting cell survival and functional benefits after transplantation into the ischemic rat brain. Exp Neurol. 2008;210(2):656–70.

47. Francis KR, Wei L. Human embryonic stem cell neural differentiation and enhanced cell survival promoted by hypoxic preconditioning. Cell Death Dis. 2010;1(2):e22.

48. Bishop ET, Bell GT, Bloor S, Broom IJ, Hendry NF, Wheatley DN. An in vitro model of angiogenesis: basic features. Angiogenesis. 1999;3(4):335–44.

49. Horie N, Pereira MP, Niizuma K, Sun G, Keren-Gill H, Encarnacion A, Shamloo M, Hamilton SA, Jiang K, Huhn S, Palmer TD, Bliss TM, Steinberg GK. Transplanted stem cell-secreted vascular endothelial growth factor effects poststroke recovery, inflammation, and vascular repair. Stem Cells 2011;29(2):274–85.

50. Wang L, Chopp M, Gregg SR, Zhang RL, Teng H, Jiang A, Feng YF, Zhang ZG. Neural progenitor cells treated with EPO induce angiogenesis through the production of VEGF. J Cerebr Blood Flow Met. 2008;28(7):1361–8.

51. Wang YM, Kilic E, Kilic U, Weber B, Bassetti CL, Marti HH, Hermann DM. VEGF overexpression induces post-ischaemic neuroprotection, but facilitates haemodynamic steal phenomena. Brain. 2005;128:52–63.

52. Ohab JJ, Fleming S, Blesch A, Carmichael ST. A neurovascular niche for neurogenesis after stroke. J Neurosci. 2006;26(50):13007–16.

2

Anti-inflammatory effects of minocycline are mediated by retinoid signaling

Vera Clemens[*], Francesca Regen, Nathalie Le Bret, Isabella Heuser and Julian Hellmann-Regen

Abstract

Background: Minocycline is a lipophilic tetracycline of increasing appeal in neuroscience as it inhibits microglial activation, a mechanism involved in numerous neuropsychiatric disorders. Own data point towards retinoid-mediated effects of minocycline in murine brain and skin, and towards a vicious cycle of neuroinflammation which is driven by microglial activation-induced breakdown of local retinoids such as retinoic acid (RA). We therefore sought to study minocycline's anti-inflammatory effects on human microglial-like monocyte-derived cells in the context of retinoid signaling.

Results: As hypothesized, minocycline exposure resulted in a substantial increase of RA levels in the human monocytic cell line THP-1. While pro-inflammatory stimulation with lipopolysaccharides resulted in increased tryptophane-degrading indoleamine-2,3-dioxygenase IDO-expression and TNF-α levels in primary human monocyte-derived microglial-like cells, this effect was attenuated by minocycline only in the presence of retinoids. The anti-inflammatory effects of minocycline on TNF-α expression were completely abolished by a pharmacological blockage of retinoic acid receptors (RARs) using BMS-493 and unaffected by selectively blocking retinoid-X-receptors using UVI-3003.

Conclusions: Our data indicate for the first time a RA-dependent, anti-inflammatory effect for minocycline in human microglial-like cells via inhibition of local RA turnover. The RA-dependent mode of action for minocycline appears to be predominantly mediated through RAR-signaling.

Keywords: Minocycline, Retinoic acid, Neuroinflammation, Microglia, Cytokines

Background

Minocycline is a well-established lipophilic tetracycline and has recently gained much attention in the neuroscience context due to its potent ability to block microglial activation [1–6], a mechanism involved in numerous neuropsychiatric disorders [7] including major depressive disorder [8, 9], schizophrenia [10], autism [11, 12] and Alzheimer's Disease [13, 14].

Being the main immune cell of the central nervous system, microglia are the central actors in neuroinflammation [7]. By synthesizing pro-inflammatory cytokines like IL-1 β [15], TNF-α or IL-6 [16, 17] as well as superoxide radicals [18], this multi-facetted cell type has been demonstrated to affect neurotransmitter metabolism, various

neuroendocrine functions and various aspects of neural plasticity [19]. Under normal conditions, microglia keep brain homeostasis in balance. However, upon sensing pathological stimuli, such as proinflammatory cytokines, alterations in pH or hypoxia, a transformation of the cells, often termed "activation", occurs that may result in a chronically sustained, vicious circle of "sub-threshold" inflammation. This subtle, yet chronically maintained pro-inflammatory condition is discussed to be the neurobiological correlate underlying the neuropsychiatric phenotype [20]. Furthermore, cytokines stimulate indoleamine-2,3-dioxygenase (IDO), the key enzyme of the kynurenine pathway (KP), that degrades the serotonin precursor tryptophan [21], resulting not only in a decreased serotonin synthesis but also in a microglial-mediated increase of the neurotoxic NMDA-receptor agonist quinolinic acid [22]. The kynurenine pathway represents not only a measure for inflammatory stimulation, but furthermore sets an important bridge between

*Correspondence: vera.clemens@charite.de
Section Clinical Neurobiology, Department of Psychiatry
and Psychotherapy, Campus Benjamin Franklin, Charité - University
Medicine Berlin, Hindenburgdamm 30, 12203 Berlin, Germany

neuro-inflammation and transmitter imbalances that are known for several neuropsychiatric disorders.

For these reasons, microglial activation represents a promising target for the treatment of numerous neuropsychiatric diseases. Preclinical evidence points towards an inhibition of microglial activation by minocycline [1–6], and clinical research indicates efficacy of minocycline in schizophrenia [23–27] and major depression [28–32], disorders where microglial activation is discussed as part of an underlying neuropathology. The mechanisms underlying these promising effects of minocycline, however, remain incompletely understood.

While own previous research points towards effects of minocycline on the homeostasis of endogenous neuroprotective and anti-inflammatory retinoic acid (RA) [33, 34], RA itself is known to inhibit microglial activation [35]. Moreover, in the clinical setting, RA exposure appears to trigger CNS side effects similar to those that are known for minocycline treatment, namely an increased intracranial pressure (pseudotumor cerebri; PTC) [36]. The risk to develop PTC can even be potentiated upon simultaneous exposure to RA and minocycline or other tetracycline derivatives [37]. This association had previously led us to hypothesize an interaction between minocycline and RA at the level of local RA degradation, the crucial step in the regulation of local tissue levels of RA [36–38]. Based on these findings, we hypothesized a potential role of RA signaling in minocycline's anti-inflammatory actions.

Therefore, we aimed to assess the potential of minocycline in inhibiting microglial activation with and without the presence of retinoids and therefore to further analyze the role of RA signaling in minocycline's pleiotropic properties.

Methods
Materials
All chemicals were purchased from Biochrom (Berlin, Germany), unless otherwise stated.

THP-1 cell culture
Human THP-1 monocyte cell line (provided by Dr. Ulrike Erben) was cultured in Dulbecco's Modified Eagle's Medium (DMEM) containing 10% fetal calf serum (FCS) and 1% penicillin (100 U/mL) and streptomycin (100 µg/mL). Cells were seeded in 96-well plates at an initial density of 8×10^4 per well and allowed to attach for 24 h.

To assess the inhibition of RA-degradation by minocycline, cells were treated with 1 µM all-trans RA (Sigma-Aldrich, St. Louis, USA) and minocycline (Minocyclinhydrochlorid, Hovione, Loures, Portugal) at concentrations of 0, 10 and 100 µM.

To further investigate the effects of inflammatory activation on RA degradation, and to quantify the impact on minocycline on the latter, cells were treated with 100 ng/mL lipopolysaccharide, a pro-inflammatory stimuli (LPS; *Escherichia coli*, Sigma-Aldrich). Vehicle or minocycline were added at 10 and 100 µM. After an incubation period of 24 h, all-trans RA was added to a final concentration of 1 µM.

Quantification and HPLC analysis of retinoids
For protein denaturation, precipitation and retinoid extraction, 2 vol of acetonitrile (200 µL) were added to each well of the 96-well cell culture plates. Plates were immediately frozen and stored at −80 °C until further analysis. Within 2 weeks, all samples were further processed by thawing plates on ice, followed by transfer to a microcentrifuge tube and centrifugation at 14,000 rpm, 4 °C, for 15 min. 100 µL of the resulting supernatant were transferred to glass vials and subjected to reversed-phase HPLC analysis (Agilent 1100 model liquid chromatography system equipped with a 1290 Infinity diode array detector; Agilent Technologies, Böblingen, Germany). Analysis of retinoids was performed as previously published [33]. In brief, retinoids and degradation products were separated on a Supelco Suplex column (5 µm, 2.1×250 mm; Sigma-Aldrich, Taufkirchen, Germany) using a mobile phase composed of acetonitrile, 2% (w/v) ammonium acetate in water, methanol, glacial acetic acid and n-butanol in a ratio of 69:16:10:3:2 vol. Isocratic elution was performed at a flow rate of 0.65 ml/min and resulted in complete separation of the all-trans RA isomer from 13-, 9-, and 9-, 13-di-cis isomers within a total analysis time of 12 min. All compounds were frequently verified by authentic standards, intra-assay variability, as assessed for the concentration range between 10 and 100 nM was well below 5% CV. Peak purity was monitored by online spectral analysis.

Primary macrophages
Human peripheral blood mononuclear cells (PBMCs) were obtained from healthy controls and prepared by traditional density gradient cell separation using Histopaque (Sigma-Aldrich) and according to the manufacturer's instructions. PBMCs were counted and seeded at an initial density of 5×10^5 cells per well.

To generate microglia-like cells, PBMCs were first grown in RPMI-1640 containing 10 µg/mL human cytokine M-CSF (Miltenyi Biotec, Bergisch Gladbach, Germany), 10% FCS, 1% penicillin (100 U/mL) and streptomycin (100 µg/mL) at 37 °C in 5% CO_2 in a humidified atmosphere. After 7 days, all non-adherent cells were discarded and adherent monocytes were washed in phosphate-buffered saline (PBS) once. Cells were further differentiated in DMEM, also supplemented with 10 µg/mL M-CSF, 1% FCS and 1% penicillin and streptomycin for additional 3 days.

In all subsequent experiments, cell cultures were first treated with a 20-fold stock solution containing either vehicle, all-trans RA, retinol, minocycline or a combination of minocycline plus retinoids at the concentrations resulting in the desired final concentrations of each compound.

Moreover, for all experiments aimed at measuring gene expression changes, cell cultures were supplemented with metabolically competent rat cortex-derived synaptosomes (50 µg/mL). These were added to simulate the metabolic features of a brain-like microenvironment and were prepared from rat brain tissue as previously described [34].

After a 24 h incubation period, pro-inflammatory stimulation was performed by adding LPS to a final concentration of 1 ng/mL. Further analyses were performed 2.5 h after LPS-treatment.

For RA receptor blockage, medium alone, pan-RXR receptor antagonist UVI-3003 (1 µM) or pan-RAR receptor antagonist BMS-493 (1 µM; both from R&D Systems, Minneapolis, USA) were added to the cell culture prior to the addition of minocycline and/or retinoids.

The study was approved by the ethics committee of the Charité—University Medicine Berlin. Written informed consent was obtained from the participants.

RNA extraction and quantitative PCR

For RNA extraction, TRIzol LS Reagent (Thermo Fisher Scientific, Waltham, USA) was added to the cell culture after medium was removed and cell culture was rinsed twice with PBS. cDNA was synthesized using the RevertAid™ RT Reverse Transcription Kit (Thermo Fisher Scientific) according to manufacturer's instructions. Polymerase chain reaction (PCR) amplification was performed using a real time PCR cycler and monitoring of SYBR Green I fluorescence (Thermo Fisher Scientific). Relative gene expression levels in treated samples were assessed as gene expression relative to housekeeping gene expression and relative to the control condition according to the − ΔΔCt method. For each data point, three independent samples were used, and each sample was run in duplicate. The following primers were used: human GAPDH (forward: TTGCCATCAATGACCCCT TCA, reverse: CGCCCCACTTGATTTTGGA), human indoleamine 2,3-dioxygenase (forward: ACCACAAGT CACAGCGCC, reverse: CCCAGCAGGACGTCAAAG) and human kynurenine 3-monooxygenase (forward: GAT GAGGAAGATAAGCTGAGGC, reverse: CTTAAGGTT TCTTCCCCCTCTC). To ensure specificity of the amplified PCR products, for each run a post-amplification

melting curve analysis was performed using the second derivate maximum method.

HTRF cytokine measurements

For measurement of intracellular protein expression, supernatant was removed and cells were lysed in HTRF lysis buffer (PBS + 0.5% Triton-X). TNF-α and IL-6 levels were assessed using the respective HTRF assays (Cisbio Bioassays, Codolet, France), which were performed according to manufacturer's instructions. Assay fluorescence was read on the Clariostar™ HTRF-compatible fluorescence reader (Clariostar, BMG Labtech, Ortenberg, Germany). Cytokine expression levels were normalized to total protein content of each sample. Total protein concentrations were assessed via BCA-Assay.

Statistical analyses

Statistical analyses were performed using the statistical software GraphPad Prism (Ver. 5.04, GraphPad Software, La Jolla, USA). Differences between group means were analyzed via one-way ANOVA followed by Tukey's post hoc test where appropriate. Values are presented as means + standard deviations. P values < 0.05 were considered as statistically significant.

Results

Minocycline inhibits RA degradation in human monocytes

Exposure of human THP-1 monocytes to the tetracycline antibiotic minocycline results in a substantial inhibition of the degradation of RA. RA was added to a final concentration of 1 µM subsequent to a 24 h treatment period with minocycline. After an additional 24 h incubation, RA levels and primary RA oxidation products (4-oxo- and 4-hydroxy-RA) were measured by HPLC. Vehicle-treated monocyte cultures exhibited a high rate of basal degradation of RA, as evidenced by decreasing RA levels and increasing levels of oxidation products. Treatment with minocycline effectively blocked this process in a concentration dependent manner (Fig. 1).

Following up on own previous findings in murine microglia on inflammation-induced increase in RA-turnover [39], we sought to assess the same in human monocytic cells and to investigate the effects of minocycline on inflammation-induced RA-turnover. Minocycline- or vehicle-pretreated human monocytic cells were exposed to vehicle or LPS and allowed to degrade RA (1 µM) over a period of 24 h. RA levels were determined in cell culture supernatants after the incubation period, revealing a strong, concentration-dependent effect of minocycline in blocking the LPS-induced increase in RA turnover (Fig. 2).

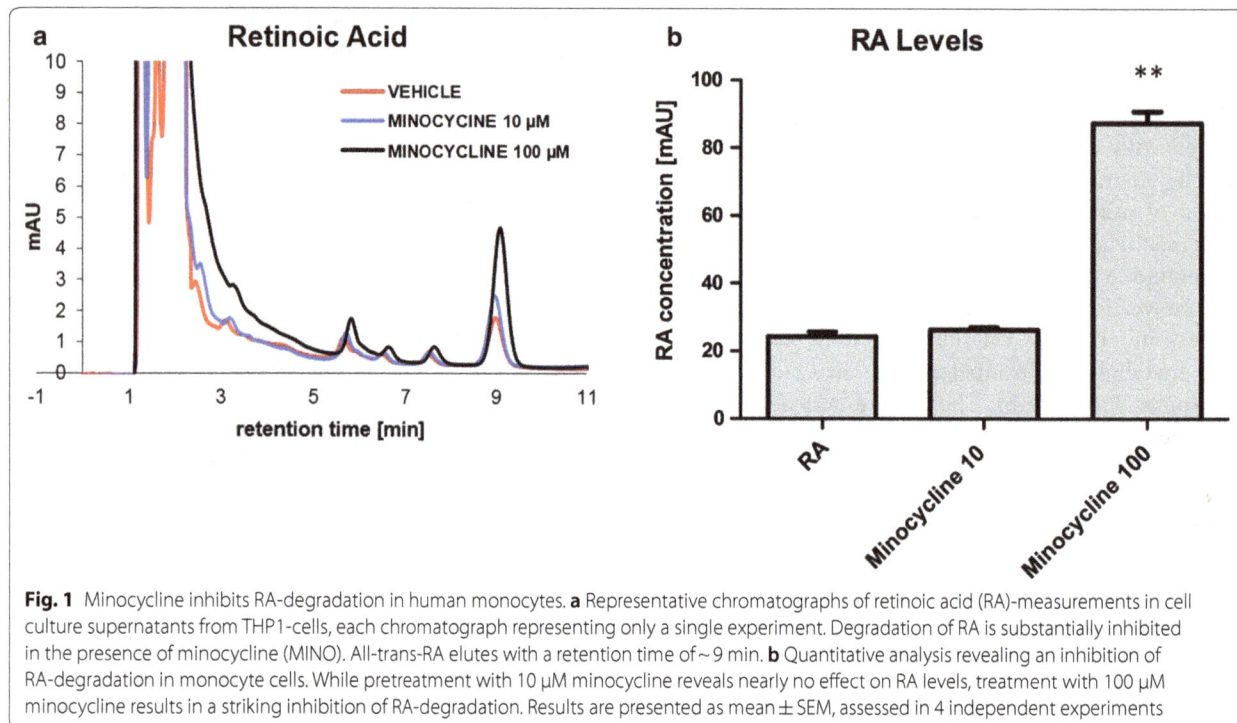

Fig. 1 Minocycline inhibits RA-degradation in human monocytes. **a** Representative chromatographs of retinoic acid (RA)-measurements in cell culture supernatants from THP1-cells, each chromatograph representing only a single experiment. Degradation of RA is substantially inhibited in the presence of minocycline (MINO). All-trans-RA elutes with a retention time of ~9 min. **b** Quantitative analysis revealing an inhibition of RA-degradation in monocyte cells. While pretreatment with 10 μM minocycline reveals nearly no effect on RA levels, treatment with 100 μM minocycline results in a striking inhibition of RA-degradation. Results are presented as mean ± SEM, assessed in 4 independent experiments

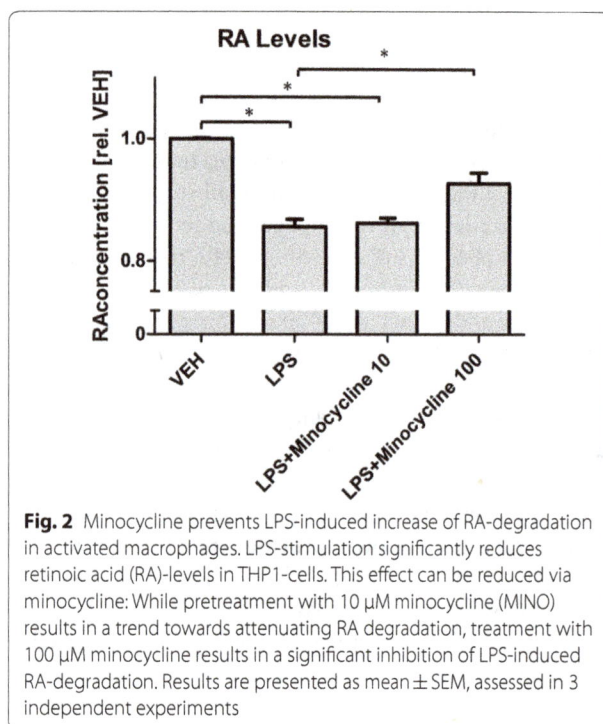

Fig. 2 Minocycline prevents LPS-induced increase of RA-degradation in activated macrophages. LPS-stimulation significantly reduces retinoic acid (RA)-levels in THP1-cells. This effect can be reduced via minocycline: While pretreatment with 10 μM minocycline (MINO) results in a trend towards attenuating RA degradation, treatment with 100 μM minocycline results in a significant inhibition of LPS-induced RA-degradation. Results are presented as mean ± SEM, assessed in 3 independent experiments

Minocycline-induced inhibition of IDO expression is retinoid-dependent

In order to assess a role for retinoid signaling in

minocycline's anti-inflammatory effects, we next examined the effects of minocycline on LPS-induced activation in the presence and absence of retinoids. We chose to quantify the expression of indoleamine-dioxygenase (IDO) and Kynurenine 3-monooxygenase (KMO) as relevant inflammation-associated enzymes that additionally play a key role in the kynurenine pathway, a process potentially related to the neuropsychiatric aftermath of chronically activated microglial cells.

As demonstrated in Fig. 3, LPS-induced activation of human monocytic, microglial-like cells results in a robust increase of kynurenine pathway-related enzymes IDO and KMO, with a statistically significant increase for IDO and a trend towards increased expression for KMO (Fig. 3). Interestingly, pretreatment with both, retinol and minocycline alone resulted in an overall increased IDO and KMO expression with a stronger increase for minocycline, an effect that was more pronounced for IDO than for KMO expression. The combined treatment with minocycline and retinol, however, resulted in a striking, statistically significant decrease in IDO, and a slight trend towards reduced expression also for the KMO.

Minocycline-induced inhibition of proinflammatory cytokines is retinoid-dependent

To assess whether the retinoid-dependent effects of minocycline on IDO expression may extend to more general, and functionally more relevant pro-inflammatory

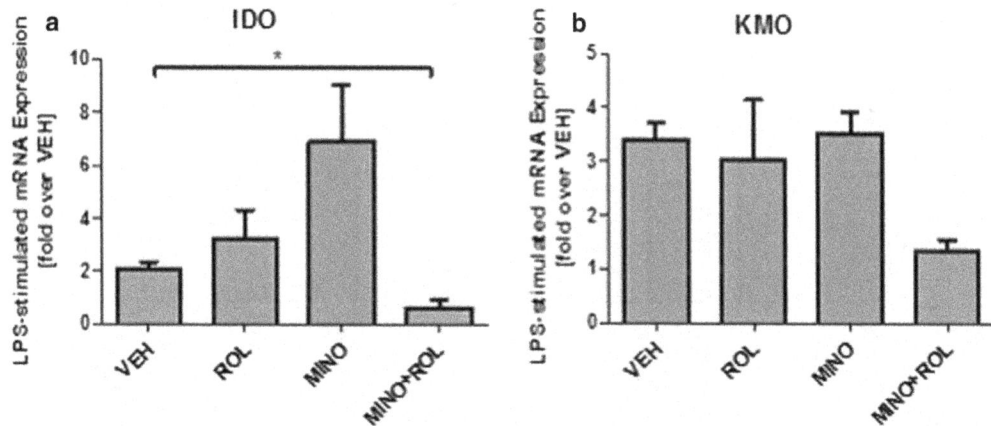

Fig. 3 Expression of IDO and KMO after LPS-induced pro-inflammatory stimulation of human microglial-like cells. LPS induces an increase of the expression of the kynurenine pathway-enzymes IDO (**a**) and KMO (**b**). Minocycline (MINO) potently inhibits stimulation of indoleamine-2,3-dioxygenase (IDO) expression only in the presence of retinol (ROL) (**a**). For Kynurenine-3-monooxygenase (KMO), the same trend can be observed, however reaching no statistical significance (**b**). Results are given as fold over vehicle (VEH), mRNA expression was calculated relative to GAPDH housekeeping gene expression (ΔΔCT-Method). Results are presented as means +/- SEM from 4 healthy controls, assessed in 4 independent experiments

processes, we next studied the protein expression of the proinflammatory cytokines TNF-α and IL-6 using the same cell culture model based on human primary microglial-like monocytes.

As expected, LPS treatment resulted in significantly increased cytokine levels of both, TNF-α and IL-6. Surprisingly, however, no inhibitory effect of minocycline, neither with nor without retinoids was observed (Fig. 4a, c). Based on the hypothesis that minocycline may promote its medium- to long-term anti-inflammatory actions indirectly via attenuating the homeostatic process of constant degradation of intracellular RA, we systematically added metabolically competent synaptosomal preparations from rat brain as a natural source of RA-degrading enzymes to cell culture media.

After the supplementation of cell culture media with synaptosomal preparations, co-treatment with minocycline and retinol again resulted in decreased TNF-α and IL-6 levels, while minocycline alone exhibited no influence on cytokine expression (Fig. 4b, d). Treatment with retinol alone resulted in a significant decrease of TNF-α expression (Fig. 4b). For IL-6 expression, without reaching statistical significance, the same trend was observed (Fig. 4d).

Minocycline's anti-inflammatory effects are mediated through RAR signaling

In order to identify the receptors involved in contributing to the anti-inflammatory effects of minocycline, we used a pharmacological approach based on the two well-established inhibitors of the two major retinoid receptors, the retinoic acid receptors (RAR) and the retinoid-X-receptors (RXR).

Using TNF-α protein levels as primary outcome parameter, human microglial-like cells were again treated with minocycline, retinoids and LPS as before, but prior to the addition of minocycline/retinoids, cells were treated either with the pan-RXR antagonist UVI-3003 (UVI) or the pan-RAR antagonist BMS-493 (BMS). Interestingly, pre-treatment with UVI remained without effect on the anti-inflammatory actions of minocycline + retinoids, and basically led to the same results that were seen in absence of the antagonist. Conversely, treatment with the pan-RAR antagonist BMS completely blocked the inhibitory effect of minocycline and RA (Fig. 5).

Discussion

The potential contribution of microglia-driven neuroinflammation to the pathogenesis of neuropsychiatric disorders gains more and more attention, and so are strategies that are aimed to specifically target this process. While microglial activation has been reported in a plethora of neuropsychiatric disorders, is appears to specifically play a role in those disorders that have been demonstrated to be associated, and hypothesised to be triggered by, chronic inflammatory processes. This has mainly been shown for primarily neurodegenerative Alzheimer's disease, but also for major depressive disorder (MDD) and for negative symptoms in schizophrenia [23–32]. In MDD, an inflammatory pathogenesis is

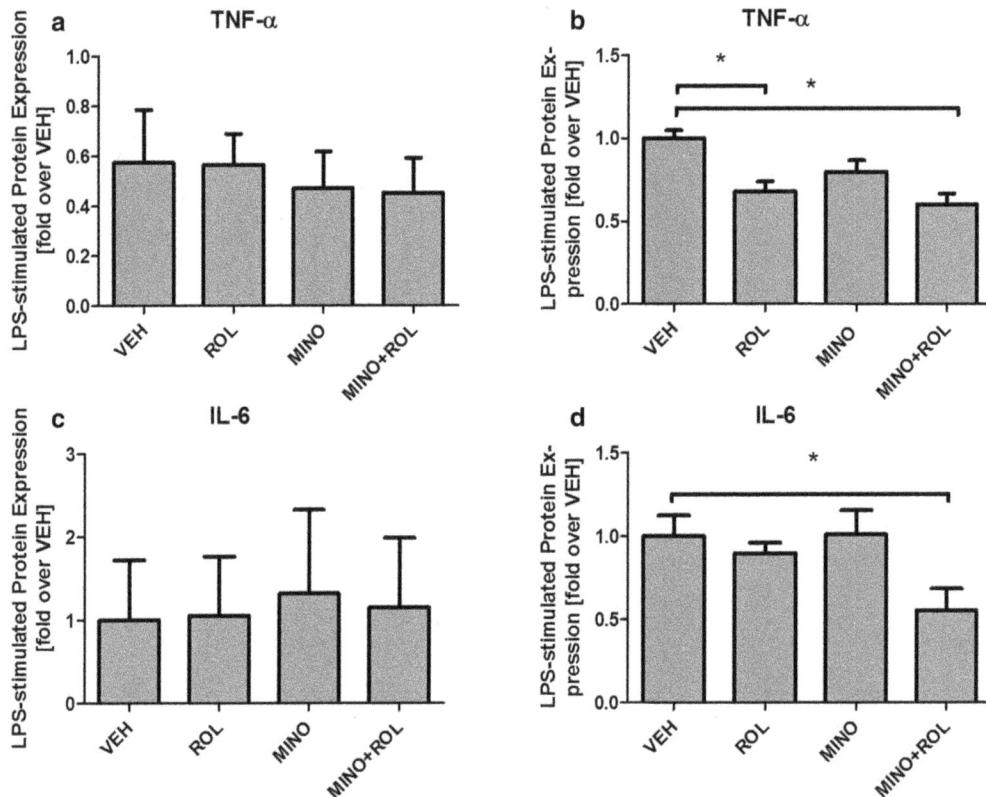

Fig. 4 TNF-α and IL-6 synthesis after LPS-induced pro-inflammatory stimulation of human microglial-like cells. LPS-stimulated cytokine expression of human microglial-like cells: Minocycline inhibits the synthesis of pro-inflammatory cytokines TNF-α (**a**, **b**) and IL-6 (**c**, **d**) only in combination with retionids. Cytokine levels are presented relative to protein concentration. Tested conditions included vehicle (VEH), retinol (ROL), minocycline (MINO) and a combination of ROL and MINO, given as differences between LPS-stimulated and the unstimulated conditions. Values are given as mean ± SEM from at least four healthy controls in independent experiments

specifically hypothesized for those subjects that appear to be "treatment refractory" [17], so that novel strategies are warranted for both, diagnostic and therapeutic approaches.

Interestingly minocycline, a well-established tetracycline antibiotic, is also known from preclinical studies in rodents to act as a potent inhibitor of (chronic) microglial activation. Minocycline still enjoys great popularity in anti-acne therapy, likely for reasons of pleiotropic, anti-inflammatory actions [33], and also in other indications such as rheumatoid arthritis, minocycline treatment is discussed as an alternative treatment strategy in certain clinically severe cases [40].

With respect to possibly microglia-mediated neuropsychiatric conditions such as negative symptoms in schizophrenia, there is first evidence from controlled clinical trials, suggesting efficacy of minocycline [41] and our own clinical trial on the efficacy of minocycline in otherwise "treatment-resistant major depression" is currently ongoing (Clintrials.org ID: NCT02456948). We have previously demonstrated a link between

minocycline's mode of action and retinoid signaling [33, 34, 42].

While minocycline can readily block the degradation of RA in murine skin and brain tissue [33, 34], this mechanism has never been studied in human tissue before, and, more importantly, the suggestive evidence pointing towards a role for this mechanism in minocycline's anti-inflammatory actions has not been investigated before. Additionally, most research on minocycline's anti-inflammatory mechanisms has been conducted in non-primate cell systems.

RA is a CNS morphogen that is not only crucial for brain development, but also known to inhibit microglial activation [39] and neuro-inflammation [35, 43]. RA is a potent neuroprotective agent and known to play a key role in synaptic scaling [44]. Synaptic scaling is one of the major synaptic plasticity-associated mechanisms in the adult brain. In sum, all of these mechanisms are known to be affected in neuropsychiatric disorders. Moreover, there is a large body of direct evidence for an involvement of retinoid signaling in the

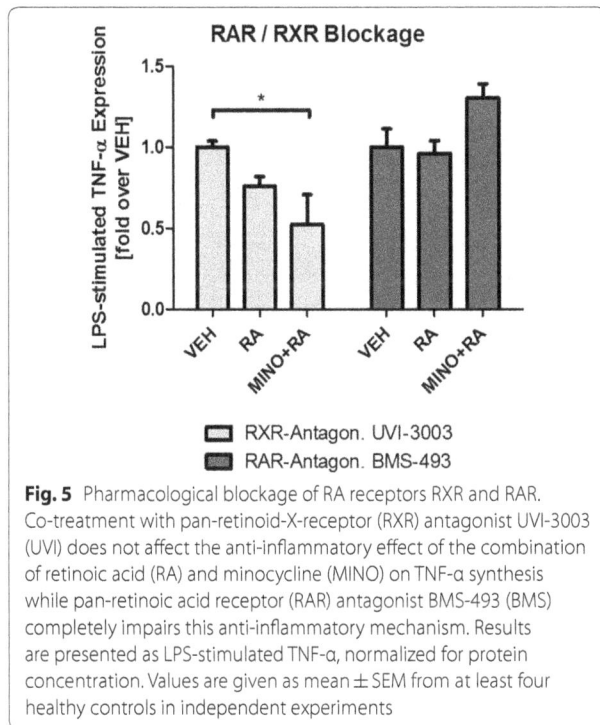

Fig. 5 Pharmacological blockage of RA receptors RXR and RAR. Co-treatment with pan-retinoid-X-receptor (RXR) antagonist UVI-3003 (UVI) does not affect the anti-inflammatory effect of the combination of retinoic acid (RA) and minocycline (MINO) on TNF-α synthesis while pan-retinoic acid receptor (RAR) antagonist BMS-493 (BMS) completely impairs this anti-inflammatory mechanism. Results are presented as LPS-stimulated TNF-α, normalized for protein concentration. Values are given as mean ± SEM from at least four healthy controls in independent experiments

pathogenesis of affective [45] and of other neuropsychiatric disorders [46], suggesting that local brain RA may function as an "endogenous antidepressant". Furthermore, the catabolism of RA [47] is inhibited by the widely-used and well-established antidepressant fluoxetine, suggesting that fluoxetine's neuroprotective, its anti-inflammatory—and potentially its anti-depressant properties may all together be mediated through RA signaling [48].

For the very first time, our data show a significant inhibition of RA degradation by minocycline in human monocytic THP-1 cells. Own previous data revealed the same effect of minocycline in human SH-SY5Y neuroblastoma cells [33, 34], underlining the hypothesis that neuroprotective and anti-inflammatory RA may be the "effector" for minocycline's pleiotropic anti-inflammatory actions. Furthermore, our results reveal that inflammatory stimulation with LPS leads to an enhanced RA-degradation and consequently lower RA-levels in monocytes. Based on previous findings in other tissues such as murine microglial cells, this mechanism was not completely unexpected [39]. Finding the same effects in human cells, however, suggests that degradation of local RA may be a significant contributor to a pro-inflammatory microenvironment. With our demonstration of minocycline significantly blocking the inflammation-enhanced RA catabolism, we have identified a mechanism that might underlie minocycline's pleiotropic

effects, namely its inhibition of monocytic/microglial activation.

Subsequent experiments were thus designed to functionally assess an involvement of retinoid signaling in minocycline's anti-inflammatory mechanisms in the human cell culture system. Pro-inflammatory conditions were simulated by using the established stimulation of cell cultures with LPS. As a readout, we chose key pro-inflammatory cytokines and enzymes of the kynurenine-pathway, a pathway that may be considered a central, inflammation-responsive pathway in activated brain macrophages. As a cellular model, we used primary human monocyte-derived macrophages that were differentiated using a set of selected cytokines, into more mature macrophages closely resembling the differentiation state of microglia. While most microglial cells in the adult CNS are thought to be derived from primitive yolk sac macrophages that have entered the brain during the embryologic period [49], microglia-like cells are also recruited from circulating monocytes [50] and continue to express numerous macrophagal receptors [51]. This makes patient specific macrophages an appealing model for studying the various aspects of monocytic/microglial cells that are claimed to be associated with psychiatric disorders. The use of peripheral monocytic cells and subsequent differentiation exhibits the advantage of easy accessibility and full genetic as well as epigenetic background of the patient. Nevertheless, it has to be pointed out that this is an in vitro model. Even though many physiological processes can be studied at a patient-specific level in vitro, there are numerous limitations to in vitro versus in vivo studies. A specific limitation concerns the cell line that was used to carry out the retinoid metabolism assays. This cell line certainly differs from the primary cells that were used for studying the inflammatory responses. Retinoid metabolism assays, however, only require intact human enzymes, for which the selected cell line represents an excellent source.

Our data reveal that LPS robustly induces the expression of IDO and KMO, the key enzymes in the kynurenine pathway, as well as inflammatory cytokine levels of TNF-α and IL-6, processes that have been associated with the pathogenesis of various neuro-inflammatory processes [7], and that have been linked to the pathogenesis of several neuropsychiatric diseases. TNF-α is known to be increased in anxiety disorder [52], posttraumatic stress disorder [53, 54] and major depression, where TNF-α and IL-6 are also associated with a smaller chance to respond to treatment with SSRIs [55]. Treatment with LPS, on the other hand, results in sickness behaviour that in many aspects resembles depressive symptoms [56], again pointing towards the relevance of these neuro-inflammatory processes. Pharmacological blockage of RAR/RXR retinoid receptors revealed that minocycline's anti-inflammatory effects are likely mediated via RAR-receptors, since blockage of RXR receptors remained without effect, blockage of RAR-receptors however completely impaired minocycline's anti-inflammatory effects as assessed by measuring TNF-α expression after LPS-stimulation.

The end product of microglial kynurenine pathway, quinolinic acid, is not only known to be a neurotoxic NMDA-receptor agonist [22] but furthermore to be elevated in the cerebrospinal fluid of suicide victims [57]. Cytokines [58] and LPS [59, 60] are known to induce key enzymes of the kynurenine pathway, resulting in increased quinolinic acid levels. Based on these findings, microglial activation is an interesting target for future treatment strategies in neuropsychiatric diseases [49] and minocycline is one promising substance to target this mechanism [61]. Nevertheless, despite the promising results of minocycline to inhibit microglial activation in in vivo models [1–6], our results reveal that minocycline alone does not inhibit LPS-stimulated increased IDO and KMO expression and cytokine levels, but requires the presence of retinoids to exert its anti-inflammatory actions. Furthermore, inhibitory effects of retinoids and minocycline were dependent on the presence of synaptosomal preparations in the assay. Based on previous findings of minocycline affecting RA metabolism [33–35], the added synaptosomal preparations represented the source of RA metabolism in the assay. This way we were able to precisely control for retinoid metabolism, indirectly demonstrating that the magnitude of minocycline's anti-inflammatory effects was indeed dependent on the presence of RA metabolic enzymes.

Conclusions

Taken together, our data suggest that retinoids may be required for minocycline's anti-inflammatory effects on human microglial-like cells in vitro. Furthermore, our data may point towards an inhibition of local RA turnover and consequently increased levels of anti-inflammatory RA as the underlying mechanism. The RA-dependent mode of action for minocycline appears to be predominantly mediated through RAR-signaling.

Abbreviations
BMS: BMS-493; DMEM: Dulbecco's modified Eagle's medium; FCS: fetal calf serum; IDO: indoleamine-2,3-dioxygenase; KMO: kynurenine 3-monooxygenase; LPS: lipopolysaccharide; MDD: major depressive disorder; PBMC: peripheral blood mononuclear cells; PTC: pseudotumor cerebri; RA: retinoic acid; RAR: retinoic acid receptor; RXR: retinoid-X-receptor; UVI: UVI-3003.

Acknowledgements
We thank the healthy volunteers for participation and Mrs. Meike Terborg and Mrs. Rita Benz for their technical support.

Authors' contributions
VC carried out most of the experiments and performed analysis of data, drafted and revised the manuscript. FR contributed to analyses and interpretation of data and revised the manuscript. NLB contributed to the experiments and revised the manuscript. IH contributed to the interpretation of data and the revision of the manuscript. JHR participated in the design, data-collection and coordination of the study and contributed to the revision of the manuscript. All authors read and approved the final manuscript.

Competing interests
The authors declare that they have no competing interests.

Funding
JHR is participant in the Charité Clinical Scientist Program funded by the Charité Universitätsmedizin Berlin and the Berlin Institute of Health. This work was further supported by the Deutsche Forschungsgemeinschaft (Grand No. he 6939) and the Bundesministerium für Bildung und Forschung (Grand No. 01EE1401F). Funding was used for acquisition of material. The funding by no means had any influence on the design of the study and collection, analysis, and interpretation of data and in writing the manuscript.

References
1. Levkovitz Y, Levi U, Braw Y, Cohen H. Minocycline, a second-generation tetracycline, as a neuroprotective agent in an animal model of schizophrenia. Brain Res. 2007;1154:154–62.
2. Levkovitz Y, Fenchel D, Kaplan Z, Zohar J, Cohen H. Early post-stressor intervention with minocycline, a second-generation tetracycline, attenuates post-traumatic stress response in an animal model of PTSD. Eur Neuropsychopharmacol. 2015;25:124–32.
3. Tikka TM, Koistinaho JE. Minocycline provides neuroprotection against N-methyl-D-aspartate neurotoxicity by inhibiting microglia. J Immunol. 2001;166:7527–33.
4. Yang Y, Salayandia VM, Thompson JF, Yang LY, Estrada EY, Yang Y. Attenuation of acute stroke injury in rat brain by minocycline promotes blood-brain barrier remodeling and alternative microglia/macrophage activation during recovery. J Neuroinflammation. 2015;12:26.
5. Seki Y, Kato TA, Monji A, Mizoguchi Y, Horikawa H, Sato-Kasai M, Yoshiga D, Kanba S. Pretreatment of aripiprazole and minocycline, but not haloperidol, suppresses oligodendrocyte damage from interferon-gamma-stimulated microglia in co-culture model. Schizophr Res. 2013;151:20–8.
6. Yune TY, Lee JY, Jung GY, Kim SJ, Jiang MH, Kim YC, Oh YJ, Markelonis GJ, Oh TH. Minocycline alleviates death of oligodendrocytes by inhibiting pro-nerve growth factor production in microglia after spinal cord injury. J Neurosci. 2007;27:7751–61.

7. Reus GZ, Fries GR, Stertz L, Badawy M, Passos IC, Barichello T, Kapczinski F, Quevedo J. The role of inflammation and microglial activation in the pathophysiology of psychiatric disorders. Neuroscience. 2015;300:141–54.

8. Setiawan E, Wilson AA, Mizrahi R, Rusjan PM, Miler L, Rajkowska G, Suridjan I, Kennedy JL, Rekkas PV, Houle S, Meyer JH. Role of translocator protein density, a marker of neuroinflammation, in the brain during major depressive episodes. JAMA Psychiatry. 2015;72:268–75.

9. Torres-Platas SG, Cruceanu C, Chen GG, Turecki G, Mechawar N. Evidence for increased microglial priming and macrophage recruitment in the dorsal anterior cingulate white matter of depressed suicides. Brain Behav Immun. 2014;42:50–9.

10. Laskaris LE, Di Biase MA, Everall I, Chana G, Christopoulos A, Skafidas E, Cropley VL, Pantelis C. Microglial activation and progressive brain changes in schizophrenia. Br J Pharmacol. 2016;173:666–80.

11. Kern JK, Geier DA, Sykes LK, Geier MR. Relevance of neuroinflammation and encephalitis in autism. Front Cell Neurosci. 2015;9:519.

12. Takano T. Role of microglia in autism: recent advances. Dev Neurosci. 2015;37:195–202.

13. Calsolaro V, Edison P. Neuroinflammation in Alzheimer's disease: current evidence and future directions. Alzheimers Dement. 2016;12:719–32.

14. Guerriero F, Sgarlata C, Francis M, Maurizi N, Faragli A, Perna S, Rondanelli M, Rollone M, Ricevuti G. Neuroinflammation, immune system and Alzheimer disease: searching for the missing link. Aging Clin Exp Res. 2016;29:821–31.

15. Song C, Halbreich U, Han C, Leonard BE, Luo H. Imbalance between pro- and anti-inflammatory cytokines, and between Th1 and Th2 cytokines in depressed patients: the effect of electroacupuncture or fluoxetine treatment. Pharmacopsychiatry. 2009;42:182–8.

16. Li Z, Ma L, Kulesskaya N, Voikar V, Tian L. Microglia are polarized to M1 type in high-anxiety inbred mice in response to lipopolysaccharide challenge. Brain Behav Immun. 2014;38:237–48.

17. Miller AH, Maletic V, Raison CL. Inflammation and its discontents: the role of cytokines in the pathophysiology of major depression. Biol Psychiatry. 2009;65:732–41.

18. Takaki J, Fujimori K, Miura M, Suzuki T, Sekino Y, Sato K. L-Glutamate released from activated microglia downregulates astrocytic L-glutamate transporter expression in neuroinflammation: the 'collusion' hypothesis for increased extracellular L-glutamate concentration in neuroinflammation. J Neuroinflammation. 2012;9:275.

19. Miller AH, Maletic V, Raison CL. Inflammation and Its discontents: the role of cytokines in the pathophysiology of major depression. Biol Psychiatry. 2009;65:732–41.

20. Dantzer R, O'Connor JC, Freund GG, Johnson RW, Kelley KW. From inflammation to sickness and depression: when the immune system subjugates the brain. Nat Rev Neurosci. 2008;9:46–56.

21. Hochstrasser T, Ullrich C, Sperner-Unterweger B, Humpel C. Inflammatory stimuli reduce survival of serotonergic neurons and induce neuronal expression of indoleamine 2,3-dioxygenase in rat dorsal raphe nucleus organotypic brain slices. Neuroscience. 2011;184:128–38.

22. Schwarcz R, Bruno JP, Muchowski PJ, Wu HQ. Kynurenines in the mammalian brain: when physiology meets pathology. Nat Rev Neurosci. 2012;13:465–77.

23. Giovanoli S, Engler H, Engler A, Richetto J, Feldon J, Riva MA, Schedlowski M, Meyer U. Preventive effects of minocycline in a neurodevelopmental two-hit model with relevance to schizophrenia. Transl Psychiatry. 2016;6:e772.

24. Chaudhry IB, Hallak J, Husain N, Minhas F, Stirling J, Richardson P, Dursun S, Dunn G, Deakin B. Minocycline benefits negative symptoms in early schizophrenia: a randomised double-blind placebo-controlled clinical trial in patients on standard treatment. J Psychopharmacol. 2012;26:1185–93.

25. Levkovitz Y, Mendlovich S, Riwkes S, Braw Y, Levkovitch-Verbin H, Gal G, Fennig S, Treves I, Kron S. A double-blind, randomized study of minocycline for the treatment of negative and cognitive symptoms in early-phase schizophrenia. J Clin Psychiatry. 2010;71:138–49.

26. Khodaie-Ardakani MR, Mirshafiee O, Farokhnia M, Tajdini M, Hosseini SM, Modabbernia A, Rezaei F, Salehi B, Yekehtaz H, Ashrafi M, et al. Minocycline add-on to risperidone for treatment of negative symptoms in patients with stable schizophrenia: randomized double-blind placebo-controlled study. Psychiatry Res. 2014;215:540–6.

27. Kelly DL, Sullivan KM, McEvoy JP, McMahon RP, Wehring HJ, Gold JM, Liu F, Warfel D, Vyas G, Richardson CM, et al. Adjunctive minocycline in clozapine-treated schizophrenia patients with persistent symptoms. J Clin Psychopharmacol. 2015;35:374–81.

28. Molina-Hernandez M, Tellez-Alcantara NP, Perez-Garcia J, Olivera-Lopez JI, Jaramillo-Jaimes MT. Antidepressant-like actions of minocycline combined with several glutamate antagonists. Prog Neuropsychopharmacol Biol Psychiatry. 2008;32:380–6.

29. Miyaoka T, Wake R, Furuya M, Liaury K, Ieda M, Kawakami K, Tsuchie K, Taki M, Ishihara K, Araki T, Horiguchi J. Minocycline as adjunctive therapy for patients with unipolar psychotic depression: an open-label study. Prog Neuropsychopharmacol Biol Psychiatry. 2012;37:222–6.

30. Molina-Hernandez M, Tellez-Alcantara NP, Perez-Garcia J, Olivera-Lopez JI, Jaramillo-Jaimes MT. Desipramine or glutamate antagonists synergized the antidepressant-like actions of intra-nucleus accumbens infusions of minocycline in male Wistar rats. Prog Neuropsychopharmacol Biol Psychiatry. 2008;32:1660–6.

31. Arakawa S, Shirayama Y, Fujita Y, Ishima T, Horio M, Muneoka K, Iyo M, Hashimoto K. Minocycline produced antidepressant-like effects on the learned helplessness rats with alterations in levels of monoamine in the amygdala and no changes in BDNF levels in the hippocampus at baseline. Pharmacol Biochem Behav. 2012;100:601–6.

32. Zheng LS, Kaneko N, Sawamoto K. Minocycline treatment ameliorates interferon-alpha- induced neurogenic defects and depression-like behaviors in mice. Front Cell Neurosci. 2015;9:5.

33. Regen F, Hildebrand M, Le Bret N, Herzog I, Heuser I, Hellmann-Regen J. Inhibition of retinoic acid catabolism by minocycline: evidence for a novel mode of action? Exp Dermatol. 2015;24:473–6.

34. Regen F, Le Bret N, Hildebrand M, Herzog I, Heuser I, Hellmann-Regen J. Inhibition of brain retinoic acid catabolism: a mechanism for minocycline's pleiotropic actions? World J Biol Psychiatry. 2015;256:1–7.

35. Hellmann-Regen J, Kronenberg G, Uhlemann R, Freyer D, Endres M, Gertz K. Accelerated degradation of retinoic acid by activated microglia. J Neuroimmunol. 2013;256:1–6.

36. Friedman DI. Medication-induced intracranial hypertension in dermatology. Am J Clin Dermatol. 2005;6:29–37.

37. Moskowitz Y, Leibowitz E, Ronen M, Aviel E. Pseudotumor cerebri induced by vitamin A combined with minocycline. Ann Ophthalmol. 1993;25:306–8.

38. Hellmann-Regen J, Herzog I, Fischer N, Heuser I, Regen F. Do tetracyclines and erythromycin exert anti-acne effects by inhibition of P450-mediated degradation of retinoic acid? Exp Dermatol. 2014;23:290–3.

39. Hellmann-Regen J, Kronenberg G, Uhlemann R, Freyer D, Endres M, Gertz K. Accelerated degradation of retinoic acid by activated microglia. J Neuroimmunol. 2013;256:1–6.

40. McEvoy T. Minocycline: rheumatoid Arthritis. Hosp Pharm. 2016;51:535–8.

41. Oya K, Kishi T, Iwata N. Efficacy and tolerability of minocycline augmentation therapy in schizophrenia: a systematic review and meta-analysis of randomized controlled trials. Hum Psychopharmacol. 2014;29:483–91.

42. Regen F, Heuser I, Herzog I, Hellmann-Regen J. Striking growth-inhibitory effects of minocycline on human prostate cancer cell lines. Urology. 2014;83(509):e501–6.

43. van Neerven S, Nemes A, Imholz P, Regen T, Denecke B, Johann S, Beyer C, Hanisch UK, Mey J. Inflammatory cytokine release of astrocytes in vitro is reduced by all-trans retinoic acid. J Neuroimmunol. 2010;229:169–79.

44. Maghsoodi B, Poon MM, Nam CI, Aoto J, Ting P, Chen L. Retinoic acid regulates RARalpha-mediated control of translation in dendritic RNA granules during homeostatic synaptic plasticity. Proc Natl Acad Sci USA. 2008;105:16015–20.

45. Bremner JD, McCaffery P. The neurobiology of retinoic acid in affective disorders. Prog Neuropsychopharmacol Biol Psychiatry. 2008;32:315–31.

46. van Neerven S, Kampmann E, Mey J. RAR/RXR and PPAR/RXR signaling in neurological and psychiatric diseases. Prog Neurobiol. 2008;85:433–51.

47. Wietrzych-Schindler M, Szyszka-Niagolov M, Ohta K, Endo Y, Perez E, de Lera AR, Chambon P, Krezel W. Retinoid x receptor gamma is implicated in docosahexaenoic acid modulation of despair behaviors and working memory in mice. Biol Psychiatry. 2011;69:788–94.

48. Hellmann-Regen J, Uhlemann R, Regen F, Heuser I, Otte C, Endres M, Gertz K, Kronenberg G. Direct inhibition of retinoic acid catabolism by fluoxetine. J Neural Transm (Vienna). 2015;122:1329–38.

49. Prinz M, Priller J. Microglia and brain macrophages in the molecular age: from origin to neuropsychiatric disease. Nat Rev Neurosci. 2014;15:300–12.

50. Lawson LJ, Perry VH, Gordon S. Turnover of resident microglia in the normal adult mouse brain. Neuroscience. 1992;48:405–15.

51. Kettenmann H, Hanisch UK, Noda M, Verkhratsky A. Physiology of microglia. Physiol Rev. 2011;91:461–553.

52. Vieira MMM, Ferreira TB, Pacheco PAF, Barros PO, Almeida CRM, Araújo-Lima CF, Silva-Filho RG, Hygino J, Andrade RM, Linhares UC, et al. Enhanced Th17 phenotype in individuals with generalized anxiety disorder. J Neuroimmunol. 2010;229:212–8.

53. Gill JM, Saligan L, Woods S, Page G. PTSD is associated with an excess of inflammatory immune activities. Perspect Psychiatr Care. 2009;45:262–77.

54. Gola H, Engler H, Sommershof A, Adenauer H, Kolassa S, Schedlowski M, Groettrup M, Elbert T, Kolassa IT. Posttraumatic stress disorder is associated with an enhanced spontaneous production of pro-inflammatory cytokines by peripheral blood mononuclear cells. BMC Psychiatry. 2013;13:40.

55. O'Brien SM, Scully P, Fitzgerald P, Scott LV, Dinan TG. Plasma cytokine profiles in depressed patients who fail to respond to selective serotonin reuptake inhibitor therapy. J Psychiatr Res. 2007;41:326–31.

56. Reichenberg A, Yirmiya R, Schuld A, Kraus T, Haack M, Morag A, Pollmacher T. Cytokine-associated emotional and cognitive disturbances in humans. Arch Gen Psychiatry. 2001;58:445–52.

57. Erhardt S, Lim CK, Linderholm KR, Janelidze S, Lindqvist D, Samuelsson M, Lundberg K, Postolache TT, Traskman-Bendz L, Guillemin GJ, Brundin L. Connecting inflammation with glutamate agonism in suicidality. Neuropsychopharmacology. 2013;38:743–52.

58. Larsson MK, Faka A, Bhat M, Imbeault S, Goiny M, Orhan F, Oliveros A, Stahl S, Liu XC, Choi DS, et al. Repeated LPS injection induces distinct changes in the kynurenine pathway in mice. Neurochem Res. 2016;41:2243–55.

59. O'Connor JC, Lawson MA, Andre C, Moreau M, Lestage J, Castanon N, Kelley KW, Dantzer R. Lipopolysaccharide-induced depressive-like behavior is mediated by indoleamine 2,3-dioxygenase activation in mice. Mol Psychiatry. 2009;14:511–22.

60. Salazar A, Gonzalez-Rivera BL, Redus L, Parrott JM, O'Connor JC. Indoleamine 2,3-dioxygenase mediates anhedonia and anxiety-like behaviors caused by peripheral lipopolysaccharide immune challenge. Horm Behav. 2012;62:202–9.

61. Dean OM, Data-Franco J, Giorlando F, Berk M. Minocycline: therapeutic potential in psychiatry. CNS Drugs. 2012;26:391–401.

3

Mapping visuospatial attention: the greyscales task in combination with repetitive navigated transcranial magnetic stimulation

Katrin Giglhuber[1,2], Stefanie Maurer[1,2], Claus Zimmer[3], Bernhard Meyer[1] and Sandro M. Krieg[1,2]*

Abstract

Background: Visuospatial attention is executed by the frontoparietal cortical areas of the brain. Damage to these areas can result in visual neglect. We therefore aimed to assess a combination of the greyscales task and repetitive navigated transcranial magnetic stimulation (rTMS) to identify cortical regions involved in visuospatial attention processes. This pilot study was designed to evaluate an approach in a cohort of healthy volunteers, with the future aim of using this technique to map brain tumor patients before surgery. Ten healthy, right-handed subjects underwent rTMS mapping of 52 cortical spots in both hemispheres. The greyscales task was presented tachistoscopically and was time-locked to rTMS pulses. The task pictures showed pairs of horizontal rectangles shaded continuously from black at one end to white at the other, mirror-reversed. On each picture the subject was asked to report which of the two greyscales appeared darker overall. The responses were categorized into "leftward" and "rightward," depending on whether the subject had chosen the rectangle with the darker end on the left or the right. rTMS applied to cortical areas involved in visuospatial attention is supposed to affect lateral shifts in spatial bias. These shifts result in an altered performance on the greyscales task compared to the baseline performance without rTMS stimulation.

Results: In baseline conditions, 9/10 subjects showed classic pseudoneglect to the left. Leftward effects also occurred more often in mapping conditions. Yet, calculated rightward deviations were strikingly greater in magnitude ($p < 0.0001$). Overall, the right hemisphere was found to be more suggestible than the left hemisphere. Both rightward and leftward deviation scores were higher for the rTMS of this brain side ($p < 0.0001$). Right hemispheric distributions accord well with current models of visuospatial attention (Corbetta et al. Nat Neurosci 8(11):1603–1610, 2005). We observed leftward deviations triggered by rTMS within superior frontal and posterior parietal areas and rightward deviations within inferior frontal areas and the temporoparietal junction (TPJ).

Conclusion: The greyscales task, in combination with rTMS, yields encouraging results in the examination of the visuospatial attention function. Future clinical implications should be evaluated.

Keywords: Cortical mapping, Greyscales task, Neglect, Repetitive navigated transcranial magnetic stimulation, Tachistoscopic testing, Visuospatial attention

*Correspondence: Sandro.Krieg@tum.de
[1] Department of Neurosurgery, Klinikum rechts der Isar, Technische Universität München, Ismaninger Str. 22, 81675 Munich, Germany
Full list of author information is available at the end of the article

Background

Visuospatial attention is processed in particular brain areas and fiber tract connections [2, 3]. The complexity of interactions becomes apparent by regarding the corresponding pathology at malfunction: visual neglect. Visual neglect describes a neurological syndrome of various forms, degrees, and recovery potential, accompanied by a significantly reduced functional outcome [4–6]. Classically observed as a consequence of right hemispheric parietal lesions, it has also been reported after left hemispheric, frontal, temporal, subcortical, and combined brain lesions [7, 8]. Research on detecting and understanding the underlying mechanisms is essential. In tumor patients, mapping prior to resection may prevent functional deficits [9, 10]. In stroke patients, mapping and timely counteraction may prevent chronification [1, 11–13].

To learn more about the visuospatial attention function, it proved insightful to study the conditions of healthy adults. As frequently reported, and also meta-analyzed by Jewell and McCourt in 2000, neurologically healthy individuals show slight but significant leftward errors in line bisection tasks [14–19]. Bowers and Heilman described this phenomenon first, calling it "pseudoneglect" [20]. Common models ascribe this observation to a right-hemispheric dominance in spatial attention processing. Imaging studies show preferential activity of the right hemisphere during visuospatial task performance [16, 21]. Other projects have examined the effect of inactivating the right hemisphere and have reported both activity shifts to the left hemisphere and a resultantly reduced leftward bias [14, 22, 23]. In 2011, Thiebaut de Schotten et al. confirmed anatomical correlates. They were able to link pseudoneglect to a larger network of frontoparietal fiber tracts within the right hemisphere compared to the left hemisphere [24]. Conclusively, Varnava et al. studied the predictability of visuospatial deficits depending on the extent and direction of pseudoneglect in the initial state. Reasoning from their findings, pseudoneglect and neglect originate from common or at least coupled mechanisms [25].

Conventional neglect screening in patients is usually undertaken using paper-and-pencil tests (e.g., line bisection). However, to measure biases in perceptual attention sensitively, task and setting must be selected appropriately [26]. As for measuring pseudoneglect in healthy volunteers, the greyscales task by Mattingley et al. consistently obtained promising results. First describing the test in 1994, they proved its sensitivity in several studies and developed an electronic version [27–30]. The task consists of tachistoscopic forced-choice decisions on the luminance of two greyscales. Analysis results in a score reflecting the spatial bias. The score ranges from − 1.00,

reflecting a maximal leftward bias, to 1.00, for the right side, respectively.

Repetitive navigated transcranial magnetic stimulation (rTMS) affords an opportunity to accurately and noninvasively detect cortical areas. rTMS pulses applied to an eloquent cortical spot effect a so-called virtual lesion and thus temporary inactivation. As a result, we can observe performance changes on concurrently conducted neuropsychological tasks. The method is increasingly used to map neuropsychological functions such as language and calculation; recently, our group also reported its usefulness for the mapping of visuospatial attention [31–37]. To further pursue this objective, we combined rTMS with the aforementioned greyscales task in the same cohort of healthy volunteers as investigated before [36]. We assumed our subjects present with a basic spatial bias that reflects their individual processing balance between the left and the right hemisphere. This bias might be indexed by the greyscales task. In the presence of pseudoneglect, we would obtain leftward baseline scores. Our next thought was that temporary inactivation of eloquent cortical spots ought to effect an inter-hemispheric misbalancing and therefore drive lateral shifts in spatial bias. These again might be indexed by the greyscales task. We expected particularly significant effects for rTMS applied to cortical spots of the right hemisphere. Based on the idea of a dominantly active right hemisphere in healthy adults with pseudoneglect, we supposed that inactivation of spots within this hemisphere would reduce the basic leftward bias. Hence we would obtain rightward deviation scores on the greyscales task.

Summarizing, the presented pilot study aims to assess a combination of the greyscales task and rTMS in healthy volunteers by examining the following hypotheses:

(1) The greyscales task in tachistoscopic test conditions is appropriate and sensitive for testing visuospatial attention function via rTMS.
(2) The resulting brain maps are in accordance with current models of visuospatial attention.

Methods
Subjects

The study included five women and five men. All subjects were healthy at state and without any history of neurological or neuropsychological deficit. Their ages ranged from 21 to 31 years (median age: 24 years). Inclusion criteria were pure right-handedness (Edinburgh inventory score > 40) and German as a first language. Exclusion criteria were general TMS and MRI exclusion criteria (pacemaker, cochlea-implant, deep brain stimulation) [38]. As mentioned in the introduction, this cohort has been examined before [36].

Navigated rTMS

MRI dataset

For MR imaging, we used a 3 Tesla MRI scanner with eight-channel phased-array head coil (Achieva 3T, Philips Medical Systems, Amsterdam, The Netherlands B.V.). Our protocol was comprised of two sequences: a T2-weighted FLAIR sequence (TR: 12,000 ms, TE: 140 ms, voxel size: $0.9 \times 0.9 \times 4$ mm^3, acquisition time: 3 min) and a T1-weighted 3D gradient echo sequence (no intravenous contrast administration, TR: 9 ms, TE: 4 ms, 1 mm^3 isovoxel covering the whole head, acquisition time: 6 min 58 s). The 3D dataset was transferred to our rTMS system by DICOM standard.

Mapping setup

For rTMS mapping, we used a Nexstim eXimia System Version 4.3 with NEXSPEECH® module (Nexstim Plc., Helsinki, Finland). This system uses a stereotactic camera to link the subject's 3-D MRI dataset with its head via anatomical landmarks and a registered "tracker" headband. This meant we were able to visualize the stimulation coil's real-time position or, rather, the induced electric field in the 3D MRI reconstruction and to selectively and accurately stimulate the brain regions [33, 34, 39, 40]. Through the use of NEXSPEECH software, we were able to stimulate the selected brain regions and time-locked present task pictures on a video screen [41].

Mapping parameter

In each subject we determined resting motor thresholds (RMT) for the right and left abductor pollicis brevis muscles and individually adjusted the stimulation intensity for the respectively contralateral hemisphere [42]. Mapping was performed at 100% RMT. rTMS pulses were applied as a train of 10 stimuli at a repetition frequency of 5 Hz, equaling stimulation trains of 1800 ms. To reach a maximal field induction, we placed the coil in anterior–posterior field orientation strictly tangentially to the skull, as previously reported [36, 41, 43].

Mapping targets

We tested 52 cortical spots on each hemisphere and distributed them to brain areas using the cortical parcellation system created by Corina (CPS; Fig. 1, Table 1) [44]. We anatomically identified the spots in each subject's 3D MRI reconstruction and marked them as stimulation targets. First we selected the targets of the left hemisphere. We probed each target five times in a block. The order of selecting was randomly chosen by the examiner. Next we examined the right hemisphere, respectively. We redid this procedure once. According to this protocol each target was probed 10 times in total. Though, due to difficulties in adjusting the stereotactic camera during the mapping, some spots got addressed more, some less frequent. Certain brain areas had to be omitted: Stimulation of the polar and anterior frontal gyri (polFG, aSFG, aMFG), the orbital part of the inferior frontal gyrus (orIFG), the polar temporal gyri (polTG), and the

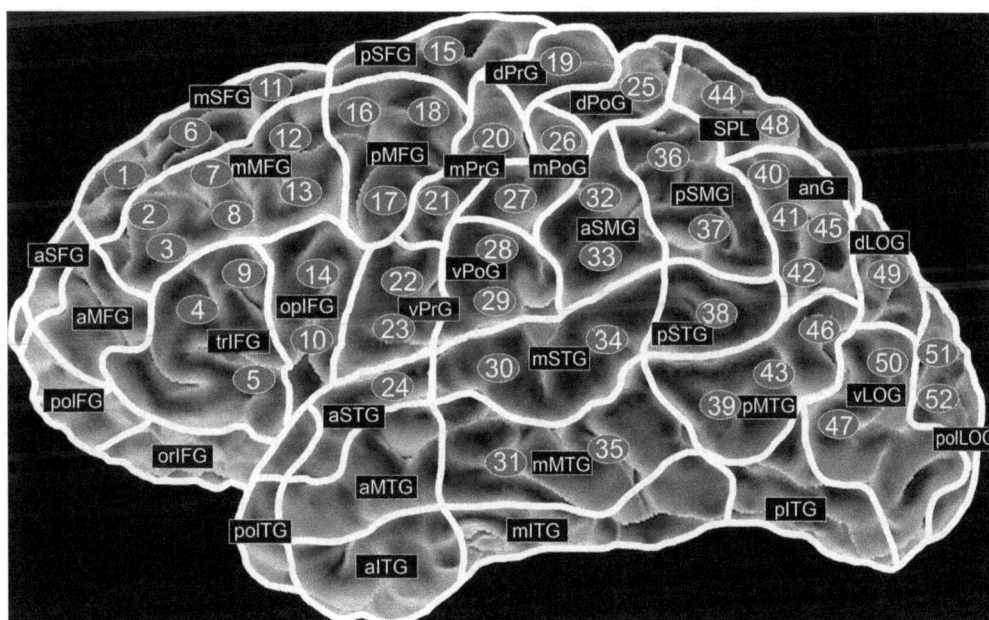

Fig. 1 Mapping targets. Brain areas and cortical spots no. 1–52 according to the cortical parcellation system [44]

Table 1 Anatomical names and abbreviations of the cortical parcellation system

Abbreviation	Anatomy
aITG	Anterior inferior temporal gyrus
aMFG	Anterior middle frontal gyrus
aMTG	Anterior middle temporal gyrus
anG	Angular gyrus
aSFG	Anterior superior frontal gyrus
aSMG	Anterior supramarginal gyrus
aSTG	Anterior superior temporal gyrus
dLOG	Dorsal lateral occipital gyrus
dPoG	Dorsal post-central gyrus
dPrG	Dorsal pre-central gyrus
mITG	Middle inferior temporal gyrus
mMFG	Middle middle frontal gyrus
mMTG	Middle middle temporal gyrus
mPoG	Middle post-central gyrus
mPrG	Middle pre-central gyrus
mSFG	Middle superior frontal gyrus
mSTG	Middle superior temporal gyrus
opIFG	Opercular inferior frontal gyrus
orIFG	Orbital part of the inferior frontal gyrus
pITG	Posterior inferior temporal gyrus
pMFG	Posterior middle frontal gyrus
pMTG	Posterior middle temporal gyrus
polFG	Polar frontal gyri
polTG	Polar temporal gyri
polLOG	Polar lateral occipital gyrus
pSFG	Posterior superior frontal gyrus
pSMG	Posterior supramarginal gyrus
pSTG	Posterior superior temporal gyrus
SPL	Superior parietal lobe
trIFG	Triangular inferior frontal gyrus
vLOG	Ventral lateral occipital gyrus
vPoG	Ventral post-central gyrus
vPrG	Ventral pre-central gyrus

Anatomical names and abbreviations according to the cortical parcellation system [44]

anterior middle temporal gyrus (aMTG) is known to be too painful to provide reliable results due to muscle contractions. Stimulation of the inferior temporal gyrus (ITG) is known to be incomparably effective because the increased range between the skull and brain tissue causes decreased stimulation intensities [39, 45].

The greyscales task
Task setup
During rTMS mapping, the subjects had to perform a visuospatial attention task. More specifically, they had to handle one task picture during each rTMS stimulation train. A video screen (38.1 cm in diameter) was placed at viewing distance (about 60 cm nose to screen) in front of the examination chair. As evaluated before, we delivered rTMS pulses and task pictures synchronously and without delay between rTMS-stimulus-onset and picture-display [46]. The inter-picture interval was set to 3000 ms.

Task design
Our visuospatial attention task follows the greyscales task by Mattingley et al. [30]. Task pictures were conceived as pairs of horizontal rectangles arranged vertically, one above another (Fig. 2). They were shaded continuously from black at one end to white at the other, shown on a grey background, and framed by a black line of 0.7 mm. The rectangles of each pair were identical in length and shading, solely depicted as mirror images. Uniformly 30 mm in height, the rectangles varied in length from 180 to 330 mm (in 30 mm steps). Six lengths per two shading orientations each made a task set of 12 different task pictures. Pictures were displayed tachistoscopically for 50 ms, as reported earlier [18, 36, 47]. The order of presentation was randomized by the software. On each picture the subject was asked to report which of the two greyscales appeared darker overall by saying aloud "top" or "bottom." There was no third option to select "no difference." The responses were categorized into "leftward" and "rightward," depending on whether the subject had chosen the rectangle with the darker end on the left or the right. Subjects performed a baseline session of 72 pictures without stimulation prior to the rTMS mapping session. Both sessions were videotaped for later analysis [41, 48].

Evaluation of discomfort
After rTMS mapping, the subjects were asked to evaluate discomfort, separately for the temporal muscle area ("temporal") and for the remainder of the head surface ("convexity"). The meter was the visual analogue scale (range 0–10): 0 signifying no pain and 10 signifying maximal pain.

Data analysis
Data analysis comprised several steps. First we went over the subject's video records and labeled each response as "leftward" or "rightward" (as outlined in 2.4.2). Next we related responses and stimulated cortical spots. For each spot we counted the number of effective rTMS stimulations and, among these, the number of leftward and rightward responses. Stimulation was deemed effective if a complete train of 10 rTMS pulses had been applied and if the electric field strength at the cortical level had been above 55 V/m the entire time [34]. Then scores were computed as

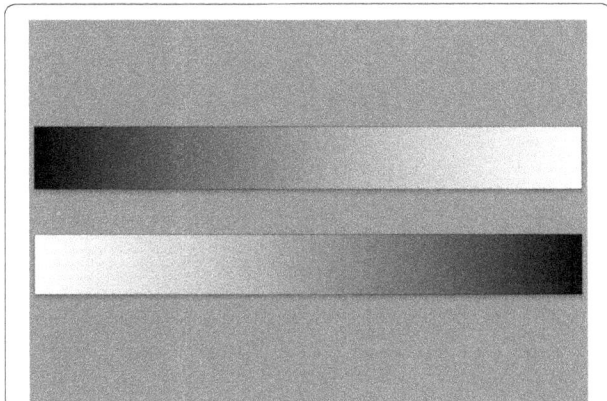

Fig. 2 Sample picture from the greyscales task. Greyscales task sample. For each picture the subject was asked to report which of the two greyscales appeared to be darker overall. The responses were categorized into "leftward" and "rightward," depending on whether the subject had chosen the rectangle with the darker end on the left or the right, as first described by Mattingley et al. [30]

the difference between the rightward and leftward responses divided by the number of effective stimulations (between a range of -1.00 and 1.00). The subject's task performance in baseline conditions was documented as the baseline score. Their performance in mapping conditions was documented for each particular spot as the particular deviation score (i.e., the spot's computed score minus the subject's baseline score). The deviation scores, in turn, were categorized as "leftward" or "rightward," depending on whether the scores were negative or positive. Then we pooled the information of all the subjects per cortical spot as follows:

(1) We calculated the number of subjects with leftward deviation scores and the mean of their scores, i.e., the mean of all leftward deviation scores.
(2) We calculated the number of subjects with rightward deviation scores and the mean of their scores, i.e., the mean of all rightward deviation scores.

For clearer comparison, we handled all mean deviation scores in terms of their magnitude.

Statistics

The results are listed as mean ± standard deviation plus median and range where applicable. Inter-spot comparisons were made by the Mann–Whitney U test for independent samples. For single-spot analysis (concerning "leftward" vs. "rightward" effects), we used the Wilcoxon matched-pairs signed rank test. All tests were regarded as significant at a p value < 0.05 (GraphPad Prism 6.0, La Jolla, CA, USA).

Results
Subject characteristics

The subject characteristics are listed in Table 2. We determined a mean RMT of $33.1 \pm 6.4\%$ maximal stimulator output, in terms of the left hemisphere, and of $32.9 \pm 5.9\%$, in terms of the right hemisphere ($p = 0.9564$). Without stimulation, 9 out of 10 subjects presented with a leftward basic bias; one subject showed a rightward basic bias. Taken together, the baseline score averaged -0.59 ± 0.51. rTMS mapping was tolerated well, and discomfort was comparable for both hemispheres. All subjects were purely right-handed and showed left-hemispheric dominance.

Number and size of deviations

Tables 3 and 4 provide all computed deviation scores on mapping conditions. Additional subject-related scores are available as an online resource (Additional files 1, 2). First we had a look at the number and size of leftward and rightward deviations.

Leftward deviations

Regarding the frequency, leftward deviations occurred significantly more often than rightward deviations within both the left ($p = 0.0077$) and the right hemisphere ($p < 0.0001$). Analyzing the results of both hemispheres together, we found that inter-hemispherically, their number was comparable ($p = 0.6397$). Regarding the effect size, rTMS of the right hemisphere elicited significantly stronger leftward deviations than rTMS of the left hemisphere ($p < 0.0001$; Fig. 3). Altogether, i.e. for both hemispheres, the mean leftward deviation scores ranged from 0.06 to 0.40 in magnitude.

Rightward deviations

Consequently, rightward deviations were more rarely observed than leftward deviations. Their number was comparable for the two hemispheres ($p = 0.6352$). However, rightward deviations were strikingly greater in magnitude, namely, compared to leftward deviations ($p < 0.0001$) and according to inter-hemispheric comparison of the right rather than the left hemisphere ($p < 0.0001$; Fig. 3). The mean rightward deviation scores ranged from 0.06 to 1.26 in magnitude.

Cortical distribution of deviations

In what follows we outline the cortical distribution of deviations. Figure 4 depicts the leftward deviations in blue color and the rightward deviations in red.

Table 2 Subject characteristics

Subject	RMT		Pain score temporal		Pain score convexity		Greyscales task baseline score
	Left hemis-phere	Right hemis-phere	Left hemis-phere	Right hemis-phere	Left hemis-phere	Right hemis-phere	
1	29	29	2	3	1	1	− 0.61
2	34	29	2	2	1	1	0.78
3	29	33	3	6	1	1	− 0.81
4	43	39	4	4	1	1	− 0.94
5	36	35	3	3	1	1	− 0.94
6	30	28	2	2	0	0	− 0.97
7	45	45	6	6	1	1	− 0.75
8	31	36	4	6	1	3	− 0.47
9	28	26	4	2	3	1	− 0.67
10	26	29	2	4	1	3	− 0.53
Mean	33.1	32.9	3.2	3.8	1.1	1.3	− 0.59
SD	6.4	5.9	1.3	1.7	0.7	0.9	0.51
Median	30.5	31	3	3.5	1	1	− 0.71
MIN	26	26	2	2	0	0	− 0.97
MAX	45	45	6	6	3	3	0.78
	$p = 0.9564$		$p = 0.5493$		$p = 0.8375$		

Subject characteristics. Resting motor threshold (RMT) as % of stimulator output. Pain score according to the visual analogue scale (VAS), range from 0 (no pain) to 10 (maximal pain). Greyscales task baseline score determined on 72 pictures without stimulation, range from − 1.00 (leftward bias) to 1.00 (rightward bias)

Leftward deviations

Regarding the left hemisphere, we observed strong leftward effects within parietal areas (vPoG, anG; spots no. 28, 40; Fig. 4a). Regarding the right hemisphere, the parietal areas (SPL, anG; spots no. 41, 45, 48) were as prominent as the middle middle temporal gyrus (mMTG; spot no. 35), and as a wide frontal area (mSFG, mMFG, pMFG; spots no. 8, 11, 13, 16–18, Fig. 4b).

Rightward deviations

Rightward deviations within the left hemisphere were distributed to the posterior superior frontal gyrus (pSFG; spot no. 15) and to occipital areas (dLOG, vLOG; spots no. 49–50; Fig. 4c). The right hemisphere showed a number of striking spots, including the posterior supramarginal gyrus (pSMG; spot no. 37), the ventral lateral occipital gyrus (vLOG; spots no. 47, 50), temporal areas (mSTG, pMTG; spots no. 34, 43, 46), and frontal areas (mMFG, trIFG, opIFG; spots no. 4, 5, 9, 13–14; Fig. 4d).

Raw data

We provide our subjects' raw data as an online resource (Additional files 3, 4). Cortical spots of the left hemisphere were stimulated 9.8 ± 0.2 times on average, and cortical spots of the right hemisphere were stimulated 9.7 ± 0.3 times. The number of effective stimulations per spot ranged from 5 to 15 for the left hemisphere and from 4 to 12 for the right hemisphere.

Discussion

General aims and limitations

We have already reported on the usability of navigated rTMS to mimic visual neglect and map corresponding cortical areas in another study [36]. While searching for preferably sensitive visuospatial tasks, we also came across literature on the greyscales task and, thus, designed the pilot study presented in this manuscript. We mainly focused on general feasibility and the broad-ranging examination of both hemispheres, which involved accepting a number of limitations. To assess new setups and to understand the anatomical correlates of pathologies, it is crucial to examine healthy subjects. Our volunteers formed a small and homogenous healthy cohort, which may be seen as a benefit [49]. At the same time, it may be seen as a restriction, and the generalizability of our findings certainly must be further assessed in relation to a higher number of subjects of all ages. Moreover, we should be aware of limitations due to our rTMS protocol. We tested a wide range of brain areas using a fixed mapping template. We stimulated at a frequency of 5 Hz and with strict anterior–posterior field orientation. Several protocol changes, for example, varying coil angulations, could have modified our results [50]. However, we proceeded comparably to all current mapping standards that have been used before [36, 37, 45]. Some cortical spots showed a quite small number of effective stimulations. However, the mean number of stimulations per spot was

Table 3 Deviation scores per cortical spot for the left hemisphere

Cortical spot	"Leftward" deviation scores		"Rightward" deviation scores	
	Number of subjects	Mean of these subjects' scores	Number of subjects	Mean of these subjects' scores
1	2	−0.06	8	0.26
2	5	−0.13	5	0.15
3	2	−0.09	8	0.27
4	2	−0.06	8	0.40
5	3	−0.23	7	0.34
6	4	−0.11	6	0.33
7	5	−0.22	5	0.30
8	2	−0.26	8	0.34
9	5	−0.19	5	0.29
10	3	−0.24	7	0.33
11	4	−0.13	6	0.28
12	4	−0.16	6	0.31
13	5	−0.13	5	0.23
14	7	−0.17	3	0.31
15	7	−0.26	3	0.88
16	6	−0.16	4	0.52
17	7	−0.15	3	0.36
18	4	−0.14	6	0.25
19	7	−0.12	3	0.40
20	5	−0.22	5	0.42
21	6	−0.19	4	0.46
22	7	−0.18	3	0.06
23	6	−0.22	4	0.20
24	9	−0.23	1	0.55
25	8	−0.23	2	0.29
26	7	−0.24	3	0.17
27	9	−0.20	1	0.47
28	5	−0.38	5	0.13
29	6	−0.31	4	0.20
30	6	−0.15	4	0.52
31	6	−0.29	4	0.21
32	5	−0.18	5	0.36
33	7	−0.26	3	0.78
34	6	−0.21	4	0.58
35	5	−0.32	5	0.61
36	4	−0.22	6	0.33
37	6	−0.28	4	0.81
38	4	−0.22	6	0.46
39	6	−0.15	4	0.62
40	6	−0.36	4	0.71
41	6	−0.15	4	0.39
42	7	−0.22	3	0.44
43	7	−0.29	3	0.42
44	5	−0.18	5	0.67

Table 3 (continued)

Cortical spot	"Leftward" deviation scores		"Rightward" deviation scores	
	Number of subjects	Mean of these subjects' scores	Number of subjects	Mean of these subjects' scores
45	8	−0.18	2	0.44
46	8	−0.18	2	0.45
47	7	−0.24	3	0.38
48	7	−0.18	3	0.81
49	7	−0.18	2	0.88
50	7	−0.24	3	0.85
51	8	−0.22	2	0.48
52	6	−0.18	4	0.14
Mean	6	−0.20	4	0.42
SD	2	−0.07	2	0.20
MIN	2	−0.06	1	0.06
MAX	9	−0.38	8	0.88

Results for stimulation of the left hemisphere. Number of subjects with negative deviation scores ("leftward") and mean of their scores. Number of subjects with positive deviation scores ("rightward") and mean of their scores. Outline per cortical spot (no. 1–52) plus mean, standard deviation (SD), minimum (MIN), and maximum (MAX)

over 9.1 for all subjects with a consistently small variance. As a last point, we can neither offer any test–retest evaluation in the form of a second examination, nor any sham-stimulation controls to exclude factors such as concentration deficits or unintended remote rTMS effects. This should be the next step following this feasibility study. With all this in mind, our findings should clearly be carefully considered. Nevertheless, as a first step in an evaluation, we may rate them as useful and encouraging for a further pursuit of this approach.

The greyscales task

Neglect patients are known to develop various mechanisms to compensate for existent pathologies. Hence, a true diagnosis requires precise and challenging task selections [26]. The greyscales task serves as a sensitive tool to measure perceptual biases in healthy subjects and in patients and has even been used to uncover deficits in patients without apparent visual neglect in conservative testing [27, 30]. In this study we chose a computerized and tachistoscopic application and conclusively can approve this setting. It proved to be applicable and highly sensitive. Tachistoscopic task display prevents effects such as fixation or eye scanning. As originally conducted, our subjects had to respond verbally. We had to take into account the fact that left-hemisphere-activation by speaking might affect the inter-hemispheric processes of visuospatial attention. On the other hand manual demands have also been reported as affecting results—for example, depending on the hand being used to perform [18]. A key advantage of the greyscales task is that there are no errors to make or be detected, but each response contributes to the overall result, representing the subject's fully individual tendency with regard to visuospatial attention processing. By determining a basic bias prior to the rTMS examination and considering all subsequent results in relation to this value, there is no usability limitation accompanying the already existent deficits. Here we examined a collective of healthy men, but our setting may be applied to patients as well. Moreover, the adaptability does not depend on the presence or form of pseudoneglect. Our baseline findings are consistent with reports on the prevalence of pseudoneglect among young adults: 9 out of our 10 subjects naturally tended to the left rather than the right [18, 20, 22, 27]. With advancing age, pseudoneglect is known to shift rightwards [51, 52]. This fact should be kept in mind for future analysis of patient data, but as stated above, it does not restrict the applicability. Besides, we should mention that Friedrich et al. analyzed the age factor of pseudoneglect by means of the greyscales task and found that healthy elderly people presented with an even stronger leftward bias than their younger participants [53].

rTMS mapping

Across the literature, visuospatial attention is described as highly individually distributed, balanced, and suggestible [1, 54–56]. However, we assume that a scaffold of cortical spots exists connected anatomically, that they are thus available by order of visuospatial function, and that they are at least available to be recruited if necessary. As already addressed in 4.1, our rTMS results certainly should not be considered absolute. There were cortical spots with outstanding deviation scores averaged over less than half of our subjects; the other subjects were either not suggestible (but by chance showed small deviation scores in the opposite direction) or alternatively were suggestible but, as a matter of fact, in the opposite direction (Tables 3, 4; Additional files 1, 2, 3, 4). One more factor we should mention is the experiment's fairly long time span. A natural leftward bias on baseline performance is known to decline in the course of visuospatial task demands. Due to diminished alertness and neural fatigue, biases shift rightward naturally over time [57–59]. We examined the two hemispheres in the order left–right–left–right, i.e., in two turns. To prevent a time-on-task effect, we took breaks after every examination of one hemisphere, and we periodically animated our subjects to maintain concentration for the time span in between. An increasing rightward shift over time should have resulted in a higher total number of rightward

deviations for the right hemisphere compared to the left hemisphere. Fortunately, we could not find any pattern of time-effects. The number of rightward deviations was comparable for both hemispheres (see "Rightward deviations" section).

To get a better measure of our findings, we performed a principal analysis of deviation numbers and sizes, as outlined in 3.2. Leftward deviations were recorded significantly more often and were significantly smaller in magnitude than rightward deviations. The higher frequency may be based on pre-existent pseudoneglect and might solely reflect right hemisphere activity during visuospatial task demands, especially as the score values tended to be small. On the other hand, an already leftward baseline score limited the attainable magnitude of negative deviation scores per se. In contrast, rightward deviations were found to be strikingly great in magnitude and significantly stronger than leftward deviations (Fig. 3; Tables 3, 4). Once more referring to the baseline performance, we could categorize these rightward deviations as a reduction or cancellation of the natural leftward bias, i.e., of pseudoneglect. This pseudoneglect "ceiling effect" has been described before [14, 17]. Furthermore these rightward deviations parallel the classic symptom of left visual neglect. In clinical routine, visual neglect is described as being both the most common and most pronounced phenomenon after right hemispheric damage [7, 8, 27, 60]. Accordingly, we found the right hemisphere to be significantly more suggestible by rTMS than the left hemisphere (Figs. 3, 4). This is also in line with our initial assumption that rTMS of the right hemisphere ought to strikingly misbalance the base state of processing in which the right hemisphere takes the dominant part. To summarize, we may reaffirm that rTMS affords a useful opportunity to map visuospatial attention function at the cortical level, most convincingly for the right hemisphere and—when examining healthy men with pseudoneglect—for attention processing to the right.

Cortical distributions with reference to the current literature

The unquestionably best-known form of visual neglect is the combination of right hemispheric parietal damage followed by contralesional left deficits. Notwithstanding, there are more and more reports of other lesion locations and clinical manifestations, up to reports on the concurrent occurrence of ipsi- and contralesional deficits [47, 61–64]. As a side note, the greyscales study by Mattingley et al. [27] also included two right-parietal patients with an extreme leftward bias and thus ipsilesional neglect. As introduced above, studies on pseudoneglect in healthy adults have additionally helped to explain processing mechanisms [14–18, 20, 22–25]. However, a comparative

Table 4 Deviation scores per cortical spot for the right hemisphere

Cortical spot	"Leftward" deviation scores		"Rightward" deviation scores	
	Number of subjects	Mean of these subjects' scores	Number of subjects	Mean of these subjects' scores
1	4	−0.21	6	0.56
2	6	−0.29	4	0.63
3	7	−0.22	3	0.73
4	7	−0.24	3	0.96
5	7	−0.18	3	0.93
6	7	−0.17	3	0.62
7	7	−0.24	3	0.33
8	5	−0.40	5	0.32
9	7	−0.26	3	1.15
10	6	−0.28	4	0.72
11	6	−0.38	4	0.73
12	7	−0.27	3	0.44
13	7	−0.34	3	1.15
14	7	−0.26	3	0.95
15	6	−0.23	4	0.48
16	7	−0.33	3	0.52
17	6	0.34	4	0.43
18	5	−0.40	5	0.73
19	6	−0.23	4	0.58
20	4	−0.30	6	0.44
21	4	−0.23	6	0.44
22	5	−0.26	5	0.80
23	4	−0.18	5	0.72
24	6	−0.21	4	0.68
25	3	−0.19	6	0.57
26	5	−0.22	5	0.58
27	5	−0.25	5	0.65
28	5	−0.21	5	0.46
29	5	−0.27	5	0.61
30	4	−0.23	6	0.80
31	5	−0.23	5	0.65
32	4	−0.28	6	0.49
33	4	−0.26	6	0.63
34	6	−0.20	4	1.04
35	4	−0.35	6	0.41
36	5	−0.20	5	0.73
37	7	−0.24	3	0.90
38	7	−0.18	3	0.77
39	4	−0.21	6	0.43
40	6	−0.23	4	0.53
41	4	−0.36	6	0.59
42	5	−0.21	5	0.38
43	6	−0.15	4	1.04
44	6	−0.24	4	0.79

Table 4 (continued)

Cortical spot	"Leftward" deviation scores		"Rightward" deviation scores	
	Number of subjects	Mean of these subjects' scores	Number of subjects	Mean of these subjects' scores
45	7	−0.33	3	0.58
46	6	−0.19	4	0.87
47	7	−0.26	3	1.26
48	5	−0.38	5	0.65
49	7	−0.22	3	0.56
50	7	−0.26	3	0.91
51	7	−0.27	3	0.59
52	4	−0.16	6	0.41
Mean	6	−0.25	4	0.67
SD	1	−0.06	1	0.22
MIN	3	−0.15	3	0.32
MAX	7	−0.40	6	1.26

Results for stimulation of the right hemisphere. Number of subjects with negative deviation scores ("leftward") and mean of their scores. Number of subjects with positive deviation scores ("rightward") and mean of their scores. Outline per cortical spot 1–52 plus mean, standard deviation (SD), minimum (MIN), and maximum (MAX)

discussion of results proves difficult because of the heterogeneity of approaches. Studies use different tasks to measure visuospatial deficits, focus on different locations, and interpret their results from different angles. One fact upon which they all agree, which has persisted over the course of decades, is that the right hemisphere at least plays a somewhat special role, whether dominant or controlling [65, 66]. This idea also provides the basis for explaining the high prevalence of pseudoneglect in healthy adults [15, 16, 21–24, 51]. Regarding cortical distributions, there is the widely accepted idea of subcortical fiber tracts connecting frontal areas with parietal areas and the temporoparietal junction (TPJ) [2, 3, 24, 54, 55, 65, 67]. Corbetta and Shulman assume two networks: a dorsal network including superior parietal and frontal areas represented on both hemispheres, and a ventral network including the TPJ and inferior frontal areas represented dominantly on the right hemisphere and supervising the dorsal network [3]. To class our findings with these models, we have to differentiate between the left and the right hemisphere. Within the left hemisphere occasional spots of frontal, parietal, and lateral occipital areas presented with strong deviation effects (Fig. 4a, c), though we cannot distribute them distinctly to the stated networks and must suggest forming careful conclusions from these findings. Yet, rTMS-lesioning of the right hemisphere detected cortical spots that accorded well with the introduced models. Interestingly,

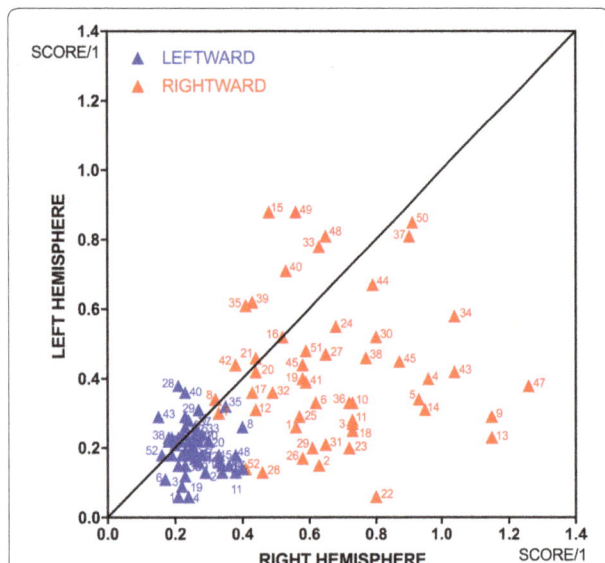

Fig. 3 Inter-hemispheric comparison of deviations. Deviation sizes in comparison. Plotted are mean deviation scores per cortical spot (no. 1–52), as always, for the left hemisphere (y-coordinate; Table 3) and the right hemisphere (x-coordinate; Table 4). Leftward deviations in blue, rightward deviations in red

we found leftward deviations (corresponding to ipsilesional neglect) to mainly be distributed to posterior parietal and superior frontal areas, according to the proposed dorsal network (Fig. 4b; Table 4). The observation of leftward instead of rightward deviations does not go in line with the basic responsibilities Corbetta and Shulmann intended for their networks [3]. However, supposing equal neuronal structures and thus rTMS-effects for dorsal or ventral brain regions, we should contemplate subtler task allocations within the dorsal network. There are several publications on the occurrence of ipsilesional neglect after right-hemispheric damage [62, 63, 68, 69]. Chokron et al. [70] even reported right visual neglect in patients with left hemianopia plus neglect. Especially the role of frontal and subcortical areas is discussed, albeit, so far, there is no generally accepted explanation that could be integrated into the model of Corbetta and Shulmann [61, 64]. On the contrary, rightward deviations (corr. to contralesional neglect) could be triggered best at inferior frontal spots and at a pool of spots within the area of the TPJ (Fig. 4d; Table 4). In turn, these observations comply with both localization and function of a ventral network.

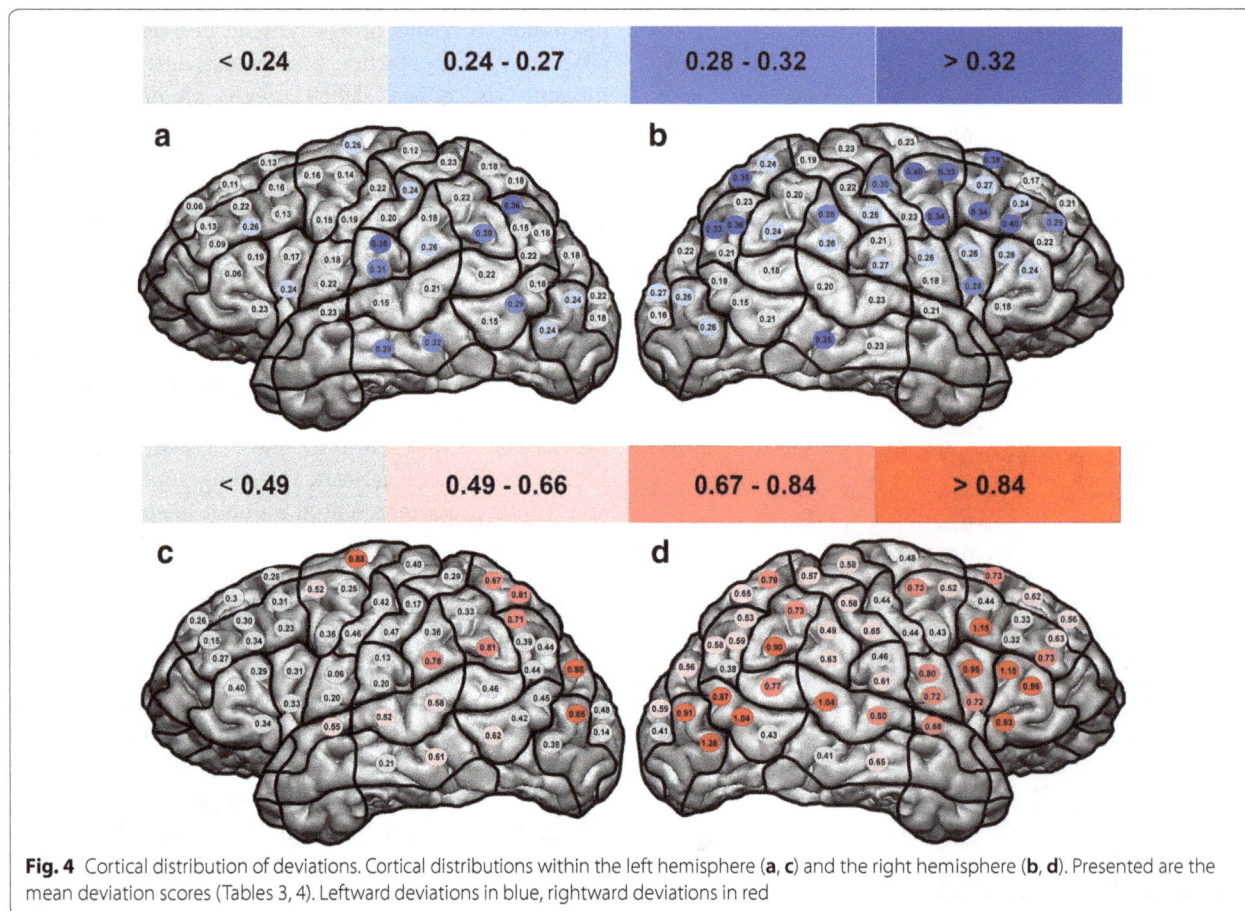

Fig. 4 Cortical distribution of deviations. Cortical distributions within the left hemisphere (**a**, **c**) and the right hemisphere (**b**, **d**). Presented are the mean deviation scores (Tables 3, 4). Leftward deviations in blue, rightward deviations in red

At this point we also want to mention our group's first work on neglect, which was a combination of rTMS and a classical landmark task [36]. We successfully showed the feasibility of mapping visuospatial attention, yet the landmark task solely provided information in the form of right-or-wrong answers, and the resulting error rates among our healthy volunteers tended to be rather small. The study presented here can be seen as a second approach to gather more and better comparable data using the greyscales task. As already outlined, the greyscales task takes into account any recorded answer and allows interpretations independently from any existent deficits. Since the two tasks use quite different ways of measuring visuospatial attention and respectively different forms of analysis, and since both approaches conformed to pilot studies' inclusive limitations, we decided not to compare single results. However, we may summarize that the findings of both go well together, embedded in the generally acknowledged model of visuospatial processing. Regarding the right hemisphere, we found consistent distributions in the area of the TPJ and for spots of the middle frontal gyrus. For clinical purposes the greyscales task design stands out by being quite easily applicable and bearable while achieving sensitive results. To reach similar sensitivity for the landmark task, we would have had to increase its difficulty, for example, by shortening the line differences between the left and right segments. Yet, all our healthy subjects reported the landmark task as being particularly demanding, which is why we seriously doubt its feasibility at a higher difficulty level, let alone in elderly patients.

Future prospects

Obviously, the acting and interacting of networks responsible for visuospatial attention has not yet been understood to the fullest extent. Research increasingly concentrates on the subcortical level [71–73]. However, several options are conceivable to integrate cortical mapping using rTMS. For example, a combination with fMRI enables the detection of unintended remote stimulation effects and potentially accountable white matter connections [74]. Furthermore, seminal approaches are made by diffusion tensor imaging fiber tracking. The combination of diffusion tensor imaging fiber tracking and rTMS language mapping recently obtained highly promising results for the imaging of subcortical language pathways and may be assessed similarly for the rTMS-mapped visuospatial attention function [75–78]. Basic research naturally aims to yield a clinical advantage. It could be shown that neurosurgeons profit by presurgical maps by preventing functional deficits while allowing maximal resection [9, 79]. In patients with certain tumor locations,

we should consider adding maps of visuospatial attention function to the individual preoperative assessment. On the other hand, dealing with already existent deficits, neurologists currently develop new treatment regimes. In light of visual neglect being the result of damage accompanied by a misbalancing of large-scale brain networks, recovery correlates with rebalancing [1, 11, 80]. Once more, the presented combination of the greyscales task and rTMS may be advantageous in terms of generating individual and accurate cortical maps for therapeutic interventions.

Conclusion

Referring to our initial hypotheses, we can conclude that the greyscales task on tachistoscopic test conditions, in combination with rTMS, is appropriate, sensitive, and accurate in mapping visuospatial attention function on a cortical level.

Additional files

Additional file 1. Subject-related deviation scores per cortical spot for the left hemisphere. Results for stimulation of the left hemisphere. Deviation scores of subject 1–10. Number of subjects with negative deviation scores ("leftward") and mean of their scores. Number of subjects with positive deviation scores ("rightward") and mean of their scores. Outline per cortical spot (no. 1–52) plus mean, standard deviation (SD), minimum (MIN), and maximum (MAX).

Additional file 2. Subject-related deviation scores per cortical spot for the right hemisphere Results for stimulation of the right hemisphere. Deviation scores of subject 1–10. Number of subjects with negative deviation scores ("leftward") and mean of their scores. Number of subjects with positive deviation scores ("rightward") and mean of their scores. Outline per cortical spot (no. 1–52) plus mean, standard deviation (SD), minimum (MIN), and maximum (MAX).

Additional file 3. Raw data per cortical spot for the left hemisphere. Results for stimulation of the left hemisphere. Raw data of each subject. Number of effective stimulations, "leftward" answers and "rightward" answers. Outline per cortical spot (no. 1–52) plus mean, standard deviation (SD), minimum (MIN), and maximum (MAX).

Additional file 4. Raw data per cortical spot for the right hemisphere. Results for stimulation of the right hemisphere. Raw data of each subject. Number of effective stimulations, "leftward" answers and "rightward" answers. Outline per cortical spot (no. 1–52) plus mean, standard deviation (SD), minimum (MIN), and maximum (MAX).

Abbreviations

fMRI: functional magnetic resonance imaging; MRI: magnetic resonance imaging; RMT: resting motor threshold; rTMS: repetitive navigated transcranial magnetic stimulation; TMS: transcranial magnetic stimulation; TPJ: temporoparietal junction.

Authors' contributions
KG was responsible for the recruitment of participants, data acquisition and analysis, literature research and manuscript draft. SM performed pretests, participated in interpreting the data and corrected the final manuscript. CZ and BM were part of the conception planning and critically revised the final manuscript. SK is responsible for concept and design of the study, performed literature research, handled the acquired data and drafted the manuscript. All authors agreed to be accountable for all aspects of the work. All authors read and approved the final manuscript.

Authors' information
KG is a medical student, SM is a neurosurgical resident. They are performing a high number of rTMS studies in healthy subjects and brain tumor patients. CZ is chairman of the section of neuroradiology. BM is chairman of the department of neurosurgery. SK is attending neurosurgeon. BM and SK are involved in the treatment of brain tumors in a specialized neurooncological center, including preoperative mapping, intraoperative neuroimaging and awake surgery.

Author details
[1] Department of Neurosurgery, Klinikum rechts der Isar, Technische Universität München, Ismaninger Str. 22, 81675 Munich, Germany. [2] TUM-Neuroimaging Center, Klinikum rechts der Isar, Technische Universität München, Munich, Germany. [3] Section of Neuroradiology, Department of Radiology, Klinikum rechts der Isar, Technische Universität München, Ismaninger Str. 22, 81675 Munich, Germany.

Acknowledgements
The first author gratefully acknowledges the support of the TUM Graduate School.

Competing interests
All authors declare that they have no conflict of interest affecting this study, the materials or methods used, or the findings specified in this paper. SK is a consultant for Brainlab AG (Munich, Germany) and for Nexstim Plc. (Helsinki, Finland).

Funding
This study was funded by institutional grants from the Department of Neurosurgery and the Section of Neuroradiology.

References
1. Corbetta M, Kincade MJ, Lewis C, Snyder AZ, Sapir A. Neural basis and recovery of spatial attention deficits in spatial neglect. Nat Neurosci. 2005;8(11):1603–10.
2. Duecker F, Sack AT. The hybrid model of attentional control: new insights into hemispheric asymmetries inferred from TMS research. Neuropsychologia. 2014;74:21–9.
3. Corbetta M, Shulman GL. Spatial neglect and attention networks. Annu Rev Neurosci. 2011;34(1):569–99.
4. Jehkonen M, Ahonen JP, Dastidar P, Koivisto AM, Laippala P, Vilkki J, Molnar G. Visual neglect as a predictor of functional outcome one year after stroke. Acta Neurol Scand. 2000;101(3):195–201.
5. Jehkonen M, Laihosalo M, Kettunen JE. Impact of neglect on functional outcome after stroke—a review of methodological issues and recent research findings. Restor Neurol Neurosci. 2006;24(4–6):209–15.
6. Katz N, Hartman-Maeir A, Ring H, Soroker N. Functional disability and rehabilitation outcome in right hemisphere damaged patients with and without unilateral spatial neglect. Arch Phys Med Rehabil. 1999;80(4):379–84.
7. Sack AT. Using non-invasive brain interference as a tool for mimicking spatial neglect in healthy volunteers. Restor Neurol Neurosci. 2010;28(4):485–97.
8. Suchan J, Rorden C, Karnath HO. Neglect severity after left and right brain damage. Neuropsychologia. 2012;50(6):1136–41.
9. Ottenhausen M, Krieg SM, Meyer B, Ringel F. Functional preoperative and intraoperative mapping and monitoring: increasing safety and efficacy in glioma surgery. Neurosurg Focus. 2015;38(1):E3.
10. Sanai N, Martino J, Berger MS. Morbidity profile following aggressive resection of parietal lobe gliomas. J Neurosurg. 2012;116(6):1182–6.
11. Fierro B, Brighina F, Bisiach E. Improving neglect by TMS. Behav Neurol. 2006;17(3):169–76.
12. Koch G, Bonni S, Giacobbe V, Bucchi G, Basile B, Lupo F, Versace V, Bozzali M, Caltagirone C. Theta-burst stimulation of the left hemisphere accelerates recovery of hemispatial neglect. Neurology. 2012;78(1):24–30.
13. Ruohonen J, Karhu J. Navigated transcranial magnetic stimulation. Neurophysiol Clin. 2010;40(1):7–17.
14. Benwell CS, Learmonth G, Miniussi C, Harvey M, Thut G. Non-linear effects of transcranial direct current stimulation as a function of individual baseline performance: Evidence from biparietal tDCS influence on lateralized attention bias. Cortex. 2015;69:152–65.
15. Brooks JL, Della Sala S, Darling S. Representational pseudoneglect: a review. Neuropsychol Rev. 2014;24(2):148–65.
16. Cicek M, Deouell LY, Knight RT. Brain activity during landmark and line bisection tasks. Front Hum Neurosci. 2009;3:7.
17. Goedert KM, Leblanc A, Tsai SW, Barrett AM. Asymmetrical effects of adaptation to left- and right-shifting prisms depends on pre-existing attentional biases. J Int Neuropsychol Soc. 2010;16(5):795–804.
18. Jewell G, McCourt ME. Pseudoneglect: a review and meta-analysis of performance factors in line bisection tasks. Neuropsychologia. 2000;38(1):93–110.
19. Manning L, Halligan PW, Marshall JC. Individual variation in line bisection: a study of normal subjects with application to the interpretation of visual neglect. Neuropsychologia. 1990;28:647–55.
20. Bowers D, Heilman KM. Pseudoneglect: effects of hemispace on a tactile line bisection task. Neuropsychologia. 1980;18(4–5):491–8.
21. Longo MR, Trippier S, Vagnoni E, Lourenco SF. Right hemisphere control of visuospatial attention in near space. Neuropsychologia. 2015;70:350–7.
22. Loftus AM, Nicholls ME. Testing the activation-orientation account of spatial attentional asymmetries using transcranial direct current stimulation. Neuropsychologia. 2012;50(11):2573–6.
23. Petitet P, Noonan MP, Bridge H, O'Reilly JX, O'Shea J. Testing the interhemispheric competition account of visual extinction with combined TMS/fMRI. Neuropsychologia. 2015;74:63–73.
24. Thiebaut de Schotten M, Dell'Acqua F, Forkel SJ, Simmons A, Vergani F, Murphy DG, Catani M. A lateralized brain network for visuospatial attention. Nat Neurosci. 2011;14(10):1245–6.
25. Varnava A, Dervinis M, Chambers CD. The predictive nature of pseudoneglect for visual neglect: evidence from parietal theta burst stimulation. PLoS ONE. 2013;8(6):e65851.
26. Bonato M. Neglect and extinction depend greatly on task demands: a review. Front Hum Neurosci. 2012;6:195.
27. Mattingley JB, Berberovic N, Corben L, Slavin MJ, Nicholls MER, Bradshaw JL. The greyscales task: a perceptual measure of attentional bias following unilateral hemispheric damage. Neuropsychologia. 2004;42(3):387–94.
28. Nicholls ME, Bradshaw JL, Mattingley JB. Free-viewing perceptual assymetries for the judgement of brightness, numerosity and size. Neuropsychologia. 1998;37(3):307–14.
29. Nicholls ME, Roberts GR. Can free-viewing perceptual asymmetries be explained by scanning, pre-motor or attentional biases? Cortex. 2002;38(2):113–36.
30. Mattingley JB, Bradshaw JL, Nettleton NC, Bradshaw JA. Can task specific perceptual bias be distinguished from unilateral neglect? Neuropsychologia. 1994;32(7):805–17.

31. Krieg SM, Sollmann N, Hauck T, Ille S, Meyer B, Ringel F. Repeated mapping of cortical language sites by preoperative navigated transcranial magnetic stimulation compared to repeated intraoperative DCS mapping in awake craniotomy. BMC Neurosci. 2014;15:20.

32. Ille S, Sollmann N, Hauck T, Maurer S, Tanigawa N, Obermueller T, Negwer C, Droese D, Zimmer C, Meyer B, et al. Combined noninvasive language mapping by navigated transcranial magnetic stimulation and functional MRI and its comparison with direct cortical stimulation. J Neurosurg. 2015;123(1):212–25.

33. Tarapore PE, Findlay AM, Honma SM, Mizuiri D, Houde JF, Berger MS, Nagarajan SS. Language mapping with navigated repetitive TMS: proof of technique and validation. NeuroImage. 2013;82:260–72.

34. Picht T, Krieg SM, Sollmann N, Rosler J, Niraula B, Neuvonen T, Savolainen P, Lioumis P, Makela JP, Deletis V, et al. A comparison of language mapping by preoperative navigated transcranial magnetic stimulation and direct cortical stimulation during awake surgery. Neurosurgery. 2013;72(5):808–19.

35. Talacchi A, Squintani GM, Emanuele B, Tramontano V, Santini B, Savazzi S. Intraoperative cortical mapping of visuospatial functions in parietal low-grade tumors: changing perspectives of neurophysiological mapping. Neurosurg Focus. 2013;34(2):E4.

36. Giglhuber K, Maurer S, Zimmer C, Meyer B, Krieg SM. Evoking visual neglect-like deficits in healthy volunteers—an investigation by repetitive navigated transcranial magnetic stimulation. Brain Imaging Behav. 2016. https://doi.org/10.1007/s11682-016-9506-9.

37. Maurer S, Tanigawa N, Sollmann N, Hauck T, Ille S, Boeckh-Behrens T, Meyer B, Krieg S. Non-invasive mapping of calculation function by repetitive navigated transcranial magnetic stimulation. Brain Struct Funct. 2015. https://doi.org/10.1007/s00429-015-1136-2.

38. Rossi S, Hallett M, Rossini PM, Pascual-Leone A. Safety, ethical considerations, and application guidelines for the use of transcranial magnetic stimulation in clinical practice and research. Clin Neurophysiol. 2009;120(12):2008–39.

39. Krieg SM, Sollmann N, Hauck T, Ille S, Foerschler A, Meyer B, Ringel F. Functional language shift to the right hemisphere in patients with language-eloquent brain tumors. PLoS ONE. 2013;8(9):e75403.

40. Sollmann N, Tanigawa N, Ringel F, Zimmer C, Meyer B, Krieg SM. Language and its right-hemispheric distribution in healthy brains: an investigation by repetitive transcranial magnetic stimulation. NeuroImage. 2014;102(Part 2):776–88.

41. Lioumis P, Zhdanov A, Makela N, Lehtinen H, Wilenius J, Neuvonen T, Hannula H, Deletis V, Picht T, Makela JP. A novel approach for documenting naming errors induced by navigated transcranial magnetic stimulation. J Neurosci Methods. 2012;204(2):349–54.

42. Krieg SM, Shiban E, Buchmann NH, Gempt J, Foerschler A, Meyer B, Ringel F. Utility of presurgical navigated transcranial magnetic brain stimulation for the resection of tumors in eloquent motor areas. J Neurosurg. 2012;116(5):994–1001.

43. Epstein CM. Optimum stimulus parameters for lateralized suppression of speech with magnetic brain stimulation. Neurology. 1996;47(6):1590–3.

44. Corina DP, Gibson EK, Martin R, Poliakov A, Brinkley J, Ojemann GA. Dissociation of action and object naming: evidence from cortical stimulation mapping. Hum Brain Mapp. 2005;24(1):1–10.

45. Hauck T, Tanigawa N, Probst M, Wohlschlaeger A, Ille S, Sollmann N, Maurer S, Zimmer C, Ringel F, Meyer B, et al. Stimulation frequency determines the distribution of language positive cortical regions during navigated transcranial magnetic stimulation. BMC Neurosci. 2015;16:5.

46. Krieg SM, Tarapore PE, Picht T, Tanigawa N, Houde J, Sollmann N, Meyer B, Vajkoczy P, Berger MS, Ringel F, et al. Optimal timing of pulse onset for language mapping with navigated repetitive transcranial magnetic stimulation. NeuroImage. 2014;100:219–36.

47. Salatino A, Poncini M, George MS, Ricci R. Hunting for right and left parietal hot spots using single-pulse TMS: modulation of visuospatial perception during line bisection judgment in the healthy brain. Front Psychol. 2014;5:1238.

48. Sollmann N, Tanigawa N, Tussis L, Hauck T, Ille S, Maurer S, Negwer C, Zimmer C, Ringel F, Meyer B, et al. Cortical regions involved in semantic processing investigated by repetitive navigated transcranial magnetic stimulation and object naming. Neuropsychologia. 2015;70:185–95.

49. Friston K. Ten ironic rules for non-statistical reviewers. NeuroImage. 2012;61(4):1300–10.

50. Sollmann N, Ille S, Obermueller T, Negwer C, Ringel F, Meyer B, Krieg SM. The impact of repetitive navigated transcranial magnetic stimulation coil positioning and stimulation parameters on human language function. Eur J Med Res. 2015;20:47.

51. Benwell CS, Thut G, Grant A, Harvey M. A rightward shift in the visuospatial attention vector with healthy aging. Front Aging Neurosci. 2014;6:113.

52. Learmonth G, Benwell CSY, Thut G, Harvey M. Age-related reduction of hemispheric lateralisation for spatial attention: an EEG study. NeuroImage. 2017;153:139–51.

53. Friedrich TE, Hunter PV, Elias LJ. Developmental trajectory of pseudoneglect in adults using the greyscales task. Dev Psychol. 2016;52(11):1937–43.

54. de Haan B, Karnath HO, Driver J. Mechanisms and anatomy of unilateral extinction after brain injury. Neuropsychologia. 2012;50(6):1045–53.

55. Karnath HO, Rorden C. The anatomy of spatial neglect. Neuropsychologia. 2012;50(6):1010–7.

56. Vallar G. Spatial hemineglect in humans. Trends Cogn Sci. 1998;2(3):87–97.

57. Benwell CSY, Harvey M, Gardner S, Thut G. Stimulus- and state-dependence of systematic bias in spatial attention: additive effects of stimulus-size and time-on-task. Cortex. 2013;49(3):827–36.

58. Dufour A, Touzalin P, Candas V. Time-on-task effect in pseudoneglect. Exp Brain Res. 2007;176(3):532–7.

59. Manly T, Dobler VB, Dodds CM, George MA. Rightward shift in spatial awareness with declining alertness. Neuropsychologia. 2005;43(12):1721–8.

60. Stone SP, Patel P, Greenwood RJ, Halligan PW. Measuring visual neglect in acute stroke and predicting its recovery: the visual neglect recovery index. J Neurol Neurosurg Psychiatry. 1992;55(431):436.

61. Kim M, Na DL, Kim GM, Adair JC, Lee KH, Heilman KM. Ipsilesional neglect: behavioural and anatomical features. J Neurol Neurosurg Psychiatry. 1999;67(35):38.

62. Kwon JC, Ahn S, Kim S, Heilman KM. Ipsilesional 'where' with contralesional 'what' neglect. Neurocase. 2011;18(5):415–23.

63. Roux FE, Dufor O, Lauwers-Cances V, Boukhatem L, Brauge D, Draper L, Lotterie JA, Demonet JF. Electrostimulation mapping of spatial neglect. Neurosurgery. 2011;69(6):1218–31.

64. Sacchetti DL, Goedert KM, Foundas AL, Barrett AM. Ipsilesional neglect: behavioral and anatomical correlates. Neuropsychology. 2015;29(2):183–90.

65. Bartolomeo P, de Schotten MT, Chica AB. Brain networks of visuospatial attention and their disruption in visual neglect. Front Hum Neurosci. 2012;6:110.

66. Heilman KM. Right hemisphere dominance for attention: the mechanism underlying hemispheric asymmetries of inattention (neglect). Neurology. 1980;30(3):327.

67. Corbetta M, Shulman GL. Control of goal-directed and stimulus-driven attention in the brain. Nat Rev Neurosci. 2002;3(3):201–15.

68. Na DL, Adair JC, Choi SH, Seo DW, Kang Y, Heilman KM. Ipsilesional versus contralesional neglect depends on attentional demands. Cortex. 2000;36(4):455–67.

69. Robertson IH, Halligan PW, Bergego C, Hömberg V, Pizzamiglio L, Weber E, Wilson BA. Right neglect following right hemisphere damage? Cortex. 1994;30(2):199–213.

70. Chokron S, Peyrin C, Perez C. Ipsilesional deficit of selective attention in left homonymous hemianopia and left unilateral spatial neglect. Neuropsychologia. 2018. https://doi.org/10.1016/j.neuropsychologia.2018.03.013.

71. Lunven M, Thiebaut De Schotten M, Bourlon C, Duret C, Migliaccio R, Rode G, Bartolomeo P. White matter lesional predictors of chronic visual neglect: a longitudinal study. Brain J Neurol. 2015;138(Pt 3):746–60.

72. Suchan J, Umarova R, Schnell S, Himmelbach M, Weiller C, Karnath HO, Saur D. Fiber pathways connecting cortical areas relevant for spatial orienting and exploration. Hum Brain Mapp. 2014;35(3):1031–43.

73. Umarova RM, Reisert M, Beier TU, Kiselev VG, Kloppel S, Kaller CP, Glauche V, Mader I, Beume L, Hennig J, et al. Attention-network specific alterations of structural connectivity in the undamaged white matter in acute neglect. Hum Brain Mapp. 2014;35(9):4678–92.

74. Ricci R, Salatino A, Li X, Funk AP, Logan SL, Mu Q, Johnson KA, Bohning DE, George MS. Imaging the neural mechanisms of TMS neglect-like bias in

healthy volunteers with the interleaved TMS/fMRI technique: preliminary evidence. Front Hum Neurosci. 2012;6:326.

75. Negwer C, Ille S, Hauck T, Sollmann N, Maurer S, Kirschke JS, Ringel F, Meyer B, Krieg SM. Visualization of subcortical language pathways by diffusion tensor imaging fiber tracking based on rTMS language mapping. Brain Imaging Behav. 2016. https://doi.org/10.1007/s11682-016-9563-0.

76. Sollmann N, Kubitscheck A, Maurer S, Ille S, Hauck T, Kirschke JS, Ringel F, Meyer B, Krieg SM. Preoperative language mapping by repetitive navigated transcranial magnetic stimulation and diffusion tensor imaging fiber tracking and their comparison to intraoperative stimulation. Neuroradiology. 2016;58(8):807–18.

77. Sollmann N, Negwer C, Ille S, Maurer S, Hauck T, Kirschke JS, Ringel F, Meyer B, Krieg SM. Feasibility of nTMS-based DTI fiber tracking of language pathways in neurosurgical patients using a fractional anisotropy threshold. J Neurosci Methods. 2016;267:45–54.

78. Sollmann N, Negwer C, Tussis L, Hauck T, Ille S, Maurer S, Giglhuber K, Bauer JS, Ringel F, Meyer B, et al. Interhemispheric connectivity revealed by diffusion tensor imaging fiber tracking derived from navigated transcranial magnetic stimulation maps as a sign of language function at risk in patients with brain tumors. J Neurosurg. 2016. https://doi.org/10.3171/2016.1.JNS152053.

79. Duffau H. The huge plastic potential of adult brain and the role of connectomics: new insights provided by serial mappings in glioma surgery. Cortex. 2013;58:325–37.

80. Brighina F, Bisiach E, Oliveri M, Piazza A, La Bua V, Daniele O, Fierro B. 1 Hz repetitive transcranial magnetic stimulation of the unaffected hemisphere ameliorates contralesional visuospatial neglect in humans. Neurosci Lett. 2003;336(2):131–3.

4

The effect of intracerebroventricular administration of orexin receptor type 2 antagonist on pentylenetetrazol-induced kindled seizures and anxiety in rats

Saeedeh Asadi[1], Ali Roohbakhsh[2], Ali Shamsizadeh[3], Masoud Fereidoni[1], Elham Kordijaz[1] and Ali Moghimi[1*] ⓘ

Abstract

Background: Current antiepileptic drugs are not able to prevent recurrent seizures in all patients. Orexins are excitatory hypothalamic neuropeptides that their receptors (Orx1R and Orx2R) are found almost in all major regions of the brain. Pentylenetetrazol (PTZ)-induced kindling is a known experimental model for epileptic seizures. The purpose of this study was to evaluate the effect of Orx2 receptor antagonist (TCS OX2 29) on seizures and anxiety of PTZ-kindled rats.

Results: Our results revealed that similar to valproate, administration of 7 μg/rat of TCS OX2 29 increased the latency period and decreased the duration time of 3rd and 4th stages of epileptiform seizures. Besides, it significantly decreased mean of seizure scores. However, TCS OX2 29 did not modulate anxiety induced by repeated PTZ administration.

Conclusion: This study showed that blockade of Orx2 receptor reduced seizure-related behaviors without any significant effect on PTZ-induced anxiety.

Keywords: Anxiety, Kindling, Orexin, Orx2 receptor, PTZ, Seizure

Background

Epilepsy is a chronic neurological disorder that its main characteristic is the recurrent appearance of spontaneous seizures [1]. Research on experimental models of this disease indicates that there is an imbalance between the inhibitory GABAergic and excitatory glutamatergic neurotransmission in the central nervous system (CNS) [2]. At present, various antiepileptics are available. However, dose-related neurotoxicity, a range of drug interactions, and systemic side effects are the major problems caused by current antiepileptic drugs [3].

Orexins (orexin A and B) are hypothalamic excitatory neuropeptides [4]. Orexinergic neurons are located in the lateral hypothalamic area, perifornical area, dorsomedial hypothalamus, and posterior hypothalamus, which project to different parts of the brain [5]. The physiological functions of the orexins are mediated by two G-protein coupled receptors: orexin receptor type 1 (Orx1R) and orexin receptor type 2 (Orx2R). The affinity of Orx1R for orexin A is higher than orexin B, whereas Orx2R has a similar affinity for both neuropeptides [6]. Stimulation of these receptors increases intracellular Ca^{2+} through Gq/11 activation in orexin responsive cells [7]. It was demonstrated that the activation of orexin receptors provoked cortical pyramidal cells and enhanced cortical excitability [8, 9]. Orexin A was reported to be involved in long-term potentiation of synaptic transmission in the CA1 region of the hippocampus. This effect was dependent on ionotropic and metabotropic GABAergic,

*Correspondence: moghimi@um.ac.ir
[1] Department of Biology, Rayan Center for Neuroscience and Behavior, Faculty of Science, Ferdowsi University of Mashhad, P.O. Box 9177948974, Mashhad, Iran
Full list of author information is available at the end of the article

glutamatergic, as well as cholinergic and noradrenergic receptors implying the active role of the orexinergic system in learning and memory [10]. Similarly, Riahi et al. [11] showed that administration of orexin A in the lateral ventricle of the rats increased electrical activity of the hippocampal pyramidal neurons.

Orexins regulate the release of serotonin, gamma-aminobutyric acid (GABA), and glutamate [12, 13]. These neurotransmitters are involved in the regulation of sleep and wakefulness, pain, food intake, reward, multiple sclerosis, and stress [5, 14]. As mentioned, orexins have excitatory effects in the CNS. There is evidence implying that orexins may be involved in the generation and propagation of seizures. For example, it was reported that intracortical and intracerebroventricular injections of orexins caused seizure-related behaviors in rats [15, 16]. Both orexin A and B enhanced the excitability of the central nervous system following administration of penicillin G [17]. In accordance, it was revealed that during pilocarpine-induced epileptic activity, the expression of orexin B was increased in the rat hippocampus [18].

Chemical kindled seizure is an animal model of temporal lobe epilepsy induced by repeated administration of an initially subconvulsive chemical stimulus such as pentylenetetrazol (PTZ) that results in behavioral signs of tonic and clonic seizures [19]. Injection of such chemicals decreases seizure threshold and culminates in a generalized seizure [20]. In other words, PTZ increases seizure susceptibility. The molecular mechanism(s) behind this phenomenon has not been well understood. Some studies have offered that inhibition of main inhibitory systems of the CNS including GABAA-mediated actions and activation of stimulatory systems such as NMDA, AMPA, and kainate receptors are part of a complex network that culminates in the development of kindling [21, 22]. Kindling has been introduced as a reliable experimental model for complex partial epilepsy in patients [23] and has been considered as a drug-resistant model of epilepsy [24].

On the other hand, anxiety is a common comorbidity that is related to epilepsy [25]. It has been demonstrated that the orexinergic system and the hypothalamic–pituitary–adrenal axis contribute together in the modulation of stress responses [26]. Moreover, orexins exert anxiety both in mice and rats [27, 28]. Using optogenetic approaches, Sears et al. [29] showed that stimulation of orexin fibers in the locus coeruleus increased threat memory formation induced via an auditory stimulus. Also, it was demonstrated that orexin A levels in the amygdala were increased following social interaction, positive emotions, and anger in narcoleptic patients [30]. Another study showed that there was a positive relation between orexin levels and childhood maltreatment [31]. All these studies imply that orexinergic system has

an important role in the modulation of anxiety both in rodents and human. On the other hand, orexin is an important neuropeptide with significant effects on food intake. It increases appetite and consequently food intake. As nutrition has been reported to be involved in anxiety [32], it is a possibility that orexins and their antagonits, through alteration of appetite, modulate anxiety.

On the basis of these findings, we hypothesized that blockade of Orx2 receptors might be useful for the prevention of epilepsy and concomitant anxiety. Accordingly, we aimed to assess the effect of an Orx2R antagonist (TCS OX2 29) on PTZ-induced chemical kindling and anxiety.

Methods
Drugs
Orexin antagonist (TCS OX2 29) was purchased from Tocris (Bristol, UK). Its chemical name is (2S)-1-(3,4-Dihydro-6,7-dimethoxy-2(1H)-isoquinolinyl)-3,3-dimethyl-2-[(4-pyridinylmethyl)amino]-1-butanone hydrochloride. This drug was first introduced by Hirose et al. in 2003. After that, the drug has been used widely as a selective Orx2R antagonist. It promoted sleep [33], decreased heart rate, and blood pressure [34], reduced morphine place preference [35], prevented analgesia, and reduced alcohol self administration [36].

Pentylenetetrazol and sodium valproate were purchased from Sigma (India) and Sanofi-aventis (France), respectively. PTZ and sodium valproate were dissolved in 0.9% sterile saline. TCS OX2 29 was dissolved in dimethyl sulfoxide (DMSO), tween 80 and sterile 0.9% saline (10/10/80% v/v respectively).

Animals
Adult male Wistar rats (200–250 g) were used in this study. The animals were bred in the experimental animal house of Ferdowsi University. All animals were maintained under normal conditions (12/12 h light/dark cycle, temperature: 23 ± 2 °C), with ad libitum availability of food and water. Each experimental group included seven animals.

Stereotaxic surgery and microinjections
Rats were anesthetized with an intraperitoneal (IP) administration of ketamine (100 mg/kg) and xylazine (4 mg/kg). They were fixed on a stereotaxic apparatus (Narishige, Tokyo, Japan). Enrofloxacin was injected to prevent infections and ketoprofen was administrated for post-operative analgesia. Stainless steel guide cannula (22-gauge) fitted with the infusion cannula (27-gauge, 1 mm longer) was implanted into the left lateral ventricle (AP = 0.8 mm, ML = 1.6 mm and D = 4 mm) according to Paxinos and Watson's stereotaxic atlas [37]. Acrylic

dental cement and surgical screws were used to fix the guide cannula. Six days after recovery from the stereotaxic surgery, different solutions (TCS OX2 29, valproate and vehicle) were injected into the left lateral ventricle (2 µl/rat) of awake and freely moving rats. Intracerebroventricular (ICV) injections were done using an infusion pump (Stoelting, USA) at the rate of 2 µl/min. At the end of experiments, 0.5 µl of methylene blue was injected through the guide cannula. After that, the rats were killed and the brain slices prepared using microtome checked under a stereo microscope to ensure the placement of cannula.

Induction of kindling and experimental design

For induction of kindling, PTZ (32 mg/kg) was injected intraperitoneally every other day for 23 days [38].

The vehicle (2 µl/rat), TCS OX2 29 (1, 3.5 and 7 µg/rat) and valproate (as the control drug, 26 µg/rat), were administered ICV 30 min before PTZ injections. The doses for TCS OX2 29 and valproate were selected according to previous studies [4, 39]. After injection of PTZ, seizure-related behaviors were recorded for 30 min. The intensity of seizure behaviors was recorded on the following scale: 0 = no response; 1 = vibrissae twitching, mouth and facial jerks; 2 = myoclonic body jerks or head nodding; 3 = forelimb clonus; 4 = rearing, falling down, forelimb tonus and hindlimb clonus; and 5 = tonic extension of the hindlimb, status epilepticus [40, 41]. Accordingly, we recorded the following parameters: (1) Median of seizure scores (2) Latency to the first forelimb clonus (S3L) (3) Duration of forelimb clonuses (4) Latency to the first sign of scale 4 behaviors (S4L) (5) Duration of scale 4 behaviors (S4D).

Elevated plus-maze (EPM)

EPM test is a standard method that has been employed for determining the anxious behaviors in rodents [42]. Hereafter, anxious behaviors in rats referred to as anxiety. It consists of two open and two closed arms as a plus sign. The percentage of open arm entries (%OAE) and the percentage of time spent on the open arms (%OAT), as standard indices of anxiety, were recorded for 5 min. Total arm entries were also recorded as a measure of spontaneous locomotor activity. A significant increase in %OAT and %OAE represent a lower anxiety response [43].

On the last day of the experiments (30 min after PTZ injection), animals were placed on the EPM. To compare the effect of PTZ on anxiety, an extra control group of animals received TCS OX2 29 vehicle (2 µl/rat, ICV) and saline (6 ml/rat, IP) and were tested in the EPM.

Statistical analysis

The data for seizure stages were expressed as median ± interquartiles. The stages were analyzed using Kruskal–Wallis non-parametric one-way analysis of variance (ANOVA) followed by 2-tailed Mann–Whitney's U test. Other data were expressed as mean ± SEM. Differences between groups were analyzed by one-way analysis of variance which was followed by Tukey as post-test. The minimum level of significance was set at $P < 0.05$.

Results

The effects of TCS OX2 29 on chemical kindling

The results showed that administration of TCS OX2 29 at the dose of 7 µg/rat significantly decreased median of seizure scores ($P < 0.01$). However, TCS OX2 29 at the doses of 1 and 3.5 µg/rat and valproate did not significantly change the median of seizure scores (Fig. 1).

Furthermore, TCS OX2 29 at the dose of 7 µg/rat decreased the duration of the 3rd stage of seizure (S3 duration, $P < 0.01$) and increased the stage 3 latency (S3 latency, $P < 0.01$), in comparison with the control group. However, valproate failed to show such protective effects either on S3 duration or S3 latency (Figs. 2, 3).

TCS OX2 29 at dose of 7 µg/rat also decreased the duration of the 4th stage of seizure (S4 duration, $P < 0.05$) and increased the stage 4 latency (S4 latency, $P < 0.01$). Similarly, valproate decreased S4 duration ($P < 0.05$) and increased S4 latency ($P < 0.01$). TCS OX2 29 at doses of 1 and 3.5 µg/rat had no significant effect on either S4 duration or S4 latency (Figs. 4, 5).

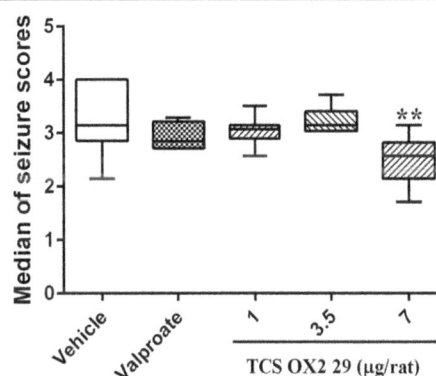

Fig. 1 The effect of intracerebroventricular injection of TCS OX2 29 (1, 3.5 and 7 µg/rat) and valproate (26 µg/rat) on median of seizure scores in pentylenetetrazol-kindled rats. TCS OX2 29 at the dose of 7 µg/rat reduced median of seizure scores. Each bar represents median ± interquartiles. **$P < 0.01$ compared to vehicle-treated rats. In each group n = 7

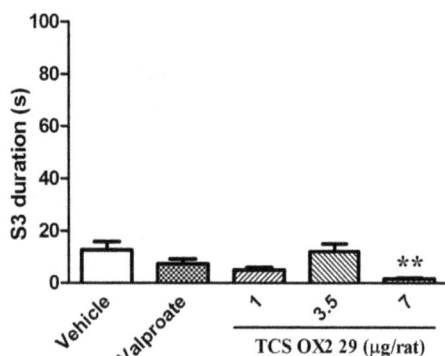

Fig. 2 The effect of intracerebroventricular injection of TCS OX2 29 (1, 3.5 and 7 µg/rat) and valproate (26 µg/rat) on stage 3 duration in pentylenetetrazol-kindled rats. TCS OX2 29 at the dose of 7 µg/rat reduced the stage 3 duration. Each bar represents mean ± SEM. **P < 0.01 compared to vehicle-treated rats. In each group n = 7

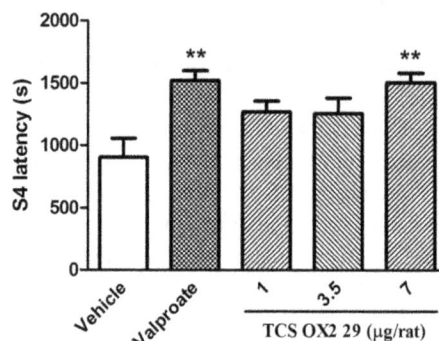

Fig. 3 The effect of intracerebroventricular injection of TCS OX2 29 (1, 3.5 and 7 µg/rat) and valproate (26 µg/rat) on stage 3 latency in pentylenetetrazol-kindled rats. TCS OX2 29 at the dose of 7 µg/rat increased latency of 3th stage of seizures. Each bar represents mean ± SEM. **P < 0.01 compared to vehicle-treated rats. In each group n = 7

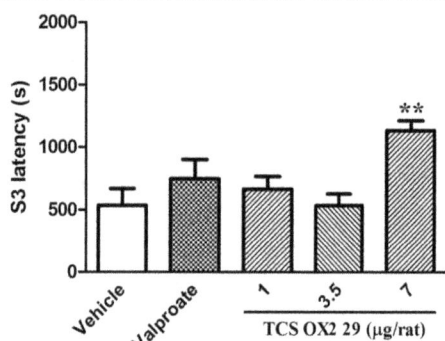

Fig. 4 The effect of intracerebroventricular injection of TCS OX2 29 (1, 3.5 and 7 µg/rat) and valproate (26 µg/rat) on stage 4 duration in pentylenetetrazol-kindled rats. TCS OX2 29 at the dose of 7 µg/rat and valproate at the dose of 26 µg/rat decreased duration of 4th stage of seizures. Each bar represents mean ± SEM. *P < 0.05 compared to vehicle-treated rats. In each group n = 7

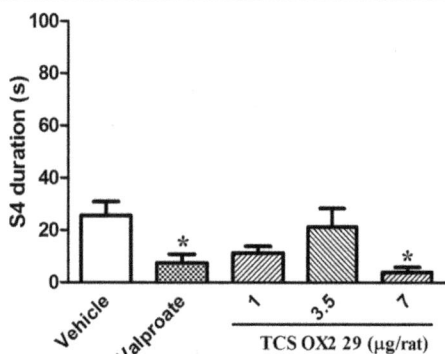

Fig. 5 The effect of intracerebroventricular injection of TCS OX2 29 (1, 3.5 and 7 µg/rat) and valproate (26 µg/rat) on stage 4 latency in pentylenetetrazol-kindled rats. TCS OX2 29 at the dose of 7 µg/rat and valproate at the dose of 26 µg/rat increased the latency period of stage 4 seizures. Each bar represents mean ± SEM. **P < 0.01 compared to vehicle-treated rats. In each group n = 7

The effects of TCS OX2 29 on PTZ-induced anxiety

The results of EPM test showed that kindling induced anxiety that was manifested as the diminished percentage of time spent on the open arms (P < 0.05) in vehicle/PTZ-treated rats. In these animals, the locomotor activity was not different from the control group implying that PTZ induced an anxiety. However, administration of either valproate or TCS OX2 29 (1, 3.5 and 7 µg/rat) did not change the anxiety of PTZ-kindled rats (Fig. 6a–c).

Discussion

The results of this study showed that similar to valproate, intracerebroventricular administration of TCS OX2 29 at the highest dose (7 µg/rat) induced significant anti-seizure effects on generalized convulsions in PTZ-kindled rats. For the first time, the results of our study revealed that Orx2R antagonists have the potential to be used in the prevention of partial seizures with secondary generalization. However, Orx2R antagonist failed to resolve concomitant anxiety.

It is presumed that blockade of the GABAergic system and increased activity of the glutamatergic system are neuronal processes involved in the kindling [19, 44]. Previous studies revealed that orexin A and orexin B have stimulatory effects on the neuronal system. For example, Stanley and Fadel showed that injection of orexin A into the CA1 area of the hippocampus increased glutamate release [45]. Similarly, it was demonstrated that following orexins injection into the cerebrospinal fluid, glutamate level in the hippocampus was increased, and it was reduced after administration of Orx1R antagonist. Similar to these findings, Goudarzi et al. [46] showed that TCS OX2 29 reduced convulsive stages and duration. There is

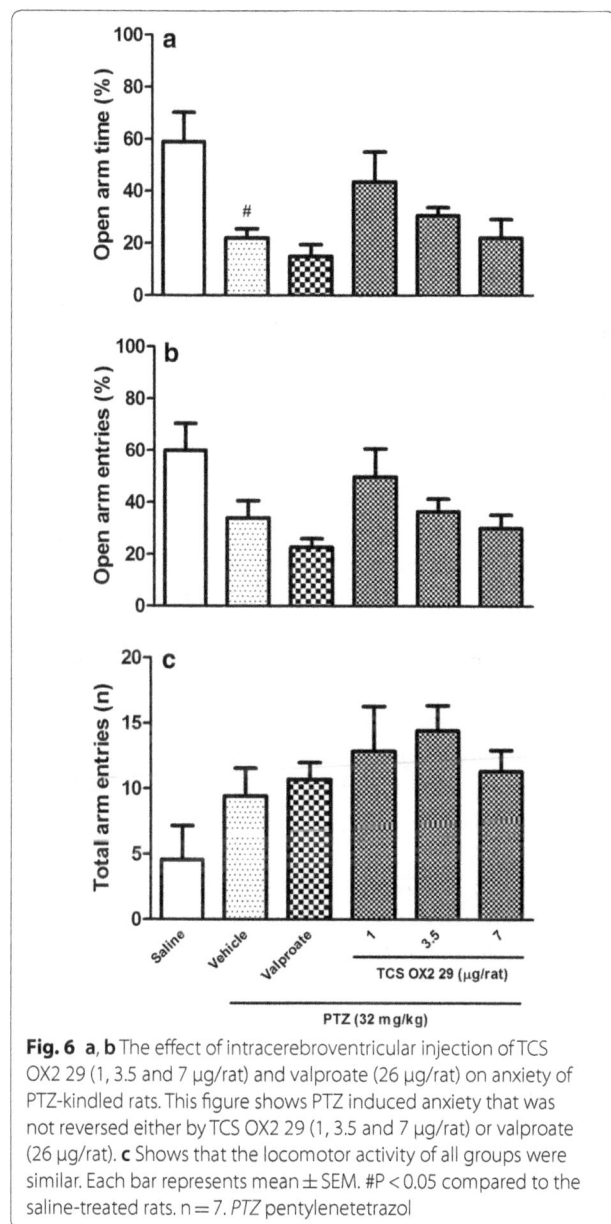

Fig. 6 a, b The effect of intracerebroventricular injection of TCS OX2 29 (1, 3.5 and 7 µg/rat) and valproate (26 µg/rat) on anxiety of PTZ-kindled rats. This figure shows PTZ induced anxiety that was not reversed either by TCS OX2 29 (1, 3.5 and 7 µg/rat) or valproate (26 µg/rat). **c** Shows that the locomotor activity of all groups were similar. Each bar represents mean ± SEM. #$P < 0.05$ compared to the saline-treated rats. n = 7. *PTZ* pentylenetetrazol

according to the previous evidence, orexin may also induce its stimulatory effects through the modulation of the GABAergic system. It is known that orexin affects the release of GABA [51] and upregulates mechanisms responsible for the synthesis and the release of glutamate [52]. In accordance, Goudarzi et al. [46] showed that following hippocampal Orx1R but not Orx2R blockade, the release of GABA was increased. Similarly, a dual orexin receptor antagonist increased the activity of GABAergic systems in the basal forebrain [51]. On the other hand, glutamate and GABA increase and decrease the activity of orexinergic neurons, respectively [53].

Another possibility that explains the effects of TCS OX2 29 on seizure is the activation of two distinct pathways by Orx2R. It was revealed that orexinergic receptors are present on different cortical GABAergic interneurons [54, 55] and neocortical pyramidal cells [56]. Here, we suggest that there are connections between some cortical inhibitory interneurons and cortical pyramidal neurons (e.g., hippocampus). In our proposed mechanism, in spite of inhibitory actions of interneurons on pyramidal neurons, during activation of orexin receptors present on both neurons, pyramidal neurons will have normal outputs. In this study, TCS OX2 29 at the dose of 1 µg/rat reduced the pyramidal neurons output after which the seizure threshold increased. However, TCS OX2 29 at the dose of 3.5 µg/rat inhibited pyramidal neurons but exerted more inhibitory effects on the interneurons, so the output of pyramidal neurons increased followed by increased susceptibility to convulsions. This suggestion may be confirmed by Tang et al. [57] study that showed the concentration dependent inhibition of Gq or Gi proteins by Orx2R antagonists, which induced different effects. Hence, at the dose of 3.5 µg/rat of the Orx2R antagonist, stronger inhibition of interneurons may be explained by more coupling of orexin receptors with Gi rather than Gq. At the dose of 7 µg/rat, the antagonist may increase the tendency of interneurons receptors for coupling with Gq (instead of Gi) that will diminish pyramidal neurons outputs and convulsive behaviors. It is possible that orexins, by activation of either Orx1R or Orx2R, modulate the function of neurotransmitters other than GABA and glutamate. Such interaction was reported just recently for endocannabinoids as TCS OX2 29 enhanced the effect of a cannabinoid receptor antagonist in the conditioned place preference paradigm [58].

Although we choose the dose of valproate as a standard antiepileptic drug according to a previous report [39], it did not induce a robust anti-seizure effect in the 3rd stage of seizure in the this study. In clinical practice, valproate has been used extensively for the treatment of

more evidence to support our results; in a recent study, it was demonstrated that administration of TCS OX2 29 reduced the severity of seizures and neuronal damage in the hippocampus of the rats following PTZ administration and sleep deprivation [4]. Also, the orexinergic system influenced the function of the limbic structures and the neocortex which are involved in controlling the incidence of seizures and epilepsy through their projections to the neuromodulatory centers located in the brain stem [47, 48]. The high-density expression of Orx2R in CA3 area of the hippocampus [49], can be a reason for the pro-convulsant effect of the orexins [50]. Furthermore,

various kinds of epilepsy including partial seizures. Valproate, via diverse pharmacological actions including the modulation of Na^+ channels, inhibition of Ca^{2+} channels, inhibition of GABA transaminase, and increase in GABA concentration induces anticonvulsant effects [59]. However, there are reports showing that valproate has lower efficacy than carbamazepine, as an standard antiepileptic drug, in the treatment of partial and secondary generalized tonic–clonic seizures. This may explain the low efficacy of valproate in this study [60, 61]. Stanojlović and colleagues showed that valproate rapidly reduced mean seizure score and audiogenic convulsions in metaphit-treated Wistar rats. However, the drug did not exhibit significant effect on electrocortical activity. So, they concluded that valproate is an anticonvulsant rather than antiepileptic drug [62]. By comparison, it may be suggested that TCS OX2 29 had a higher potency than valproate.

Epileptic patients also suffer from anxiety [25]. So, finding medications that are able to treat both disorders are of great interest and importance. Our obtained results revealed that PTZ induced anxiety in the elevated plus-maze. In parallel with our results, it was demonstrated that PTZ, by activation of the glutamatergic system, induced convulsion and caused anxiety [63]. We presumed that orexinergic system is a target that modulates both anxiety and seizure. It has been reported that orexinergic system overactivation is an important factor in maintaining arousal and anxiety [64]. It was reported that depressive behaviors were higher in mice with lower hippocampal orexin [65]. In addition, knocking down of Orx2R in the basolateral amygdala increased anxious behaviors in mice [66]. Approval of suvorexant, as a dual receptor antagonist, for the treatment of insomnia [67] shows the importance of the orexinergic system in sleep and wake cycle. There are numerous orexinergic terminals in areas associated with stress and anxiety including the middle prefrontal cortex of cingulate cortex. Also, ICV injection of orexin A induced anxiety in different experimental models of anxiety [28]. Similarly, it was reported that injection of orexin A and B in the paraventricular nuclei of the thalamus caused anxiety [27]. This evidence implies that orexinergic system is an important target in the modulation of stress and anxiety [68]. However, it should be mentioned that previous studies showed that Orx1R has a more important role than Orx2R in the modulation of anxiety [64]. According to our results, TCS OX2 29 failed to overcome PTZ-induced anxiety. This finding is possibly in accordance with previous studies showing that the anxiogenic effect of orexins is mediated mainly by Orx1R [69]. However, we cannot rule out the effect of TCS OX2 29 on anxiety at higher doses. Our results also revealed that the motor

activity of the animals that received TCS OX2 29 was not different from the vehicle-treated group on the EPM. This finding may imply that the anticonvulsant effect of TCS OX2 29 at the dose of 7 µg/rat was not influenced by changes in muscle tone. One of the limitations of this study is that we used an animal model of anxiety that did not have a social component. For example, social interaction test would be more applicable in such kind of studies. As the second limitation, electrical kindling has been reported with minor advantages over chemical kindling that makes it a better method for evaluation of the potential anticonvulsant drugs [70]. Finally, it is a possibility that orexin and its antagonists modulate epilepsy and anxiety via metabolic changes. For example, hyperhomocysteinemia is reported to be affected by different dietary patterns [71]. Hyperhomocysteinemia has been related to anxiety-like behaviors in rats [72] and human [73]. On the other hand, low levels of homocysteine may induce epilepsy [74]. Considering the very important role of orexinergic system in feeding and nutrition, it is a possibility that this system modulates anxiety and/or epilepsy via metabolic changes.

Our study showed that TCS OX2 29, as a selective Orx2R antagonist, reduced the severity of the seizures of the PTZ-kindled rats. However, it did not affect PTZ-induced anxiety.

Conclusion

It may be suggested that the orexinergic system has the potential to be considered as an important target in the treatment of epilepsy.

Authors' contributions
SA and EK did the experiments including the stereotaxic surgery, induction of kindling and behavioral assessment. AS and AR designed the experiments and did the statistical analysis. MF and AM interpreted the data, drafted, and wrote the manuscript. SA and AR did a critical revision of the manuscript. All authors read and approved the final manuscript.

Author details
Department of Biology, Rayan Center for Neuroscience and Behavior, Faculty of Science, Ferdowsi University of Mashhad, P.O. Box 9177948974, Mashhad, Iran. [2] Pharmaceutical Research Center, Pharmaceutical Technology Institute, Mashhad University of Medical Sciences, Mashhad, Iran. [3] Physiology-Pharmacology Research Center, Rafsanjan University of Medical Sciences, Rafsanjan, Iran.

Acknowledgements
The authors acknowledge the vice president of the Ferdowsi University of Mashhad in research and technology and research council of Mashhad University of Medical Sciences for their official and financial supports.

Competing interests
The authors declare that they have no competing interests.

Funding

Authors are grateful for financial and instrumental supports of the Mashhad University of Medical Sciences (Grant No. 922445) and also the Ferdowsi University of Mashhad for partially financial support (Grant No. 3/37138).

References

1. Blumcke I, Beck H, Lie AA, Wiestler OD. Molecular neuropathology of human mesial temporal lobe epilepsy. Epilepsy Res. 1999;36:205–23.
2. Mehta A, Prabhakar M, Kumar P, Deshmukh R, Sharma PL. Excitotoxicity: bridge to various triggers in neurodegenerative disorders. Eur J Pharmacol. 2013;698:6–18.
3. Reynolds EH, Trimble MR. Adverse neuropsychiatric effects of anticonvulsant drugs. Drugs. 1985;29:570–81.
4. Ni LY, Zhu MJ, Song Y, Liu XM, Tang JY. Pentylenetetrazol-induced seizures are exacerbated by sleep deprivation through orexin receptor-mediated hippocampal cell proliferation. Neurol Sci. 2014;35:245–52.
5. Sakurai T. The role of orexin in motivated behaviours. Nat Rev Neursci. 2014;15:719–31.
6. Sakurai T, Amemiya A, Ishii M, Matsuzaki I, Chemelli RM, Tanaka H, et al. Orexins and orexin receptors: a family of hypothalamic neuropeptides and G protein-coupled receptors that regulate feeding behavior. Cell. 1998;92:13.
7. Gotter AL, Webber AL, Coleman PJ, Renger JJ, Winrow CJ. International Union of Basic and Clinical Pharmacology. LXXXVI. Orexin receptor function, nomenclature and pharmacology. Pharmacol Rev. 2012;64:389–420.
8. Li B, Chen F, Ye J, Chen X, Yan J, Li Y, et al. The modulation of orexin A on HCN currents of pyramidal neurons in mouse prelimbic cortex. Cereb Cortex. 2009. https://doi.org/10.1093/cercor/bhp241.
9. Yan J, He C, Xia J-X, Zhang D, Hu Z-A. Orexin-A excites pyramidal neurons in layer 2/3 of the rat prefrontal cortex. Neurosci Lett. 2012;520:92–7.
10. Selbach O, Doreulee N, Bohla C, Eriksson KS, Sergeeva OA, Poelchen W, et al. Orexins/hypocretins cause sharp wave- and theta-related synaptic plasticity in the hippocampus via glutamatergic, gabaergic, noradrenergic, and cholinergic signaling. Neuroscience. 2004;127:519–28.
11. Riahi E, Arezoomandan R, Fatahi Z, Haghparast A. The electrical activity of hippocampal pyramidal neuron is subjected to descending control by the brain orexin/hypocretin system. Neurobiol Learn Mem. 2015;119:93–101.
12. Liu RJ, van den Pol AN, Aghajanian GK. Hypocretins (orexins) regulate serotonin neurons in the dorsal raphe nucleus by excitatory direct and inhibitory indirect actions. J Neurosci. 2002;22:9453–64.
13. van den Pol AN, Gao XB, Obrietan K, Kilduff TS, Belousov AB. Presynaptic and postsynaptic actions and modulation of neuroendocrine neurons by a new hypothalamic peptide, hypocretin/orexin. J Neurosci. 1998;18:7962–71.
14. Fatemi I, Shamsizadeh A, Roohbakhsh A, Ayoobi F, Sanati MH, Motevalian M. Increased mRNA level of orexin1 and 2 receptors following induction of experimental autoimmune encephalomyelitis in mice. Iran J Allergy Asthma. 2016;15:20–6.
15. Erken HA, Erken G, Genc O, Kortunay S, Sahiner M, Turgut G, et al. Orexins cause epileptic activity. Peptides. 2012;37:161–4.
16. Ida T, Nakahara K, Katayama T, Murakami N, Nakazato M. Effect of lateral cerebroventricular injection of the appetite-stimulating neuropeptide, orexin and neuropeptide Y, on the various behavioral activities of rats. Brain Res. 1999;821:526–9.
17. Kortunay S, Erken HA, Erken G, Genc O, Sahiner M, Turgut S, et al. Orexins increase penicillin-induced epileptic activity. Peptides. 2012;34:419–22.
18. Morales A, Bonnet C, Bourgoin N, Touvier T, Nadam J, Laglaine A, et al. Unexpected expression of orexin-B in basal conditions and increased levels in the adult rat hippocampus during pilocarpine-induced epileptogenesis. Brain Res. 2006;1109:164–75.
19. Szyndler J, Maciejak P, Turzynska D, Sobolewska A, Walkowiak J, Plaznik A. The effects of electrical hippocampal kindling of seizures on amino acids and kynurenic acid concentrations in brain structures. J Neural Transm (Vienna). 2012;119:141–9.
20. Hansen SL, Sperling BB, Sanchez C. Anticonvulsant and antiepileptogenic effects of GABAA receptor ligands in pentylenetetrazole-kindled mice. Prog Neuropsychopharmacol Biol Psychiatry. 2004;28:105–13.
21. Morimoto K, Fahnestock M, Racine RJ. Kindling and status epilepticus models of epilepsy: rewiring the brain. Prog Neurobiol. 2004;73:1–60.
22. Morimoto K. Seizure-triggering mechanisms in the kindling model of epilepsy: collapse of GABA-mediated inhibition and activation of NMDA receptors. Neurosci Biobehav Rev. 1989;13:253–60.
23. Kupferberg H. Animal models used in the screening of antiepileptic drugs. Epilepsia. 2001;42(Suppl 4):7–12.
24. Loscher W, Rundfeldt C, Honack D. Pharmacological characterization of phenytoin-resistant amygdala-kindled rats, a new model of drug-resistant partial epilepsy. Epilepsy Res. 1993;15:207–19.
25. Wlaz P, Poleszak E, Serefko A, Wlaz A, Rundfeldt C. Anxiogenic- and antidepressant-like behavior in corneally kindled rats. Pharmacol Rep. 2015;67:349–52.
26. Sakamoto F, Yamada S, Ueta Y. Centrally administered orexin-A activates corticotropin-releasing factor-containing neurons in the hypothalamic paraventricular nucleus and central amygdaloid nucleus of rats: possible involvement of central orexins on stress-activated central CRF neurons. Regul Pept. 2004;118:183–91.
27. Li Y, Li S, Wei C, Wang H, Sui N, Kirouac GJ. Orexins in the paraventricular nucleus of the thalamus mediate anxiety-like responses in rats. Psychopharmacology. 2010;212:251–65.
28. Suzuki M, Beuckmann CT, Shikata K, Ogura H, Sawai T. Orexin-A (hypocretin-1) is possibly involved in generation of anxiety-like behavior. Brain Res. 2005;1044:116–21.
29. Sears RM, Fink AE, Wigestrand MB, Farb CR, de Lecea L, Ledoux JE. Orexin/hypocretin system modulates amygdala-dependent threat learning through the locus coeruleus. Proc Natl Acad Sci USA. 2013;110:20260–5.
30. Blouin AM, Fried I, Wilson CL, Staba RJ, Behnke EJ, Lam HA, et al. Human hypocretin and melanin-concentrating hormone levels are linked to emotion and social interaction. Nat Commun. 2013;4:1547.
31. Ozsoy S, Olguner Eker O, Abdulrezzak U, Esel E. Relationship between orexin A and childhood maltreatment in female patients with depression and anxiety. Soc Neurosci. 2017;12:330 6.
32. Agarwal U, Mishra S, Xu J, Levin S, Gonzales J, Barnard ND. A multicenter randomized controlled trial of a nutrition intervention program in a multiethnic adult population in the corporate setting reduces depression and anxiety and improves quality of life: the GEICO study. Am J Health Promot. 2015;29:245–54.
33. Kummangal BA, Kumar D, Mallick HN. Intracerebroventricular injection of orexin-2 receptor antagonist promotes REM sleep. Behav Brain Res. 2013;237:59–62.
34. Xiao F, Jiang M, Du D, Xia C, Wang J, Cao Y, et al. Orexin A regulates cardiovascular responses in stress-induced hypertensive rats. Neuropharmacology. 2013;67:16–24.
35. Sadeghi B, Ezzatpanah S, Haghparast A. Effects of dorsal hippocampal orexin-2 receptor antagonism on the acquisition, expression, and extinction of morphine-induced place preference in rats. Psychopharmacology. 2016;233:2329–41.
36. Walker LC, Lawrence AJ. The role of orexins/hypocretins in alcohol use and abuse. Curr Top Behav Neurosci. 2017;33:221–46.
37. Paxinos G, Watson CR, Emson PC. AChE-stained horizontal sections of the rat brain in stereotaxic coordinates. J Neurosci Methods. 1980;3:129–49.
38. Ben J, de Oliveira PA, Gonçalves FM, Peres TV, Matheus FC, Hoeller AA, et al. Effects of pentylenetetrazole kindling on mitogen-activated protein kinases levels in neocortex and hippocampus of mice. Neurochem Res. 2014;39:2492–500.
39. Serralta A, Barcia JA, Ortiz P, Duran C, Hernandez ME, Alos M. Effect of intracerebroventricular continuous infusion of valproic acid versus single i.p. and i.c.v. injections in the amygdala kindling epilepsy model. Epilepsy Res. 2006;70:15–26.
40. Jain S, Bharal N, Khurana S, Mediratta PK, Sharma KK. Anticonvulsant and antioxidant actions of trimetazidine in pentylenetetrazole-induced kindling model in mice. Naunyn Schmiedebergs Arch Pharmacol. 2011;383:385–92.
41. Rezvani ME, Roohbakhsh A, Mosaddegh MH, Esmailidehaj M, Khaloobagheri F, Esmaeili H. Anticonvulsant and depressant effects of aqueous extracts of *Carum copticum* seeds in male rats. Epilepsy Behav. 2011;22:220–5.
42. Rahimi A, Hajizadeh Moghaddam A, Roohbakhsh A. Central administra-

tion of GPR55 receptor agonist and antagonist modulates anxiety-related behaviors in rats. Fund Clin Pharm. 2015;29:185–90.

43. Roohbakhsh A, Moghaddam AH, Delfan KM. Anxiolytic-like effect of testosterone in male rats: GABAC receptors are not involved. Iran J Basic Med Sci. 2011;14:376–82.

44. Doi T, Ueda Y, Nagatomo K, Willmore LJ. Role of glutamate and GABA transporters in development of pentylenetetrazol-kindling. Neurochem Res. 2009;34:1324–31.

45. Stanley EM, Fadel JR. Aging-related alterations in orexin/hypocretin modulation of septo-hippocampal amino acid neurotransmission. Neuroscience. 2011;195:70–9.

46. Goudarzi E, Elahdadi Salmani M, Lashkarbolouki T, Goudarzi I. Hippocampal orexin receptors inactivation reduces PTZ induced seizures of male rats. Pharmacol Biochem Behav. 2015;130:77–83.

47. Bonnavion P, de Lecea L. Hypocretins in the control of sleep and wakefulness. Curr Neurol Neurosci Rep. 2010;10:174–9.

48. Sakurai T. The neural circuit of orexin (hypocretin): maintaining sleep and wakefulness. Nat Rev Neurosci. 2007;8:171–81.

49. Trivedi P, Yu H, MacNeil DJ, Van der Ploeg LH, Guan XM. Distribution of orexin receptor mRNA in the rat brain. FEBS Lett. 1998;438:71–5.

50. Zhu F, Wang XQ, Chen YN, Yang N, Lang SY, Zuo PP, et al. Changes and overlapping distribution in the expression of CB1/OX1-GPCRs in rat hippocampus by kainic acid-induced status epilepticus. Brain Res. 2015;1597:14–27.

51. Vazquez-DeRose J, Schwartz MD, Nguyen AT, Warrier DR, Gulati S, Mathew TK, et al. Hypocretin/orexin antagonism enhances sleep-related adenosine and GABA neurotransmission in rat basal forebrain. Brain Struct Funct. 2016;221:923–40.

52. Akbari N, Salmani ME, Goudarzvand M, LashkarBoluki T, Goudarzi I, Abrari K. Unilateral hypothalamus inactivation prevents PTZ kindling development through hippocampal orexin receptor 1 modulation. Basic Clin Neurosci. 2014;5:66–73.

53. Akanmu MA, Honda K. Selective stimulation of orexin receptor type 2 promotes wakefulness in freely behaving rats. Brain Res. 2005;1048:138–45.

54. Aracri P, Banfi D, Pasini ME, Amadeo A, Becchetti A. Hypocretin (orexin) regulates glutamate input to fast-spiking interneurons in layer V of the Fr2 region of the murine prefrontal cortex. Cereb Cortex. 2015;25:1330–47.

55. Mieda M, Hasegawa E, Kisanuki YY, Sinton CM, Yanagisawa M, Sakurai T. Differential roles of orexin receptor-1 and-2 in the regulation of non-REM and REM sleep. J Neursci. 2011;31:6518–26.

56. Leonard C, Kukkonen J. Orexin/hypocretin receptor signalling: a functional perspective. Br J Pharmacol. 2014;171:294–313.

57. Tang J, Chen J, Ramanjaneya M, Punn A, Conner AC, Randeva HS. The signalling profile of recombinant human orexin-2 receptor. Cell Signal. 2008;20:1651–61.

58. Yazdi F, Jahangirvand M, Pirasteh A-H, Moradi M, Haghparast A. Functional interaction between OX2 and CB1 receptors in the ventral tegmental area and the nucleus accumbens in response to place preference induced by chemical stimulation of the lateral hypothalamus. Pharmacol Biochem Behav. 2015;139:39–46.

59. Brunton L, Knollmann B, Hilal-Dandan R. Goodman and Gilman's the pharmacological basis of therapeutics. New York: McGraw Hill Medical; 2018.

60. Mattson RH, Cramer JA, Collins JF. A comparison of valproate with carbamazepine for the treatment of complex partial seizures and secondarily generalized tonic-clonic seizures in adults. The Department of Veterans Affairs Epilepsy Cooperative Study No. 264 Group. N Engl J Med. 1992;327:765–71.

61. Hu Y, Huang Y, Quan F, Hu Y, Lu Y, Wang XF. Comparison of the retention rates between carbamazepine and valproate as an initial monotherapy in Chinese patients with partial seizures: a ten-year follow-up, observational study. Seizure. 2011;20:208–13.

62. Stanojlovic OP, Hrncic DR, Zivanovic DP, Susic VT. Anticonvulsant, but not antiepileptic, action of valproate on audiogenic seizures in metaphit-treated rats. Clin Exp Pharmacol Physiol. 2007;34:1010–5.

63. Cavalli J, Bertoglio LJ, Carobrez AP. Pentylenetetrazole as an unconditioned stimulus for olfactory and contextual fear conditioning in rats. Neurobiol Learn Mem. 2009;92:512–8.

64. Flores A, Saravia R, Maldonado R, Berrendero F. Orexins and fear: implications for the treatment of anxiety disorders. Trends Neurosci. 2015;38:550–9.

65. Arendt DH, Ronan PJ, Oliver KD, Callahan LB, Summers TR, Summers CH. Depressive behavior and activation of the orexin/hypocretin system. Behav Neurosci. 2013;127:86–94.

66. Arendt DH, Hassell J, Li H, Achua JK, Guarnieri DJ, Dileone RJ, et al. Anxiolytic function of the orexin 2/hypocretin A receptor in the basolateral amygdala. Psychoneuroendocrinology. 2014;40:17–26.

67. Patel KV, Aspesi AV, Evoy KE. Suvorexant a dual orexin receptor antagonist for the treatment of sleep onset and sleep maintenance insomnia. Ann Pharmacother. 2015;49:477–83.

68. Palotai M, Telegdy G, Jaszberenyi M. Orexin A-induced anxiety-like behavior is mediated through GABA-ergic, alpha- and beta-adrenergic neurotransmissions in mice. Peptides. 2014;57:129–34.

69. Sears RM, Fink AE, Wigestrand MB, Farb CR, De Lecea L, LeDoux JE. Orexin/hypocretin system modulates amygdala-dependent threat learning through the locus coeruleus. Proc Natl Acad Sci. 2013;110:20260–5.

70. Kumar A, Nidhi S, Manveen B, Sumitra S. A review on chemical induced kindling models of epilepsy. J Vet Med Res. 2016;3:1–6.

71. Appel LJ, Miller ER 3rd, Jee SH, Stolzenberg-Solomon R, Lin PH, Erlinger T, et al. Effect of dietary patterns on serum homocysteine: results of a randomized, controlled feeding study. Circulation. 2000;102:852–7.

72. Hrncic D, Mikic J, Rasic-Markovic A, Velimirovic M, Stojkovic T, Obrenovic R, et al. Anxiety-related behavior in hyperhomocysteinemia induced by methionine nutritional overload in rats: role of the brain oxidative stress. Can J Physiol Pharmacol. 2016;94:1074–82.

73. Chung KH, Chiou HY, Chen YH. Associations between serum homocysteine levels and anxiety and depression among children and adolescents in Taiwan. Sci Rep. 2017;7:8330.

74. Hrncic D, Rasic-Markovic A, Bjekic-Macut J, Susic V, Djuric D, Stanojlovic O. Paradoxical sleep deprivation potentiates epilepsy induced by homocysteine thiolactone in adult rats. Exp Biol Med (Maywood). 2013;238:77–83.

5

Effects of transcranial focused ultrasound on human primary motor cortex using 7T fMRI

Leo Ai[1], Priya Bansal[1], Jerel K. Mueller[1] and Wynn Legon[1,2]* [ID]

Abstract

Background: Transcranial focused ultrasound (tFUS) is a new non-invasive neuromodulation technique that uses mechanical energy to modulate neuronal excitability with high spatial precision. tFUS has been shown to be capable of modulating EEG brain activity in humans that is spatially restricted, and here, we use 7T MRI to extend these findings. We test the effect of tFUS on 7T BOLD fMRI signals from individual finger representations in the human primary motor cortex (M1) and connected cortical motor regions. Participants (N = 5) performed a cued finger tapping task in a 7T MRI scanner with their thumb, index, and middle fingers to produce a BOLD signal for individual M1 finger representations during either tFUS or sham neuromodulation to the thumb representation.

Results: Results demonstrated a statistically significant increase in activation volume of the M1 thumb representation for the tFUS condition as compared to sham. No differences in percent BOLD changes were found. This effect was spatially confined as the index and middle finger M1 finger representations did not show similar significant changes in either percent change or activation volume. No effects were seen during tFUS to M1 in the supplementary motor area or the dorsal premotor cortex.

Conclusions: Single element tFUS can be paired with high field MRI that does not induce significant artifact. tFUS increases activation volumes of the targeted finger representation that is spatially restricted within M1 but does not extend to functionally connected motor regions.

Keywords: Ultrasound, Neuromodulation, Human, 7T fMRI, Motor cortex, BOLD

Introduction

Transcranial focused ultrasound (tFUS) is a noninvasive, low energy technique that uses mechanical energy for neuromodulation at high spatial resolutions [1]. tFUS has been shown to be capable of modulating neural activity in mice [2–4], rabbit [5], swine [6], and monkeys [7]. tFUS has also been shown to be a safe and effective method to modulate human cortical activity [1, 8–13]. In Legon et al. [1], we demonstrated the spatial selectivity of tFUS neuromodulation though the spatial resolution of

EEG is not ideal for this. The pairing of tFUS with functional MRI is advantageous as it provides complimentary high spatial resolution with whole brain coverage. Previous reports have shown ultrasound to elicit a blood oxygen level dependent (BOLD) response. In craniotomized rabbits, Yoo et al. [5] showed focused ultrasound directed at the somatomotor area to result in a well-defined BOLD response commensurate with the focus of sonication. In a recent study in humans, Lee et al. [11] delivered focused ultrasound to the primary visual cortex and showed BOLD activity around the sonication focus in visual cortices but also for ultrasound to activate spatially distinct functionally connected regions of the visual system. We have also previously tested the ability of tFUS to produce a reliable BOLD signal in humans at 3T and

*Correspondence: wlegon@virginia.edu
2 Department of Neurological Surgery, School of Medicine, University of Virginia, 409 Lane Rd. Rm 1031, Charlottesville, VA 22901, USA
Full list of author information is available at the end of the article

report variable effects [8]. Here, we extend these findings and pair tFUS with high field 7T fMRI in humans to improve signal to noise ratios and the ability to discriminate small spatially restricted changes in activity from tFUS. Specifically, we apply tFUS to the human primary motor cortex (M1) and test the effect of tFUS on specific finger BOLD signals as well as on functionally connected regions including the supplementary motor area (SMA) and dorsal premotor cortex (PMd).

Methods

Participants

Five participants [ages 20–25 (mean 22.8 ± 2.2 years); 3 male, 2 females; 4 right handed, 1 left handed] were included in the study. This study was approved by University of Minnesota's Institutional Review Board and all participants gave written informed consent to participate. Participants were physically and neurologically healthy and had no history of neurological disorders. Participants were also screened for medications contraindicated for other forms of non-invasive neuromodulation [14].

Experimental procedures

The study consisted of two magnetic resonance imaging (MRI) scanning sessions on separate days. The first session included a T1 anatomical scan and a functional scan with the finger tapping task (see below) to identify M1 thumb, index and middle finger representations. The thumb representation was then used as the target for the application of tFUS for the second session. In the second session, participants performed the same finger tapping task during either tFUS or sham neuromodulation. The order of tFUS and sham conditions was counterbalanced across participants.

Finger tapping task

Participants performed a visually cued finger tapping task using either the thumb, index, and middle fingers with their self-reported dominant hand. Participants lay supine in the MRI with their dominant arm supported with foam to ensure a comfortable position to tap their fingers on their thigh while limiting proximal arm and shoulder movement. Visual cues indicating the timing for tapping were presented using Cogent (www.vislab.ucl.ac.uk/cogent.php) for Matlab (MathWorks, Natick, MA, USA) and delivered using a projector to a screen that participants could see while inside of the bore of the MRI machine. The visual cues displayed the text ('thumb', 'index', or 'middle') with white block letter on a black background in the center of the screen with a large font, indicating the finger to be tapped paced at 1 Hz. This task used a block design with a single finger to be tapped for the duration of a block at the 1 Hz pace. Each finger was

tapped for three blocks for a total of nine 30 s blocks, with 30 s rest blocks separating each finger tapping block (Fig. 1a). The ordering for the finger to be tapped per block was pseudo-randomly generated for each MRI scan where no finger would be tapped for three contiguous blocks.

Prior to scanning, participants practiced the finger tapping task to familiarize themselves with the task demands. To standardize movement range, participants were instructed to follow the visual prompts by extending and flexing the cued finger at the proximal phalanx while limiting movement of other fingers. Participants performed this practice session with feedback from the study staff to ensure the task would be performed properly while inside the scanner. Ultrasonic waveforms were delivered every two repetition times (TR, 2750 ms) for a total of 6 stimulations per 30 s block (54 total stimulations per scan). The tFUS condition involved acoustically coupling the active face of the ultrasound transducer to the scalp at the pre-determined neuronavigation (see below) site. To achieve acoustic coupling to the head, the volunteer's hair was parted to expose the scalp and ultrasound gel was used to keep the hair out of the way and ensure proper coupling with the tFUS transducer. The

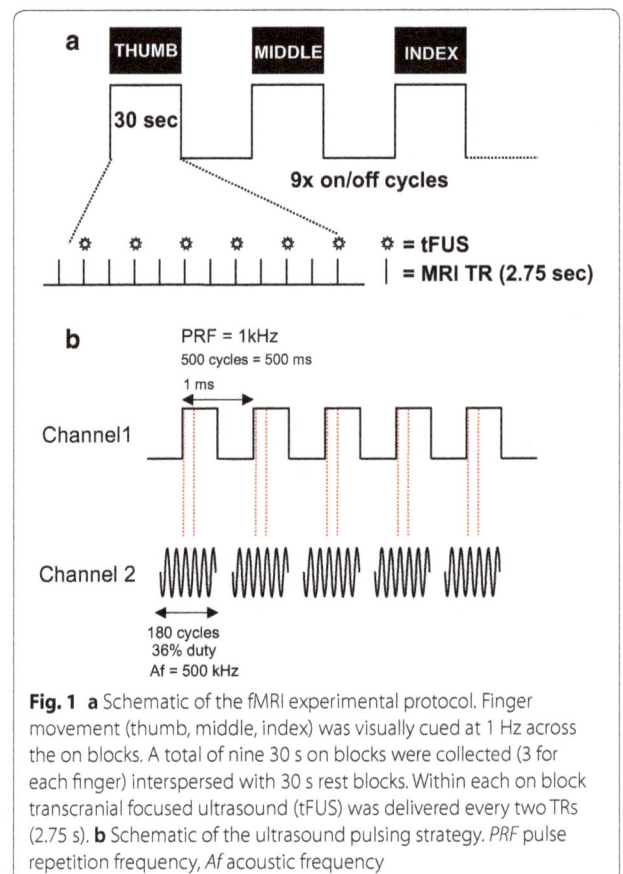

Fig. 1 **a** Schematic of the fMRI experimental protocol. Finger movement (thumb, middle, index) was visually cued at 1 Hz across the on blocks. A total of nine 30 s on blocks were collected (3 for each finger) interspersed with 30 s rest blocks. Within each on block transcranial focused ultrasound (tFUS) was delivered every two TRs (2.75 s). **b** Schematic of the ultrasound pulsing strategy. *PRF* pulse repetition frequency, *Af* acoustic frequency

transducer was also prepped with ultrasound gel on the surface that met the head, and was then placed on the exposed scalp and held in place using a secure head band. The sham condition involved turning off the transducer so that it would not deliver stimulation. Participants reported no auditory or tactile sensation from either the tFUS or sham condition as has previously been reported in similar setups outside of the MRI environment [1, 9].

tFUS waveform and delivery

The ultrasound transducer was a custom made [15] 30 mm diameter 7T MRI compatible single element focused 500 kHz with a focal length of 30 mm. The waveform used was the same as previously described [1]. This waveform was generated using a two-channel 2-MHz function generator (BK Precision Instruments, CA, USA). Channel 1 was set to deliver tFUS at a pulse repetition frequency (PRF) at 1 kHz and channel 2 was set to drive the transducer at 500 kHz in burst mode while using channel 1 as the trigger for channel 2. Channel 2 was set to deliver 180 cycles per pulse, and channel 1 was set to deliver 500 pulses, resulting in a 500 ms duration (Fig. 1b). Channel 2 output was sent to a 100 W linear amplifier (2100L Electronics & Innovation Ltd, NY, USA), with the output of the amplifier sent to the custom made tFUS transducer while using a Mini-Circuits (New York City, NY) 50-ohm low pass filter (1.9 MHz cutoff frequency) between the amplifier and the transducer at the patch panel to reduce radio frequency noise [16] and an "L" matching network to match the impedance of the RF amplifier and the transducer consisting of an inductor and capacitor arranged in the low pass form to also suppress higher order harmonics in the driving source [17].

Quantitative acoustic field mapping

The acoustic intensity profile of the waveform was measured in an acoustic test tank filled with deionized, degassed, and filtered water (Precision Acoustics Ltd., Dorchester, Dorset, UK). A calibrated hydrophone (HNR-0500, Onda Corp., Sunnyvale, CA, USA) mounted on a motorized stage was used to measure the acoustic intensity profile from the ultrasound transducer in the acoustic test tank at a 0.5 mm spatial resolution. Intensity parameters were derived from measured values of pressure using the approximation of plane progressive acoustic radiation waves. The ultrasound transducer was positioned in the tank using opto-mechanical components (Edmund Optics Inc., Barrington, NJ and Thorlabs Inc., Newton, NJ). Acoustic field scans were performed in the free water of the tank. Measurements in the acoustic tank revealed an spatial peak pulse average intensity (I_{sppa}) of 16.95 W/cm^2 and a mechanical index (MI) of 0.97 from the ultrasonic neuromodulation waveform in water. The -3 dB pressure field was 3.83 mm in the X axis, 3.98 mm in the Y axis and 33.6 mm in the Z axis (Fig. 2). We have previously modelled the acoustic field through human skulls overlying the motor cortex demonstrating the skull to reduce peak pressure produced by the transducer in free water by a factor of 6–7, and it can be expected for the targeted region of the brain to experience pressure to be reduced as such [18]. In addition, the brain tissue and skull do not alter the beam path significantly [18, 19] or result in appreciable heating of the skin or skull bone [19].

tFUS targeting

The target for tFUS was chosen based on the isolated thumb fMRI representations found in the first MRI session (Fig. 3b). The thumb BOLD representation was loaded into a stereotaxic neuronavigation system (BrainSight; Rogue Research Inc, Montreal, Quebec, CA), and targets were created to guide tFUS based on the strongest BOLD signals in M1 with an approximate depth of $\sim$30 mm (based on the focal length of the transducer) from the scalp on a per subject basis (Fig. 3b).

Quantitative modelling of ultrasound wave propagation

To better quantify the intracranial pressure in primary motor cortex from tFUS, a computational model was run to visualize and evaluate the wave propagation of tFUS across an example skull. The model was run using a magnetic resonance (MR) imaging and computerized tomography (CT) dataset taken from the Visible Human Project® [20]. The transducer was placed on the scalp site overlying the hand knob of the primary motor cortex. Simulations were performed using the k-Wave MATLAB toolbox [21] and modelling parameters and methods are detailed in [18]. The modelled beam is overlaid on an individual subject MRI image to show the ultrasound beam location relative to the thumb functional activity (Fig. 3a) and also to show the lateral resolution of the modelled beam relative to fMRI finger activations (Fig. 3c).

MRI acquisition parameters

All MRI scans were performed at the University of Minnesota's Center for Magnetic Resonance Research on a 7T Siemens MRI scanner (Siemens Medical Solutions, Erlangen, Germany) using a Nova Medical 1 × 32 head coil (Wilmington, MA, USA). The fMRI scans were acquired using a gradient echo, echo planar image pulse sequence with the following parameters: repetition time (TR) = 2750 ms, echo time (TE) = 22 ms, flip angle = 70, field of view (FOV) = 192 mm × 192 mm, number of slices = 108, voxel size = 1.05 × 1.05 × 1.05 mm^3, integrated parallel imaging technique (iPAT) = 3.

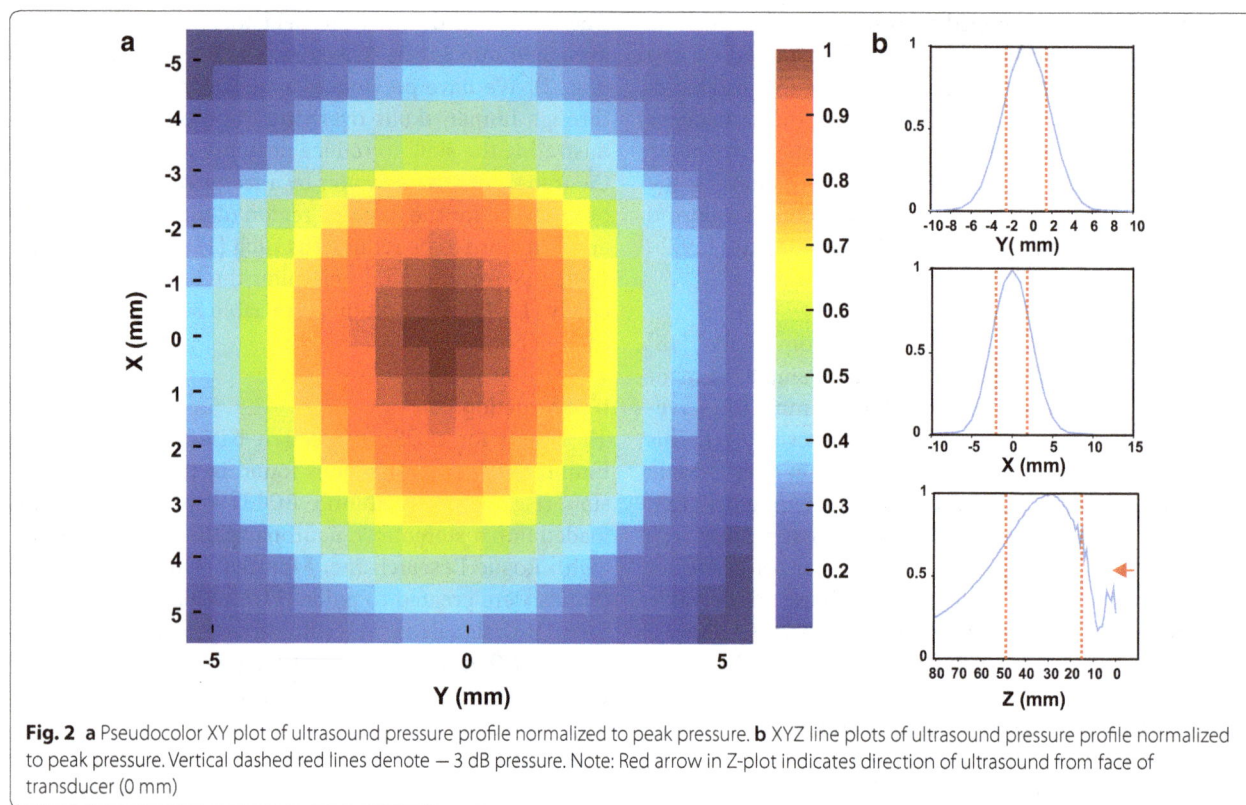

Fig. 2 a Pseudocolor XY plot of ultrasound pressure profile normalized to peak pressure. **b** XYZ line plots of ultrasound pressure profile normalized to peak pressure. Vertical dashed red lines denote − 3 dB pressure. Note: Red arrow in Z-plot indicates direction of ultrasound from face of transducer (0 mm)

Additionally, T1 anatomical scans were performed with the following parameters: TR = 3000 ms, TE = 3.28 ms, flip angle = 6, FOV = 192 mm × 216 mm, number of slices = 256, voxel size = $1 \times 1 \times 1$ mm^3.

BOLD fMRI data analysis

The fMRI data was processed in Analysis of Functional NeuroImages (AFNI) [22]. The data had 3D motion correction, linear and quadratic trends removed, a Gaussian filter with full width half maximum of 3 mm applied, slice timing correction, and distortion correction applied. A general linear model analysis was utilized to generate a statistical parametric map with a reference function generated by convolving the hemodynamic response function with the task function. This process was performed for all subjects' fMRI data to isolate the individual representations of the thumb, index, and middle fingers using a threshold of t = 5 (p = 1e−6 uncorrected). To measure volume changes, a region of interest (ROI) was drawn around the pre-central gyrus (M1) to the depth of the central sulcus. Activated voxels (t = 5; p = 1e−6) in this ROI were used to calculate the activation volume in M1 due to the finger movement being performed for both the tFUS and sham condition. To test for differences between tFUS and sham neuromodulation, the total number of

voxels that met this threshold within this ROI was subjected to a paired student's t test.

For percent signal change analysis, we concentrated on a brain volume at the measured focal volume of the ultrasound beam (see Fig. 3). These coordinates were found for each subject and an ROI of 125 mm^3 ($5 \times 5 \times 5$ mm) was drawn to encompass partial volume of the ultrasound pressure field. Based upon free water field ultrasound beam measurements, the FWHM volume of the beam was ~ 230 mm^3. Percent signal change between tFUS and sham conditions were compared with a paired t test (N = 5). To further investigate the spatial selectivity of the tFUS effect, a $5 \times 5 \times 5$ mm ROI was also placed at the region of strongest M1 activations for the index and middle finger representations in each participant to examine if tFUS has effects on these representations despite not being directly targeted for stimulation. Similar group (N = 5) paired t-tests were performed separately for the index and middle finger representations.

To test for potential downstream motor network effects as has previously been shown [11], we also examined the effect of tFUS to M1 on the SMA and ipsilateral PMd. The SMA and PMd were defined according to anatomical landmarks. Specifically, SMA included the volume between the precentral and central sulci down to the cingulate sulcus and laterally

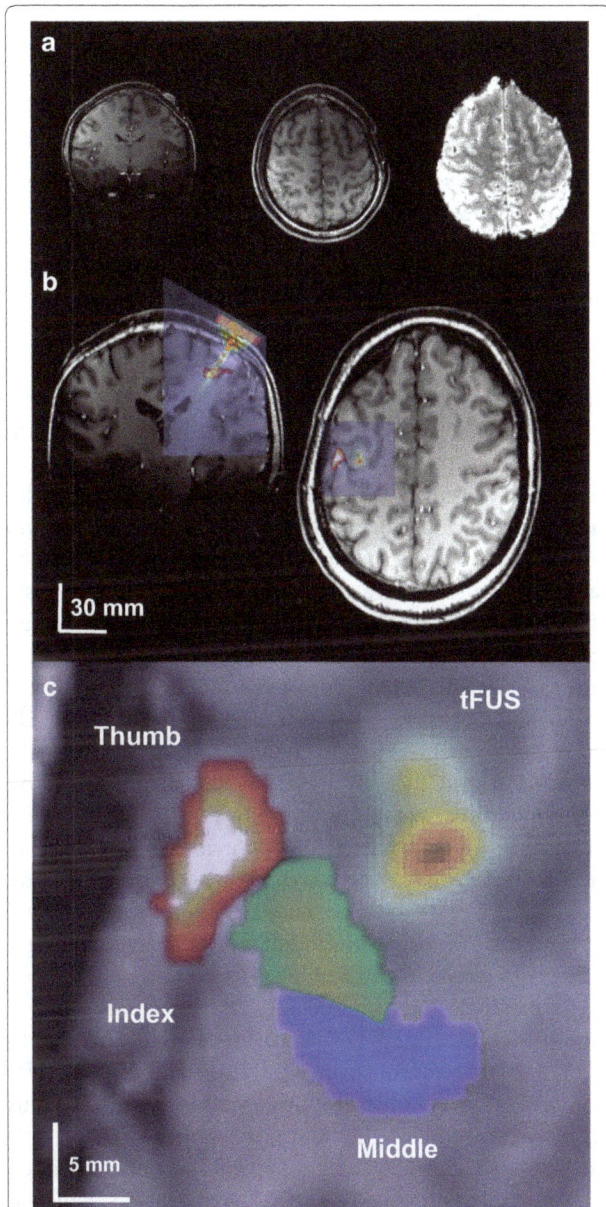

Fig. 3 a 7T anatomical T1 (left, middle) and functional EPI image showing ultrasound transducer. **b** Overlay of functional MRI thumb activation and acoustic model of the ultrasound beam on subject anatomical T1 scan. Note in right image ultrasound beam is purposefully displaced from the fMRI thumb activation to better show relative size compared to fMRI activation. **c** Blowup of single subject fMRI BOLD finger representations with overlaid acoustic model that is purposefully displaced to show relative size of ultrasound beam to fMRI activations. For experiments, tFUS would have been placed directly over the thumb activation

such that the ROI borders M1 and PMd. The PMd ROI included parts of the superior frontal gyrus and middle frontal gyrus lateral to the SMA and anterior to the precentral sulcus. Data from the entire scanning session (9 on blocks; thumb, middle and index finger movement;

54 tFUS stimulations) was used in this analysis. We examined both volume and average percent signal from both the SMA and PMd volumes for each participant and each region was tested in a separate group (N = 5) paired t-test to assess differences between the tFUS and sham condition.

Results
M1 thumb volumes
The application of tFUS at the thumb BOLD representation resulted in larger activation volumes for all five participants (Fig. 4a). The group average M1 thumb activation volume was 703 ± 334 mm^3 for the tFUS condition and 375 ± 167 mm^3 for the sham condition. The paired t-test revealed a significant increase in BOLD volume for the tFUS condition as compared to sham ($t_4 = 3.01$, $p = 0.039$) (Fig. 4b). Table 1 shows the individual subject activation volumes found in M1.

The calculated percent changes at the ultrasound beam focus location showed no statistically significant differences between tFUS and sham (Sham: $1.84\% \pm 1.36\%$ vs. tFUS: $1.98\% \pm 1.17\%$; $t_4 = 0.7$, $p = 0.47$). See Table 1 for individual participant results.

Spatial selectivity of tFUS within M1
Based upon previous results that demonstrated high spatial selectivity of ultrasound neuromodulation [1] we explored the effect of tFUS on adjacent contiguous volumes within M1. The average Euclidian distance between the center of gravity for the index and middle finger representations were (thumb to index: 10.08 mm $\pm$ 5.05 mm; thumb to middle: 10.49 mm $\pm$ 6.46 mm). For context, the full-width half maximum lateral resolution of the pressure field is ~ 5.5–6 mm thus the tFUS pressure field can resolve the spatial resolution of the finger representations. While directing tFUS at the thumb representation we found no differences in activation volumes of the index finger representation (572 ± 999 mm^3 vs. 665 ± 1428 mm^3; $t_4 = 0.46$, $p = 0.67$) or the middle finger representation (948 ± 738 mm^3 vs. 761 ± 793 mm^3; $t_4 = 0.47$, $p = 0.80$). In addition to BOLD volume changes, we tested for percent signal change and found no differences for either finger representation. The average index finger percent changes were $1.16 \pm 1.06\%$ and $2.15 \pm 1.79\%$ during the tFUS and sham conditions respectively ($t_4 = 0.46$, $p = 0.67$) and $2.47 \pm 1.53\%$ and $2.69 \pm 1.95\%$ for the middle finger representation during the tFUS and sham conditions respectively ($t_4 = 0.46$, $p = 0.67$). See Table 1 for individual subject activation volumes and percent changes for the index and middle fingers.

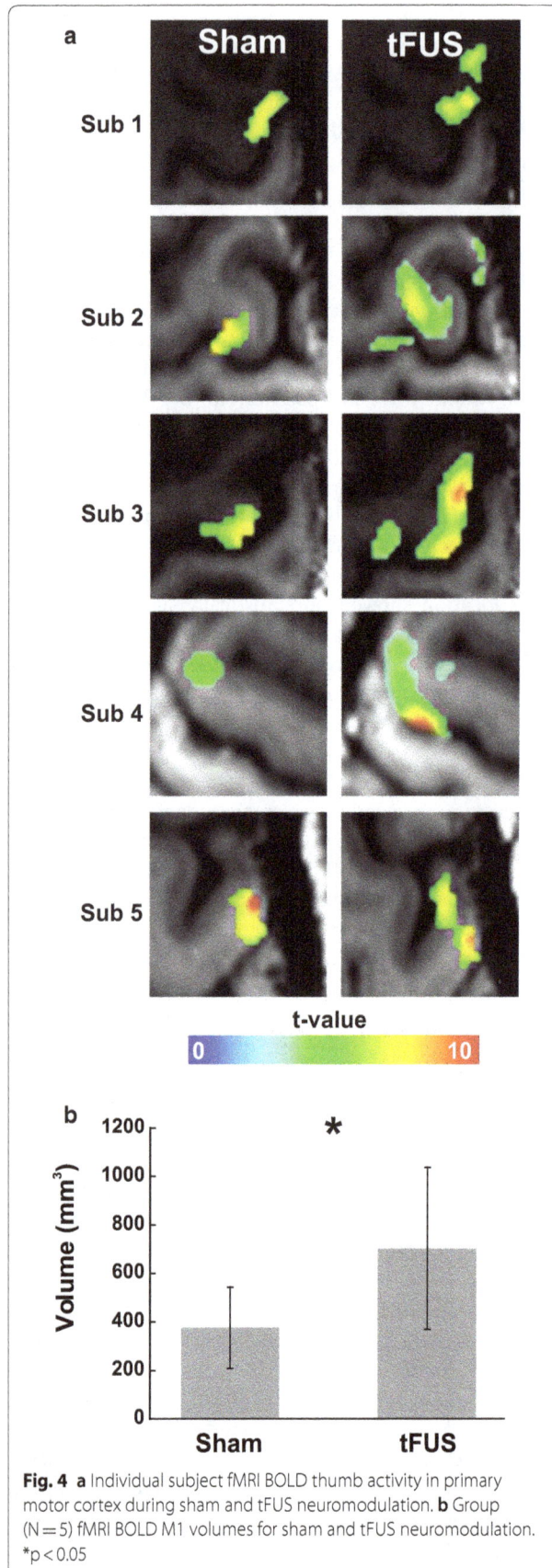

Fig. 4 **a** Individual subject fMRI BOLD thumb activity in primary motor cortex during sham and tFUS neuromodulation. **b** Group (N = 5) fMRI BOLD M1 volumes for sham and tFUS neuromodulation. *p < 0.05

PMd and SMA

No significant changes were found in SMA between the tFUS and sham conditions for either activation volumes (3191 ± 2966 mm³ vs. 2903 ± 2839 mm³; $t_4 = 1.35$, p = 0.25) or percent signal change (1.92 ± 0.37% vs. 1.87 ± 0.36%; $t_4 = 0.73$, p = 0.51). No significant changes were found in PMd between the tFUS and sham condition for activation volumes (202 ± 292 mm³ vs. 85 ± 168 mm³; $t_4 = 1.86$, p = 0.14) or percent signal change (0.65 ± 0.60% vs. 0.66 ± 1.00%; $t_4 = 0.04$, p = 0.97).

Discussion

This is the first study to combine tFUS with 7T fMRI in humans in addition to targeting individual finger representations within M1. The results show that single element 0.5 MHz tFUS targeted at the dominant thumb representation of contralateral M1 increases BOLD activation volumes generated during a cued tapping task. This increase in volume was spatially confined to the sonicated area as it only affected the thumb representation as both adjacent middle and index finger representations did not show any effect. The application of tFUS did not affect percent signal change as compared to sham stimulation and did not have any detectable effect on functionally connected motor regions including the SMA and PMd. These results extend previous results testing the effect of tFUS to elicit a BOLD response [5, 8, 11] and provide for a more detailed perspective on the spatial resolution of tFUS for neuromodulation of individual finger representations within a single gyrus.

The original study by Yoo et al. [5] in craniotomized rabbits demonstrated 690 kHz focused ultrasound to elicit a BOLD response in M1. The volume of activation was in good spatial approximation with the focus of the pressure field. They did not report any other activation sites suggesting only a local BOLD effect limited to the application site. This BOLD activity was achieved at a relatively low intensity of 3.3 W/cm² and interestingly did not scale with increasing intensity. Double the intensity resulted in a similar increase in percent signal change of around 1.5% from baseline. In Lee et al. [11] they applied 270 kHz focused tFUS to primary visual cortex (V1) in humans at intensities ranging from∼ 1 to 10 W/cm² and reported induced V1 BOLD activity that approximated the pressure field but also reported tFUS to induce activity in functionally connected visual regions. Here, we did not find any evidence for an effect of tFUS on percent signal change in contrast to the above studies or a downstream effect. This is most likely due to differences in experimental design, but also could be related to differences in tFUS parameters. Based upon our previous research that has largely shown inhibition

Table 1 Individual participant fMRI activation

Subject	Volume (mm³)		Percent Change (%)	
	tFUS	Sham	tFUS	Sham
Thumb				
1	725	542	1.19	1.09
2	906	311	3.3	3.67
3	1136	553	3.03	2.57
4	382	300	0.01	0.78
5	364	171	1.65	1.8
Mean	703	375	1.84	1.98
SD	334	167	1.36	1.17
Index finger				
1	0	39	0	2.18
2	21	20	1.13	4.96
3	2346	3219	2.43	1.65
4	253	0	0.24	0
5	238	48	1.98	1.94
Mean	572	665	1.16	2.15
SD	999	1428	1.06	1.79
Middle finger				
1	473	108	3.14	2.7
2	2145	1429	1.79	3.88
3	1157	1800	4.82	5.1
4	630	168	0.93	0.05
5	335	301	1.69	1.71
Mean	948	761	2.47	2.69
SD	738	793	1.53	1.95

[1, 23], we hypothesized tFUS to also result in inhibition of the BOLD response. As such, we experimentally induced a BOLD signal through a functional motor task and tested the effect of tFUS on this existing signal. It is possible that we did not detect an increase in percent signal change as the motor task had already significantly activated the region and tFUS did not have an additive effect or was undetectable in relation to the strong effect of the motor task. Yoo et al. [5] reported percent signal changes in the range of 1.5% from ultrasound as compared to resting baseline, though we did not detect any significant increase over our 'baseline' that was already at ~1.8–2.0% above rest blocks due to the motor task. We cannot compare our % signal change to Lee et al. [11] as these values were not presented for the ultrasound versus sham contrast. Unfortunately, we did not test ultrasound during a resting condition in this study to directly compare results with these previous findings for tFUS to induce a BOLD activation. We have previously reported preliminary results in human M1 that showed tFUS to variably induce 3T BOLD activity in 3 of 6 participants though these findings were not robust or statistically significant at the group level [8]. In this study, we were specifically interested in how tFUS affects existing activity and had the specific hypothesis that tFUS would result in inhibition. We assumed that inhibition would translate to a reduction in percent BOLD signal change similar to evoked potential studies where ultrasound attenuated the amplitude of these evoked potentials [1]. However, this was not the case. We found an increase in signal volume and no differences in percent signal change. An increase in signal volume is presumptive of an increase in activity and this could be evidence of the ability of tFUS to produce excitation though it also may be that this increase in volume is a function of increased inhibition. We previously found in Legon et al. [1] for tFUS to have preferential effects in the gamma band when delivered to primary somatosensory cortex and that this may be a mechanism for the neuromodulatory effect of tFUS. In consideration of the effects found here, a small but very interesting finding in Legon et al. [1] was for tFUS to increase gamma power when delivered to the precentral gyrus (M1). This somewhat overlooked finding becomes relevant as the gamma frequency band is thought to largely contribute to the BOLD signal [24, 25] and this could explain why we saw an increase in signal volume and would also explain why we did not find an increase in percent signal change. As such, the increase in signal volume we found for all participants in this study could be an indicator of tFUS to preferentially target inhibitory inter-neuronal populations that largely contribute to gamma power [26, 27]. This account fits well with data from our lab but is difficult to reconcile with other existing literature that has demonstrated tFUS to motor cortex to elicit peripheral motor responses [2, 5, 28] which would be de facto excitation of pyramidal cells. Here, and in a previous report [8] we do not report any peripheral muscle activity. These discrepancies may be the result of differences in the specific parameters used and/or due to differences in cranial volume or other non-neuronal considerations [29]. In this study, we delivered a total of 54 0.5 s stimulations every 2 TRs (5.5 s). This is a higher inter-stimulus interval compared to Yoo et al. [5] who delivered 3 stimulations every 21 s and Lee et al. [11] that delivered stimulation every 13 s though it is unclear how many total sonications were delivered in that study as it is not expressly stated. We employed 500 kHz tFUS which is between what Yoo et al. [5] and Lee et al. [11] used though the intensities are similar. These differences may be critical as slight differences in parameters may have a significant impact on the neuronal results as different groups have demonstrated changes in amplitude, duration or duty cycle to affect the neuronal effect [3, 5, 30]. Theoretical accounts of the neuronal effect of ultrasound also predict thresholds for changes in neuronal excitation to inhibition based upon duty cycle and intensity.

In the neuronal intramembrane cavitation excitation (NICE) model of the effects of ultrasound our lower duty cycle (36% vs. 50%) and intensity values may leave us in the transition zone between excitation and inhibition or result only in inhibition [31]. Despite this theoretical model, and the work in small animal models, the effect of tFUS parameters on neuronal excitation in humans is not well understood empirically and indeed the basic putative mechanisms of how mechanical energy affects neuronal excitability is still largely theoretical [31–33]. There is evidence for US to affect certain mechanosensitive channels [34, 35] but the proliferation and density of these channels in human central nervous system is not well understood and the contribution of these channels to pyramidal excitation and neurovascular coupling is also unclear.

Another important difference between animal studies that show motor excitation and our results is cranial volume. We have previously demonstrated that skull size relative to the ultrasound beam size plays an important role in the intracranial propagation of ultrasound such that smaller skulls or cranial volumes lead to greater interaction of the sound field and higher pressures [18] that could increase the ultrasound effect and produce excitation. Higher amplitude or intensity is theoretically related to excitation [31] and empirical work in oocytes [34] and mice [3] has shown excitation to be a function of amplitude. The waveform we used here measured ~ 17 W/cm^2 in free water and is estimated from empirical observations through hydrated human skull and through detailed acoustic models to attenuate 4–6 times depending on specific properties of the skull [1, 18]. Unfortunately, we were not able to collect computed tomography scans of the subjects here to accurately model and estimate intracranial pressures though the above estimates are in a similar range to previous human studies [1, 10]. In general, ultrasound for neuromodulation follows the safety guidelines of the FDA for diagnostic ultrasound that include derated limits of a spatial peak pulse average intensity (Isppa) of 190 W/cm^2, a spatial peak temporal average of 720 mW/cm^2 and a mechanical index of 1.9. Several previous studies have reported no adverse events or evidence of anatomical damage [1, 9–12] and a recent in-depth survey of the safety of ultrasound for human neuromodulation did not find any evidence of serious events in a large cohort of participants [36].

In addition to assessing the effect of tFUS on existing BOLD activity, we were also interested in the spatial selectivity of this effect. To examine this, we had participants perform a cued finger tapping task with one of three digits (thumb, index, middle) and only delivered tFUS to the thumb representation during each finger movement. This allowed us to explore the effect of tFUS to not only the targeted thumb region but also on the adjacent non-stimulated index and middle finger regions. We did not find similar index and middle finger volume expansions while tFUS was directed at the thumb representation indicating local spatial effects like those found by Yoo et al. [5].

We did not find any evidence that application of tFUS to M1 is able to significantly affect downstream functionally connected regions of the motor system. This finding is at odds with Lee et al. [11] that reported tFUS directed at primary visual cortex (V1) to also result in activity in functionally connected regions of the human visual system. Again, differences in experimental design and/or stimulation parameters likely contribute to these differences. The task we used indeed activated both the SMA and the ipsilateral PMd and we do see a weak trend for volume changes in PMd but perhaps the local mechanisms that results in volume increases are limited to the immediate spatial vicinity and are not robust enough to affect downstream regions. One possibility is for the ultrasound effect to be too spatially restricted in that we may have "missed" the targets or not activated enough volume for downstream modulation. Indeed, the effect of non-invasive neuromodulation looks to be spatially and functionally specific as Opitz et al. [37] showed that depending upon transcranial magnetic stimulation (TMS) current direction to the dorsal lateral pre-frontal cortex different functionally connected networks were activated despite similar spatial locations [37]. As such, due to the spatial restriction of tFUS it is possible that we were not in the ideal spot to effect SMA and PMd activity. It is also possible that again, the motor task sufficiently activated these regions and tFUS did not have an appreciable effect above this level of activity.

Finally, an important consideration when pairing tFUS with MRI and BOLD is for the possibility that the detected response is a result of mechanical energy acting directly on the microvasculature and not on neuronal populations to induce neurovascular coupling. This is likely not the case as pressure levels used here are too low to affect the vasculature. Kaye et al. [38] demonstrated that focused ultrasound delivered up to 620 W/cm^2 results in tissue displacement on the order of micrometers, and that this displacement was not detectable in an EPI magnitude MRI image [38].

Conclusion

This study demonstrated that single element focused ultrasound can be paired with high field 7T fMRI to target individual finger representations within primary motor cortex. With continued research, the pairing of ultrasound with MRI can prove to be a valuable combination for high resolution mapping of discrete brain circuits both cortically and sub-cortically.

Abbreviations

BOLD: blood oxygen level dependent; EEG: electroencephalography; FOV: field of view; Isppa: spatial peak pulse average intensity; M1: primary motor cortex; MI: mechanical index; MHz: megahertz; MRI: magnetic resonance imaging; PMd: dorsal premotor cortex; PRF: pulse repetition frequency; ROI: region of interest; SMA: supplementary motor area; tFUS: transcranial focused ultrasound; TE: echo time; TR: repetition time; TMS: transcranial magnetic stimulation; V1: primary visual cortex.

Authors' contributions

LA, JKM and WL were responsible for experimental design, collection, analysis and manuscript preparation. PB was responsible for participant recruitment, collection and manuscript preparation. All authors read and approved the final manuscript.

Author details

[1] Division of Physical Therapy and Division of Rehabilitation Science, Department of Rehabilitation Medicine, Medical School, University of Minnesota, 426 Church St. SE Rm 361, Minneapolis, MN 55455, USA. [2] Department of Neurological Surgery, School of Medicine, University of Virginia, 409 Lane Rd. Rm 1031, Charlottesville, VA 22901, USA.

Acknowledgements

None.

Competing interests

The authors declare that they have no competing interests.

Funding

Funding for this study was provided by the Department of Rehabilitation Medicine and MNDrive at the University of Minnesota.

References

1. Legon W, Sato TF, Opitz A, Mueller J, Barbour A, Williams A, Tyler WJ. Transcranial focused ultrasound modulates the activity of primary somatosensory cortex in humans. Nat Neurosci. 2014;17(2):322–9.
2. Tufail Y, Matyushov A, Baldwin N, Tauchmann ML, Georges J, Yoshihiro A, Tillery SI, Tyler WJ. Transcranial pulsed ultrasound stimulates intact brain circuits. Neuron. 2010;66(5):681–94.
3. King RL, Brown JR, Newsome WT, Pauly KB. Effective parameters for ultrasound-induced in vivo neurostimulation. Ultrasound Med Biol. 2013;39(2):312–31.
4. Mehic E, Xu JM, Caler CJ, Coulson NK, Moritz CT, Mourad PD. Increased anatomical specificity of neuromodulation via modulated focused ultrasound. PLoS ONE. 2014;9(2):e86939.
5. Yoo SS, Bystritsky A, Lee JH, Zhang Y, Fischer K, Min BK, McDannold NJ, Pascual-Leone A, Jolesz FA. Focused ultrasound modulates region-specific brain activity. Neuroimage. 2011;56(3):1267–75.
6. Dallapiazza RF, Timbie KF, Holmberg S, Gatesman J, Lopes MB, Price RJ, Miller GW, Elias WJ. Noninvasive neuromodulation and thalamic mapping with low-intensity focused ultrasound. J Neurosurg. 2017;128:1–10.
7. Deffieux T, Younan Y, Wattiez N, Tanter M, Pouget P, Aubry JF. Low-intensity focused ultrasound modulates monkey visuomotor behavior. Curr Biol. 2013;23(23):2430–3.
8. Ai L, Mueller J, Grant A, Eryaman Y, Legon W. Transcranial focused ultrasound for BOLD fMRI signal modulation in humans. In: 2016 38th annual international conference of the IEEE Engineering in Medicine and Biology Society (EMBC), Orlando, FL, USA, 16–20 August 2016, p. 1758–61. https://doi.org/10.1109/embc.2016.7591057.
9. Legon W, Ai L, Bansal P, Mueller JK. Neuromodulation with single-element transcranial focused ultrasound in human thalamus. Hum Brain Mapp. 2018;00:1–12.
10. Lee W, Kim H, Jung Y, Song IU, Chung YA, Yoo SS. Image-guided transcranial focused ultrasound stimulates human primary somatosensory cortex. Sci Rep. 2015;5:8743.
11. Lee W, Kim HC, Jung Y, Chung YA, Song IU, Lee JH, Yoo SS. Transcranial focused ultrasound stimulation of human primary visual cortex. Sci Rep. 2016;6:34026.
12. Lee W, Chung YA, Jung Y, Song IU, Yoo SS. Simultaneous acoustic stimulation of human primary and secondary somatosensory cortices using transcranial focused ultrasound. BMC Neurosci. 2016;17(1):68.
13. Legon W, Bansal P, Tyshynsky R, Ai L, Mueller JK. Transcranial focused ultrasound neuromodulation of the human primary motor cortex. Sci Rep. 2018;8:10007. https://doi.org/10.1038/s41598-018 28230-1.
14. Rossi S, Hallett M, Rossini PM, Pascual-Leone A. Safety of TMS Consensus Group: safety, ethical considerations, and application guidelines for the use of transcranial magnetic stimulation in clinical practice and research. Clin Neurophysiol. 2009;120(12):2008–39.
15. Kim Y, Maxwell AD, Hall TL, Xu Z, Lin KW, Cain CA. Rapid prototyping fabrication of focused ultrasound transducers. IEEE Trans Ultrason Ferroelectr Freq Control. 2014;61(9):1559–74.
16. Bungert A, Chambers CD, Long E, Evans CJ. On the importance of specialized radiofrequency filtering for concurrent TMS/MRI. J Neurosci Methods. 2012;210(2):202–5.
17. Garcia-Rodriguez M, Garcia-Alvarez J, Yanez Y, Garcia-Hernandez J, Salazar A, Turo A, Chavez JA. Low cost matching network for ultrasonic transducers. Phys Procedia. 2010;3(1):1025.
18. Mueller JK, Ai L, Bansal P, Legon W. Numerical evaluation of the skull for human neuromodulation with transcranial focused ultrasound. J Neural Eng. 2017. https://doi.org/10.1088/1741-2552/aa843e.
19. Mueller JK, Ai L, Bansal P, Legon W. Computational exploration of wave propagation and heating from transcranial focused ultrasound for neuromodulation. J Neural Eng. 2016;13(5):056002-2560/13/5/056002.
20. Spitzer VM, Whitlock DG. The Visible Human Dataset: the anatomical platform for human simulation. Anat Rec. 1998;253(2):49–57.
21. Treeby BE, Cox BT. k-Wave: MATLAB toolbox for the simulation and reconstruction of photoacoustic wave fields. J Biomed Opt. 2010;15(2):021314.
22. Cox RW. AFNI: software for analysis and visualization of functional magnetic resonance neuroimages. Comput Biomed Res. 1996;29(3):162–73.
23. Mueller J, Legon W, Opitz A, Sato TF, Tyler WJ. Transcranial focused ultrasound modulates intrinsic and evoked EEG dynamics. Brain Stimul. 2014;7(6):900–8.
24. Nir Y, Fisch L, Mukamel R, Gelbard-Sagiv H, Arieli A, Fried I, Malach R. Coupling between neuronal firing rate, gamma LFP, and BOLD fMRI is related to interneuronal correlations. Curr Biol. 2007;17(15):1275–85.
25. Scheeringa R, Fries P, Petersson KM, Oostenveld R, Grothe I, Norris DG, Hagoort P, Bastiaansen MC. Neuronal dynamics underlying high- and low-frequency EEG oscillations contribute independently to the human BOLD signal. Neuron. 2011;69(3):572–83.
26. Bartos M, Vida I, Jonas P. Synaptic mechanisms of synchronized gamma oscillations in inhibitory interneuron networks. Nat Rev Neurosci. 2007;8(1):45–56.

27. Buzsaki G, Wang XJ. Mechanisms of gamma oscillations. Annu Rev Neurosci. 2012;35:203–25.

28. Lee W, Lee SD, Park MY, Foley L, Purcell-Estabrook E, Kim H, Fischer K, Maeng LS, Yoo SS. Image-guided focused ultrasound-mediated regional brain stimulation in sheep. Ultrasound Med Biol. 2016;42(2):459–70.

29. Guo H, Hamilton M, Offutt S, Gloeckner C, Li T, Kim Y, Legon W, Alford JK, Lim HH. Ultrasound produces extensive brain activation via a cochlear pathway. Neuron. 2018;98(5):1020–30.e4. https://doi.org/10.1016/j.neuron.2018.04.036.

30. Kim H, Chiu A, Lee SD, Fischer K, Yoo SS. Focused ultrasound-mediated non-invasive brain stimulation: examination of sonication parameters. Brain Stimul. 2014;7(5):748–56.

31. Plaksin M, Kimmel E, Shoham S. Cell-type-selective effects of intramembrane cavitation as a unifying theoretical framework for ultrasonic neuromodulation. eNeuro. 2016. https://doi.org/10.1523/eneuro.0136-15.2016 **(eCollection 2016 May–Jun)**.

32. Tyler WJ. Noninvasive neuromodulation with ultrasound? A continuum mechanics hypothesis. Neuroscientist. 2011;17(1):25–36.

33. Krasovitski B, Frenkel V, Shoham S, Kimmel E. Intramembrane cavitation as a unifying mechanism for ultrasound-induced bioeffects. Proc Natl Acad Sci USA. 2011;108(8):3258–63.

34. Kubanek J, Shi J, Marsh J, Chen D, Deng C, Cui J. Ultrasound modulates ion channel currents. Sci Rep. 2016;6:24170.

35. Prieto ML, Butrus KF, Khuri-Yakub T, Maduke M. Mechanical activation of piezo1 but not Nav1.2 channels by ultrasound. biorxiv 2017.

36. Legon W, Bansal P, Ai L, Mueller JK, Meekins G, Gillick B. Safety of transcranial focused ultrasound for human neuromodulation. Bioarxiv 2018.

37. Opitz A, Fox MD, Craddock RC, Colcombe S, Milham MP. An integrated framework for targeting functional networks via transcranial magnetic stimulation. Neuroimage. 2016;127:86–96.

38. Kaye EA, Chen J, Pauly KB. Rapid MR-ARFI method for focal spot localization during focused ultrasound therapy. Magn Reson Med. 2011;65(3):738–43.

6

Mice lacking galectin-3 (*Lgals3*) function have decreased home cage movement

Tammy R. Chaudoin and Stephen J. Bonasera[*]

Abstract

Background: Galectins are a large family of proteins evolved to recognize specific carbohydrate moieties. Given the importance of pattern recognition processes for multiple biological tasks, including CNS development and immune recognition, we examined the home cage behavioral phenotype of mice lacking galectin-3 (*Lgals3*) function. Using a sophisticated monitoring apparatus capable of examining feeding, drinking, and movement at millisecond temporal and 0.5 cm spatial resolutions, we observed daily behavioral patterns from 10 wildtype male C57BL/6J and 10 *Lgals3* constitutive knockout (*Lgals3$^{-/-}$*; both cohorts aged 2–3 months) mice over 17 consecutive days. We performed a second behavioral assessment of this cohort at age 6–7 months.

Results: At both ages, *Lgals3$^{-/-}$* mice demonstrated less movement compared to wildtype controls. Both forward locomotion and movement-in-place behaviors were decreased in *Lgals3$^{-/-}$* mice, due to decreased bout numbers, initiation rates, and durations. We additionally noted perturbation of behavioral circadian rhythms in *Lgals3$^{-/-}$* mice, with mice at both ages demonstrating greater variability in day-to-day performance of feeding, drinking, and movement (as assessed by Lomb-Scargle analysis) compared to wildtype.

Conclusion: Carbohydrate recognition tasks performed by *Lgals3* may be required for appropriate development of CNS structures involved in the generation and control of locomotor behavior.

Keywords: Circadian rhythm, Galectin-3, Ingestive behavior, *Lgals3*, Locomotor behavior

Background

Galectins are an evolutionarily ancient family of proteins sharing a high binding affinity for carbohydrates with β-galactoside linkages. In the extracellular space, galectins interact (through a conserved carbohydrate recognition domain, *aka* CRD) with glycosylated proteins to mediate both cell-to-cell interactions and cell-to-matrix adhesion. Galectins are thus pattern recognition molecules specialized to distinguish carbohydrate moieties.

Within the galectin family, galectin-3 (also known as *Lgals3*) has unique properties. Its preferred ligand is N-acetyllactosamine [1]. It is also the only galectin containing a conserved N-domain as well as a single CRD domain. This N-domain allows *Lgals3* not bound to a carbohydrate target to form multimeric complexes [2].

In this manner, low extracellular *Lgals3* concentrations tend to inhibit extracellular interactions and adhesion [3], while high *Lgals3* extracellular concentrations facilitate cellular adhesion [4, 5]. *Lgals3* affinity for ECM substrates is also modulated by phosphorylation at its Ser6 residue [6].

Lgals3 is an NFκB target gene [7]; *Lgals3* protein is widely distributed throughout most tissue sites (as demonstrated by the TiGER Tissue specific gene expression and regulation database; [8]). Furthermore, within specific tissues, *Lgals3* protein expression is widespread, with extracellular [9], membrane bound, cytoplasmic, and nuclear localizations (for review, see [10]).

Given these varied *Lgals3* tissue and cellular distributions, it is not surprising to find that cellular functions attributed to *Lgals3* are numerous and diverse: (1) context-sensitive cell adhesion [11] or dehiscence [12], (2) receptor for advanced glycation (AGE) and advanced lipoxygenation (ALE) end products [13], (3) regulating

*Correspondence: sbonasera@unmc.edu
Division of Geriatrics, Department of Internal Medicine, University of Nebraska Medical Center, 3028 Durham Research Center II, Omaha, NE 68198-5039, USA

clathrin-independent endocytosis [14], (4) regulating intracellular signal transduction by spacing apart membrane-bound signaling complexes [15], (5) modulating Wnt/β-catenin signaling [16], (6) influencing TTF-1 and STAT transcription factor activities [17, 18], (6) regulating mRNA maturation through their effects on spliceosome function [19], (7) repairing DNA damage [20], (8) inducing late G_1 cell cycle arrest [21], (9) promoting cell proliferation [22], and (10) promoting cell survival through the anti-apoptotic effects of Bcl2 [23]. *Lgals3* also participates in immune function. It contributes to innate immunity through its abilities to opsonize cellular debris [24], facilitate generation of respiratory burst enzymes [25], function as a MerTK-specific eat-me signal [26], and act as a CNS alarmin [27]; moreover, it contributes to acquired immunity through its regulation of T cell activation [15].

Finally, there is an increasing recognition that proteins capable of molecular pattern recognition play significant roles in CNS synapse formation, pruning, and maintenance [28]. Already, many different classes of pattern recognition molecules have been implicated in these processes: major histocompatibility genes [29, 30], complement [31], paired immunoglobulin-like receptors [32], and toll-like receptors [33]. These pattern recognition receptors all have highly conserved glycosylation sites (MHC-I [34]; C3 [35]; PirB [36]; Tlr2 [37]), making them potential *Lgals3* interaction partners. *Lgals3*-mediated recognition of specific N-acetyllactosamine sites may be required for CNS developmental events. For example, prior studies demonstrate that altered *Lgals3* expression has a role in age-related synaptic changes accompanying functional loss [38].

Objectives
We thus assessed baseline behaviors in a mouse model to evaluate *Lgals3* influence on important behaviors of clinical interest, including metabolism, feeding, drinking, movement, and circadian rhythm. We measured metabolism using indirect calorimetry with correction for mouse adiposity. We used a sophisticated home cage monitoring approach to assess mouse feeding, drinking, activity, and circadian rhythm in a noninvasive manner over more than 2 weeks of observation. Surprisingly, despite the large number of molecular interactions involving *Lgals3*, and well-documented *Lgals3* CNS expression (in neurons, microglia, and astrocytes), we found only two significant behavioral deficits accompanying constitutive *Lgals3* loss: decreased locomotor movement, and diminished fidelity of circadian feeding, drinking, and movement patterns.

Methods
Ethical statement
All studies were performed in full concordance with both institutional and federal regulations regarding animal care and use; our research protocol was approved by the University of Nebraska Medical Center (UNMC) Institutional Animal Care and Use Committee (IACUC).

Animal models and husbandry
We evaluated cohorts of C57BL/6J male mice (stock number 000664) and mice carrying a constitutive *Lgals3* mutation (*Lgals3*$^{-/-}$; B6.Cg-*Lgals3*^{tm1Poi}/J; stock number 006338), both obtained from Jackson Laboratories. Briefly, these mice were created through homologous recombination removing the native *Lgals3* exons II, III, and IV and replacing them with a neomycin resistance cassette. Homozygous mutant offspring derived from this targeted lesion expressed only the 3.4 kb predicted *Eco*RI fragment, and did not have the 6.4 kb WT fragment [39]. Mice obtained from Jackson have undergone 7 backcrosses to C57BL/6J from the original chimeric mouse. Upon initial receipt at our vivarium, mice were housed in a microisolator system (Lab Products, Seaford DE) at a density of ≤ 5 mice per cage. No mice were used for breeding purposes. The facility maintained a 12:12 circadian lighting schedule with lights on at 06:00 CST; vivarium temperatures ranged between 20 and 23 °C. All mice had ad libitum access to food (Envigo Teklad #7012), water, and environmental enrichment (Crinkle Paper Pouches, WF Fisher). Animal health was checked on a daily basis by UNMC Comparative Medicine staff. Mice remained in the vivarium for 14 days prior to start of testing. While mice were housed in the vivarium, cage bedding, food, and water were changed every 14 days. Mice were returned to the vivarium and kept singly-housed between the two longitudinal assessments. Following testing, mice were sacrificed by CO_2 inhalation followed by cervical dislocation.

Body mass composition
We performed dual X-ray absorptiometry (DEXA) imaging to measure mouse adiposity. We performed a longitudinal assessment of 10 WT and 10 *Lgals3*$^{-/-}$ mice; we first tested mice at 2–3 months old, followed by repeat assessment at 6–7 months old. Investigators were not blinded to mouse genotype. Mice received DEXA imaging in a random manner. DEXA testing occurred between 10:00 and 16:00. Animals were lightly anesthetized with isoflurane at 1–3 vol%, and imaged with a Piximus I (Inside/Outside, Fitchburg WI). Before data acquisition, the system was calibrated by imaging a phantom with

defined radiological characteristics. We used vendor supplied software (Piximus I, GE Lunar) to identify regions of interest (ROIs) encompassing the mouse chest/abdomen/pelvis for determination of bone mass density (BMD), bone mineral content (BMC), bone area (BArea), tissue area (TArea), ratio of soft tissue attenuation (R_{ST}), total tissue mass (TTM), and percent adiposity (% fat). Data was analyzed by repeated measures analysis of variance (ANOVA, implemented in MATLAB 2011b) with genotype and mouse age as primary factors, and a genotype × age interaction.

Indirect calorimetry to assess basal and activity-associated metabolism

We performed a longitudinal assessment of 10 WT and 10 $Lgals3^{-/-}$ mice; we first tested mice at 2–3 months old, followed by repeat assessment at 6–7 months old. Investigators were not blinded to mouse genotype. Mice were assigned to calorimetry enclosures in a random manner. Animals were fasted overnight, then placed into 8 hermetically-sealed metabolic cages (Oxymax, Columbus Instruments). Mice were tested between 10:00 and 17:00; each measurement of gas tension required 2 min, so each animal had its metabolic parameters assessed every 16 min during the testing period. We used vendor supplied software (Oxymax for Windows 4.49) to determine maximum oxygen uptake ($\dot{V}O_2$), global oxygen delivery (DO_2), oxygen output (O_2out), maximum CO_2 production, ($\dot{V}CO_2$), global CO_2 removal (DCO_2), CO_2 output (CO_2out), and heat generated. Basal metabolic rates were determined by averaging measurements obtained during the 3 epochs displaying the least activity (as measured by photobeam brackets spanning the length of the metabolic chamber); similarly, activity-associated metabolic rates were determined by averaging measurements obtained during the 3 epochs displaying the most activity. Metabolic parameters were then adjusted for mouse adiposity and mouse lean body mass using ANCOVA [40, 41]. Full description of our metabolic testing apparatus is provided in [42]. Mice were weighed using a Scout Pro SP401 (Ohaus, Parsippany NJ) before indirect calorimetry, home cage behavioral monitoring, and on a weekly basis between the two longitudinal assessments and following the last assessment.

Home cage behavioral monitoring

Details describing our home cage behavioral monitoring system have been previously published [43, 44]. Briefly, we measure mouse feeding, drinking, and movement at high temporal and spatial precision in a custom-designed home cage over extended periods of time. Feeding is quantified by the number of times a mouse breaks a photobeam while accessing a food hopper (ms resolution).

Drinking is quantified by a capactive lickometer (ms resolution). Movement is quantified by solving exact equations of torque measured at three load cells and knowing mouse body weight (ms temporal, 0.5 cm spatial resolution). Data undergoes rigorous automated quality control, followed by behavioral classification and analysis [43]. We performed a longitudinal assessment of 10 WT and 10 $Lgals3^{-/-}$ mice; we first tested mice at 2–3 months old, followed by repeat assessment at 6–7 months old. Mice were randomly assigned to one of 64 home cage behavioral assessment arenas. Each arena contained a niche modeled to approximate dimensions of a mouse burrow to organize mouse resting location, and a nestlet (NES3600, Ancare) for nesting materials. Powdered chow and water were available to all mice ad libitum; behavioral testing room lighting schedule was 12:12 with lights on at 0600 h CST. Room temperature ranged between 20 and 23 °C; facility relative humidity ranged between 35 and 51%. The arena floor was layered with absorbent bedding (200 ml Teklad Sani-chips (Envigo, Huntington UK), 300 ml ALPHA-Dri®+PLUS (Shepherd Specialty Papers, Watertown TN)). Mice were allowed to habituate to the home cage monitoring system for 5 days before start of data collection. Investigators were not blinded regarding mouse genotype. We then collected 17 consecutive days of data for each mouse (to ensure that we had at least 14 full days of data after quality control) at each longitudinal assessment time point.

Mouse behavioral data quality control, classification, and analysis

We employed automated data quality control checks to identify outliers and epochs where there may be questions regarding data integrity (in particular, blocked photobeams and sipper tube leaks). These epochs constituted less than 1% of total data collected, and were removed from the dataset. Following data quality control, individual mouse feeding, drinking, and movement events were classified to determine active and inactive state properties (in a manner similar to human actigraphy), and to fit these behaviors to a Gaussian mixture model that would allow us to compare bout structures across genotypes. Theory and implementation of these processes has been published in [42, 43 (both manuscript and data supplement), 44].

Following data classification, we performed false-discovery rate (FDR) analysis over 665 different outcomes that assessed differences in major behavioral categories including overall feeding/drinking/movement, time budget, active and inactive state structure, intake and movement bout structure, within-bout structure, and periodicity. These results are provided as Additional file 1: Table 1. For significant behaviors identified by this analysis, we quantified genotypic differences in mouse behavior by one-way ANOVA with genotype as primary factor. In these analyses, multiple comparisons were addressed by Bonferroni correction.

Periodicity analysis

We examined circadian periodicities using Lomb-Scargle analysis, which detects multiple periodicities within a time series [45, 46]. A major advantage of this approach is that it remains robust in the setting of incompletely sampled data streams. Feeding, drinking, and movement data were binned into 6-min epochs, and significant periodicities (up to 60 h duration) were calculated using an implementation described by [47] and coded in MATLAB 2011b (MathWorks, Natick MA).

Results

FDR analysis suggests that $Lgals3^{-/-}$ mice demonstrate significant movement deficits

In 2–3 months old mice at $\alpha = 0.10$, we identified 20 behaviors that significantly differed between the WT and $Lgals3^{-/-}$ cohort, 16 of which related to movement (Additional file 1: Table 1, first tab, column 29). By χ^2 test, movement-related behaviors were overrepresented within this set (16 observed, 7 expected, $p < 0.009$ with critical $p < 0.016$). Similarly, in 6–7 months old mice at $\alpha = 0.05$, we identified 82 behaviors that significantly differed between the WT and $Lgals3^{-/-}$ cohort, 62 of which were related to movement (Additional file 1: Table 1, second tab, column 29). By χ^2 test, movement-related behaviors were again highly overrepresented within this set (62 observed, 29 expected, $p < 1.0 \times 10^{-6}$ with critical $p < 0.016$). These results suggest that $Lgals3^{-/-}$ mice have a deficit in motor function that progresses with age.

Movement deficits in $Lgals3^{-/-}$ mice

As is evident in Fig. 1a, both 2–3 months old and 6–7 months old $Lgals3^{-/-}$ mice demonstrate significantly less total movement compared to WT mice. This phenotype is particularly prominent during the circadian dark cycle, when mice are most active. In an effort to determine the underlying cause of this decreased movement, we subdivide movement into locomotion (consisting of movements performed at high gait speeds with small turning angles) and movement-in-place (consisting of movements performed at low gait speeds with large turning angles). For 2–3 months old mice, we note no significant genotypic differences in any locomotor bout properties (Fig. 1b, top left). However, for 2–3 months old mice we note significant genotypic differences in movement-in-place bout properties of total movement, bout rate, active state bout rate, bout number, and bout duration (Fig. 1b, top right, also see Table 1). In 2–3 months

old $Lgals3^{-/-}$ mice, movement-in-place bouts were also statistically more likely to be the first behavior performed within new dark cycle active states (WT probability 0.09 ± 0.01; $Lgals3^{-/-}$ probability 0.13 ± 0.01, $p < 0.007$ with critical $p < 0.0125$).

The above movement phenotype was more prominent in 6–7 months old mice. We noted genotypic differences in locomotor bout total distance, overall bout rate, active state bout rate, bout number, and bout duration (Fig. 1b bottom left, also Table 2). These differences led to a statistically significant decrease in the percent time devoted to locomotion within a 24 h time budget ($3.8 \pm 1.0\%$ WT, $2.5 \pm 0.4\%$ $Lgals3^{-/-}$, $p < 0.002$ with critical $p < 0.01$). Older $Lgals3^{-/-}$ mice demonstrated changes in movement-in-place bouts similar to those observed in younger mice, with genotypic differences in bout total distance, bout rate, bout active state rate, bout number, and per-bout duration (Fig. 1b bottom right, also Table 2). Finally, we again noticed that movement-in-place bouts were statistically overrepresented as the first behavior performed within newly started dark cycle active states (WT probability 0.11 ± 0.01; $Lgals3^{-/-}$ probability 0.18 ± 0.01, $p < 0.004$ with critical $p < 0.0125$).

$Lgals3^{-/-}$ mice have greater day-to-day heterogeneity in circadian rhythms for movement, food, and water intake

In both 2–3 months and 6–7 months old mouse cohorts, we note significant decreases in normalized power of the 24-h spectral components for feeding, drinking, and movement behaviors in $Lgals3^{-/-}$ mice (Fig. 2). These decreases suggest an increase in the variability of feeding, drinking, and movement over 6 min time windows extending through the duration of our 16 day long observation. We did not appreciate any significant advance or retreat of the daily activity onset and offset times, nor did we find any statistically significant difference in overall active phase duration.

6–7 months old $Lgals3^{-/-}$ mice have greater body weights than WT cohorts

We found no genotypic differences in neither body weight nor body mass composition between 2 and 3 months old WT and $Lgals3^{-/-}$ mice. Similarly, we found no genotypic differences in basal metabolic or activity-associated metabolic rates between 2 and 3 months old WT and $Lgals3^{-/-}$ mice. However, 6–7 months old $Lgals3^{-/-}$ mice were heavier than their WT counterparts (27.0 ± 1.2 g WT, 28.4 ± 1.3 g $Lgals3^{-/-}$, $p < 0.02$). Body mass over the study time period is shown in Fig. 3, and suggests that the two cohorts diverge around 6–7 months of age. Body mass composition parameters noted with this weight change included greater adiposity ($14.1 \pm 2.1\%$ WT, $16.1 \pm 2.0\%$ $Lgals3^{-/-}$, $p < 0.03$), greater total tissue

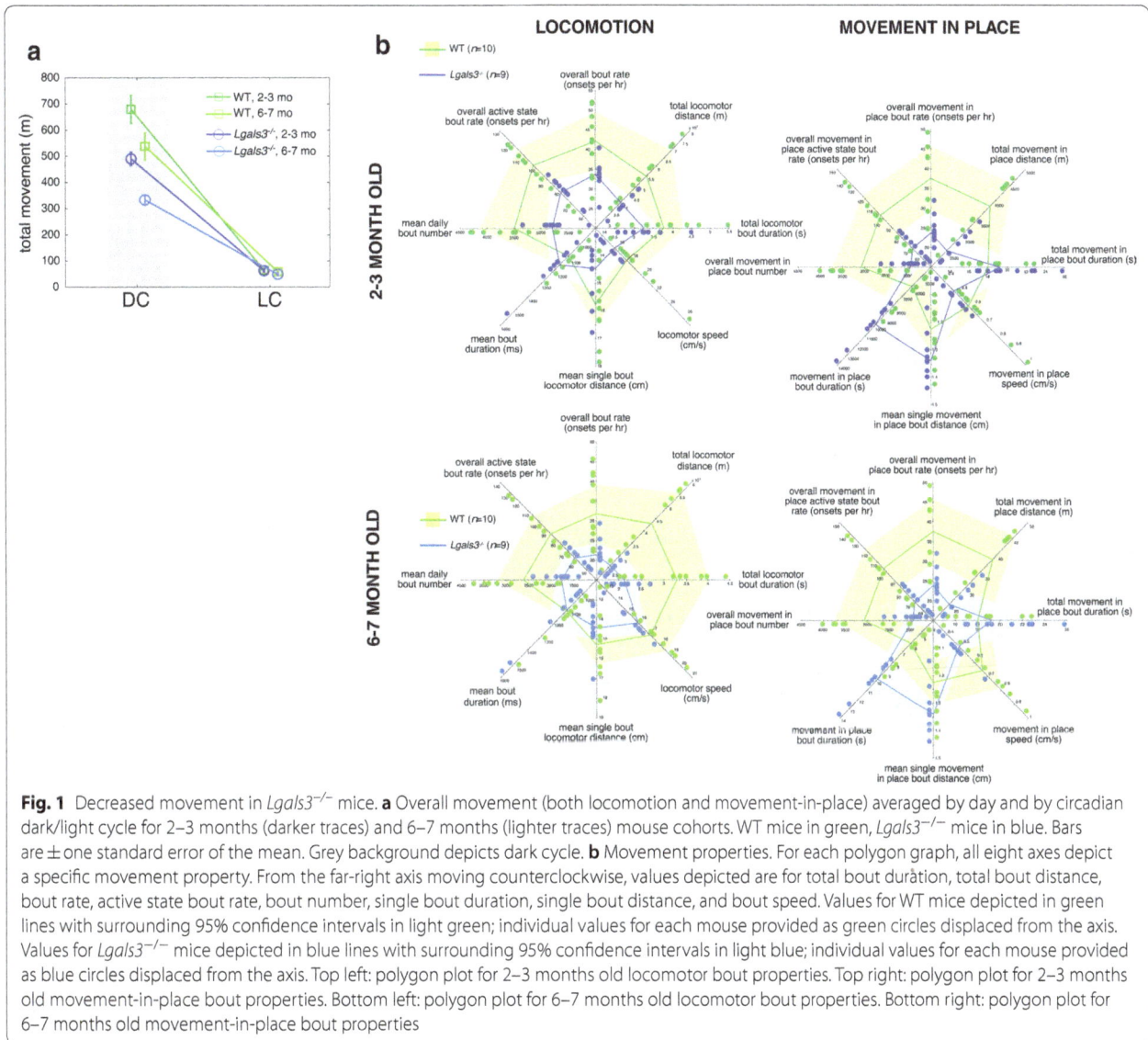

Fig. 1 Decreased movement in *Lgals3*$^{-/-}$ mice. **a** Overall movement (both locomotion and movement-in-place) averaged by day and by circadian dark/light cycle for 2–3 months (darker traces) and 6–7 months (lighter traces) mouse cohorts. WT mice in green, *Lgals3*$^{-/-}$ mice in blue. Bars are ± one standard error of the mean. Grey background depicts dark cycle. **b** Movement properties. For each polygon graph, all eight axes depict a specific movement property. From the far-right axis moving counterclockwise, values depicted are for total bout duration, total bout distance, bout rate, active state bout rate, bout number, single bout duration, single bout distance, and bout speed. Values for WT mice depicted in green lines with surrounding 95% confidence intervals in light green; individual values for each mouse provided as green circles displaced from the axis. Values for *Lgals3*$^{-/-}$ mice depicted in blue lines with surrounding 95% confidence intervals in light blue; individual values for each mouse provided as blue circles displaced from the axis. Top left: polygon plot for 2–3 months old locomotor bout properties. Top right: polygon plot for 2–3 months old movement-in-place bout properties. Bottom left: polygon plot for 6–7 months old locomotor bout properties. Bottom right: polygon plot for 6–7 months old movement-in-place bout properties

Table 1 Movement bout properties, 2–3 months old cohort

Behavior	WT (mean ± SD)	*Lgals3*$^{-/-}$ (mean ± SD)	p
Movement in place total distance (m)	43.8 ± 7.6	26.9 ± 3.7	< 0.02
Movement in place bout rate (onsets/h)	45.0 ± 9.1	24.7 ± 3.8	< 0.02
Movement in place bout active rate	106.0 ± 20.2	68.6 ± 11.0	< 0.01
Movement in place total number bouts	3736 ± 758	2031 ± 308	< 0.02
Movement in place mean bout duration (s)	6.5 ± 1.7	10.1 ± 1.4	< 0.01

mass (23.8 ± 1.0 g WT, 25.3 ± 1.3 g *Lgals3*$^{-/-}$, $p < 0.01$), and greater bone mineral density (0.051 ± 0.003 OD/cm^2 WT, 0.0054 ± 0.002 OD/cm^2 *Lgals3*$^{-/-}$, $p < 0.008$) in 6–7 months old *Lgals3*$^{-/-}$ compared to WT mice. No differences in either basal or activity-associated metabolic rates were appreciated between 6 and 7 months old WT and *Lgals3*$^{-/-}$ mice.

Table 2 Movement bout properties, 6–7 months old cohort

Behavior	WT (mean ± SD)	Lgals3$^{-/-}$ (mean ± SD)	p
Locomotor total distance (m)	422.9 ± 135.5	261.5 ± 29.3	< 0.003
Locomotor bout rate (onsets/h)	33.2 ± 8.6	22.2 ± 3.5	< 0.002
Locomotor bout active state rate	90.5 ± 23.9	61.5 ± 11.0	< 0.004
Locomotor total number bouts	2726 ± 704	1821 ± 289.6	< 0.002
Locomotor total bout duration (s)	3123.5 ± 833.3	2123.4 ± 306.1	< 0.004
Movement in place total distance (m)	37.3 ± 8.5	26.9 ± 4.5	< 0.004
Movement in place bout rate (onsets/h)	37.0 ± 9.2	24.7 ± 3.6	< 0.002
Movement in place bout active rate	100.5 ± 24.9	68.6 ± 11.8	< 0.003
Movement in place total number bouts	3032 ± 759	2031 ± 298	< 0.002
Movement in place mean bout duration (s)	6.4 ± 1.8	10.1 ± 2.0	< 0.0006

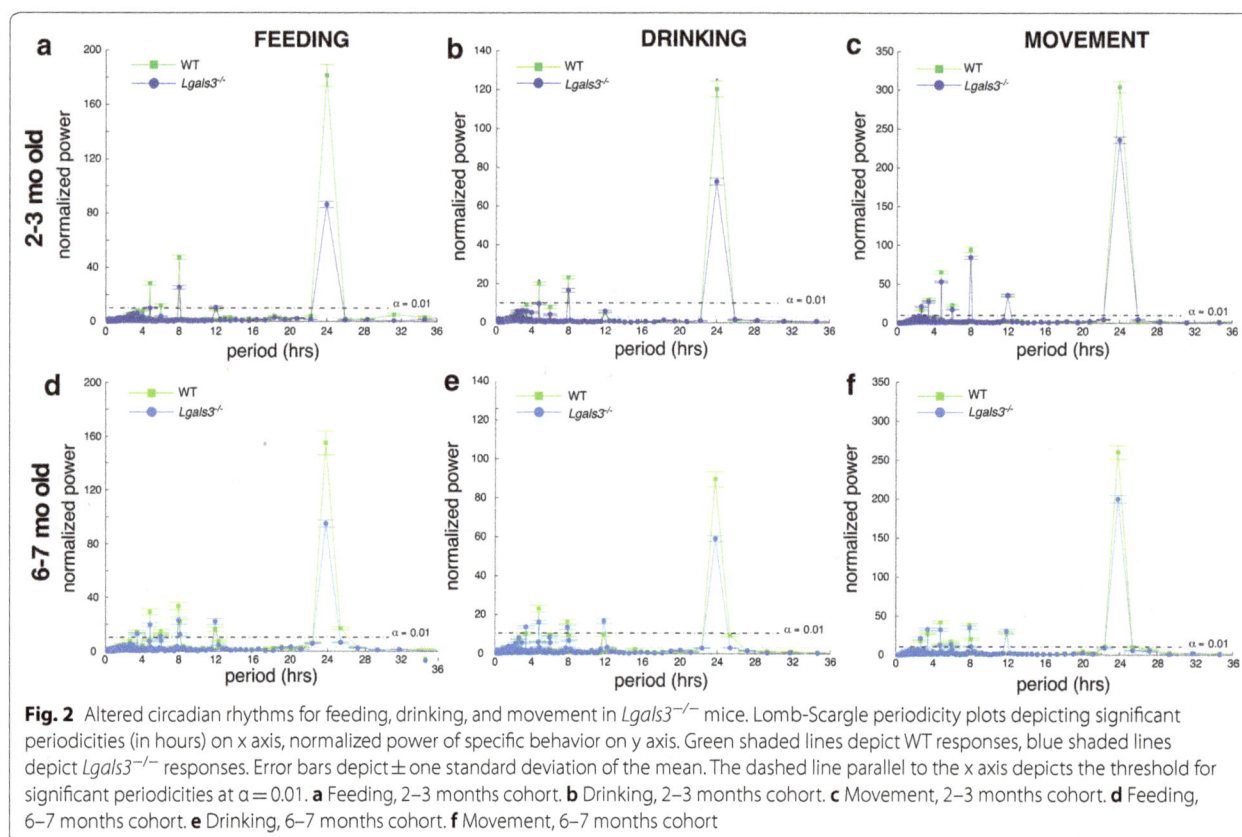

Fig. 2 Altered circadian rhythms for feeding, drinking, and movement in Lgals3$^{-/-}$ mice. Lomb-Scargle periodicity plots depicting significant periodicities (in hours) on x axis, normalized power of specific behavior on y axis. Green shaded lines depict WT responses, blue shaded lines depict Lgals3$^{-/-}$ responses. Error bars depict ± one standard deviation of the mean. The dashed line parallel to the x axis depicts the threshold for significant periodicities at α = 0.01. **a** Feeding, 2–3 months cohort. **b** Drinking, 2–3 months cohort. **c** Movement, 2–3 months cohort. **d** Feeding, 6–7 months cohort. **e** Drinking, 6–7 months cohort. **f** Movement, 6–7 months cohort

Phenotypes with no difference between WT and Lgals3$^{-/-}$ cohorts in both 2–3 and 6–7 months old mice

Regarding home cage phenotypes, we noted no significant differences in overall food or water ingestion between WT and Lgals3$^{-/-}$ mice. Except for the previously-noted difference in time allocated to locomotion seen across the 6–7 month old cohorts, there were no significant differences in the 24 h time budgets for feeding, drinking, locomotion, movement-in-place, and resting. There were also no differences in the percentage of time within an active state devoted to feeding, drinking, locomotion, and movement-in-place. We noted no significant differences (overall, or in either circadian dark or light cycles) in active or inactive state properties, including state onset rates, state durations, state transition probabilities, and total numbers of states. Finally, we

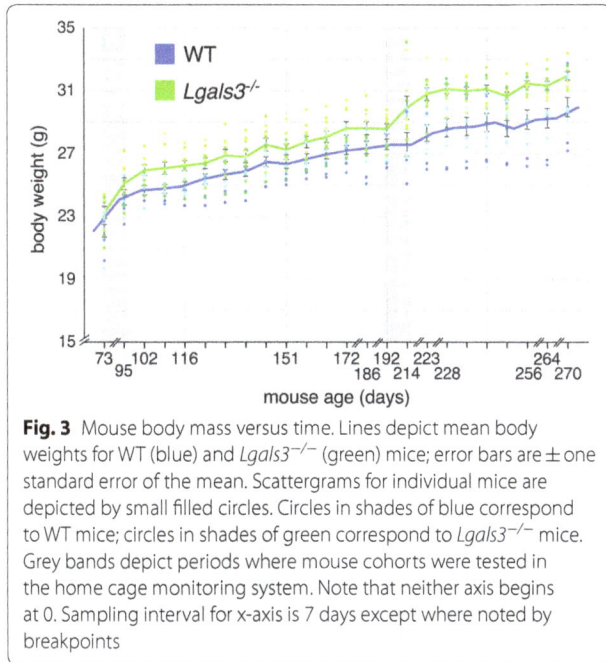

Fig. 3 Mouse body mass versus time. Lines depict mean body weights for WT (blue) and *Lgals3*$^{-/-}$ (green) mice; error bars are ± one standard error of the mean. Scattergrams for individual mice are depicted by small filled circles. Circles in shades of blue correspond to WT mice; circles in shades of green correspond to *Lgals3*$^{-/-}$ mice. Grey bands depict periods where mouse cohorts were tested in the home cage monitoring system. Note that neither axis begins at 0. Sampling interval for x-axis is 7 days except where noted by breakpoints

noted no differences in bout properties of feeding and drinking, including the circadian patterns of total bout intake, bout onset, bout probability, bout duration, bout intensity, and per-bout intake.

Discussion

There are currently few published studies examining the behavioral consequences of *Lgals3* loss. The Consortium for Functional Glycomics (CFG) spearheaded an impressive effort to obtain baseline behavioral profiles for a wide variety of genes involved in carbohydrate biology, including *Lgals3*. Their results suggested that *Lgals3*$^{-/-}$ mice had diminished freezing in a contextual fear assay, and were more aggressive both in response to an approaching object and in a paired social encounter [48, 49]. *Lgals3* has also been implicated in regulation of energy balance status and development of obesity [50]. Loss of *Lgals3* function was associated with accelerated development of obesity, increased adiposity, insulin resistance, metabolic syndrome, and type II diabetes in mice receiving a high fat diet ([51, 52]; however, data from [53, 54] suggest low *Lgals3* expression as potentially protective against type II DM). *Lgals3* also has been shown to regulate adipose tissue development and function [55–57], and may be an important molecule mediating how diet influences hepatic steatosis [58, 59]. Finally, impaired cognition in older adults has been associated with specific *Lgals3* polymorphisms (rs4644, rs4652, and rs1009977; [60]).

Comparing the above studies to our work, we first note that the CFG investigators observed no genotypic

differences in body weight, dark and light cycle metabolic rates, and locomotion. Similarly, we did not find any genotypic differences in food consumption or basal/activity-associated metabolic rates in either 2–3 months old or 6–7 months old mouse cohorts. Values for $\dot{V}O_2$ reported by CFG for both light and dark cycle epochs were consistent with our measured basal and activity-associated $\dot{V}O_2$. We also noted no genotypic differences in body weight between 2 and 3 months WT and *Lgals3*$^{-/-}$ mice. However, 6–7 months old mice (slightly older than the oldest reported in [48]) had increased body weight and greater adiposity in *Lgals3*$^{-/-}$ compared to WT cohorts. Since the Teklad 7012 diet is 17% fat, and mouse dietary requirements are estimated at 5% fat [61], it is reasonable to suggest that the increase in *Lgals3*$^{-/-}$ body weight/adiposity we observe in part replicates prior findings of high-fat-diet-induced obesity.

We provide the first data suggesting *Lgals3* involvement in motor system development and/or performance. Specifically, we noted an overall ~30% decrease in *Lgals3*$^{-/-}$ movement (both locomotion and movement in place) compared to WT mice. This decrease was observed in an acclimated home cage over 16 days, and thus does not assess the same construct reported by the CFG investigators, who found no change in open field locomotion over 30 min. *Lgals3*$^{-/-}$ mice therefore display decreased home cage locomotion with no change in novelty-evoked locomotion. The moderate increase in *Lgals3*$^{-/-}$ body weight may slightly increase the behavioral cost of movement, and thus decrease total movement. However, the prominent differences in movement-in-place bout rate, active state bout rate, bout duration, and bout number observed in 2–3 months old mice, as well as the large differences in both locomotion and movement-in-place bout rate, active state bout rate, bout duration, and bout number observed in 6–7 months old mice, suggest that *Lgals3* constitutive loss evokes functional deficits in underlying motor substrates. Both gene (ebi.ac.uk/gxa, informatics.jax.org/expression.shtml) and protein expression (emouseatlas.org, proteinatlas.org) atlases suggest that *Lgals3* expression (at low-to-moderate levels) occurs in both pre-and post-natal brain, and has been localized to regions involved in motor behavior generation, including the cortex, striatum, cerebellum, and spinal cord. We thus argue that *Lgals3* loss alters mouse motor function, either through its impact on motor development or through altered neuronal signaling in CNS regions that regulate or produce motor behavior. Further studies examining the consequences of *Lgals3* loss at synaptic, neuronal, ensemble, and tissue levels of organization will be required to determine the precise mechanisms underlying this functional loss.

As mentioned earlier, *Lgals3* has been implicated in a large number of physiological tasks at both a cellular and organwide level of organization. It is thus notable that mice with complete loss of *Lgals3* function demonstrate relatively few behavioral differences when compared to wildtype C57BL/6J mice. This finding suggests that, at least in the mouse, there is some genetic redundancy regarding *Lgals3* function. Studies of galectin evolution focusing on intron/exon organization as well as sequence identity suggest that duplication of ancestral galectin genes in animal lineages preceding the first teleost fish [62] provided the precursors for what has become a large vertebrate protein family [63]. There is also data suggesting that galectins may be able to substitute for one another in specific circumstances. For example, Lgals1 may compensate for *Lgals3* loss at the spliceosome [64]. Extracellular Lgals1 also regulates T cell apoptosis in a manner similar to that of extracellular *Lgals3* [65]. The behavioral phenotype arising from *Lgals3* functional loss thus identifies neuronal loci and processes where there is no compensation for gene loss.

Finally, these findings support the hypothesis that loss of molecules with specific pattern recognition properties (in this case, for β-galactosidase linkages) evokes behavioral phenotypes potentially arising from inappropriate neuronal synaptogenesis, pruning, and/or maintenance. There is already clear evidence that molecules able to recognize specific protein regions play crucial roles during CNS development [66, 67]. This study further implies that molecules able to recognize specific carbohydrate regions may have parallel roles during CNS development. Further efforts to understand carbohydrate recognition in the developing brain are thus clearly justified, and may provide important and clinically relevant insights into significant psychiatric conditions, including autism spectrum disorders [68] and schizophrenia [69].

Conclusions

This study provides the first data describing home cage feeding, drinking, movement, and circadian rhythm in mice cohorts constitutively lacking *Lgals3* function. We performed a longitudinal assay of these behaviors at 2–3 and 6–7 months of age. At both ages, *Lgals3*$^{-/-}$ mice showed less home cage movement compared to WT. This decrease was due to decreases in both forward locomotion and movement-in-place. These differences grew more pronounced with age. In older mice, we could further determine that decreased movement was a result of lower bout initiation rates (for both locomotor and

movement-in-place bouts), with similar distances traversed per bout. Lower bout initiation rates also led to lower total numbers of locomotion and movement-in place bouts. *Lgals3*$^{-/-}$ mice at both ages also had more heterogeneous circadian patterns of feeding, drinking, and movement compared to WT mice.

Abbreviations
Lgals3: galectin-3; CRD: carbohydrate recognition domain; DEXA: dual energy X-ray absorptiometry; BMD: bone mass density; BMC: bone mineral content; BArea: bone area; TArea: tissue area; R_{ST}: ratio of soft tissue attenuation; TTM: total tissue mass; $\dot{V}O_2$: maximum oxygen uptake; DO_2: global oxygen delivery; O_2out: oxygen output; $\dot{V}CO_2$: maximum CO_2 production; DCO_2: global CO_2 removal; CO_2out: CO_2 output; FDR: false discovery rate; WT: wildtype.

Authors' contributions
TRC performed experiments, data analysis, manuscript preparation; SJB performed data analysis, manuscript preparation. Both authors have read and approved the final manuscript.

Acknowledgements
We thank Carol A. Casey, Ph.D. and Nicholas W. DeKorver, Ph.D. for their critique of earlier versions of this manuscript.

Competing interests
The authors declare that they have no competing interests.

Funding
This work was supported by the National Institutes of Health/National Institute on Aging (AG031158 to SJB).

References
1. Agrwal N, Sun Q, Wang SY, Wang JL. Carbohydrate-binding protein 35. I. Properties of the recombinant polypeptide and the individuality of the domains. J Biol Chem. 1993;268(20):14932–9.
2. Massa SM, Cooper DN, Leffler H, Barondes SH. L-29, an endogenous lectin, binds to glycoconjugate ligands with positive cooperativity. Biochemistry. 1993;32(1):260–7.
3. Song S, Mazurek N, Liu C, Sun Y, Ding QQ, Liu K, Hung MC, Bresalier RS. Galectin-3 mediates nuclear β-catenin accumulation and Wnt signaling in human colon cancer cells by regulation of glycogen synthase kinase-3β activity. Can Res. 2009;69(4):1343–9.
4. Hughes RC. Galectins as modulators of cell adhesion. Biochimie. 2001;83:667–76.
5. Matarrese P, Fusco O, Tinari N, Natoli C, Liu FT, Semeraro ML, Malorni W, Iacobelli S. Galectin-3 overexpression protects from apoptosis by improving cell adhesion properties. Int J Cancer. 2000;85(4):545–54.
6. Mazurek N, Conklin J, Byrd JC, Raz A, Bresalier RS. Phosphorylation of the β-galactoside-binding protein galectin-3 modulates binding to its ligands. J Biol Chem. 2000;275(46):36311–5.

7. Hsu DK, Hammes SR, Kuwabara I, Greene WC, Liu FT. Human T lymphotropic virus-I infection of human T lymphocytes induces expression of the beta-galactoside-binding lectin, galectin-3. Am J Pathol. 1996;148(5):1661–70.

8. Liu X, Yu X, Zack DJ, Zhu H, Qian J. TiGER: a database for tissue-specific gene expression and regulation. BMC Bioinform. 2008;9:271.

9. Cherayil BJ, Chaitovitz S, Wong C, Pillai S. Molecular cloning of a human macrophage lectin specific for galactose. Proc Natl Acad Sci USA. 1990;87(18):7324–8.

10. Haudek KC, Spronk KJ, Voss PG, Patterson RJ, Wang JL, Arnoys EJ. Dynamics of galectin-3 in the nucleus and cytoplasm. Biochim Biophys Acta (BBA) Gener Subj. 2010;1800(2):181–9.

11. Friedrichs J, Torkko JM, Helenius J, Teräväinen TP, Füllekrug J, Muller DJ, Simons K, Manninen A. Contributions of galectin-3 and-9 to epithelial cell adhesion analyzed by single cell force spectroscopy. J Biol Chem. 2007;282(40):29375–83.

12. Friedrichs J, Manninen A, Muller DJ, Helenius J. Galectin-3 regulates integrin α2β1-mediated adhesion to collagen-I and-IV. J Biol Chem. 2008;283(47):32264–72.

13. Pricci F, Leto G, Amadio L, Iacobini C, Romeo G, Cordone S, Gradini R, Barsotti P, Liu FT, Di Mario U, Pugliese G. Role of galectin-3 as a receptor for advanced glycosylation end products. Kidney Int. 2000;58:S31–9.

14. Lakshminarayan R, Wunder C, Becken U, Howes MT, Benzing C, Arumugam S, Sales S, Ariotti N, Chambon V, Lamaze C, Loew D. Galectin-3 drives glycosphingolipid-dependent biogenesis of clathrin-independent carriers. Nat Cell Biol. 2014;16(6):592–603.

15. Demetriou M, Granovsky M, Quaggin S, Dennis JW. Negative regulation of T-cell activation and autoimmunity by Mgat5 N-glycosylation. Nature. 2001;409(6821):733–9.

16. Shimura T, Takenaka Y, Tsutsumi S, Hogan V, Kikuchi A, Raz A. Galectin-3, a novel binding partner of β-catenin. Can Res. 2004;64(18):6363–7.

17. Paron I, Scaloni A, Pines A, Bachi A, Liu FT, Puppin C, Pandolfi M, Ledda L, Di Loreto C, Damante G, Tell G. Nuclear localization of Galectin-3 in transformed thyroid cells: a role in transcriptional regulation. Biochem Biophys Res Commun. 2003;302(3):545–53.

18. Jeon SB, Yoon HJ, Chang CY, Koh HS, Jeon SH, Park EJ. Galectin-3 exerts cytokine-like regulatory actions through the JAK–STAT pathway. J Immunol. 2010;185(11):7037–46.

19. Dagher SF, Wang JL, Patterson RJ. Identification of galectin-3 as a factor in pre-mRNA splicing. Proc Natl Acad Sci USA. 1995;92(4):1213–7.

20. Carvalho RS, Fernandes VC, Nepomuceno TC, Rodrigues DC, Woods NT, Suarez-Kurtz G, Chammas R, Monteiro AN, Carvalho MA. Characterization of LGALS3 (galectin-3) as a player in DNA damage response. Cancer Biol Ther. 2014;15(7):840–50.

21. Kim HR, Lin HM, Biliran H, Raz A. Cell cycle arrest and inhibition of anoikis by galectin-3 in human breast epithelial cells. Can Res. 1999;59(16):4148–54.

22. Inohara H, Akahani S, Raz A. Galectin-3 stimulates cell proliferation. Exp Cell Res. 1998;245(2):294–302.

23. Yang RY, Hsu DK. Liu FT. Expression of galectin-3 modulates T-cell growth and apoptosis. Proc Natl Acad Sci USA. 1996;93(13):6737–42.

24. Karlsson A, Christenson K, Matlak M, Björstad Å, Brown KL, Telemo E, Salomonsson E, Leffler H, Bylund J. Galectin-3 functions as an opsonin and enhances the macrophage clearance of apoptotic neutrophils. Glycobiology. 2008;19(1):16–20.

25. Yamaoka A, Kuwabara I, Frigeri LG, Liu FT. A human lectin, galectin-3 (epsilon bp/Mac-2), stimulates superoxide production by neutrophils. J Immunol. 1995;154(7):3479–87.

26. Caberoy NB, Alvarado G, Bigcas JL, Li W. Galectin-3 is a new MerTK-specific eat-me signal. J Cell Physiol. 2012;227(2):401–7.

27. Yip PK, Carrillo-Jimenez A, King P, Vilalta A, Nomura K, Chau CC, Egerton AM, Liu ZH, Shetty AJ, Tremoleda JL, Davies M. Galectin-3 released in response to traumatic brain injury acts as an alarmin orchestrating brain immune response and promoting neurodegeneration. Sci Rep. 2017;7:41689.

28. Schafer DP, Stevens B. Synapse elimination during development and disease: immune molecules take centre stage. Biochem Soc Trans. 2010;38(2):476–81.

29. Huh GS, Boulanger LM, Du H, Riquelme PA, Brotz TM, Shatz CJ. Functional requirement for class I MHC in CNS development and plasticity. Science. 2000;290(5499):2155–9.

30. Glynn MW, Elmer BM, Garay PA, Liu XB, Needleman LA, El-Sabeawy F, McAllister AK. MHCI negatively regulates synapse density during the establishment of cortical connections. Nat Neurosci. 2011;14(4):442–51.

31. Stevens B, Allen NJ, Vazquez LE, Howell GR, Christopherson KS, Nouri N, Micheva KD, Mehalow AK, Huberman AD, Stafford B, Sher A, Litke AM, Lambris JD, Smith SJ, John SWM, Barres BA. The classical complement cascade mediates CNS synapse elimination. Cell. 2007;131(6):1164–78.

32. Djurisic M, Vidal GS, Mann M, Aharon A, Kim T, Santos AF, Zuo Y, Hübener M, Shatz CJ. PirB regulates a structural substrate for cortical plasticity. Proc Natl Acad Sci USA. 2013;110(51):20771–6.

33. DeKorver NW, Chaudoin TR, Bonasera SJ. Toll-like receptor 2 is a regulator of circadian active and inactive state consolidation in C57BL/6 mice. Front Aging Neurosci. 2017;9:219.

34. Ryan SO, Cobb BA. Roles for major histocompatibility complex glycosylation in immune function. In: Lowe J, editor. Seminars in immunopathology 2012 May 1, Vol. 34, No. 3. Berlin: Springer, p. 425–441. https://link.springer.com/journal/281/34/3/page/1

35. Janssen BJ, Halff EF, Lambris JD, Gros P. Structure of compstatin in complex with complement component C3c reveals a new mechanism of complement inhibition. J Biol Chem. 2007;282(40):29241–7.

36. Hayami K, Fukuta D, Nishikawa Y, Yamashita Y, Inui M, Ohyama Y, Hikida M, Ohmori H, Takai T. Molecular cloning of a novel murine cell-surface glycoprotein homologous to killer cell inhibitory receptors. J Biol Chem. 1997;272(11):7320–7.

37. Weber AN, Morse MA, Gay NJ. Four N-linked glycosylation sites in human toll-like receptor 2 cooperate to direct efficient biosynthesis and secretion. J Biol Chem. 2004;279(33):34589–94.

38. Bonasera SJ, Arikkath J, Boska MD, Chaudoin TR, DeKorver NW, Goulding EH, Hoke TA, Mojtahedzedah V, Reyelts CD, Sajja B, Schenk AK. Age-related changes in cerebellar and hypothalamic function accompany non-microglial immune gene expression, altered synapse organization, and excitatory amino acid neurotransmission deficits. Aging (Albany NY). 2016;8(9):2153.

39. Colnot C, Fowlis D, Ripoche MA, Bouchaert I, Poirier F. Embryonic implantation in galectin 1/galectin 3 double mutant mice. Dev Dyn. 1998;211(4):306–13.

40. Tschöp MH, Speakman JR, Arch JR, Auwerx J, Brüning JC, Chan L, Eckel RH, Farese RV Jr, Galgani JE, Hambly C, Herman MA. A guide to analysis of mouse energy metabolism. Nat Methods. 2012;9(1):57–63.

41. Even PC, Nadkarni NA. Indirect calorimetry in laboratory mice and rats: principles, practical considerations, interpretation and perspectives. Am J Physiol Regul Integr Comp Physiol. 2012;303(5):R459–76.

42. Bonasera SJ, Chaudoin TR, Goulding EH, Mittek M, Dunaevsky A. Decreased home cage movement and oromotor impairments in adult Fmr1-KO mice. Genes Brain Behav. 2017;16(5):564–73.

43. Goulding EH, Schenk AK, Juneja P, MacKay AW, Wade JM, Tecott LH. A robust automated system elucidates mouse home cage behavioral structure. Proc Natl Acad Sci USA. 2008;105(52):20575–82.

44. Parkison SA, Carlson JD, Chaudoin TR, Hoke TA, Schenk AK, Goulding EH, Pérez LC, Bonasera SJ. A low-cost, reliable, high-throughput system for rodent behavioral phenotyping in a home cage environment. In: 2012 annual international conference of the IEEE on engineering in medicine and biology society (EMBC), IEEE, p. 2392–2395.

45. Lomb NR. Least-squares frequency analysis of unequally spaced data. Astrophys Space Sci. 1976;39(2):447–62.

46. Scargle JD. Studies in astronomical time series analysis. II-Statistical aspects of spectral analysis of unevenly spaced data. Astrophys J. 1982;263:835–53.

47. Van Dongen HP, Olofsen E, Van Hartevelt JH, Kruyt EW. A procedure of multiple period searching in unequally spaced time-series with the Lomb-Scargle method. Biol Rhythm Res. 1999;30(2):149–77.

48. Orr SL, Le D, Long JM, Sobieszczuk P, Ma B, Tian H, Fang X, Paulson JC, Marth JD, Varki N. A phenotype survey of 36 mutant mouse strains with gene-targeted defects in glycosyltransferases or glycan-binding proteins. Glycobiology. 2013;23(3):363–80.

49. www.functionalglycomics.org:80/glycomics/behavior/jsp/searchBehaviorResults.jsp?searchType=0&expId=%25&criteria0=is&searchResultsType=download&criteria2=is&targetGene=Gal-3&sideMenu=no. Accessed 17 April 2018.

50. Menini S, Iacobini C, Blasetti Fantauzzi C, Pesce CM, Pugliese G. Role of galectin-3 in obesity and impaired glucose homeostasis. Oxid Med Cell Longev. 2016;2016:9618092.

51. Pejnovic NN, Pantic JM, Jovanovic IP, Radosavljevic GD, Milovanovic MZ, Nikolic IG, Zdravkovic NS, Djukic AL, Arsenijevic NN, Lukic ML. Galectin-3 deficiency accelerates high-fat diet-induced obesity and amplifies inflammation in adipose tissue and pancreatic islets. Diabetes. 2013;62(6):1932–44.

52. Pang J, Rhodes DH, Pini M, Akasheh RT, Castellanos KJ, Cabay RJ, Cooper D, Perretti M, Fantuzzi G. Increased adiposity, dysregulated glucose metabolism and systemic inflammation in Galectin-3 KO mice. PLoS ONE. 2013;8(2):e57915.

53. Saksida T, Nikolic I, Vujicic M, Nilsson UJ, Leffler H, Lukic ML, Stojanovic I, Stosic-Grujicic S. Galectin-3 deficiency protects pancreatic islet cells from cytokine-triggered apoptosis in vitro. J Cell Physiol. 2017;228(7):1568–76.

54. Yilmaz H, Cakmak M, Inan O, Darcin T, Akcay A. Increased levels of galectin-3 were associated with prediabetes and diabetes: new risk factor? J Endocrinol Invest. 2015;38(5):527–33.

55. Kiwaki K, Novak CM, Hsu DK, Liu FT, Levine JA. Galectin-3 stimulates preadipocyte proliferation and is up-regulated in growing adipose tissue. Obesity. 2007;15(1):32–9.

56. Rhodes DH, Pini M, Castellanos KJ, Montero-Melendez T, Cooper D, Perretti M, Fantuzzi G. Adipose tissue-specific modulation of galectin expression in lean and obese mice: evidence for regulatory function. Obesity. 2013;21(2):310–9.

57. Baek JH, Kim SJ, Kang HG, Lee HW, Kim JH, Hwang KA, Song J, Chun KH. Galectin-3 activates PPARγ and supports white adipose tissue formation and high-fat diet-induced obesity. Endocrinology. 2015;156(1):147–56.

58. Pejnovic N, Jeftic I, Jovicic N, Arsenijevic N, Lukic ML. Galectin-3 and IL-33/ST2 axis roles and interplay in diet-induced steatohepatitis. World J Gastroenterol. 2016;22(44):9706.

59. Jeftic I, Jovicic N, Pantic J, Arsenijevic N, Lukic ML, Pejnovic N. Galectin-3 ablation enhances liver steatosis, but attenuates inflammation and IL-33-dependent fibrosis in obesogenic mouse model of nonalcoholic steatohepatitis. Mol Med. 2015;21(1):453.

60. Trompet S, Jukema W, Mooijaart SP, Ford I, Stott DJ, Westendorp RG, de Craen AJ. Genetic variation in galectin-3 gene associates with cognitive function at old age. Neurobiol Aging. 2012;33(9):2232-e1.

61. Reeves PG, Shaw HA, Smith JE, Steele RD. Nutrient requirements of the mouse. From: Nutrient requirements of laboratory animals. 4th ed. Washington: National Academies Press; 1995.

62. Houzelstein D, Gonçalves IR, Fadden AJ, Sidhu SS, Cooper DN, Drickamer K, Leffler H, Poirier F. Phylogenetic analysis of the vertebrate galectin family. Mol Biol Evol. 2004;21(7):1177–87.

63. Cooper DN, Barondes SH. God must love galectins; He made so many of them. Glycobiology. 1999;9(10):979–84.

64. Patterson RJ, Wang W, Wang JL. Understanding the biochemical activities of galectin-1 and galectin-3 in the nucleus. Glycoconj J. 2002;19(7):499–506.

65. Stillman BN, Hsu DK, Pang M, Brewer CF, Johnson P, Liu FT, Baum LG. Galectin-3 and galectin-1 bind distinct cell surface glycoprotein receptors to induce T cell death. J Immunol. 2006;176(2):778–89.

66. Cebrián C, Loike JD, Sulzer D. Neuronal MHC-I expression and its implications in synaptic function, axonal regeneration and Parkinson's and other brain diseases. Front Neuroanat. 2014;8:114.

67. Zabel MK, Kirsch WM. From development to dysfunction: microglia and the complement cascade in CNS homeostasis. Ageing Res Rev. 2013;12(3):749–56.

68. Bauman ML, Kemper TL. Neuroanatomic observations of the brain in autism: a review and future directions. Int J Dev Neurosci. 2005;23(2):183–7.

69. Nimgaonkar VL, Prasad KM, Chowdari KV, Severance EG, Yolken RH. The complement system: a gateway to gene-environment interactions in schizophrenia pathogenesis. Mol Psychiatry. 2017;22;1554.

7

Effect of pulsed transcranial ultrasound stimulation at different number of tone-burst on cortico-muscular coupling

Ping Xie[*] [iD], Sa Zhou, Xingran Wang, Yibo Wang and Yi Yuan[*]

Abstract

Background: Pulsed transcranial ultrasound stimulation (pTUS) can modulate the neuronal activity of motor cortex and elicit muscle contractions. Cortico-muscular coupling (CMC) can serve as a tool to identify interaction between the oscillatory activity of the motor cortex and effector muscle. This research aims to explore the neuromodulatory effect of low-intensity, pTUS with different number of tone burst to neural circuit of motor-control system by analyzing the coupling relationship between motor cortex and tail muscle in mouse. The motor cortex of mice was stimulated by pulsed transcranial ultrasound with different number of tone bursts (NTB = 100 150 200 250 300). The local field potentials (LFPs) in tail motor cortex and electromyography (EMG) in tail muscles were recorded simultaneously during pTUS. The change of integral coupling strength between cortex and muscle was evaluated by mutual information (MI). The directional information interaction between them were analyzed by transfer entropy (TE).

Results: Almost all of the MI and TE values were significantly increased by pTUS. The results of MI showed that the CMC was significantly enhanced with the increase of NTB. The TE results showed the coupling strength of CMC in descending direction (from LFPs to EMG) was significantly higher than that in ascending direction (from EMG to LFPs) after stimulation. Furthermore, compared to NTB = 100, the CMC in ascending direction were significantly enhanced when NTB = 250, 300, and CMC in descending direction were significantly enhanced when NTB = 200, 250, 300.

Conclusion: These results confirm that the CMC between motor cortex and the tail muscles in mouse could be altered by pTUS. And by increasing the NTB (i.e. sonication duration), the coupling strength within the cortico-muscular circuit could be increased, which might further influence the motor function of mice. It demonstrates that, using MI and TE method, the CMC could be used for quantitatively evaluating the effect of pTUS with different NTBs, which might provide a new insight into the effect of pTUS neuromodulation in motor cortex.

Keywords: Pulsed transcranial ultrasound stimulation, Cortico-muscular coupling, Number of tone bursts, Mutual information, Transfer entropy

Background

Neuromodulation techniques have gained attention recent years for both neuroscientific research and neural engineering applications [1, 2]. Pulsed transcranial ultrasound stimulation (pTUS) [3, 4] is a promising technique for neuromodulation which has non-invasiveness, high spatial resolution (< 2 mm), and deep penetration [5–7].

As a mechanical pressure wave, pulsed ultrasound can be transmitted through the skull and facilitate or inhibit neural activities [8, 9]. By observing the cerebral blood flow [10], LFPs or EEG signals from brain [11, 12] or electromyography (EMG) signals from the muscle [13–15], etc., the effect of pTUS have been widely investigated. For instance, Legon W et al. modulated the activity of primary somatosensory cortex and spectral content of sensory-evoked brain oscillations in humans [16]. Li [10] and Guo [17] used low-intensity pTUS to modulate the brain of stroke rats and found pTUS is neuroprotective

*Correspondence: pingx@ysu.edu.cn; yuanyi513@ysu.edu.cn
Institute of Electric Engineering, Yanshan University,
Qinhuangdao 066004, Hebei, China

for ischemic brain injury. Previously, we [11] found that the focused ultrasound stimulation could modulate the phase-amplitude coupling between neuronal oscillations in the rat hippocampus. Moreover, pTUS can stimulate the motor cortex to induce muscle contraction and EMG signals [13]. These rapidly increasing body of findings provide ample evidence that ultrasound stimulation can flexibly modulate the cortical oscillatory dynamics and induce evident motor response.

As a well-established neurophysiological measure, cortico-muscular coupling (CMC) can be used to understand the communication between the oscillation of the cortical and spinal cord activities [18–20]. It is generally believed that the effective movement control depends on the synchronization of oscillatory activity between the motor cortex and effector muscle [21, 22]. By analyzing the coupling between the local field potentials (LFPs) (or magnetoencephalogram (MEG), electroencephalogram (EEG)) of the motor cortex and the electromyogram (EMG) of muscles, previous studies shown that CMC is related to the motor performance [23] and could identify the impaired neural pathway in patients [24]. As pTUS could elicit evident muscle contraction [13] and modulate neural oscillatory [11], we speculate that pTUS-induced change of information flow between motor cortex and effector muscle is subsistent, which could be evaluated by CMC. Previous studies about the effect of pTUS mainly focus on the change of neural activities in the brain [25] or the motor response in muscle [26], however, the coupling between the cortical and spinal cord activities during pTUS is still unknown. Therefore, it is important to evaluate the influence of pTUS with different parameters on neuromodulation from a cortical-muscular coupling view.

As the neural network of cortico-muscular system has nonlinear features of its parts and interactions between them [27], MI [28] and TE [29], which are model-free and sensitive to nonlinear interaction [30], are capable of quantitatively describing the cortico-muscular coupling by measuring the statistical dependencies between two variables [31–33]. In addition, the coupling between cortical and the targeted muscle is bidirectional which includes both the motor command from the cortex and feedback information from the contracting muscle [34, 35]. Because MI is symmetric, it could be used to quantify the amount coupled information of cortico-muscular [33] without the directional information between them [36]. TE which complements the non-directional defect of MI [37], can be used to evaluate the directional interaction of CMC [32].

In the present study, we introduce a novel way to assess the effect of pTUS with different NTBs by applying the cortico-muscular coupling between motor cortex and

the tail muscles in mice, thus allowing for quantification of ultrasound effect on motor command circuit. First, since low-intensity pTUS is capable of neuromodulation without thermal effects or tissue damage [8, 38], the low-intensity transcranial ultrasound (1.1 W/cm^2) was applied to stimulate the motor cortex in mice at different number of tone bursts (NTB = 100, 150, 200, 250, 300). Then, the LFPs in tail motor cortex and EMG in tail muscles were recorded simultaneously during pTUS. Finally, based on the recorded LFPs and EMG signals, the integral coupling strength between cortex and muscle induced by pTUS was evaluated by mutual information (MI), and the change of directional information interaction between them was analyzed using and transfer entropy (TE).

Methods
Data recording
Experimental system and parameter settings
The experimental system is shown in Fig. 1a, consisting of six main components: (1) two function generators (AFG3022C, Tektronix, USA), (2) a linear radio frequency power amplifier (RFA) (240L, ENI Inc., USA), (3) an unfocused ultrasound transducer (V301-SU, Olympus, Japan) with center frequency of 500 kHz and diameter of 31 mm driven by RFA, and (4) an custom conical plastic collimator (Length 50 mm, diameter 2 and 31.2 mm) filled with degassed ultrasound gel and delivering the pTUS to the cortex, (5) single-channel microelectrodes (WE50030.1B10, MicroProbe, USA) recording the LFPs and fine wire electrode recording EMG signals,(6) a dual-channel front-end amplifier (63386, A-M SYSTEMS INC., USA) that amplifying the LFPs and EMG signals, and a 16-channel neural signal processor (NSP) (Cerebus Data Acquisition System, Blackrock Microsystems, USA) converting the signals into digital signals, (7) a computer for data storage and displaying the recorded data simultaneously.

Ultrasonic parameters are illustrated in Fig. 1c, i.e., acoustic intensity (AI), the number of acoustic cycles per pulse (NC), pulse repetition frequency (PRF), the number of tone bursts (NTB), the inter trial interval (ITI) and the sonication duration. In this paper, the parameter setting is AI = 1.10 W/cm^2, NC = 250, PRF = 1 kHz, ITI = 3.6 s. The excitability or inhibition of pTUS on the neural oscillatory activity are related to the ultrasound beam and parameters of ultrasound [17], especially the pulse repetition frequency. Based on our experiments and other literatures [10, 17, 39], we used PRF = 1kHz to facilitate the motor cortical activity and evoke EMG signals in tail muscle. To explore the effect of pTUS to cortico-muscular coupling, the sonication duration was changed with different NTB (100, 150, 200, 250, 300). High-intensity and long duration ultrasound stimulation can produce

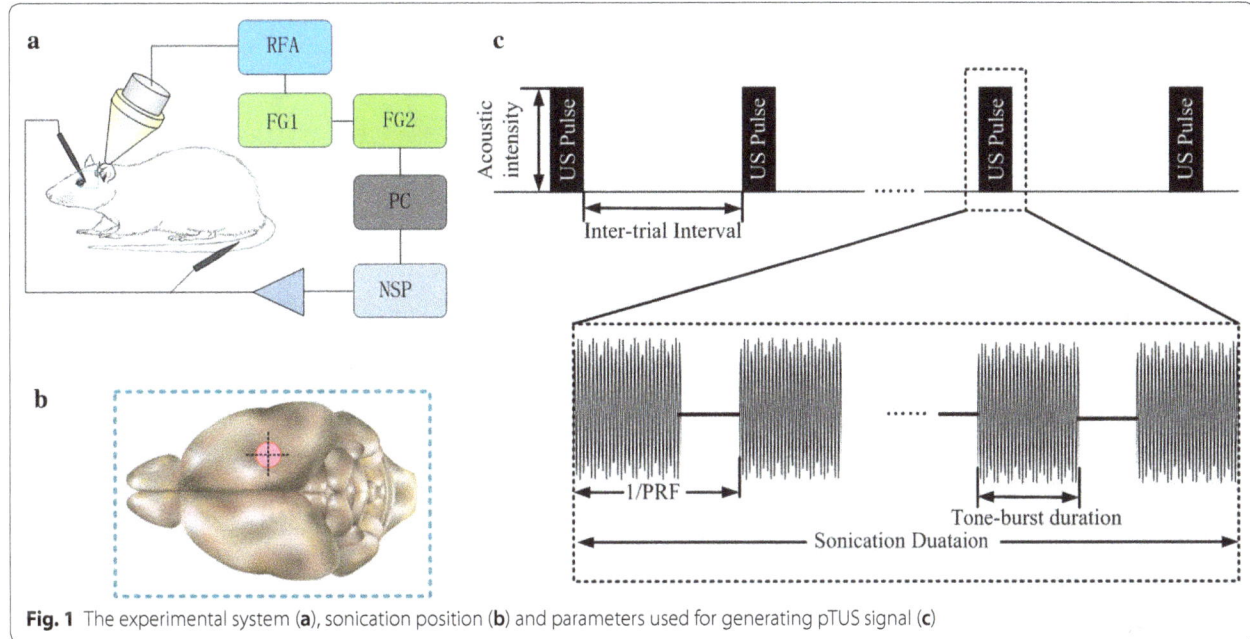

Fig. 1 The experimental system (**a**), sonication position (**b**) and parameters used for generating pTUS signal (**c**)

thermal effects and damage brain tissue [40]. Therefore, it is safe to use low-intensity pTUS with NTB = 100, 150, 200, 250, 300 in the present study [39]. The pTUS signals were digitized at a sample rate of 30 kHz.

Animal surgery and anesthesia

Nine BALB/c mice (male, body weights ∼ 20 g, Beijing Vital River Laboratory Animal Technology Co., Ltd. China) were used in this study. After anesthetized with sodium pentobarbital (1%, 5 mg/100 g, IP), mice were constrained on the stereotaxic apparatus (68002, 68030, RWD Co., China). Then, the fur covering the scalp was shaved and the skin was cleaned with physiological saline solution. The scalp of the mice was incised along the midline of the skull, and the exposed tissues and periosteum were cleaned carefully to expose the skull. Finally, the sonication site as illustrated in Fig. 1b, was determined by an atlas and a cranial window of ∼ 0.5 × 0.5 cm was drilled to expose the brain tissue in the tail motor cortex. At the end of the experiment, mice were sacrificed with an overdose anesthetic (sodium pentobarbital, 1%, 15 mg/100 g, IP). All the experiment steps were approved with the Animal Ethics and Administrative Council of Yanshan University, Hebei Province, China.

Data acquisition

After the surgery procedure, a tungsten microelectrode was inserted into the tail motor cortex to acquire the LFPs signal, a fine-wire was inserted into tail muscle to acquire the EMG signal. When the anesthesia effect in mice was over, the LFPs and EMG signals

were synchronously recorded at 2 kHz using the same device. The angle between the pTUS and microelectrode was ∼ 60°. The acoustic collimator connected with the planar ultrasound transducer was aimed at the mice tail motor cortex. The ultrasonic wave passed through the acoustic collimator to stimulate the brain tissue for non-invasive neuromodulation.

Data processing and analysis

Data preprocessing

To reject the artifacts in raw LFPs and EMG recordings, a notch filter was used to remove the power signal of 50 Hz and an adaptive high-pass filter was used to remove baseline drift. The LFPs and EMG was band-passed to 0.5–200 Hz and 10–200 Hz, respectively. Then, the EMG was rectified. Finally, the LFPs and EMG before and after stimulation were cut in trials according to the pulse of TUS. After preprocessing, the LFPs, EMG and pTUS were shown in Fig. 2, were used subsequent analysis.

Cortico-muscular coupling analysis by mutual information

In this paper, the amount coupled information of cortico-muscular under pTUS was quantitively described by mutual information [28]. The LFPs and EMG were denoted as x_t and y_t, respectively. The entropy of LFPs could be computed as following:

$$H(LFP) = -\int_x p(x) \log(p(x))dx \tag{1}$$

where $p(x)$ is the probability density function of LFPs. The entropy of EMG can be calculated as the same way.

The joint entropy of LFPs and EMG is:

$$H(LFP, EMG) = - \int\limits_{x} \int\limits_{y} p(x,y) \log(p(x,y)) dx dy$$

(2)

where $p(x, y)$ is the joint probability density function of LFPs and EMG.

The mutual information between LFPs and EMG is:

$$MI(LFP, EMG) = H(LFP) + H(EMG) - H(LFP, EMG)$$

$$= \int\limits_{x} \int\limits_{y} p(x,y) \log \frac{p(x,y)}{p(x)p(y)}$$

(3)

Cortico-muscular coupling analysis by transfer entropy

The directional interaction of CMC under pTUS was represented by transfer entropy [29]. Two time series x_t and y_t were approximated by Markov process, the transfer entropy from LFPs to EMG under pTUS can be written as follows:

$$TE_{LFP \rightarrow EMG} = H\left(y_{t+1} | y_t^n\right) - H\left(y_{t+1} | x_t^n, y_t^n\right)$$

$$= \sum_{y_{t+1}, y_t^n, x_t^m} p\left(y_{t+1}, y_t^n, x_t^m\right) \log \left(\frac{p\left(y_{t+1} | y_t^n, x_t^m\right)}{p\left(y_{t+1} | y_t^n\right)} \right)$$

(4)

where $x_t^m = (x_t, \ldots, x_{t-m+1})$ and $y_t^n = (y, \ldots, y_{t-n+1})$, m and n are the orders of Markov process. $H(y_{t+1} | y_t^n)$ is the conditional entropy of EMG depending on the past values.

The two processes LFPs and EMG are reconstructed to a higher and same dimensional space. Thus, the formula of transfer entropy for two time series can be written as follows [41]:

$$TE_{LEP \rightarrow EMG} = \sum_{y_{t+u}, y_t^d, x_t^d} p\left(y_{t+1}, y_t^d, x_t^d\right) \log \left(\frac{p\left(y_{t+u} | y_t^d, x_t^d\right)}{p\left(y_{t+u} | y_t^n\right)} \right)$$

(5)

where $x_t^d = (x_t, x_{t-\tau}, x_{t-2\tau}, \ldots, x_{t-(d-1)\tau})$ and $y_t^d = (y_t, y_{t-\tau}, y_{t-2\tau}, \ldots, y_{t-(d-1)\tau})$. The d, τ and u are the embedding dimension, embedding delay and the

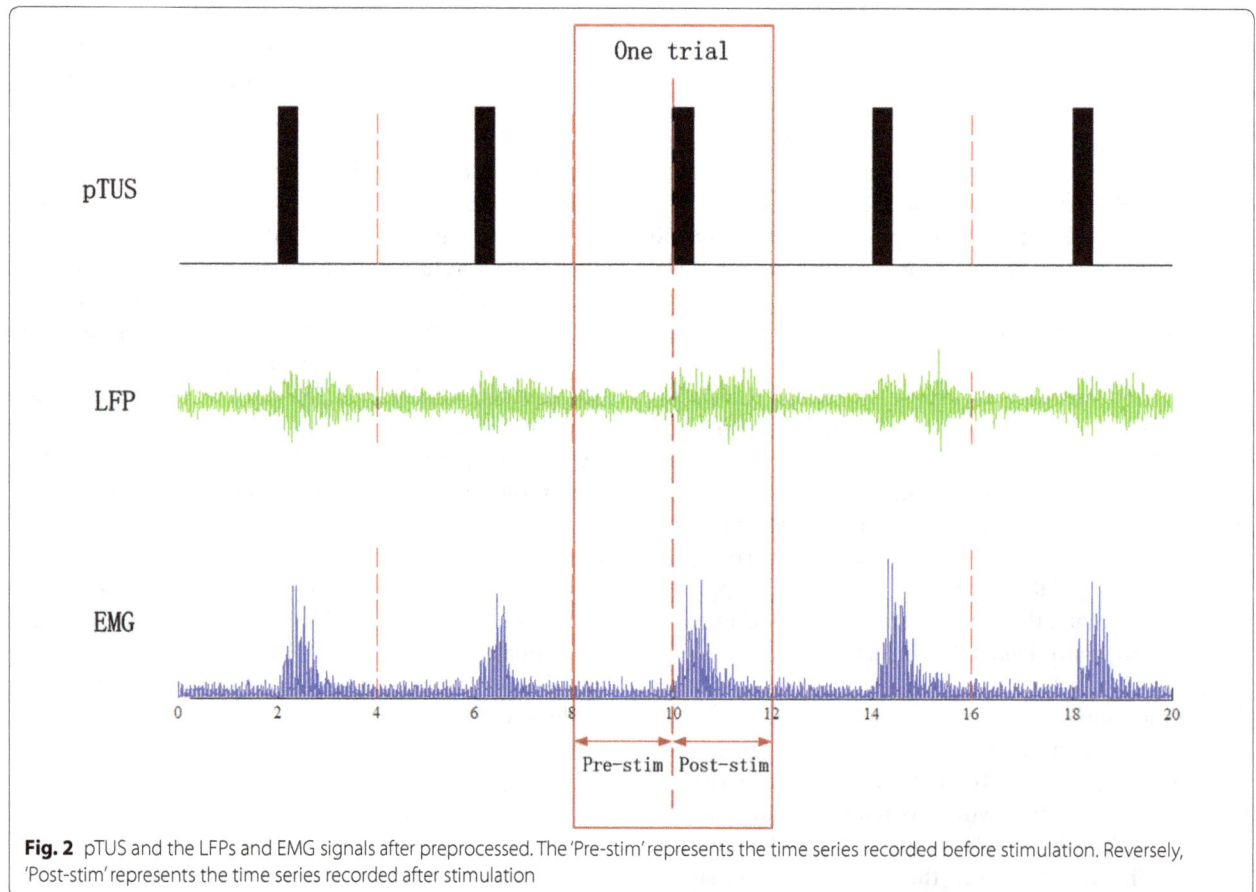

Fig. 2 pTUS and the LFPs and EMG signals after preprocessed. The 'Pre-stim' represents the time series recorded before stimulation. Reversely, 'Post-stim' represents the time series recorded after stimulation

prediction time, respectively. The transfer entropy from EMG to LFPs is $TE_{EMG \to LFP}$ computed by the same process.

In this paper, the values of mutual information and transfer entropy were calculated using TRENTOOL toolbox [42]. Specifically, The embedding delay (τ) and embedding dimension (d) for state space reconstruction were determined according to Ragwitz criterion [43]. The Kraskove-Stögbauere-Grassberger estimator and the nearest-neighbor search were applied to perform the TE estimation [44]. The number of neighbors k was set to 4 as suggested in [45]. The prediction time u was optimized in the range of [10, 49] ms according to the influence of pTUS to EMG responses latency [13].

Statistical analysis

The differences between the TE/MI values of pre-stimulation and post-stimulation were statistically analyzed based on one-way repeated measures analysis of variance (rANOVA), and the differences between the TE values of the descending direction and ascending direction also performed by one-way rANOVA. The correlations between LFPs/EMG and MI/TE values at different NTB were determined using PEARSONs Correlation coefficient. The correlation was calculated using the MI/TE values and mean values of LFPs/EMG data in each trial. Significance level was set as p < 0.05. All the results of MI and TE were expressed as mean ± S.D. SPSS 19.0 for windows (SPSS Inc., Chicago, IL, USA) was used for all statistical computations.

Results

MI result

To investigate the interaction information between motor cortex and tail muscle, the mean MI values between LFPs and EMG acquired from nine mice were calculated. Figure 3a shows the results of MI between LFPs and EMG before and after stimulation. Before the motor cortex was stimulated by the pTUS, the MI values between LFPs and EMG at different NTB were 0.0600 ± 0.0040, 0.0595 ± 0.0029, 0.0610 ± 0.0030, 0.0627 ± 0.0038, 0.0630 ± 0.0034 (mean ± S.D, n = 9). After the motor cortex was stimulated by the pTUS, the MI values were 0.0649 ± 0.0034, 0.0651 ± 0.0030, 0.0716 ± 0.0032, 0.0732 ± 0.0029, 0.0719 ± 0.0020 (mean ± S.D, n = 9). There were highly significant differences (p < 0.01, one-way ANOVA) of MI between before and after stimulation in descending direction at NTB = 200, 250, 300 cyc, while lower significant differences (p < 0.05) of MI between before and after stimulation in ascending direction at NTB = 150 cyc, and no significant difference (p > 0.05) between them when NTB = 100 cyc.

To further explore the influence of pTUS at different NTB on MI values, we performed a significant test with the post-stimulation MI results. As shown in Fig. 3b, when NTB = 200, 250, 300, the MI results were significantly increased (p < 0.05, one-way ANOVA) compared with NTB = 100.

TE result

To study the changes of directional interaction information between motor cortex and tail muscle that was

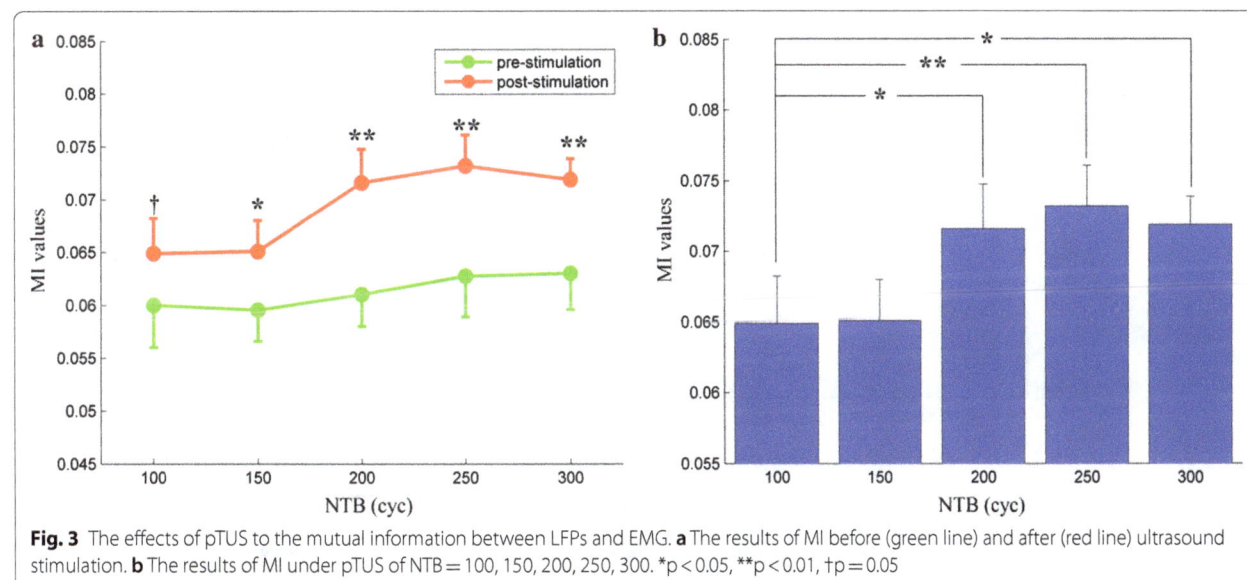

Fig. 3 The effects of pTUS to the mutual information between LFPs and EMG. **a** The results of MI before (green line) and after (red line) ultrasound stimulation. **b** The results of MI under pTUS of NTB = 100, 150, 200, 250, 300. *p < 0.05, **p < 0.01, †p = 0.05

induced by pTUS with different NTB, we calculated the transfer entropy in both descending (from LFPs to EMG) and ascending (from EMG to LFPs) directions. Figure 4 shows the TE results in descending and ascending direction before and after stimulation. Before the motor cortex was stimulated by the pTUS, the TE values from LFPs to EMG at different NTB were $0.0327 \pm 0.0016, 0.0329 \pm 0.0015, 0.0329 \pm 0.0019, 0.0335 \pm 0.0016, 0.0333 \pm 0.0015$ (mean $\pm$ S.D, n $=9$). And the TE values from EMG to LFPs at different NTB were $0.0341 \pm 0.0012, 0.0325 \pm 0.0011, 0.0342 \pm 0.0013, 0.0340 \pm 0.0014, 0.0346 \pm 0.0018$ (mean $\pm$ S.D, n $=9$).

After the motor cortex was stimulated by the pTUS, the TE values in descending direction were $0.0393 \pm 0.0021, 0.0410 \pm 0.0018, 0.0404 \pm 0.0019, 0.0426 \pm 0.0021, 0.0441 \pm 0.0026$ (mean $\pm$ S.D, n $=9$). The TE values in ascending direction were $0.0382 \pm 0.0021, 0.0377 \pm 0.0018, 0.0390 \pm 0.0019, 0.0388 \pm 0.0016, 0.0402 \pm 0.0015$ (mean $\pm$ S.D, n $=9$). Moreover, the TE values in both two directions were increased after the motor cortex was exposed to pTUS.

The significant analysis (the four lines at the top of Fig. 4) showed highly significant differences ($p < 0.01$, one-way rANOVA) of TE between before and after stimulation in descending direction (Line 4), while lower significant differences ($p < 0.05$, one-way rANOVA) of TE between before and after stimulation in ascending direction (Line 3). Additionally, there were three significant differences (NTB $= 150, 250, 300$ cyc) between the TE in descending and ascending direction after stimulation (Line 2), while no significant difference between them before stimulation (Line 1).

The effect of different parameters of pTUS to the transfer entropy between LFPs and EMG was shown in Fig. 5. In Fig. 5a, when NTB $= 200, 250, 300$ cyc, the TE values in descending direction were significantly increased ($p < 0.05$, one-way rANOVA) compared with NTB $= 100$ cyc, where the most significant increase ($p < 0.01$) was

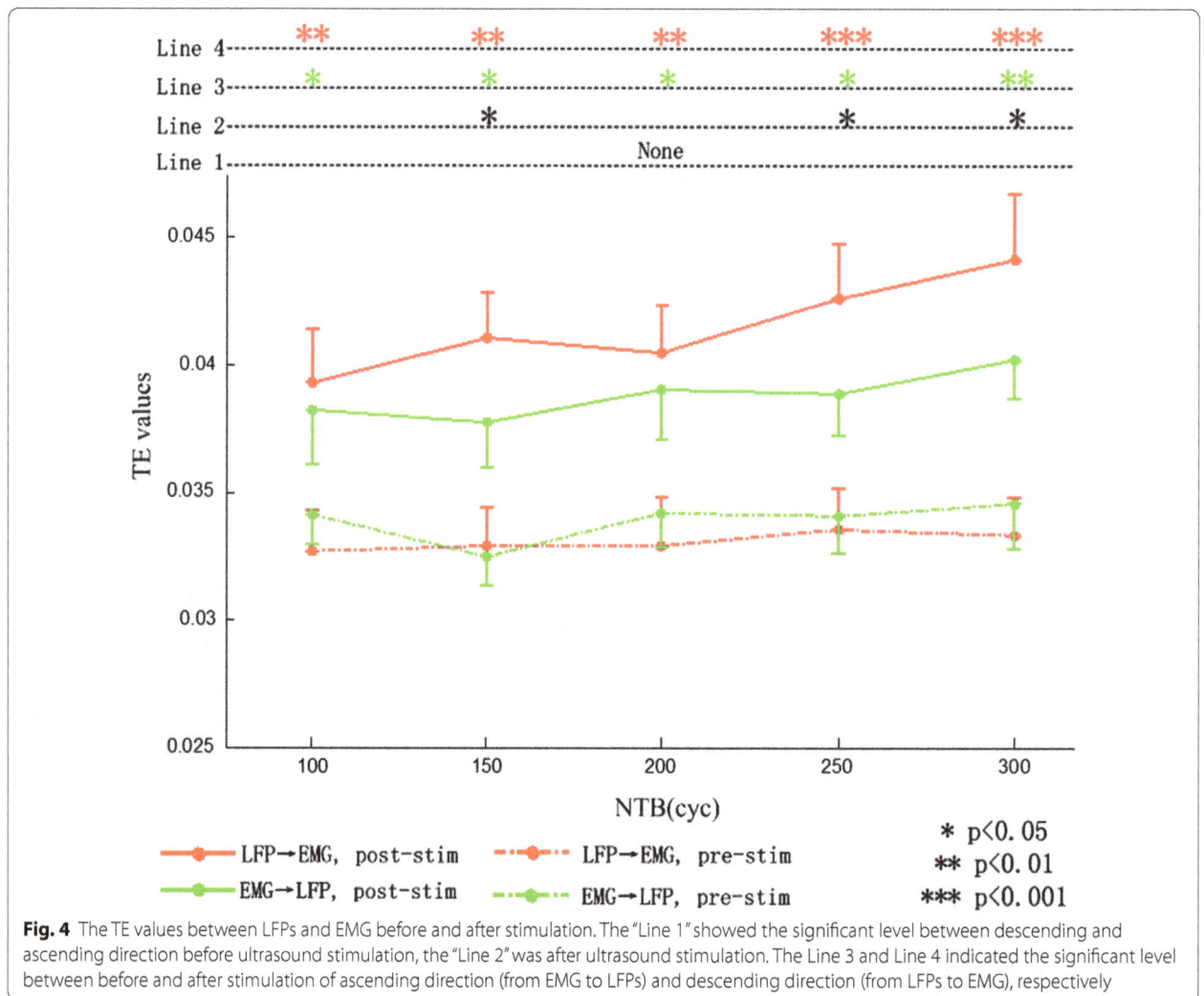

Fig. 4 The TE values between LFPs and EMG before and after stimulation. The "Line 1" showed the significant level between descending and ascending direction before ultrasound stimulation, the "Line 2" was after ultrasound stimulation. The Line 3 and Line 4 indicated the significant level between before and after stimulation of ascending direction (from EMG to LFPs) and descending direction (from LFPs to EMG), respectively

in NTB = 300 cyc. In Fig. 5b, when NTB = 250, 300 cyc, the TE values in ascending direction were significantly increased (p < 0.05) compared with NTB = 100 cyc.

Discussion

Ultrasound stimulation has emerged as a potential approach that can address the defects faced by modern neuromodulation technologies [7, 46], which can be applied noninvasively to activate or modulate the activity of targeted brain regions [16, 47, 48]. Recent years, many studies found evidently motor responses in animals by activating the primary motor cortex using the transcranial ultrasound [5, 13, 14, 49, 50], where the induced movement was all measured by EMG signals. However, both motor command from brain and feedback from muscle are involved in effective movement control [22, 23], and there is a coupled relationship between the cortical oscillation and muscle activation [51, 52]. To our knowledge, there are still a lack of evidence that assessed the neuromodulatory effect of pTUS from the neural circuit of motor-control system view. Thus, in this study, we considered applying the cortico-muscular coupling to evaluate the effect of pTUS with different number of tone bursts (NTB). Since CMC has been applied to assess the movement response induced by other neuromodulation techniques, such as transcranial magnetic stimulation (TMS), transcranial alternating current stimulation (tACS) and deep-brain stimulation (DBS) [53–55], we assume that the CMC could serve as a promising tool for the assessment of ultrasound neuromodulation.

Intention of the present study is to elucidate the effect of pTUS with different number of tone bursts (NTB) using CMC. We recorded LFPs and EMG evoked by pTUS in mice's motor cortex and tail muscle. As shown in Fig. 2, the amplitude of LFPs and EMG signals increased after stimulation. It means that the neural activity of motor cortex and the contralateral muscle could be altered by pTUS, which supports the previous studies of pTUS [5, 13, 49]. Then, we analyzed the coupling relationships between these two kind of signals using mutual information and transfer entropy.

We can see that both the TE and MI values between LFPs and EMG signals could be significantly increased with pTUS. These results indicated that the CMC between motor cortex and tail muscle could be enhanced by pTUS. Although the reason of the enhancement of CMC induced by pTUS is still unclear, the pTUS-induced EMG response [13] and the cortical excitement [56] might be related to this phenomenon, as significant correlations (p < 0.05) between the mean amplitude of the recorded signals (LFPs and EMG) and MI values could be observed when NTB = 100, 200, 250, 300 (Table 1), where the quality of the correlation was expressed by ρ, and the significant level was expressed by p.

The MI results revealed that the CMC in the sensory and motor system could be enhanced by pTUS (Fig. 3a). The TE results suggested that the CMC in descending direction could be significantly higher than that in ascending direction after stimulation (Fig. 4). It suggested that the neural pathways responded for motor command would transmit more information than the feedback pathway due to the effect of pTUS. Correlation analysis (Table 1) showed a highly significant correlation (p < 0.01) between the mean LFPs amplitude and the TE values in

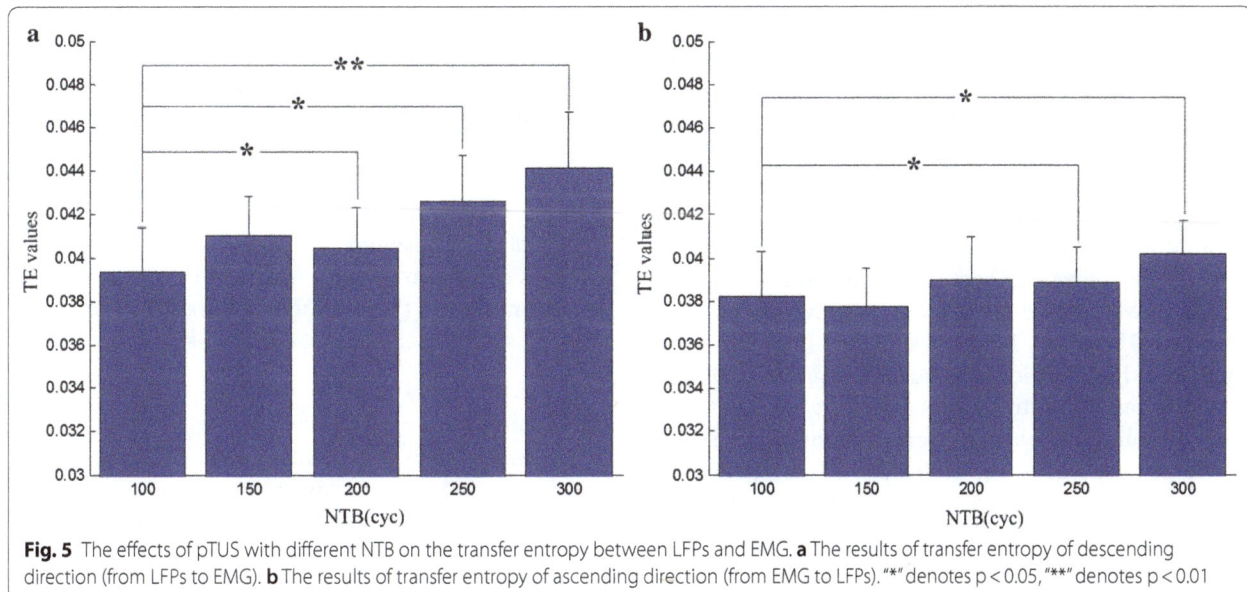

Fig. 5 The effects of pTUS with different NTB on the transfer entropy between LFPs and EMG. **a** The results of transfer entropy of descending direction (from LFPs to EMG). **b** The results of transfer entropy of ascending direction (from EMG to LFPs). "*" denotes p < 0.05, "**" denotes p < 0.01

Table 1 Results of correlation analysis

NTB	Correlation LFPs and MI	Correlation EMG and MI	Correlation LFPs and TE (LFPs → EMG)	Correlation LFPs and TE (EMG → LFPs)
100	$\rho^2 = 0.032$	$\rho^2 = 0.014$	$\rho^2 = 0.010$	$\rho^2 = 0.012$
	$p = 0.035$	$p = 0.043$	$p = 0.0061$	$p = 0.058$
150	$\rho^2 = 0.010$	$\rho^2 = 0.001$	$\rho^2 = 0.023$	$\rho^2 = 0.002$
	$p = 0.062$	$p = 0.086$	$p = 0.0046$	$p = 0.084$
200	$\rho^2 = 0.036$	$\rho^2 = 0.032$	$\rho^2 = 0.026$	$\rho^2 = 0.0001$
	$p = 0.026$	$p = 0.036$	$p = 0.0043$	$p = 0.096$
250	$\rho^2 = 0.036$	$\rho^2 = 0.036$	$\rho^2 = 0.090$	$\rho^2 = 0.003$
	$p = 0.024$	$p = 0.034$	$p = 0.0015$	$p = 0.081$
300	$\rho^2 = 0.040$	$\rho^2 = 0.023$	$\rho^2 = 0.292$	$\rho^2 = 0.026$
	$p = 0.0031$	$p = 0.0047$	$p = 0.003$	$p = 0.043$

descending direction (LFPs → EMG) (NTB = 150, 200, 250, 300), and a poor correlation (p > 0.05) in ascending direction (LFPs → EMG). The results revealed that the transferred information from the brain to muscle might be facilitated by the excitement of neural activity in motor cortex. It suggested that CMC could serve as a more useful tool for evaluating the effect of pTUS in motor cortex, which could not only assess the pTUS-induced motor responses as previous studies did by using LFP and EMG [12–14], but also reveal the information interaction between motor cortex and muscle in motor system. The mechanism of cortical excitement evoked by pTUS is still debated [57, 58]. In general, cavitation of neural membrane is known as the critical factor for eliciting neuromodulatory efficacy, which has been confirmed in cellular-scale and in vivo [50]. Recent findings revealed an indirect auditory mechanism for ultrasound-induced cortical activity and movement [57, 58]. And we speculate that the no-task experimental condition in mouse, which was different from human [35], might also result in the lower CMC in ascending direction compared with another direction. Overall, the results in this study revealed that MI could be applied to quantitatively estimate the integral CMC between motor cortex and contralateral muscle during pTUS in mouse. And TE could be used to analyze the change of directional interaction information between them. Moreover, the CMC estimated by MI and TE could increase with the increasing of NTB (NTB = 100, 150, 200, 250, 300) (Figs. 3b, 5). As the sonication duration depends a lot on the NTB, this study reveals a positive correlation between CMC and stimulus duration. It also supports that the longer stimulus duration increases the probability of motor response [26, 39].

Furthermore, previous studies showed that the motor response induce by other brain stimulation techniques such as TMS, tACS, DBS could be assessed by CMC in human [53–55], especially in patients with motor dysfunction diseases. For example, the CMC of Parkinson's disease (PD) could be modulated by DBS [59]. And pTUS had shown cerebral protection effect for stroke [10]. In this study, the CMC in descending direction is significantly increased and higher than the ascending direction after ultrasound stimulation (Fig. 5a). As it is generally believed that the impairment in neural-pathway of the descending direction is the main cause of stroke [35], applying CMC into the evaluation of pTUS neuromodulation may provide an evidence for understanding the mechanism of pTUS in stroke rehabilitation. Moreover, the MI and TE methods, which quantified CMC, could be used for measuring the effect of ultrasound stimulation and optimizing the ultrasonic duration.

Since this study only explored the influence of pTUS on the CMC in healthy mouse, we plan to extend this work to stroke or PD mice to investigate whether the abnormal CMC in those diseases can be improved by pTUS. Additionally, a previous study suggested that the ultrasound-induced EMG signals in mouse could increase as a function of both the ultrasound intensity and sonication duration [26]. Our study only investigated the effect of sonication duration to CMC, perhaps other parameters such as ultrasound intensity, frequency or number of cycles could also produce modulation effects to CMC. The influence of the ultrasound parameters to CMC could be systematically studied in the next step.

Conclusion

In this study, the neuromodulatory effect of pulsed transcranial ultrasound was analyzed by the cortico-muscular coupling between motor cortex and tail muscle in mice, which was quantified using the transfer entropy and mutual information algorithms. The results of MI and TE showed that the CMC between motor cortex and tail muscle was significantly increased by pTUS, and the CMC in descending direction could be significantly higher than that of ascending direction after ultrasound stimulation. Furthermore, by increasing the NTB, the CMC between motor cortex and tail muscle could also be significantly enhanced. Since the CMC is a promising tool for movement evaluation, it suggests that pTUS might influence the motor function of mice. This study demonstrates for the first time, using MI and TE method, the CMC can be used for quantitatively evaluating the effect of different sonication durations of pTUS-induced movement, which might provide a new insight into the effect of pTUS neuromodulation in motor cortex.

Abbreviations
pTUS: pulsed transcranial ultrasound stimulation; EMG: electromyograms; CMC: cortico-muscular coupling; NTB: number of tone bursts; MI: mutual information; TE: transfer entropy; LFPs: local field potentials; MEG: magnetoencephalogram; EEG: electroencephalogram; FG: function generators; RFA: radio frequency power amplifier; NSP: neural signal processor; AI: acoustic intensity; NC: number of acoustic cycles per pulse; PRF: pulse repetition frequency; ITI: inter trial interval; TMS: transcranial magnetic stimulation; tACS: transcranial alternating current stimulation; DBS: deep-brain stimulation; PD: Parkinson's disease.

Authors' contributions
PX, SZ and YY were responsible for experimental design, analysis and manuscript preparation. XW and YW were responsible for experimental data collection, statistical analysis and manuscript revision. All authors read and approved the final manuscript.

Acknowledgements
None.

Competing interests
The authors declare that they have no competing interests.

Funding
This work was supported by National Nature Science Foundation of China under Grants 61673336, and Natural Science Foundation of Hebei, China under Grants F2015203372. The funders do not participate in the experimental research, or preparation the manuscript.

References
1. Lewis PM, Thomson RH, Rosenfeld JV, Fitzgerald PB. Brain neuromodulation techniques: a review. Neurosci Rev J Bringing Neurobiol Neurol Psychiatry. 2016;22(4):406–21.
2. Leinenga G, Götz J. Scanning ultrasound removes amyloid-β and restores memory in an Alzheimer's disease mouse model. Sci Transl Med. 2015;7(278):278ra233.
3. Mueller JK, Ai L, Bansal P, Legon W. Numerical evaluation of the skull for human neuromodulation with transcranial focused ultrasound. J Neural Eng. 2017;14(6):066012.
4. Panczykowski DM, Rd ME, Friedlander RM. Transcranial focused ultrasound modulates the activity of primary somatosensory cortex in humans. Neurosurgery. 2014;74(6):322.
5. Yoo SS, Bystritsky A, Lee JH, Zhang Y, Fischer K, Min BK, Mcdannold NJ, Pascualleone A, Jolesz FA. Focused ultrasound modulates region-specific brain activity. Neuroimage. 2011;56(3):1267–75.
6. Bystritsky A, Korb AS, Douglas PK, Cohen MS, Melega WP, Mulgaonkar AP, Desalles A, Min BK, Yoo SS. A review of low-intensity focused ultrasound pulsation. Brain Stimul. 2011;4(3):125.
7. Naor O, Krupa S, Shoham S. Ultrasonic neuromodulation. J Neural Eng. 2016;13(3):031003.
8. Tyler WJ, Yusuf T, Michael F, Tauchmann ML, Olson EJ, Cassondra M. Remote excitation of neuronal circuits using low-intensity, low-frequency ultrasound. PLoS ONE. 2008;3(10):e3511.
9. Legon W, Bansal P, Tyshynsky R, Ai L, Mueller JK. Transcranial focused ultrasound neuromodulation of the human primary motor cortex. Sci Rep. 2018;8:10007.
10. Li H, Sun J, Zhang D, Omiremayor D, Lewin PA, Tong S. Low-intensity (400 mW/cm^2, 500 kHz) pulsed transcranial ultrasound preconditioning may mitigate focal cerebral ischemia in rats. Brain Stimul. 2017;10(3):695–702.
11. Yuan Y, Yan J, Ma Z, Li X. Noninvasive focused ultrasound stimulation can modulate phase-amplitude coupling between neuronal oscillations in the rat hippocampus. Front Neurosci. 2016;10(191):348.
12. Mueller J, Legon W, Opitz A, Sato TF, Tyler WJ. Transcranial focused ultrasound modulates intrinsic and evoked EEG dynamics. Brain Stimul. 2014;7(6):900–8.
13. Tufail Y, Matyushov A, Baldwin N, Tauchmann ML, Georges J, Yoshihiro A, Tillery SI, Tyler WJ. Transcranial pulsed ultrasound stimulates intact brain circuits. Neuron. 2010;66(5):681.
14. King RL, Brown JR, Pauly KB. Localization of ultrasound-induced in vivo neurostimulation in the mouse model. Ultrasound Med Biol. 2014;40(7):1512–22.
15. Tufail Y, Yoshihiro A, Pati S, Li MM, Tyler WJ. Ultrasonic neuromodulation by brain stimulation with transcranial ultrasound. Nat Protoc. 2011;6(9):1453.
16. Legon W, Sato TF, Opitz A, Mueller J, Barbour A, Williams A, Tyler WJ. Transcranial focused ultrasound modulates the activity of primary somatosensory cortex in humans. Nat Neurosci. 2014;17(2):322.
17. Guo T, Li H, Lv Y, Lu H, Niu J, Sun J, Yang GY, Ren C, Tong S. Pulsed transcranial ultrasound stimulation immediately after the ischemic brain injury is neuroprotective. IEEE Trans Biomed Eng. 2015;62(10):2352–7.
18. Conway BA, Halliday DM, Farmer SF, Shahani U, Maas P, Weir AI, Rosenberg JR. Synchronization between motor cortex and spinal motoneuronal pool during the performance of a maintained motor task in man. J Physiol. 1995;489(3):917.
19. Baker SN, Olivier E, Lemon RN. Coherent oscillations in monkey motor cortex and hand muscle EMG show task-dependent modulation. J Physiol. 1997;501 (Pt 1)(1):225.
20. Kakei S, Hoffman DS, Strick PL. Muscle and movement representations in the primary motor cortex. Science. 1999;285(5436):2136–9.
21. Mehrkanoon S, Breakspear M, Boonstra TW. The reorganization of corticomuscular coherence during a transition between sensorimotor states. Neuroimage. 2014;100:692–702.
22. Mima T, Matsuoka T, Hallett M. Information flow from the sensorimotor cortex to muscle in humans. Clin Neurophys Off J Int Fed Clin Neurophys. 2001;112(1):122–6.
23. Kilner JM, Baker SN, Salenius S, Hari R, Lemon RN. Human cortical muscle coherence is directly related to specific motor parameters. J Neurosci Off J Soc Neurosci. 2000;20(23):8838.

24. Von Carlowitz-Ghori K, Bayraktaroglu Z, Hohlefeld FU, Losch F, Curio G, Nikulin VV. Corticomuscular coherence in acute and chronic stroke. Clin Neurophys Off J Int Fed Clin Neurophysiol. 2014;125(6):1182–91.

25. Mehic E. Increased anatomical specificity for neuromodulation using modulated focused ultrasound. PLoS ONE. 2014;9(2):e86939.

26. King RL, Brown JR, Newsome WT, Pauly KB. Effective parameters for ultrasound-induced in vivo neurostimulation. Ultrasound Med Biol. 2013;39(2):312–31.

27. Jin SH, Lin P, Hallett M. Linear and nonlinear information flow based on time-delayed mutual information method and its application to corticomuscular interaction. Clin Neurophys Off J Int Fed Clin Neurophys. 2010;121(3):392–401.

28. Viola P, Iii WMW. Alignment by maximization of mutual information. Int J Comput Vis. 1997;24(2):137–54.

29. Schreiber T. Measuring information transfer. Phys Rev Lett. 2000;85(2):461.

30. Vicente R, Wibral M, Lindner M, Pipa G. Transfer entropy—a model-free measure of effective connectivity for the neurosciences. J Comput Neurosci. 2011;30(1):45–67.

31. Zhou S, Xie P, Chen X, Wang Y, Zhang Y, Du Y. Optimization of relative parameters in transfer entropy estimation and application to corticomuscular coupling in humans. J Neurosci Methods. 2018. https://doi.org/10.1016/j.jneumeth.2018.07.004.

32. So WK, Yang L, Jelfs B, She Q, Wong SW, Mak JN, Chan RH: Cross-frequency information transfer from EEG to EMG in grasping. In: Engineering in medicine and biology society. 2016. p. 4531.

33. Chen CC, Hsieh JC, Wu YZ, Lee PL, Chen SS, Niddam DM, Yeh TC, Wu YT. Mutual-information-based approach for neural connectivity during self-paced finger lifting task. Hum Brain Mapp. 2008;29(3):265.

34. Mima T, Steger J, Schulman AE, Gerloff C, Hallett M. Electroencephalographic measurement of motor cortex control of muscle activity in humans. Clin Neurophys Off J Int Fed Clin Neurophys. 2000;111(2):326.

35. Witham CL, Riddle CN, Baker MR, Baker SN. Contributions of descending and ascending pathways to corticomuscular coherence in humans. J Physiol. 2011;589(15):3789–800.

36. Ouyang G, Li X. Estimating coupling direction between neuronal populations. Neuroimage. 2010;52(2):497–507.

37. Vakorin VA, Bratislav M, Olga K, Randal MIA. Empirical and theoretical aspects of generation and transfer of information in a neuromagnetic source network. Front Syst Neurosci. 2011;5:96.

38. Mueller JK, Ai L, Bansal P, Legon W. Computational exploration of wave propagation and heating from transcranial focused ultrasound for neuromodulation. J Neural Eng. 2016;13(5):056002.

39. Kim H, Chiu A, Lee SD, Fischer K, Yoo SS. Focused ultrasound-mediated non-invasive brain stimulation: examination of sonication parameters. Brain Stimul. 2014;7(5):748–56.

40. Dalecki D. Mechanical bioeffects of ultrasound. Ann Rev Biomed Eng. 2004;6(1):229.

41. Wibral M, Rahm B, Rieder M, Lindner M, Vicente R, Kaiser J. Transfer entropy in magnetoencephalographic data: quantifying information flow in cortical and cerebellar networks. Prog Biophys Mol Biol. 2011;105(1–2):80–97.

42. Lindner M, Vicente R, Priesemann V, Wibral M. TRENTOOL: a Matlab open source toolbox to analyse information flow in time series data with transfer entropy. BMC Neurosci. 2011;12(1):119.

43. Ragwitz M, Kantz H. Markov models from data by simple nonlinear time series predictors in delay embedding spaces. Phys Rev E Stat Nonlinear Soft Matter Phys. 2002;65(5 Pt 2):056201.

44. Wibral M, Pampu N, Priesemann V, Siebenhühner F, Seiwert H, Lindner M, Lizier JT, Vicente R. Measuring information-transfer delays. PLOS One. 2013;8(2):e55809.

45. Kraskov A, Gbauer StH, Grassberger P. Estimating mutual information. Phys Rev E Stat Nonlinear Soft Matter Phys. 2003;69(6 Pt 2):066138.

46. Ye J, Tang S, Meng L, Li X, Wen X, Chen S, Niu L, Li X, Qiu W, Hu H, et al. Ultrasonic control of neural activity through activation of the mechano-sensitive channel MscL. Nano Lett. 2018;18(7):4148–55.

47. Lee W, Kim H, Jung Y, Song IU, Yong AC, Yoo SS. Image-guided transcranial focused ultrasound stimulates human primary somatosensory cortex. Sci Rep. 2015;5:8743.

48. Lee W, Kim HC, Jung Y, Yong AC, Song IU, Lee JH, Yoo SS. Transcranial focused ultrasound stimulation of human primary visual cortex. Sci Rep. 2016;6:34026.

49. Legon W, Ai L, Bansal P, Mueller JK. Neuromodulation with single-element transcranial focused ultrasound in human thalamus. Hum Brain Mapp. 2018;39(5):1995–2006.

50. Ye PP, Brown JR, Pauly KB. Frequency dependence of ultrasound neurostimulation in the mouse brain. Ultrasound Med Biol. 2016;42(7):1512–30.

51. Murase N, Duque J, Mazzocchio R, Cohen LG. Influence of interhemispheric interactions on motor function in chronic stroke. Ann Neurol. 2004;55(3):400.

52. Schulz H, Ubelacker T, Keil J, Müller N, Weisz N. Now I am ready-now i am not: the influence of pre-TMS oscillations and corticomuscular coherence on motor-evoked potentials. Cereb Cortex. 2014;24(7):1708–19.

53. Sağlam M, Matsunaga K, Murayama N, Hayashida Y, Huang YZ, Nakanishi R. Parallel inhibition of cortico-muscular synchronization and corticospinal excitability by theta burst TMS in humans. Clin Neurophys Off J Int Fed Clin Neurophys. 2008;119(12):2829–38.

54. Wach C, Krause V, Moliadze V, Paulus W, Schnitzler A, Pollok B. The effect of 10 Hz transcranial alternating current stimulation (tACS) on corticomuscular coherence. 2013;7(5):511.

55. Beuter A, Lefaucheur JP, Modolo J. Closed-loop cortical neuromodulation in Parkinson's disease: an alternative to deep brain stimulation? Clin Neurophys Off J Int Fed Clin Neurophys. 2014;125(5):874–85.

56. Kamimura HAS, Wang S, Chen H, Wang Q, Aurup C, Acosta C, Carneiro AAO, Konofagou EE. Focused ultrasound neuromodulation of cortical and subcortical brain structures using 1.9 MHz. Med Phys. 2016;43(10):5730.

57. Guo H, Mark Hamilton II, Offutt SJ, Gloeckner CD, Li T, Kim Y, Legon W, Alford JK, Lim HH. Ultrasound produces extensive brain activation via a cochlear pathway. Neuron. 2018;98(5):1020–30.e4.

58. Sato T, Shapiro MG, Tsao DY. Ultrasonic neuromodulation causes widespread cortical activation via an indirect auditory mechanism. Neuron. 2018;98(5):1031.

59. Airaksinen K, Mäkelä JP, Nurminen J, Luoma J, Taulu S, Ahonen A, Pekkonen E. Cortico-muscular coherence in advanced Parkinson's disease with deep brain stimulation. Clin Neurophys Off J Int Fed Clin Neurophys. 2015;126(4):748.

8

Cognitive and emotional alterations in *App* knock-in mouse models of Aβ amyloidosis

Yasufumi Sakakibara[1*], Michiko Sekiya[1], Takashi Saito[2], Takaomi C. Saido[2] and Koichi M. Iijima[1,3*] (iD)

Abstract

Background: Alzheimer's disease (AD), the most common cause of dementia, is characterized by the progressive deposition of amyloid-β (Aβ) peptides and neurofibrillary tangles. Mouse models of Aβ amyloidosis generated by knock-in (KI) of a humanized Aβ sequence provide distinct advantages over traditional transgenic models that rely on overexpression of amyloid precursor protein (APP). In *App*-KI mice, three familial AD-associated mutations were introduced into the endogenous mouse *App* locus to recapitulate Aβ pathology observed in AD: the Swedish (NL) mutation, which elevates total Aβ production; the Beyreuther/Iberian (F) mutation, which increases the Aβ42/Aβ40 ratio; and the Arctic (G) mutation, which promotes Aβ aggregation. App^{NL-G-F} mice harbor all three mutations and develop progressive Aβ amyloidosis and neuroinflammatory response in broader brain areas, whereas App^{NL} mice carrying only the Swedish mutation exhibit no overt AD-related pathological changes. To identify behavioral alterations associated with Aβ pathology, we assessed emotional and cognitive domains of App^{NL-G-F} and App^{NL} mice at different time points, using the elevated plus maze, contextual fear conditioning, and Barnes maze tasks.

Results: Assessments of emotional domains revealed that, in comparison with wild-type (WT) C57BL/6J mice, $App^{NL-G-F/NL-G-F}$ mice exhibited anxiolytic-like behavior that was detectable from 6 months of age. By contrast, $App^{NL/NL}$ mice exhibited anxiogenic-like behavior from 15 months of age. In the contextual fear conditioning task, both $App^{NL/NL}$ and $App^{NL-G-F/NL-G-F}$ mice exhibited intact learning and memory up to 15–18 months of age, whereas $App^{NL-G-F/NL-G-F}$ mice exhibited hyper-reactivity to painful stimuli. In the Barnes maze task, $App^{NL-G-F/NL-G-F}$ mice exhibited a subtle decline in spatial learning ability at 8 months of age, but retained normal memory functions.

Conclusion: $App^{NL/NL}$ and $App^{NL-G-F/NL-G-F}$ mice exhibit behavioral changes associated with non-cognitive, emotional domains before the onset of definitive cognitive deficits. Our observations consistently indicate that $App^{NL-G-F/NL-G-F}$ mice represent a model for preclinical AD. These mice are useful for the study of AD prevention rather than treatment after neurodegeneration.

Keywords: Alzheimer's disease, Amyloid precursor protein, Knock-in mouse model, Emotional behavior, Spatial learning

*Correspondence: bara@ncgg.go.jp; iijimakm@ncgg.go.jp
[1] Department of Alzheimer's Disease Research, Center for Development of Advanced Medicine for Dementia, National Center for Geriatrics and Gerontology, Obu, Aichi 474-8511, Japan
Full list of author information is available at the end of the article

Background

Alzheimer's disease (AD) is characterized by a progressive decline in cognitive functions, usually starting with memory complaints, and eventually leading to multiple cognitive, neuropsychological, and behavioral deficits [1, 2]. The neuropathology of AD begins before overt cognitive symptoms, including the accumulation of amyloid-β peptide (Aβ) as extracellular plaques, aggregation of hyperphosphorylated tau as intracellular neurofibrillary tangles (NFTs), and activation of multiple neuroinflammatory pathways [3–5]. These brain pathologies are thought to induce neuronal cell loss in the hippocampus and cerebral cortex [3–5]. However, the etiology of AD is still not fully clarified, and many fundamental questions remain unanswered.

Mouse models of AD pathology are critical research tools for testing potential therapeutic approaches to AD and investigating the molecular mechanisms underlying AD pathogenesis [6, 7]. Several transgenic mouse lines overexpressing amyloid precursor protein (APP) have been developed as experimental models for Aβ amyloidosis [8, 9]. However, non-physiological overexpression of APP results in overproduction of various APP fragments in addition to Aβ [8], making it technically difficult to distinguish the pathophysiological effects caused by Aβ from those caused by other APP fragments [8, 10, 11]. Moreover, overexpression of APP causes memory impairment without Aβ deposition in some *App* transgenic mice [8, 11], suggesting that the brains of these transgenic mouse models may have pathophysiological properties that are not relevant to AD pathogenesis.

To produce Aβ pathology without non-physiological overexpression of APP in the mouse brain, alternative mouse models have been generated utilizing an *App* knock-in (KI) strategy [12] in which the murine Aβ sequence was humanized by changing three amino acids that differ between the mouse and human proteins. In addition, three familial AD-associated mutations were introduced into the endogenous mouse *App* locus: the Swedish (NL) mutation, which elevates total Aβ production [13]; the Beyreuther/Iberian (F) mutation, which increases the Aβ42/Aβ40 ratio [14, 15]; and the Arctic (G) mutation, which promotes Aβ aggregation [16, 17]. In App^{NL-G-F} mice, which harbor all three mutations within the Aβ sequence, Aβ amyloidosis is aggressively accelerated and neuroinflammation is observed in subcortical structures and cortical regions [12, 18]. By contrast, App^{NL} mice that carry only the Swedish mutation produce significantly higher levels of Aβ40 and Aβ42 but exhibit no overt AD-related brain pathology such as extracellular Aβ plaques or neuroinflammation [12, 18]. None of these *App*-KI mice exhibit tau pathology

or severe neuron loss, suggesting that they are models of preclinical AD [11].

Recent reports demonstrated that *App*-KI mice exhibit a reduction in the number of hippocampal mushroom spines [19, 20] and disruption of neural circuit activities organized by gamma oscillations in the medial entorhinal cortex [21]. They also revealed new mechanisms underlying Aβ pathology: genetic deletion of the orphan G protein GPR3, which regulates γ-secretase activity and Aβ generation, attenuates Aβ pathology [22], whereas ablation of kallikrein-related peptidase 7 (KLK7), an astrocyte-derived Aβ-degrading enzyme, accelerates Aβ pathologies in the brains of *App*-KI mice [23]. To further understand the utility of the *App*-KI mouse models for basic and translational research, it is crucial to obtain detailed information on their behavioral phenotypes, including cognitive and non-cognitive comorbidity related to AD [7, 12, 18, 24–26].

To investigate the behavioral changes associated with Aβ pathology, we searched for alterations in cognitive and emotional domains specifically present in $App^{NL-G-F/NL-G-F}$ mice. As our experimental paradigms, we used the elevated plus maze (EPM), contextual fear conditioning (CFC), and Barnes maze (BM) tasks. Analysis with EPM revealed that $App^{NL-G-F/NL-G-F}$ mice exhibited robust anxiolytic-like behaviors, whereas $App^{NL/NL}$ mice exhibited anxiogenic-like behaviors, in comparison with wild-type (WT) C57BL/6J mice. In CFC and BM, no significant learning and memory deficits were observed in $App^{NL-G-F/NL-G-F}$ or $App^{NL/NL}$ mice, whereas $App^{NL-G-F/NL-G-F}$ mice exhibited a subtle decline in spatial learning ability in the BM. These results suggest that $App^{NL-G-F/NL-G-F}$ and $App^{NL/NL}$ mice exhibit significant changes in anxiety-related behaviors, with minimal alterations in learning ability and memory. Our results provide information about behavioral readouts in *App*-KI mice that will be useful for future basic and translational research.

Results

In $App^{NL-G-F/NL-G-F}$ mice, age-dependent cortical Aβ amyloidosis began by 2 months and saturated around 7 months of age (Additional file 1: Fig. S1) [12]. These mice also developed Aβ amyloidosis in the hippocampal and subcortical regions [12]. Despite aggressive Aβ amyloidosis in $App^{NL-G-F/NL-G-F}$ mice, neuroinflammatory responses such as astrocytosis and microgliosis were not intense at the age of 6–9 months, whereas greater reactive gliosis was observed in cortical and hippocampal regions, as well as in subcortical regions, at the age of 15–18 months (Additional file 1: Fig. S1) [12, 18]. By contrast, Aβ plaques and neuroinflammatory responses were negligible even at 18 months of age in $App^{NL/NL}$ mice, despite elevation of the Aβ level in the brain [12, 18].

Based on this neuropathological information, we carried out behavioral assays to capture cognitive (BM and CFC tasks) and emotional (EPM task) alterations in *App*-KI mice over the course of aging (Additional file 1: Fig. S1). In the experimental design, we noted that the same group of mice (Group 4) was repeatedly tested at 4, 6, and 8 months of age in the BM task (Additional file 1: Fig. S1).

App^{NL-G-F/NL-G-F} mice exhibit anxiolytic-like behavior, whereas *App*^{NL/NL} mice exhibit anxiogenic-like behavior, in comparison with control WT mice

Anxiety-related behaviors were assessed using the EPM task, in which increased exploration of open arms indicates anxiolytic-like behavior [27, 28]. In 6–9-month-old *App*^{NL-G-F/NL-G-F} mice, the amount of time on (Fig. 1a; $F[2, 21] = 4.35$, $p = 0.026$, post hoc, WT vs. *App*^{NL-G-F/NL-G-F}, $p = 0.565$) and entries into (Fig. 1b; $F[2, 21] = 2.22$, $p = 0.133$) open arms during the 10-min test were slightly increased in comparison with WT mice, although these differences were not statistically significant with our sample size. The average total number of arm entries (Fig. 1c; $F[2, 21] = 1.95$, $p = 0.167$) and the distance travelled during the 10-min test (Additional file 2: Fig. S2a and b; $F[2, 21] = 0.27$, $p = 0.766$) were also slightly increased in *App*^{NL-G-F/NL-G-F} mice, although these differences were not statistically significant. By contrast, *App*^{NL/NL} mice exhibited similar levels of the amount of time on (Fig. 1a; post hoc, WT vs. *App*^{NL/NL}, $p = 0.170$) and entries into (Fig. 1b) open arms to those of WT mice, with no alterations in general exploratory activity (Fig. 1c, Additional file 2: Fig. S2b).

However, the patterns of exploration in *App*^{NL-G-F/NL-G-F} mice differed from those observed in WT mice. When we analyzed the time course of open arm exploration by scoring the percentage of time spent on the arms in each 2-min interval (Fig. 1d), WT mice exhibited significant reductions in the time spent on the open arms as the test progressed ($F[4, 28] = 3.75$, $p = 0.014$), consistent with a previous report [28–30]. By contrast, *App*^{NL-G-F/NL-G-F} mice persistently explored the open arms throughout the test (Fig. 1d; $F[4, 28] = 0.68$, $p = 0.610$). At a later time point, *App*^{NL-G-F/NL-G-F} mice spent significantly more time on the open arms than WT mice (Fig. 1d; Time 8–10, $F[2, 21] = 6.11$, $p = 0.008$, post hoc, WT vs. *App*^{NL-G-F/NL-G-F}, $p = 0.022$). In contrast, similar to WT mice, *App*^{NL/NL} mice exhibited a decrease in open arm exploration as the test progressed (Fig. 1d; $F[4, 28] = 2.69$, $p = 0.051$). These results suggest that *App*^{NL-G-F/NL-G-F} mice have altered responses to aversive situations, such as open spaces.

Previous studies demonstrated that laboratory rodents exhibited a significant reduction of open arm exploration when re-exposed to the EPM [28, 30, 31]. This suggests that prior test experience caused a qualitative shift in emotional state, and the acquisition of a phobic state rather than an unconditioned anxiety response. To investigate whether prior test experience could alter anxiety-related behavior, we re-tested the *App*-KI and WT mice in the same EPM paradigm.

As reported previously, WT mice exhibited robust avoidance responses to the open arms in the second trial of our EPM task, reflected by reduced percentages of time spent on and entries into the arms. By contrast, 6–9-month-old *App*^{NL-G-F/NL-G-F} mice spent significantly more time on the open arms (Fig. 1e; $F[2, 21] = 5.30$, $p = 0.014$, post hoc, WT vs. *App*^{NL-G-F/NL-G-F}, $p = 0.034$) and entered them more frequently (Fig. 1f; $F[2, 21] = 6.11$, $p = 0.008$, post hoc, WT vs. *App*^{NL-G-F/NL-G-F}, $p = 0.006$) during the 10-min test period than WT mice. The time course analysis also revealed a persistent and durable exploration of open arms in *App*^{NL-G-F/NL-G-F} mice (Fig. 1h; $F[4, 28] = 0.207$, $p = 0.932$). These mice showed slightly higher preference toward the open arms in comparison with WT mice at each time point, although the differences were not statistically significant (Fig. 1h; Time

(See figure on next page.)
Fig. 1 Anxiety-related behaviors in *App*^{NL-G-F/NL-G-F} and *App*^{NL/NL} mice assessed by the elevated plus maze task. Anxiety-related behaviors were assessed at both 6–9 (**a–h**) and 15–18 (**i–p**) months of age. At 6–9 months of age, *App*^{NL-G-F/NL-G-F} mice exhibited slightly increased levels of open arm exploration than WT mice, as indicated by the percentages of time spent on (**a**) and entries into (**b**) the open arms in the first trial. *App*^{NL/NL} and WT mice showed similar levels of open arm exploration. General exploratory activity in *App*^{NL-G-F/NL-G-F} mice was also slightly increased in comparison with WT mice (**c**). *App*^{NL-G-F/NL-G-F} mice persistently explored the open arms throughout the 10-min test, in contrast to the WT and *App*^{NL/NL} mice (**d**). In the second trial, *App*^{NL-G-F/NL-G-F} mice spent more time on (**e**) and entered more often into (**f**) the open arms than WT mice, with a slight increase in general activity (**g**). WT, *App*^{NL/NL} and *App*^{NL-G-F/NL-G-F} mice did not exhibit elevated avoidance responses to the open arms throughout the test in the second trial (**h**). At 15–18 months of age, *App*^{NL-G-F/NL-G-F} mice exhibited slight increases in open arm exploration in comparison with WT mice in the first trial, whereas *App*^{NL/NL} mice exhibited reduced levels of the exploration (**i** and **j**). General exploratory activity in *App*^{NL-G-F/NL-G-F} mice was slightly increased in comparison with WT mice (**k**). WT and *App*^{NL/NL} mice exhibited elevated open arm avoidance as the test progressed, whereas *App*^{NL-G-F/NL-G-F} mice did not (**l**). In the second trial, *App*^{NL-G-F/NL-G-F} mice spent more time on (**m**) and entered more often into (**n**) the open arms than WT mice. *App*^{NL-G-F/NL-G-F} mice also exhibited an elevation in general activity during the test (**o**). WT, *App*^{NL/NL} and *App*^{NL-G-F/NL-G-F} mice did not exhibit elevated avoidance responses to the open arms throughout the test in the second trial (**p**). 6–9 month-old; n = 8 WT (B6J), n = 8 *App*^{NL/NL}, n = 8 *App*^{NL-G-F/NL-G-F}. 15–18 month-old; n = 12 WT (B6J), n = 10 *App*^{NL/NL}, n = 11 *App*^{NL-G-F/NL-G-F}. *$p < 0.05$; **$p < 0.01$; ***$p < 0.001$ versus WT (B6J); †$p < 0.05$; ††$p < 0.01$; †††$p < 0.001$ versus *App*^{NL/NL}

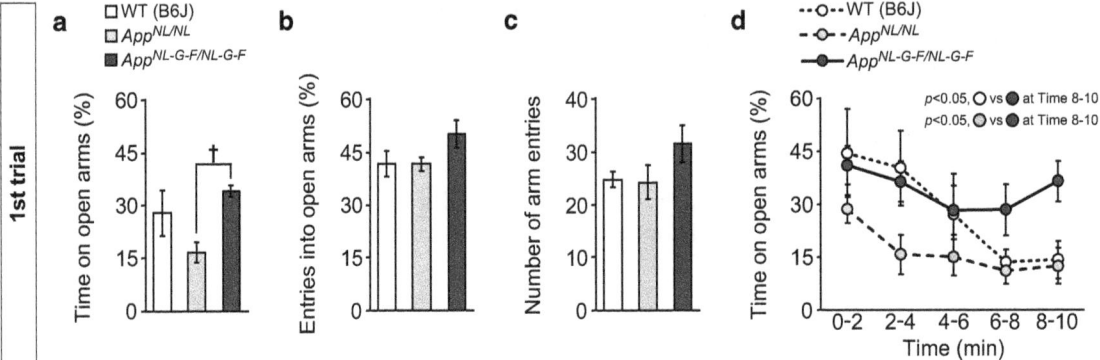

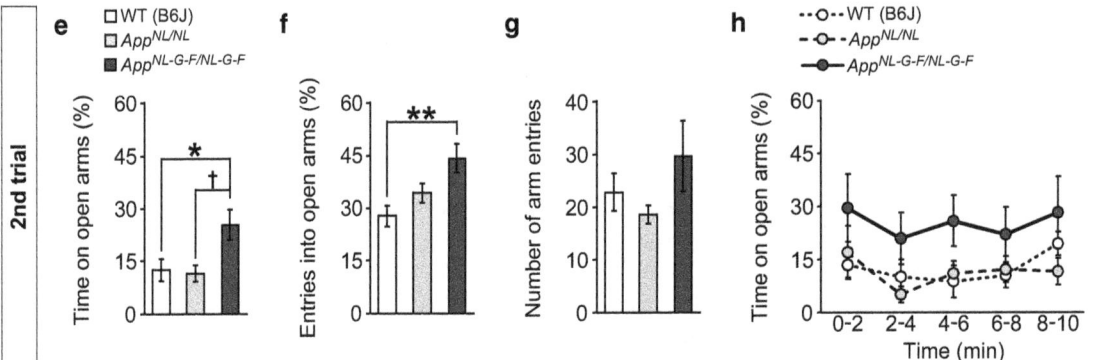

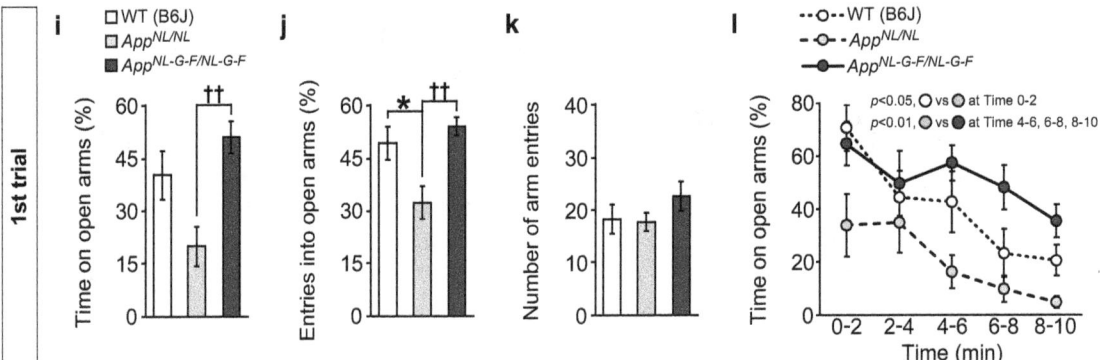

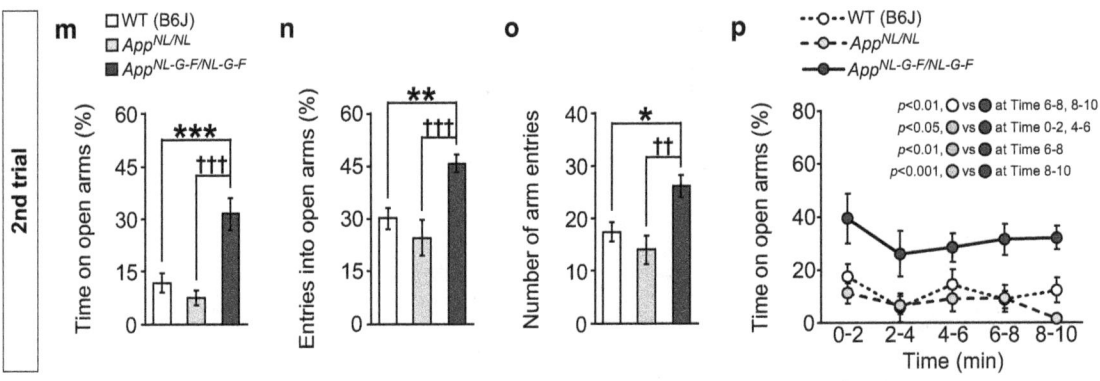

0–2, $F[2, 21] = 1.33$, $p = 0.286$; Time 2–4, $F[2, 21] = 2.44$, $p = 0.111$; Time 4–6, $F[2, 21] = 3.05$, $p = 0.069$; Time 6–8, $F[2, 21] = 1.35$, $p = 0.280$; Time 8–10, $F[2, 21] = 1.59$, $p = 0.228$). $App^{NL/NL}$ and WT mice engaged in similar levels of open arm exploration (Fig. 1e, f and h). As with the case of the first trial, $App^{NL-G-F/NL-G-F}$ mice exhibited slight increases in the average total number of arm entries (Fig. 1g; $F[2, 21] = 1.53$, $p = 0.240$) and the distance travelled during the 10-min test (Additional file 2: Fig. S2c and d; $F[2, 21] = 1.22$, $p = 0.316$), although these differences were not statistically significant with our sample size.

Taken together, these results suggest that 6–9-month-old $App^{NL-G-F/NL-G-F}$ mice exhibit robust anxiolytic-like behavior, even after they have habituated to a test environment.

To investigate whether the observed anxiolytic-like behavior in $App^{NL-G-F/NL-G-F}$ mice was maintained during aging, we performed the same EPM task at 15–18 months of age. In the first trial, $App^{NL-G-F/NL-G-F}$ mice showed a tendency to spent more time on (Fig. 1i; $F[2, 30] = 6.78$, $p = 0.004$, post hoc, WT vs. $App^{NL-G-F/NL-G-F}$, $p = 0.401$) and a slightly higher frequency of entries into (Fig. 1j; $F[2, 30] = 7.01$, $p = 0.003$, post hoc, WT vs. $App^{NL-G-F/NL-G-F}$, $p = 0.700$) the open arms during the 10-min test than WT mice, although these differences were not statistically significant. By contrast, $App^{NL/NL}$ mice tended to spend less time in the open arms (Fig. 1i; post hoc, WT vs. $App^{NL/NL}$, $p = 0.054$) and entered them significantly less frequently (Fig. 1j; post hoc, WT vs. $App^{NL/NL}$, $p = 0.021$) than WT mice, suggesting anxiogenic-like behavior in $App^{NL/NL}$ mice. General exploratory activity was slightly increased in $App^{NL-G-F/NL-G-F}$ mice, although the difference was not statistically significant with our sample size (Fig. 1k; $F[2, 30] = 1.07$, $p = 0.356$; Additional file 2: Fig. S2e and f; $F[2, 30] = 0.18$, $p = 0.836$).

As observed at 6–9 months of age, 15–18-month-old WT and $App^{NL/NL}$ mice exhibited clear avoidance of the open arms as the test progressed (Fig. 1l; WT, $F[4, 44] = 8.96$, $p < 0.001$; $App^{NL/NL}$, $F[4, 36] = 4.15$, $p = 0.007$), whereas $App^{NL-G-F/NL-G-F}$ mice did not exhibit a significant change in open arm exploration during the test ($F[4, 40] = 1.83$, $p = 0.141$). At an early time point, $App^{NL/NL}$ mice spent significantly less time on the open arms than WT mice (Fig. 1l; Time 0–2, $F[2, 30] = 4.13$, $p = 0.026$, post hoc, WT vs. $App^{NL/NL}$, $p = 0.021$). By contrast, $App^{NL-G-F/NL-G-F}$ mice exhibited slightly higher open arm exploration in the latter half of the test in comparison with WT mice, but the differences were not statistically significant (Fig. 1l; Time 4–6, $F[2, 30] = 5.30$, $p = 0.011$, post hoc, WT vs. $App^{NL-G-F/NL-G-F}$, $p = 0.466$; Time 6–8, $F[2, 30] = 5.74$, $p = 0.008$, post hoc, WT vs. $App^{NL-G-F/NL-G-F}$, $p = 0.079$; Time 8–10, $F[2, 30] = 7.94$, $p = 0.002$, post hoc,

WT vs. $App^{NL-G-F/NL-G-F}$, $p = 0.125$). These results suggest that 15–18-month-old $App^{NL-G-F/NL-G-F}$ mice exhibit alterations in the habituation process to aversive stimuli.

In the second trial, 15–18-month-old $App^{NL-G-F/NL-G-F}$ mice spent significantly more time on the open arms (Fig. 1m; $F[2, 30] = 13.87$, $p < 0.001$, post hoc, WT vs. $App^{NL-G-F/NL-G-F}$, $p < 0.001$) and entered them more often (Fig. 1n; $F[2, 30] = 9.37$, $p < 0.001$, post hoc, WT vs. $App^{NL-G-F/NL-G-F}$, $p = 0.009$) than WT mice. The time course analysis also revealed a persistent and durable exploration of open arms in $App^{NL-G-F/NL-G-F}$ mice (Fig. 1p; $F[4, 40] = 0.74$, $p = 0.570$). $App^{NL-G-F/NL-G-F}$ mice spent more time on the open arms from the beginning of the test (Fig. 1p; Time 0–2, $F[2, 30] = 5.13$, $p = 0.012$, post hoc, WT vs. $App^{NL-G-F/NL-G-F}$, $p = 0.053$; Time 2–4, $F[2, 30] = 3.31$, $p = 0.050$; Time 4–6, $F[2, 30] = 3.51$, $p = 0.043$, post hoc, WT vs. $App^{NL-G-F/NL-G-F}$, $p = 0.157$) and particularly at later time points (Time 6–8, $F[2, 30] = 7.26$, $p = 0.003$, post hoc, WT vs. $App^{NL-G-F/NL-G-F}$, $p = 0.005$; Time 8–10, $F[2, 30] = 15.14$, $p < 0.001$, post hoc, WT vs. $App^{NL-G-F/NL-G-F}$, $p = 0.003$). In addition, $App^{NL-G-F/NL-G-F}$ mice exhibited a significant increase in the total number of arm entries in comparison with WT mice (Fig. 1o; $F[2, 30] = 7.85$, $p = 0.002$, post hoc, WT vs. $App^{NL-G-F/NL-G-F}$, $p = 0.021$). We also measured the distance travelled during the test (Additional file 2: Fig. S2g and h) and noticed that $App^{NL-G-F/NL-G-F}$ mice moved longer than WT mice, though the difference was not statistically significant with our sample size ($F[2, 30] = 3.76$, $p = 0.035$, post hoc, WT vs. $App^{NL-G-F/NL-G-F}$, $p = 0.154$). In contrast to the first trial, $App^{NL/NL}$ and WT mice exhibited similar levels of open arm exploration (Fig. 1m and n), presumably due to habituation of WT mice to the test environment.

Taken together, these results suggest that 15–18-month-old $App^{NL-G-F/NL-G-F}$ mice exhibit robust anxiolytic-like behaviors, with increases in general exploratory activity, whereas $App^{NL/NL}$ mice displayed unconditioned anxious phenotypes in comparison with WT mice.

$App^{NL-G-F/NL-G-F}$ and $App^{NL/NL}$ mice exhibit normal learning and memory of contextual fear up to 15–18 months of age in comparison with WT mice

The CFC task is a commonly used procedure for inducing learned fear, which is believed to be hippocampal-dependent [32, 33]. In this paradigm, a particular context as a conditioned stimulus evokes fear through association with an aversive event, such as a footshock [34]. Conditioned fear responses are impaired in both human patients and mouse models of AD [35–38].

At 6–9 months of age, the velocities of both $App^{NL-G-F/NL-G-F}$ and $App^{NL/NL}$ mice during administration of each footshock were comparable to those of WT mice (Fig. 2a; first, $F[2,$

$18] = 0.32, p = 0.732$; second, $F[2, 18] = 0.71, p = 0.506$; third, $F[2, 18] = 1.30, p = 0.297$). In addition, $App^{NL\text{-}G\text{-}F/NL\text{-}G\text{-}F}$, $App^{NL/NL}$, and WT mice exhibited the same levels of the freezing response upon subsequent presentation of footshocks during conditioning (Fig. 2b; genotype, $F[2, 18] = 0.19$, $p = 0.830$; time, $F[1.6, 28.7] = 18.02$, $p < 0.001$). To determine whether there were any locomotor deficits that could have confounded the outcome, we compared the distance travelled during the pre-shock period (the 3-min period prior to the first footshock) among genotypes (Additional file 3: Fig. S3a and b). At these ages, $App^{NL\text{-}G\text{-}F/NL\text{-}G\text{-}F}$ mice seemed to be less active than WT mice during the pre-shock period, although the difference was not statistically significant with our sample size (Additional file 3: Fig. S3b; $F[2, 18] = 2.99$, $p = 0.076$). These results suggest that all genotypes were capable of detecting and responding to footshock stimuli at similar levels.

In the context test, min-by-min scoring of the percentage of freezing behavior revealed that all genotypes exhibited similar increases in the response as the test progressed (Fig. 2c; genotype, $F[2, 18] = 10.25$, $p = 0.371$; time, $F[2.6, 46.4] = 21.08$, $p < 0.001$). Moreover, levels of the freezing response during the total 5-min period were comparable among all genotypes (Fig. 2d; $F[2, 18] = 1.05$, $p = 0.371$). These results suggest that both $App^{NL\text{-}G\text{-}F/NL\text{-}G\text{-}F}$ and $App^{NL/NL}$ mice can learn and memorize the association between cues in the experimental chamber and footshock as effectively as WT mice.

At 15–18 months of age, $App^{NL\text{-}G\text{-}F/NL\text{-}G\text{-}F}$ mice exhibited significantly higher shock reactivity than WT mice, as revealed by an increased velocity during the second and third footshocks (Fig. 2e; first, $F[2, 19] = 0.85$, $p = 0.444$; second, $F[2, 19] = 7.36$, $p = 0.004$, post hoc, WT vs. $App^{NL\text{-}G\text{-}F/NL\text{-}G\text{-}F}$, $p = 0.007$; third, $F[2, 19] = 10.82$, $p < 0.001$, post hoc, WT vs. $App^{NL\text{-}G\text{-}F/NL\text{-}G\text{-}F}$, $p = 0.008$). This result suggests that 15–18-month-old $App^{NL\text{-}G\text{-}F/NL\text{-}G\text{-}F}$ mice have heightened sensitivity to painful stimuli. During conditioning, both $App^{NL\text{-}G\text{-}F/NL\text{-}G\text{-}F}$ and $App^{NL/NL}$ mice exhibited levels of freezing upon subsequent presentation of footshocks similar to those of WT mice (Fig. 2f; genotype,

$F[2, 19] = 0.0$, $p = 0.994$; time, $F[1.9, 36.5] = 84.15$, $p < 0.001$). We also found that $App^{NL/NL}$ mice moved significantly less than WT mice during the pre-shock period (Additional file 3: Fig. S3c and d; $F[2, 19] = 5.13$, $p = 0.017$, post hoc, WT vs. $App^{NL/NL}$, $p = 0.016$). However, a slight reduction in locomotor activity in $App^{NL/NL}$ mice does not significantly affect the behavioral outcomes of the CFC task in $App^{NL/NL}$ mice, since these mice can exhibit similar levels of shock reactivity and freezing behavior with WT mice (Fig. 2e and f). Locomotor activity during the pre-shock period was also slightly decreased in $App^{NL\text{-}G\text{-}F/NL\text{-}G\text{-}F}$ mice, but the difference was not statistically significant with our sample size (Additional file 3: Fig. S3d; post hoc, WT vs. $App^{NL\text{-}G\text{-}F/NL\text{-}G\text{-}F}$, $p = 0.092$).

In the context test, the min-by-min data for freezing behavior revealed that the time course of the freezing response was similar among all genotypes (Fig. 2g; genotype, $F[2, 19] = 0.23$, $p = 0.799$; time, $F[4, 76] = 5.06$, $p = 0.001$). During the total 5-min period of the test, both $App^{NL\text{-}G\text{-}F/NL\text{-}G\text{-}F}$ and $App^{NL/NL}$ mice exhibited levels of freezing behavior similar to those of WT mice (Fig. 2h; $F[2, 19] = 0.23$, $p = 0.800$).

Taken together, these results suggest that both $App^{NL\text{-}G\text{-}F/NL\text{-}G\text{-}F}$ and $App^{NL/NL}$ mice have intact learning and memory of contextual fear, even at 15–18 months of age.

$App^{NL\text{-}G\text{-}F/NL\text{-}G\text{-}F}$ mice exhibit alterations in spatial learning ability, with intact memory, in the BM task at 8 months of age

The BM task is a spatial memory task that requires animals to learn the location of an escape hole using spatial cues, and is therefore thought to be hippocampal-dependent [39, 40]. This task is commonly used for assessment of memory deficits in animal models of AD [41–43]. In our experiments, mice were asked to acquire the spatial location of a target hole that was connected to a dark escape box during the acquisition phase (Fig. 3a [left]). One day after the fifth session of the acquisition phase, a probe test was conducted without an escape box to investigate whether mice had learned the location of

---

(See figure on next page.)

Fig. 2 Emotional learning and fear memory in $App^{NL\text{-}G\text{-}F/NL\text{-}G\text{-}F}$ and $App^{NL/NL}$ mice, assessed by the contextual fear conditioning task. Learning and memory of contextual fear were assessed at both 6–9 (**a–d**) and 15–18 (**e–h**) months of age. At 6–9 months of age, $App^{NL\text{-}G\text{-}F/NL\text{-}G\text{-}F}$ and $App^{NL/NL}$ mice exhibited similar levels of shock reactivity, as indicated by velocity, during each presentation of footshock (**a**). During conditioning, all genotypes exhibited the same levels of freezing response to subsequent presentation of footshock (indicated by black arrows) (**b**). In the context test, all genotypes exhibited similar increases in the freezing response during the test, as revealed by the min-by-min data (**c**). Total levels of freezing response during the 5-min test period were comparable among all genotypes (**d**). At 15–18 months of age, $App^{NL\text{-}G\text{-}F/NL\text{-}G\text{-}F}$ mice exhibited higher shock reactivity than WT mice, as revealed by an increase in velocity during the second and third footshocks (**e**). During conditioning, all genotypes exhibited the same levels of freezing response to subsequent presentation of footshock (indicated by black arrows) (**f**). The time course of the freezing response in the context test was not different among genotypes (**g**). During the 5-min test period, the percentages of time spent in the frozen state by $App^{NL\text{-}G\text{-}F/NL\text{-}G\text{-}F}$ and $App^{NL/NL}$ mice were similar to that in WT mice (**h**). 6–9 month-old; n = 6 WT (B6J), n = 6 $App^{NL/NL}$, n = 9 $App^{NL\text{-}G\text{-}F/NL\text{-}G\text{-}F}$. 15–18 month-old; n = 8 WT (B6J), n = 7 $App^{NL/NL}$, n = 7 $App^{NL\text{-}G\text{-}F/NL\text{-}G\text{-}F}$

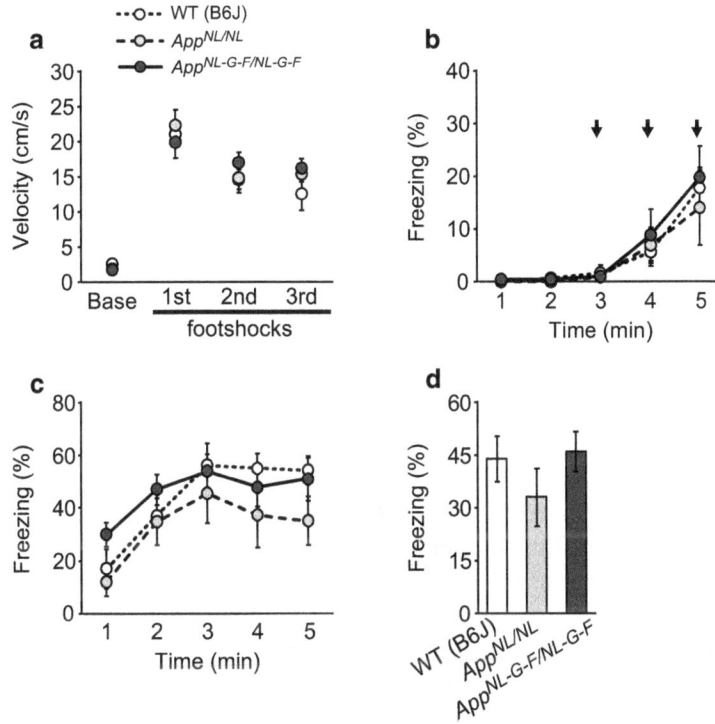

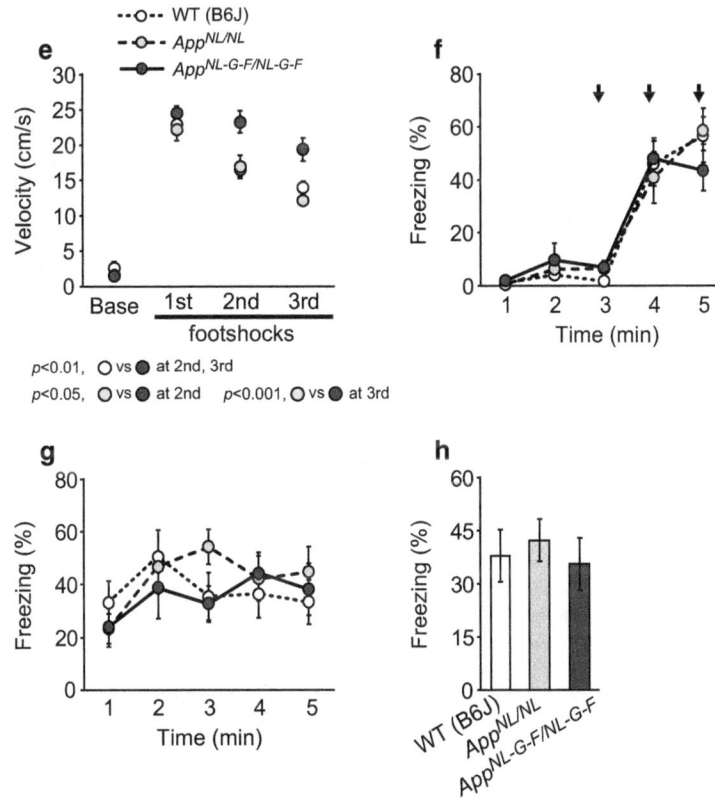

the target hole by extra-maze cues (Fig. 3a [middle]). To further assess cognitive flexibility, mice were subjected to the reversal learning task (five sessions) 1 day after the probe test (Fig. 3a [right]). And as mentioned in the experimental design above, the same group of mice was repeatedly tested at 4, 6, and 8 months of age in this BM task (Additional file 1: Fig. S1).

We found that $App^{NL/NL}$, $App^{NL-G-F/NL-G-F}$, and WT mice performed equally well in acquisition of the target hole in the BM at the ages of 4 months (Fig. 3b; $F[2, 20] = 3.12$, $p = 0.066$, Fig. 3c; $F[2, 20] = 0.48$, $p = 0.625$, Fig. 3d; $F[2, 20] = 1.10$, $p = 0.353$) and 6 months (Fig. 3g; $F[2, 20] = 1.27$, $p = 0.303$, Fig. 3h; $F[2, 20] = 2.80$, $p = 0.085$, Fig. 3i; $F[2, 20] = 0.24$, $p = 0.788$). The number of errors (Fig. 3b; $F[4, 80] = 23.21$, $p < 0.001$, Fig. 3g; $F[2.7, 54.8] = 10.07$, $p < 0.001$), latency (Fig. 3c; $F[1.9, 37.6] = 29.26$, $p < 0.001$, Fig. 3h; $F[1.7, 33.1] = 8.06$, $p = 0.002$), and distance (Fig. 3d; $F[2.3, 45.3] = 23.18$, $p < 0.001$, Fig. 3i; $F[2.8, 56.5] = 7.11$, $p = 0.001$) to reach the target hole significantly decreased as the session progressed, suggesting that all genotypes had similar learning ability.

In the probe test, all genotypes exhibited similar levels of preference toward the target quadrant that contained the target hole and the two adjacent holes at both 4 months (Fig. 3e; genotype, $F[2, 20] = 1.06$, $p = 0.365$; quadrant, $F[2.0, 40.3] = 49.06$, $p < 0.001$) and 6 months of age (Fig. 3j; genotype, $F[2, 20] = 1.56$, $p = 0.235$; quadrant, $F[1.6, 32.0] = 30.84$, $p < 0.001$). A percentage of time spent in the target quadrant for each genotype was significantly higher than chance level (25%) at both 4 months (Fig. 3e; WT, $t(14) = 6.59$, $p < 0.001$; $App^{NL/NL}$, $t(14) = 5.88$, $p < 0.001$; $App^{NL-G-F/NL-G-F}$, $t(12) = 3.28$, $p = 0.007$) and 6 months of age (Fig. 3j; WT, $t(14) = 3.91$, $p = 0.002$; $App^{NL/NL}$, $t(14) = 4.07$, $p = 0.001$; $App^{NL-G-F/NL-G-F}$, $t(12) = 3.22$, $p = 0.007$). Moreover, all genotypes exhibited similar levels of exploration of the holes in the target quadrant, with

no differences in general exploratory activity, at both 4 months (Fig. 3f; (left) $F[2, 20] = 0.05$, $p = 0.949$; (right) $F[2, 20] = 1.03$, $p = 0.375$) and 6 months of age (Fig. 3k; (left) $F[2, 20] = 0.67$, $p = 0.524$; (right) $F[2, 20] = 0.75$, $p = 0.487$). These results suggest that both $App^{NL-G-F/NL-G-F}$ and $App^{NL/NL}$ mice had intact spatial learning and memory at 4 and 6 months of age.

At 8 months of age, $App^{NL-G-F/NL-G-F}$ mice exhibited a significant increase in the number of errors (Fig. 3l; $F[2, 18] = 5.34$, $p = 0.015$, post hoc, WT vs. $App^{NL-G-F/NL-G-F}$, $p = 0.015$), latency (Fig. 3m; $F[2, 18] = 10.28$, $p = 0.001$, post hoc, WT vs. $App^{NL-G-F/NL-G-F}$, $p < 0.001$), and distance (Fig. 3n; $F[2, 18] = 6.24$, $p = 0.009$, post hoc, WT vs. $App^{NL-G-F/NL-G-F}$, $p = 0.016$) in comparison with WT mice. However, $App^{NL-G-F/NL-G-F}$ mice still exhibited a significant decrease in the number of errors (Fig. 3l; $F[2.5, 45.2] = 11.47$, $p < 0.001$), latency (Fig. 3m; $F[1.4, 25.2] = 6.91$, $p = 0.008$), and distance (Fig. 3n; $F[2.1, 38.1] = 8.35$, $p = 0.001$), and were able to solve the task proficiently (at levels comparable to those of WT mice) by the fifth training session. These results suggest that 8-month-old $App^{NL-G-F/NL-G-F}$ mice have subtle alterations in their ability to learn the spatial location of the target hole.

In the probe test, all genotypes exhibited similar levels of preference toward the target quadrant (Fig. 3o; genotype, $F[2, 18] = 1.36$, $p = 0.283$; quadrant, $F[1.8, 31.9] = 38.63$, $p < 0.001$). The percentages of time spent in the target quadrant were significantly higher above chance level for WT and $App^{NL/NL}$ mice (Fig. 3o; WT, $t(14) = 6.00$, $p < 0.001$; $App^{NL/NL}$, $t(12) = 5.07$, $p < 0.001$), but not for $App^{NL-G-F/NL-G-F}$ mice ($t(10) = 2.11$, $p = 0.062$), with our sample size. The percentage of hole exploration in the target quadrant (Fig. 3p; (left) $F[2, 18] = 3.35$, $p = 0.058$) and the total number of hole visits (Fig. 3p; (right) $F[2, 18] = 0.35$, $p = 0.712$) were similar among all genotypes.

(See figure on next page.)

Fig. 3 Spatial learning and memory in $App^{NL-G-F/NL-G-F}$ and $App^{NL/NL}$ mice assessed by the Barnes maze task. Spatial learning and memory were assessed at 4 (**b–f**), 6 (**g–k**), and 8 (**i–p**) months of age. In the acquisition phase (**a** [left]), one hole (indicated by a gray hole) was designated as the target hole with an escape box. A probe test was performed 1 day after the last training session, in which the escape box was removed (**a** [middle]). The three black arrows indicate the target hole and adjacent holes, respectively. In the reversal phase (**a** [right]), the target hole was moved to the position opposite the original 1 day after the probe test. TQ: target quadrant; OQ: opposite quadrant; RQ: right quadrant; LQ: left quadrant. At 4 and 6 months of age, $App^{NL-G-F/NL-G-F}$ and $App^{NL/NL}$ mice performed as well as WT mice in acquisition of the target hole, as revealed by similar decreases in the number of errors (**b** and **g**), latency (**c** and **h**), and distance (**d** and **i**) across the acquisition phase. In the probe test, all genotypes exhibited similar levels of preference toward the target quadrant (TQ) above chance level (25%, as indicated by dotted lines) (**e** and **j**) and similar levels of exploration of the holes in the target quadrant (**f** [left] and **k** [left]) with no differences in exploratory activity (**f** [right] and **k** [right]). At 8 months of age, $App^{NL-G-F/NL-G-F}$ mice made more errors (**l**), took more time (**m**), and travelled farther (**n**) to reach the target hole than WT mice throughout the acquisition phase. In the probe test, WT and $App^{NL/NL}$ mice exhibited significant preference toward the target quadrant (TQ) above chance level (25%, as indicated by dotted lines) (**o**). All genotypes exhibited similar levels of exploration of the holes in the target quadrant (**p** [left]), with no alterations in general activity (**p** [right]). 4 month-old; n = 8 WT (B6J), n = 8 $App^{NL/NL}$, n = 7 $App^{NL-G-F/NL-G-F}$. 6 month-old; n = 8 WT (B6J), n = 8 $App^{NL/NL}$, n = 7 $App^{NL-G-F/NL-G-F}$. 8 month-old; n = 8 WT (B6J), n = 7 $App^{NL/NL}$, n = 6 $App^{NL-G-F/NL-G-F}$. ##$p < 0.01$, ###$p < 0.001$ versus chance level

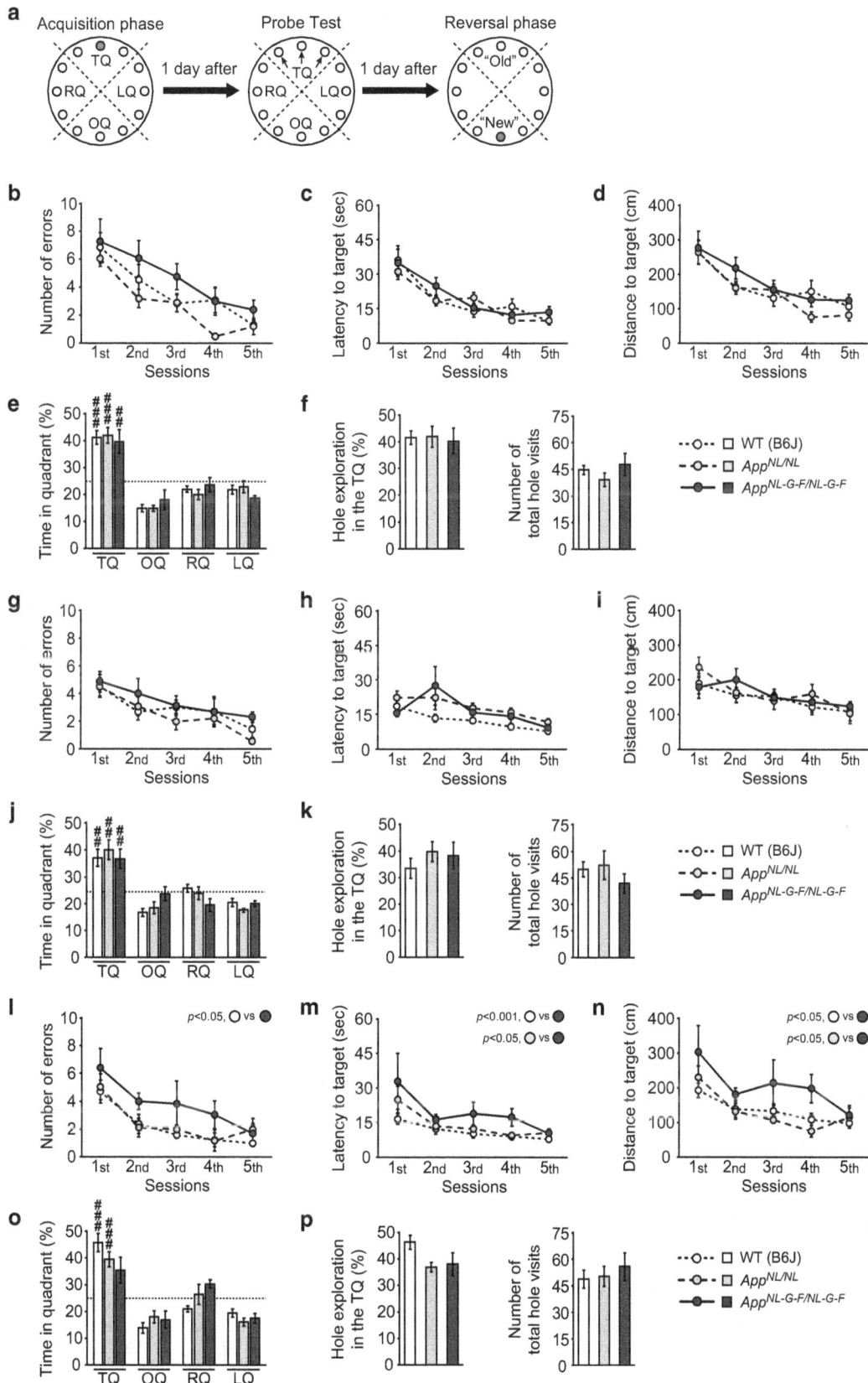

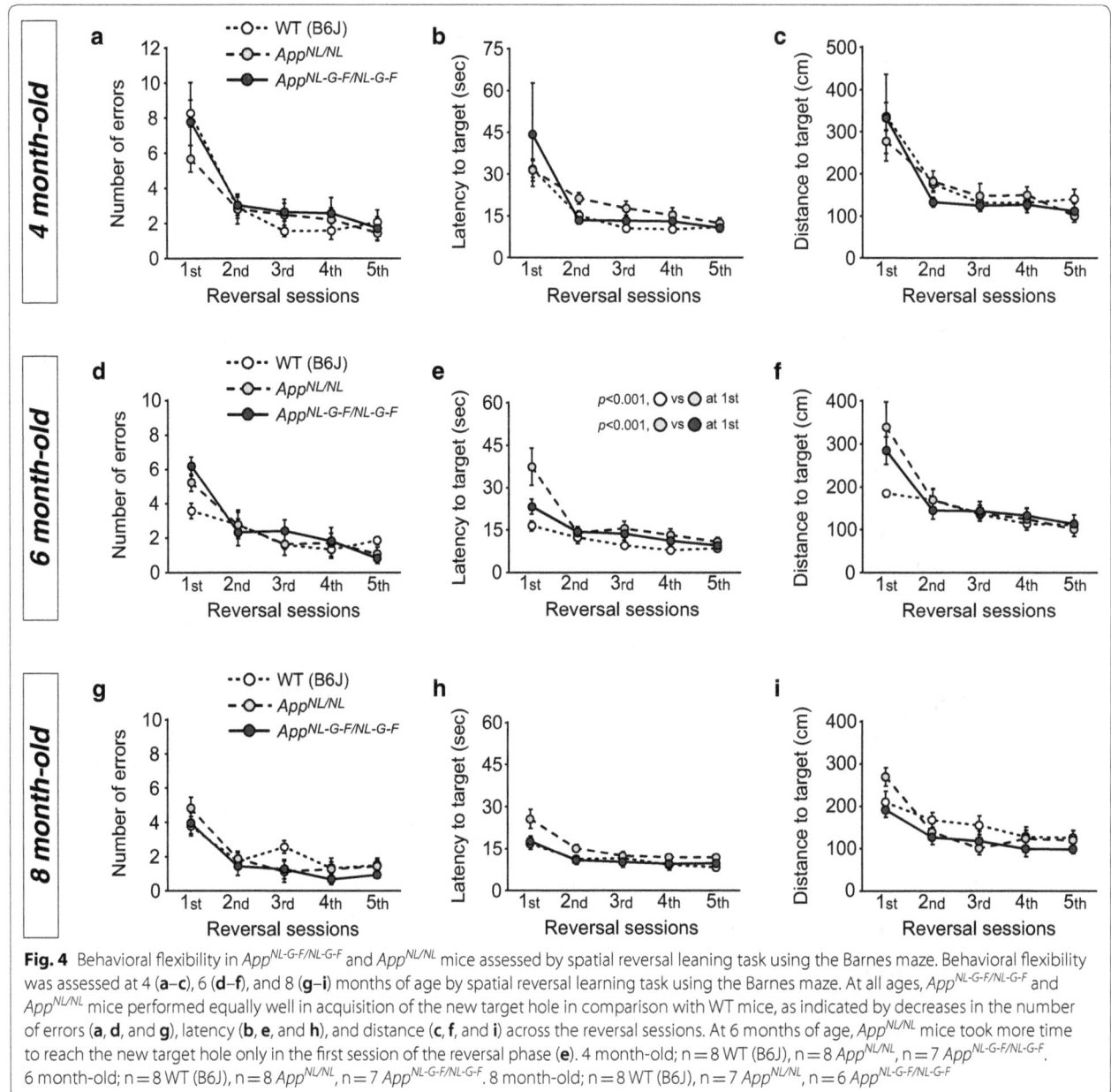

Fig. 4 Behavioral flexibility in $App^{NL-G-F/NL-G-F}$ and $App^{NL/NL}$ mice assessed by spatial reversal leaning task using the Barnes maze. Behavioral flexibility was assessed at 4 (**a–c**), 6 (**d–f**), and 8 (**g–i**) months of age by spatial reversal learning task using the Barnes maze. At all ages, $App^{NL-G-F/NL-G-F}$ and $App^{NL/NL}$ mice performed equally well in acquisition of the new target hole in comparison with WT mice, as indicated by decreases in the number of errors (**a**, **d**, and **g**), latency (**b**, **e**, and **h**), and distance (**c**, **f**, and **i**) across the reversal sessions. At 6 months of age, $App^{NL/NL}$ mice took more time to reach the new target hole only in the first session of the reversal phase (**e**). 4 month-old; n = 8 WT (B6J), n = 8 $App^{NL/NL}$, n = 7 $App^{NL-G-F/NL-G-F}$. 6 month-old; n = 8 WT (B6J), n = 8 $App^{NL/NL}$, n = 7 $App^{NL-G-F/NL-G-F}$. 8 month-old; n = 8 WT (B6J), n = 7 $App^{NL/NL}$, n = 6 $App^{NL-G-F/NL-G-F}$

Taken together, these results suggest that, at 8 months of age, $App^{NL-G-F/NL-G-F}$ mice exhibit reduced spatial learning ability in comparison with WT mice, but still retain normal spatial memory.

Both $App^{NL-G-F/NL-G-F}$ and $App^{NL/NL}$ mice exhibit normal flexibility in a reversal learning task up to 8 months of age

Reversal learning, a way to model some aspects of higher-order cognitive functions in rodents [44, 45], requires cognitive flexibility and impulse control, and thus taps into components of human executive function [46, 47]. Previous studies demonstrated that transgenic mouse models of Aβ amyloidosis are impaired in reversal learning [48–50]. To assess reversal learning using the BM, we moved the target hole to the opposite position 1 day after the probe test (Fig. 3a [right]).

We found that both $App^{NL-G-F/NL-G-F}$ and $App^{NL/NL}$ mice exhibited similar levels of performance in the reversal learning task in comparison with WT mice at 4 months (Fig. 4a; $F[2, 20] = 0.35$, $p = 0.711$, Fig. 4b; $F[2, 20] = 0.87$, $p = 0.434$, Fig. 4c; $F[2, 20] = 0.32$, $p = 0.733$), 6 months (Fig. 4d; $F[2, 20] = 0.38$, $p = 0.690$, Fig. 4e; $F[2, 20] = 6.31$, $p = 0.008$, Fig. 4f; $F[2, 20] = 1.73$, $p = 0.202$), and 8 months of age (Fig. 4g; $F[2, 18] = 0.66$, $p = 0.530$, Fig. 4h; $F[2, 18] = 3.00$, $p = 0.075$, Fig. 4i; $F[2, 18] = 1.41$, $p = 0.269$).

The number of errors (Fig. 4a; $F[1.8, 36.4] = 28.55$, $p < 0.001$, Fig. 4d; $F[2.5, 49.8] = 30.91$, $p < 0.001$, Fig. 4g; $F[2.2, 40.0] = 28.20$, $p < 0.001$), latency (Fig. 4b; $F[1.1, 22.9] = 13.28$, $p = 0.001$, Fig. 4e; $F[1.3, 25.6] = 24.78$, $p < 0.001$, Fig. 4h; $F[2.1, 38.6] = 29.80$, $p < 0.001$) and distance (Fig. 4c; $F[1.5, 29.1] = 20.47$, $p < 0.001$, Fig. 4f; $F[1.4, 28.6] = 21.32$, $p < 0.001$, Fig. 4i; $F[2.4, 42.7] = 21.93$, $p < 0.001$) to the new target hole were progressively reduced in all genotypes and at all ages, suggesting that both $App^{NL-G-F/NL-G-F}$ and $App^{NL/NL}$ mice could adjust their response to find the new location as effectively as WT mice.

We noticed that 6-month-old $App^{NL/NL}$ mice spent more time to reach the new target hole than WT mice at the first session of the reversal phase (Fig. 4e; genotype × session, $F[2.6, 25.6] = 3.47$, $p = 0.037$, simple main effect on first session, $p < 0.001$, post hoc, WT vs. $App^{NL/NL}$, $p < 0.001$). However, no significant change in the latency was detected at the second session (simple main effect on second session, $p = 0.833$). Moreover, no such difference was observed in the 8-month-old $App^{NL/NL}$ mice (Fig. 4h).

Taken together, these results suggest that both $App^{NL-G-F/NL-G-F}$ and $App^{NL/NL}$ mice exhibit normal cognitive flexibility in the reversal learning task up to 8 months of age.

Discussion

Aβ amyloidosis, tau aggregation, neuroinflammation, neurodegeneration, and cognitive deficits are defining features of AD. To date, multiple transgenic mouse models overexpressing human APP with familial AD mutations have been shown to develop age-dependent Aβ amyloidosis, neuroinflammation, and cognitive impairments in spatial memory and contextual fear memory [6, 7, 51]. However, these APP-overexpressing mouse models may have pathophysiological properties caused by non-physiological overexpression of APP, in addition to Aβ pathology [11].

To overcome this issue, several App-KI mouse models have been generated that recapitulate Aβ pathology without APP overexpression. The first reported App-KI line, App^{NLh} mice, harbor the Swedish mutation with humanized Aβ sequences in the murine App gene locus. Although App^{NLh} mice do not develop Aβ pathology, the double KI line interbred with mutant $Psen1^{P264L/P264L}$ KI line ($App^{NLh/NLh} × Psen1^{P264L/P264L}$ mice) progressively develop Aβ pathology and cognitive impairments with no alterations in locomotor activity and anxiety-related behavior [52, 53]. More recently developed App^{DSL} mice harbor three familial

AD-associated mutations (Swedish, London, and Dutch) with a humanized Aβ sequence in the murine App locus [54]. Similar to the App^{NLh} mice, App^{DSL} mice do not develop Aβ pathology independently, but do so when interbred with $Psen1^{M146V}$ KI mice. The double KI line $App^{DSL/DSL} × Psen1^{M146V/M146V}$ also exhibits elevated levels of anxiety, followed by deficits in spatial learning and memory [54]. However, these earlier App-KI mouse models required homozygous expression of familial AD mutant Psen1 alleles to obtain Aβ deposition [52, 54, 55], and the potential effects of homozygous mutation in Psen1 on observed phenotypes must be considered.

By contrast, $App^{NL-G-F/NL-G-F}$ mice exhibit progressive amyloid pathology, including microglial and astrocytic activation and loss of synaptic markers, in the absence of Psen1 mutation [12, 18]. Reports of cognitive deficits in $App^{NL-G-F/NL-G-F}$ mice have varied between laboratories [12, 25, 26], although mild impairment in spatial reversal learning and enhanced impulsivity have been detected using an automated IntelliCage apparatus [18]. These results suggest that, despite aggressive Aβ pathology and neuroinflammation, cognitive alterations in $App^{NL-G-F/NL-G-F}$ mice are modest.

Consistent with these previous studies, our results demonstrated that neither $App^{NL-G-F/NL-G-F}$ nor $App^{NL/NL}$ mice exhibited severe memory deficits in the CFC (Fig. 2) or BM tasks (Fig. 3). However, we detected a subtle decline in spatial learning ability in $App^{NL-G-F/NL-G-F}$ mice at the age of 8 months (Fig. 3). Because the learning deficits were not evident at younger ages (4 and 6 months of age), this may represent an aspect of age-dependent cognitive impairment in $App^{NL-G-F/NL-G-F}$ mice. Moreover, alterations in acquisition of spatial information may occur before the onset of memory deficit in $App^{NL-G-F/NL-G-F}$ mice. In our experimental design, the BM task was not run at a similar age range to the EPM and CFC tasks (Additional file 1: Fig. S1). To clarify whether $App^{NL-G-F/NL-G-F}$ mice show more dramatic deficits in spatial learning and memory during aging, it would be important to examine a spatial task after 8 months of age.

Several previous studies have shown that commonly used transgenic models such as the Tg2576 and $App^{Swe}/Psen1^{dE9}$ mice exhibit deficits in spatial learning in the BM [41–43]. Of particular interest, the TgCRND8 mouse model exhibit poor spatial learning in the BM task [56], while they also have deficits in attentional control [57]. Given that attentional deficits are likely to influence performance on memory tasks, it is conceivable that reduced attentional control of $App^{NL-G-F/NL-G-F}$ mice [18] might have contributed to alterations in spatial learning ability in our BM task.

In this study, we repeatedly subjected the same group of mice to the BM task until the age of 8 months (Additional file 1: Fig. S1), suggesting that mice might become familiar with the rules and environment of the maze. In fact, habituation of the testing environment and rule learning by repeated exposure to the maze resulted in the fewer errors at the age of 8 months in comparison with younger ages (Figs. 3 and 4). Thus, as suggested by a previous study in $App^{Swe}/Psen1^{dE9}$ mice using the BM task [42], these processes might be compromised in 8-month-old $App^{NL-G-F/NL-G-F}$ mice, which may lead to observed spatial learning impairment. These results also suggest that the experimental strategy testing App-KI mouse models in the BM task without prior test experience is likely to yield different results observed in this study.

In addition to cognitive deficits, 60–80% of AD cases are associated with non-cognitive neuropsychiatric symptoms [58, 59], including anxiety disturbances, depressive symptoms, activity disturbances, and aggression [60–62]. For example, some AD patients are subjected to anxiety, whereas the opposite tendency (disinhibition) has also been reported [60, 61]. Intriguingly, several APP-overexpressing mouse models exhibit anxiety disturbances [7, 24] and an increase in open arm exploration has been observed in several APP-overexpressing mouse models with parenchymal Aβ plaques, including APP23, Tg2576, and $App^{Swe}/Psen1^{dE9}$ mice [24].

A very recent study reported anxiolytic-like behavior in $App^{NL-G-F/NL-G-F}$ mice in comparison with $App^{NL/NL}$ mice, detectable from 3 months of age [25]. Similarly, we found that $App^{NL-G-F/NL-G-F}$ mice exhibited anxiolytic-like behavior in comparison with WT mice (Fig. 1). These data from App-KI mice suggest that anxiolytic-like behaviors observed in mouse models of Aβ amyloidosis are associated with Aβ-mediated pathologies [24, 53] rather than overexpression of APP. Interestingly, some mouse models with traumatic brain injury exhibit increases in open arm exploration in the EPM task, followed by elevated levels of reactive gliosis and cerebrovascular dysfunction [63–66]. Another study demonstrated that local neuroinflammation within the dorsal raphe nucleus, resulting in serotonergic hypofunction, caused the same behavioral consequences in the EPM task [67]. Because elevated levels of reactive gliosis are associated with Aβ pathology in $App^{NL-G-F/NL-G-F}$ mice [12], these pathological changes (including neuroinflammatory responses and vascular dysfunction) may play a role in the expression of anxiolytic-like behavior.

We also noticed that activity of $App^{NL-G-F/NL-G-F}$ mice was slightly higher than that of WT mice in the EPM task (Fig. 1 and Additional file 2: Fig. S2), raising a possibility that there may be a general increase in locomotor activity in $App^{NL-G-F/NL-G-F}$ mice. However, in the CFC task, $App^{NL-G-F/NL-G-F}$ mice were rather less active than WT mice during the pre-shock period (Additional file 3:

Fig. S3). These results suggest that the hyperactive phenotypes observed in the EPM task may be elicited by an aversive situation, rather than an innate behavioral trait in $App^{NL-G-F/NL-G-F}$ mice.

We also found that $App^{NL/NL}$ mice, which do not develop Aβ pathology, exhibited lower open arm durations at 15–18 months of age, suggesting elevated anxiety levels in these mice. A previous study also reported that transgenic mice overexpressing APP^{Swe} without Aβ pathology exhibited elevated anxiety levels in the same EPM paradigm [24, 68]. Increased anxiety levels in these mice are not due to overproduction of N- or C-terminal fragment-β (NTF-β or CTF-β) of APP, as demonstrated by the observation that $App^{NL-G-F/NL-G-F}$ mice exhibited anxiolytic-like behavior, whereas Tg13592 mice overexpressing CTF-β did not exhibit altered anxiety levels in comparison with their non-transgenic controls [69]. Although $App^{NL/NL}$ mice develop neither Aβ pathology nor neuroinflammatory response, they have dramatically increased levels of soluble Aβ in comparison with WT mice. Thus, higher levels of soluble Aβ may induce changes in synaptic functions, which may be responsible for emotional control in these KI mice. Hyperanxious behavior in the EPM task is often associated with alterations in several neurotransmitter systems, including γ-aminobutyric acid (GABA)ergic and serotonergic neurotransmission [70, 71]. Thus, altered neurotransmission caused by high levels of soluble Aβ may contribute to the expression of anxiogenic-like behavior in $App^{NL/NL}$ mice.

Conclusion
Our results demonstrate that $App^{NL-G-F/NL-G-F}$ and $App^{NL/NL}$ mice exhibit behavioral changes associated with non-cognitive, emotional domains before the onset of definitive cognitive deficits. These observations consistently indicate that $App^{NL-G-F/NL-G-F}$ mice represent a model for preclinical AD and that they are useful for the study of AD prevention rather than treatment after neurodegeneration. This study provides information that will be critical for both translational and basic research for AD using $App^{NL-G-F/NL-G-F}$ and $App^{NL/NL}$ mice.

Methods
Animals
The original lines of App-KI ($App^{NL-G-F/NL-G-F}$ and $App^{NL/NL}$) mice were established as C57BL/6J congenic line (a genetic background strain) by repeated backcrosses as described previously [12] and obtained from RIKEN Center for Brain Science (Wako, Japan). All experiments were performed with male $App^{NL-G-F/NL-G-F}$, $App^{NL/NL}$ and WT (C57BL/6J) mice at the Institute for Animal Experimentation in National Center for Geriatrics and Gerontology. After weaning at postnatal day

(PND) 28–35, all mice were housed socially in same-sex groups in a temperature-controlled environment under a 12-h light/dark cycle (lights on at 7:00, lights off at 19:00), with food and water available ad libitum. We prepared four independent groups of male mice with mixed genotypes ($App^{NL-G-F/NL-G-F}$, $App^{NL/NL}$, and WT) and assessed cognitive and emotional domains using three behavioral paradigms at different ages (Additional file 1: Fig. S1). All handling and experimental procedures were performed in accordance with the Guidelines for the Care of Laboratory Animals of National Center for Geriatrics and Gerontology (Obu, Japan). All animals were euthanized with intraperitoneal barbiturate overdose (sodium pentobarbital, 120 mg/kg body weight) after each behavioral experiment.

Elevated plus maze task

The apparatus consisted of two opposing open arms (25 × 5 cm) and two opposing closed arms (25 × 5 cm, surrounded by 15 cm-high transparent walls) that extended from a center platform (5 × 5 cm) forming a cross shape (O'hara & Co., Tokyo, Japan) [72]. The maze was elevated 50 cm above the floor with a light intensity on the center platform of approximately 100 lx. To avoid falls, the open arms were surrounded by a 0.3 cm-high rim. On the test day, 6–9-($n = 8$/genotype) and 15–18-($n = 10$–12/genotype) month-old mice were placed individually in the center platform facing an open arm and allowed to freely explore the apparatus for 10 min. At the end of the first trial, the mice were returned to their homecage and socially housed until the beginning of the second trial. The apparatus was cleaned with distilled water and then ethanol to remove any odor cues between subject mice. All animals were retested after 10–27 days from the first trial. Time spent on open arms (s), total distance travelled (cm) and numbers of open and closed arm entries were automatically measured by the ANY-Maze video tracking software (Stoelting Co., IL, USA) [73]. The number of open and closed arm entries was combined to yield a measure of total arm entries, which reflected general exploratory activity during the test. Open arm entries were analyzed as a percentage score by dividing the number of open arm entries by the total number of arm entries (% Entries into open arms = [Number of open arm entries/Number of total arm entries] × 100).

Contextual fear conditioning task

Mice were handled for 3 days prior to the commencement of contextual fear conditioning. The mice were trained and tested in conditioning chambers (17 × 10 × 10 cm) with a stainless-steel grid floor (0.2 cm diameter, spaced 0.5 cm apart; O'hara & Co., Tokyo, Japan) [72] surrounded by a sound-attenuating

white chest (approximately 200 lx in the chest) with a background noise (55 dB). On the conditioning day, 6–9-($n = 6$–9/genotype) and 15–18-($n = 7$–8/genotype) month-old mice were individually placed in the conditioning chamber and allowed to explore freely for 3 min. At the end of this 3-min period, a mild footshock (0.5 mA, 2 s) was presented. Two more footshocks were presented with a 1-min inter-stimulus interval, and then the mice were returned to their home cage at 30 s after the last footshock. One day after the conditioning, mice were placed in the same chamber and allowed to explore freely for 5 min without footshock administration. The chambers were cleaned with distilled water and then ethanol to remove any odor cues between subject mice. In each test, percentage of freezing time and distance travelled (cm) were calculated automatically using ImageFZ software (O'hara & Co., Tokyo, Japan). To assess sensitivity or reactivity to footshock, we also calculated the velocity during each footshock presentation and an equivalent baseline period (actual 2-s period just prior to the first footshock), based on distance travelled during a given time period, since it has been suggested to be the most sensitive aspect of shock reactivity [34, 74, 75].

Barnes maze task

The Barnes circular maze task was conducted on a white circular surface (1.0 m in diameter, with 12 holes equally spaced around the perimeter; O'hara & Co., Tokyo, Japan) [72]. The circular open field was elevated 75 cm above the floor with a light intensity on the center of the circular open field of approximately 1000 lx. A black acrylic escape box (17 × 13 × 7 cm) was located under one of the holes, and the hole above the escape box represented the target hole. The location of the target hole was consistent for a given mouse, and mice within a squad were assigned to the same target hole location across the sessions. Trials were administered in a spaced fashion so that all mice within a squad completed a given trial before subsequent trials were run. The maze was rotated 90° between trials, with the spatial location of the target hole unchanged with respect to the distal visual room cues, to prevent a bias based on olfactory or proximal cues within the maze. After each trial, the apparatus including the cylinder and escape box were cleaned carefully with distilled water and then ethanol to eliminate any potential odor cues.

One day after the habituation to familiarize mice with the maze and the escape box, they were subjected to 5 days training sessions (four trials per session). The same group of mice was repeatedly tested at 4, 6 and 8 months of age (Additional file 1: Fig. S1). During the acquisition phase, 4-($n = 7$–8/genotype), 6-($n = 7$–8/genotype) and 8-($n = 6$–8/genotype) month-old mice were individually placed in a white acrylic cylinder

(17 cm-high, 11 cm diameter) before the start of each trial, and after approximately 30 s the cylinder was removed to start the trial. Each trial ended when the mouse entered the escape box or after 5 min had elapsed. The mice that could not find the target hole were guided to the hole manually and allowed to enter the escape box to remain there for 1 min. For each trial, the number of errors, latency (s) and distance travelled (cm) to reach the target hole were automatically measured by custom-written software in MATLAB (The MathWorks, Inc., MA, USA). In our software, target zones were defined to include each separate hole and 1 cm around them. We recorded an error when a mouse touched a target zone that did not have an escape box beneath it.

One day after the last training session, a probe test was conducted without the escape box for 3 min, to confirm that this spatial task was acquired based on navigation by distal environmental cues. The time spent in each quadrant (TQ; target quadrant, OQ; opposite quadrant, RQ; right quadrant, LQ; left quadrant) (s) and numbers of the visits to the target hole and two adjacent holes (indicated by black arrows in Fig. 3a) and total hole visits during the test were measured by the software. Hole exploration in the target quadrant was defined by percentage of the visits to three holes in the target quadrant for total hole visits during the test.

For reversal leaning task (reversal phase), the target was moved to a new position opposite to the original 1 day after the probe test, and mice were retrained in 5 days reversal sessions to find the new location of the escape box. During the reversal phase, the number of errors, latency (s), and distance travelled (cm) to reach the new target were also calculated by the software.

Statistical analysis

Statistical differences between genotypes against behavioral parameters with one dependent variable were determined by repeated-measures analysis of variance (ANOVA). When necessary, Greenhouse–Geisser estimates of sphericity were used to correct for degrees of freedom. Bonferroni post hoc comparisons were used to evaluate group differences. For the comparisons of multiple means with genotypes as one independent variable, one-way ANOVA followed by the Tukey's post hoc tests was used. One-sample t test was used to compare performance on the probe test of the Barnes maze task against chance level (25%). Data are presented as means $\pm$ SEM. All alpha levels were set at 0.05.

Additional files

Additional file 1: Fig. S1. Time course of experimental procedures for assessing cognitive and emotional domains in *App*-KI mice. Based on pathological information about the brains of $App^{NL-G-F/NL-G-F}$ mice, cognitive and emotional domains in *App*-KI mice were assessed at different ages using three behavioral assays. The same group of mice (Group 4) was assessed at 4, 6 and 8 months of age for spatial learning and memory and behavioral flexibility using the Barnes maze (BM) task, and at 15–18 months of age for contextual fear memory using the contextual fear conditioning (CFC) task. Time courses of brain pathology in $App^{NL-G-F/NL-G-F}$ mice are shown based on previous studies.

Additional file 2: Fig. S2. Locomotor activity of $App^{NL-G-F/NL-G-F}$ and $App^{NL/NL}$ mice during the first and second trials in the elevated plus maze task. The distance travelled during the 10-min test of the first and second trials in the elevated plus maze task was compared among genotypes at both 6–9 (**a–d**) and 15–18 (**e–h**) months of age. Representative images of movement tracks during the first and second trials for each genotype at 6–9 (**a** and **c**) and 15–18 (**e** and **g**) months of age were shown (closed arms are indicated by shaded areas). At 6–9 months of age, $App^{NL-G-F/NL-G-F}$ mice exhibited slight increases in distance travelled during the first (**b**) and second (**d**) trials in comparison with WT mice. By contrast, locomotor activity in $App^{NL/NL}$ mice was comparable with WT mice in the two trials. At 15–18 months of age, $App^{NL-G-F/NL-G-F}$ mice exhibited a slight increase in movement compared to WT mice during the first (**f**) and second (**g**) trials. $App^{NL/NL}$ mice moved at similar levels compared with WT mice in the two trials. 6–9 month-old; n = 8 WT (B6J), n = 8 $App^{NL/NL}$, n = 8 $App^{NL-G-F/NL-G-F}$. 15–18 month-old; n = 12 WT (B6J), n = 10 $App^{NL/NL}$, n = 11 $App^{NL-G-F/NL-G-F}$. $\dagger p < 0.05$ versus $App^{NL/NL}$.

Additional file 3: Fig. S3. Locomotor activity in $App^{NL-G-F/NL-G-F}$ and $App^{NL/NL}$ mice during the pre-shock period in the contextual fear conditioning task. The distance travelled during the pre-shock period (3-min period just prior to the first footshock) in conditioning was compared among genotypes at both 6–9 (**a** and **b**) and 15–18 (**c** and **d**) months of age. Representative images of movement tracks during the pre-shock period in each genotype at 6–9 (**a**) and 15–18 (**c**) months of age were shown. At 6–9 months of age, $App^{NL-G-F/NL-G-F}$ mice exhibited a slight decrease in distance travelled during the pre-shock period in comparison with WT mice (**b**). At 15–18 months of age, $App^{NL/NL}$ mice exhibited a significant decrease in distance travelled during the pre-shock period in comparison with WT mice (**d**). Locomotor activity in $App^{NL-G-F/NL-G-F}$ mice was also slightly decreased in comparison with WT mice. 6–9 month-old; n = 6 WT (B6 J), n = 6 $App^{NL/NL}$, n = 9 $App^{NL-G-F/NL-G-F}$. 15–18 month-old; n = 8 WT (B6 J), n = 7 $App^{NL/NL}$, n = 7 $App^{NL-G-F/NL-G-F}$. $*p < 0.05$ versus WT (B6J).

Abbreviations

AD: Alzheimer's disease; APP: amyloid precursor protein; Aβ: amyloid-β; NFT: neurofibrillary tangle; KI: knock-in; WT: wild-type; EPM: elevated plus maze; CFC: contextual fear conditioning; BM: Barnes maze; ANOVA: analysis of variance; CTF-β: C-terminal fragment-β; NTF-β: N-terminal fragment-β; GABA: γ-aminobutyric acid.

Authors' contributions

YS, MS and KMI conceived the experiments, YS conducted the experiment, YS, MS and KMI analyzed and interpret the data. TS and TCS provided the *App*-KI mice and interpret the data. YS, MS and KMI wrote the paper. All authors critically reviewed the manuscript. All authors read and approved the final manuscript.

Author details
[1] Department of Alzheimer's Disease Research, Center for Development of Advanced Medicine for Dementia, National Center for Geriatrics and Gerontology, Obu, Aichi 474-8511, Japan. [2] Laboratory for Proteolytic Neuroscience, RIKEN Center for Brain Science, Wako, Saitama 351-0198, Japan. [3] Department of Experimental Gerontology, Graduate School of Pharmaceutical Sciences, Nagoya City University, Nagoya 467-8603, Japan.

Acknowledgements
We thank Drs. Yosefu Arime and Kaichi Yoshizaki for statistical advice and comments on the manuscript and Drs. Nobuyuki Kimura and Katsuhiko Yanagisawa for the comments on the data. We also thank Dr. Akihiko Takashima for letting us use the Barnes maze and Dr. Tetsuya Kimura for technical assistance on analyzing data by the MATLAB software.

Competing interests
The authors declare that they have no competing interests.

Funding
This study was supported by the Research Funding for Longevity Science from National Center for Geriatrics and Gerontology, Japan, Grant No. 28-26 and Takeda Science Foundation (JP) (to KMI).

References
1. Scheltens P, Blennow K, Breteler MM, de Strooper B, Frisoni GB, Salloway S, Van der Flier WM. Alzheimer's disease. Lancet. 2016;388(10043):505–17.
2. Winblad B, Amouyel P, Andrieu S, Ballard C, Brayne C, Brodaty H, Cedazo-Minguez A, Dubois B, Edvardsson D, Feldman H, et al. Defeating Alzheimer's disease and other dementias: a priority for European science and society. Lancet Neurol. 2016;15(5):455–532.
3. Braak H, Braak E. Demonstration of amyloid deposits and neurofibrillary changes in whole brain sections. Brain Pathol. 1991;1(3):213–6.
4. Hyman BT, Phelps CH, Beach TG, Bigio EH, Cairns NJ, Carrillo MC, Dickson DW, Duyckaerts C, Frosch MP, Masliah E, et al. National Institute on Aging–Alzheimer's Association guidelines for the neuropathologic assessment of Alzheimer's disease. Alzheimers Dement. 2012;8(1):1–13.
5. Serrano-Pozo A, Frosch MP, Masliah E, Hyman BT. Neuropathological alterations in Alzheimer disease. Cold Spring Harb Perspect Med. 2011;1(1):a006189.
6. Puzzo D, Gulisano W, Palmeri A, Arancio O. Rodent models for Alzheimer's disease drug discovery. Expert Opin Drug Discov. 2015;10(7):703 11.
7. Webster SJ, Bachstetter AD, Nelson PT, Schmitt FA, Van Eldik LJ. Using mice to model Alzheimer's dementia: an overview of the clinical disease and the preclinical behavioral changes in 10 mouse models. Front Genet. 2014;5:88.
8. Balducci C, Forloni G. APP transgenic mice: their use and limitations. Neuromolecular Med. 2011;13(2):117–37.
9. Kitazawa M, Medeiros R, Laferla FM. Transgenic mouse models of Alzheimer disease: developing a better model as a tool for therapeutic interventions. Curr Pharm Des. 2012;18(8):1131–47.
10. Gidyk DC, Deibel SH, Hong NS, McDonald RJ. Barriers to developing a valid rodent model of Alzheimer's disease: from behavioral analysis to etiological mechanisms. Front Neurosci. 2015;9:245.
11. Sasaguri H, Nilsson P, Hashimoto S, Nagata K, Saito T, De Strooper B, Hardy J, Vassar R, Winblad B, Saido TC. APP mouse models for Alzheimer's disease preclinical studies. EMBO J. 2017;36(17):2473–87.
12. Saito T, Matsuba Y, Mihira N, Takano J, Nilsson P, Itohara S, Iwata N, Saido TC. Single App knock-in mouse models of Alzheimer's disease. Nat Neurosci. 2014;17(5):661–3.
13. Citron M, Oltersdorf T, Haass C, McConlogue L, Hung AY, Seubert P, Vigo-Pelfrey C, Lieberburg I, Selkoe DJ. Mutation of the beta-amyloid precursor protein in familial Alzheimer's disease increases beta-protein production. Nature. 1992;360(6405):672–4.
14. Guardia-Laguarta C, Pera M, Clarimon J, Molinuevo JL, Sanchez-Valle R, Llado A, Coma M, Gomez-Isla T, Blesa R, Ferrer I, et al. Clinical, neuropathologic, and biochemical profile of the amyloid precursor protein I716F mutation. J Neuropathol Exp Neurol. 2010;69(1):53–9.
15. Lichtenthaler SF, Wang R, Grimm H, Uljon SN, Masters CL, Beyreuther K. Mechanism of the cleavage specificity of Alzheimer's disease gamma-secretase identified by phenylalanine-scanning mutagenesis of the transmembrane domain of the amyloid precursor protein. Proc Natl Acad Sci USA. 1999;96(6):3053–8.
16. Hashimoto T, Adams KW, Fan Z, McLean PJ, Hyman BT. Characterization of oligomer formation of amyloid-beta peptide using a split-luciferase complementation assay. J Biol Chem. 2011;286(31):27081–91.
17. Tsubuki S, Takaki Y, Saido TC. Dutch, Flemish, Italian, and Arctic mutations of APP and resistance of Aβ to physiologically relevant proteolytic degradation. Lancet. 2003;361(9373):1957–8.
18. Masuda A, Kobayashi Y, Kogo N, Saito T, Saido TC, Itohara S. Cognitive deficits in single App knock-in mouse models. Neurobiol Learn Mem. 2016;135:73–82.
19. Zhang H, Sun S, Wu L, Pchitskaya E, Zakharova O, Fon Tacer K, Bezprozvanny I. Store-operated calcium channel complex in postsynaptic spines: a new therapeutic target for Alzheimer's disease treatment. J Neurosci. 2016;36(47):11837–50.
20. Zhang H, Wu L, Pchitskaya E, Zakharova O, Saito T, Saido T, Bezprozvanny I. Neuronal store-operated calcium entry and mushroom spine loss in amyloid precursor protein knock-in mouse model of Alzheimer's disease. J Neurosci. 2015;35(39):13275–86.
21. Nakazono T, Lam TN, Patel AY, Kitazawa M, Saito T, Saido TC, Igarashi KM. Impaired in vivo gamma oscillations in the medial entorhinal cortex of knock-in Alzheimer model. Front Syst Neurosci. 2017;11:48.
22. Huang Y, Skwarek-Maruszewska A, Horre K, Vandewyer E, Wolfs L, Snellinx A, Saito T, Radaelli E, Corthout N, Colombelli J, et al. Loss of GPR3 reduces the amyloid plaque burden and improves memory in Alzheimer's disease mouse models. Sci Transl Med. 2015;7(309):309ra164.
23. Kidana K, Tatebe T, Ito K, Hara N, Kakita A, Saito T, Takatori S, Ouchi Y, Ikeuchi T, Makino M, et al. Loss of kallikrein-related peptidase 7 exacerbates amyloid pathology in Alzheimer's disease model mice. EMBO Mol Med. 2018;10:e8184.
24. Lalonde R, Fukuchi K, Strazielle C. APP transgenic mice for modelling behavioural and psychological symptoms of dementia (BPSD). Neurosci Biobehav Rev. 2012;36(5):1357–75.
25. Latif-Hernandez A, Shah D, Craessaerts K, Saido T, Saito T, De Strooper B, Van der Linden A, D'Hooge R. Subtle behavioral changes and increased prefrontal-hippocampal network synchronicity in APP(NL-G-F) mice before prominent plaque deposition. Behav Brain Res. 2017. https://doi.org/10.1016/j.bbr.2017.11.017.
26. Whyte LS, Hemsley KM, Lau AA, Hassiotis S, Saito T, Saido TC, Hopwood JJ, Sargeant IJ. Reduction in open field activity in the absence of memory deficits in the AppNL-G-F knock-in mouse model of Alzheimer's disease. Behav Brain Res. 2018;336:177–81.
27. Bourin M. Animal models for screening anxiolytic-like drugs: a perspective. Dialogues Clin Neurosci. 2015;17(3):295–303.
28. Carobrez AP, Bertoglio LJ. Ethological and temporal analyses of anxiety-like behavior: the elevated plus-maze model 20 years on. Neurosci Biobehav Rev. 2005;29(8):1193–205.
29. Calzavara MB, Patti CL, Lopez GB, Abilio VC, Silva RH, Frussa-Filho R. Role of learning of open arm avoidance in the phenomenon of one-trial tolerance to the anxiolytic effect of chlordiazepoxide in mice. Life Sci. 2005;76(19):2235–46.
30. Jurgenson M, Aonurm-Helm A, Zharkovsky A. Behavioral profile of mice with impaired cognition in the elevated plus-maze due to a

deficiency in neural cell adhesion molecule. Pharmacol Biochem Behav. 2010;96(4):461–8.

31. Bertoglio LJ, Carobrez AP. Previous maze experience required to increase open arms avoidance in rats submitted to the elevated plus-maze model of anxiety. Behav Brain Res. 2000;108(2):197–203.

32. Maren S, Phan KL, Liberzon I. The contextual brain: implications for fear conditioning, extinction and psychopathology. Nat Rev Neurosci. 2013;14(6):417–28.

33. Tovote P, Fadok JP, Luthi A. Neuronal circuits for fear and anxiety. Nat Rev Neurosci. 2015;16(6):317–31.

34. Shoji H, Takao K, Hattori S, Miyakawa T. Contextual and cued fear conditioning test using a video analyzing system in mice. J Vis Exp. 2014;85:e50871.

35. Dineley KT, Xia X, Bui D, Sweatt JD, Zheng H. Accelerated plaque accumulation, associative learning deficits, and up-regulation of alpha 7 nicotinic receptor protein in transgenic mice co-expressing mutant human presenilin 1 and amyloid precursor proteins. J Biol Chem. 2002;277(25):22768–80.

36. Hamann S, Monarch ES, Goldstein FC. Impaired fear conditioning in Alzheimer's disease. Neuropsychologia. 2002;40(8):1187–95.

37. Hoefer M, Allison SC, Schauer GF, Neuhaus JM, Hall J, Dang JN, Weiner MW, Miller BL, Rosen HJ. Fear conditioning in frontotemporal lobar degeneration and Alzheimer's disease. Brain. 2008;131(Pt 6):1646–57.

38. Knafo S, Venero C, Merino-Serrais P, Fernaud-Espinosa I, Gonzalez-Soriano J, Ferrer I, Santpere G, DeFelipe J. Morphological alterations to neurons of the amygdala and impaired fear conditioning in a transgenic mouse model of Alzheimer's disease. J Pathol. 2009;219(1):41–51.

39. Harrison FE, Reiserer RS, Tomarken AJ, McDonald MP. Spatial and nonspatial escape strategies in the Barnes maze. Learn Mem. 2006;13(6):809–19.

40. Sharma S, Rakoczy S, Brown-Borg H. Assessment of spatial memory in mice. Life Sci. 2010;87(17–18):521–36.

41. O'Leary TP, Brown RE. Visuo-spatial learning and memory deficits on the Barnes maze in the 16-month-old APPswe/PS1dE9 mouse model of Alzheimer's disease. Behav Brain Res. 2009;201(1):120–7.

42. Reiserer RS, Harrison FE, Syverud DC, McDonald MP. Impaired spatial learning in the APPSwe + PSEN1DeltaE9 bigenic mouse model of Alzheimer's disease. Genes Brain Behav. 2007;6(1):54–65.

43. Yassine N, Lazaris A, Dorner-Ciossek C, Despres O, Meyer L, Maitre M, Mensah-Nyagan AG, Cassel JC, Mathis C. Detecting spatial memory deficits beyond blindness in tg2576 Alzheimer mice. Neurobiol Aging. 2013;34(3):716–30.

44. Floresco SB, Jentsch JD. Pharmacological enhancement of memory and executive functioning in laboratory animals. Neuropsychopharmacology. 2011;36(1):227–50.

45. Humby T, Wilkinson LS. Assaying dissociable elements of behavioural inhibition and impulsivity: translational utility of animal models. Curr Opin Pharmacol. 2011;11(5):534–9.

46. Chudasama Y. Animal models of prefrontal-executive function. Behav Neurosci. 2011;125(3):327–43.

47. Stopford CL, Thompson JC, Neary D, Richardson AM, Snowden JS. Working memory, attention, and executive function in Alzheimer's disease and frontotemporal dementia. Cortex. 2012;48(4):429–46.

48. Filali M, Lalonde R, Theriault P, Julien C, Calon F, Planel E. Cognitive and non-cognitive behaviors in the triple transgenic mouse model of Alzheimer's disease expressing mutated APP, PS1, and Mapt (3xTg-AD). Behav Brain Res. 2012;234(2):334–42.

49. Papadopoulos P, Rosa-Neto P, Rochford J, Hamel E. Pioglitazone improves reversal learning and exerts mixed cerebrovascular effects in a mouse model of Alzheimer's disease with combined amyloid-beta and cerebrovascular pathology. PLoS ONE. 2013;8(7):e68612.

50. Zhuo JM, Prakasam A, Murray ME, Zhang HY, Baxter MG, Sambamurti K, Nicolle MM. An increase in Aβ42 in the prefrontal cortex is associated with a reversal-learning impairment in Alzheimer's disease model Tg2576 APPsw mice. Curr Alzheimer Res. 2008;5(4):385–91.

51. Ameen-Ali KE, Wharton SB, Simpson JE, Heath PR, Sharp P, Berwick J. Review: neuropathology and behavioural features of transgenic murine models of Alzheimer's disease. Neuropathol Appl Neurobiol. 2017;43(7):553–70.

52. Flood DG, Reaume AG, Dorfman KS, Lin YG, Lang DM, Trusko SP, Savage MJ, Annaert WG, De Strooper B, Siman R, et al. FAD mutant PS-1

53. Webster SJ, Bachstetter AD, Van Eldik LJ. Comprehensive behavioral characterization of an APP/PS-1 double knock-in mouse model of Alzheimer's disease. Alzheimers Res Ther. 2013;5(3):28.

54. Li H, Guo Q, Inoue T, Polito VA, Tabuchi K, Hammer RE, Pautler RG, Taffet GE, Zheng H. Vascular and parenchymal amyloid pathology in an Alzheimer disease knock-in mouse model: interplay with cerebral blood flow. Mol Neurodegener. 2014;9:28.

55. Reaume AG, Howland DS, Trusko SP, Savage MJ, Lang DM, Greenberg BD, Siman R, Scott RW. Enhanced amyloidogenic processing of the beta-amyloid precursor protein in gene-targeted mice bearing the Swedish familial Alzheimer's disease mutations and a "humanized" Abeta sequence. J Biol Chem. 1996;271(38):23380–8.

56. Walker JM, Fowler SW, Miller DK, Sun AY, Weisman GA, Wood WG, Sun GY, Simonyi A, Schachtman TR. Spatial learning and memory impairment and increased locomotion in a transgenic amyloid precursor protein mouse model of Alzheimer's disease. Behav Brain Res. 2011;222(1):169–75.

57. Romberg C, Horner AE, Bussey TJ, Saksida LM. A touch screen-automated cognitive test battery reveals impaired attention, memory abnormalities, and increased response inhibition in the TgCRND8 mouse model of Alzheimer's disease. Neurobiol Aging. 2013;34(3):731–44.

58. Craig D, Mirakhur A, Hart DJ, McIlroy SP, Passmore AP. A cross-sectional study of neuropsychiatric symptoms in 435 patients with Alzheimer's disease. Am J Geriatr Psychiatry. 2005;13(6):460–8.

59. Lyketsos CG, Sheppard JM, Steinberg M, Tschanz JA, Norton MC, Steffens DC, Breitner JC. Neuropsychiatric disturbance in Alzheimer's disease clusters into three groups: the Cache County study. Int J Geriatr Psychiatry. 2001;16(11):1043–53.

60. Chung JA, Cummings JL. Neurobehavioral and neuropsychiatric symptoms in Alzheimer's disease: characteristics and treatment. Neurol Clin. 2000;18(4):829–46.

61. Hart DJ, Craig D, Compton SA, Critchlow S, Kerrigan BM, McIlroy SP, Passmore AP. A retrospective study of the behavioural and psychological symptoms of mid and late phase Alzheimer's disease. Int J Geriatr Psychiatry. 2003;18(11):1037–42.

62. Shin IS, Carter M, Masterman D, Fairbanks L, Cummings JL. Neuropsychiatric symptoms and quality of life in Alzheimer disease. Am J Geriatr Psychiatry. 2005;13(6):469–74.

63. Logsdon AF, Lucke-Wold BP, Turner RC, Li X, Adkins CE, Mohammad AS, Huber JD, Rosen CL, Lockman PR. A mouse model of focal vascular injury induces astrocyte reactivity, tau oligomers, and aberrant behavior. Arch Neurosci. 2017;4(2):e44254.

64. Mannix R, Berglass J, Berkner J, Moleus P, Qiu J, Andrews N, Gunner G, Berglass L, Jantzie LL, Robinson S, et al. Chronic gliosis and behavioral deficits in mice following repetitive mild traumatic brain injury. J Neurosurg. 2014;121(6):1342–50.

65. Mouzon BC, Bachmeier C, Ojo JO, Acker CM, Ferguson S, Paris D, Ait-Ghezala G, Crynen G, Davies P, Mullan M, et al. Lifelong behavioral and neuropathological consequences of repetitive mild traumatic brain injury. Ann Clin Transl Neurol. 2018;5(1):64–80.

66. Ojo JO, Mouzon B, Algamal M, Leary P, Lynch C, Abdullah L, Evans J, Mullan M, Bachmeier C, Stewart W, et al. Chronic repetitive mild traumatic brain injury results in reduced cerebral blood flow, axonal injury, gliosis, and increased t-tau and tau oligomers. J Neuropathol Exp Neurol. 2016;75(7):636–55.

67. Howerton AR, Roland AV, Bale TL. Dorsal raphe neuroinflammation promotes dramatic behavioral stress dysregulation. J Neurosci. 2014;34(21):7113–23.

68. Savonenko AV, Xu GM, Price DL, Borchelt DR, Markowska AL. Normal cognitive behavior in two distinct congenic lines of transgenic mice hyperexpressing mutant APP SWE. Neurobiol Dis. 2003;12(3):194–211.

69. Lalonde R, Dumont M, Fukuchi K, Strazielle C. Transgenic mice expressing the human C99 terminal fragment of betaAPP: effects on spatial learning, exploration, anxiety, and motor coordination. Exp Gerontol. 2002;37(12):1401–12.

70. Cryan JF, Sweeney FF. The age of anxiety: role of animal models of anxiolytic action in drug discovery. Br J Pharmacol. 2011;164(4):1129–61.

71. Olivier JD, Vinkers CH, Olivier B. The role of the serotonergic and GABA system in translational approaches in drug discovery for anxiety disorders. Front Pharmacol. 2013;4:74.

gene-targeted mice: increased Aβ42 and Aβ deposition without APP overproduction. Neurobiol Aging. 2002;23(3):335–48.

72. Shoji H, Takao K, Hattori S, Miyakawa T. Age-related changes in behavior in C57BL/6 J mice from young adulthood to middle age. Mol Brain. 2016;9:11.

73. Sakakibara Y, Kasahara Y, Hall FS, Lesch KP, Murphy DL, Uhl GR, Sora I. Developmental alterations in anxiety and cognitive behavior in serotonin transporter mutant mice. Psychopharmacology (Berlin). 2014;231(21):4119–33.

74. Anagnostaras SG, Josselyn SA, Frankland PW, Silva AJ. Computer-assisted behavioral assessment of Pavlovian fear conditioning in mice. Learn Mem. 2000;7(1):58–72.

75. Anagnostaras SG, Wood SC, Shuman T, Cai DJ, Leduc AD, Zurn KR, Zurn JB, Sage JR, Herrera GM. Automated assessment of pavlovian conditioned freezing and shock reactivity in mice using the video freeze system. Front Behav Neurosci. 2010;4:158.

9

Transcranial direct current stimulation for the treatment of tinnitus

Tifei Yuan[1,2], Ali Yadollahpour[3*] ⓘ, Julio Salgado-Ramírez[4], Daniel Robles-Camarillo[5] and Rocío Ortega-Palacios[4]

Abstract

Background: Tinnitus is the perception of sound in the absence of any external acoustic stimulation. Transcranial direct current stimulation (tDCS) has shown promising though heterogeneous therapeutic outcomes for tinnitus. The present study aims to review the recent advances in applications of tDCS for tinnitus treatment. In addition, the clinical efficacy and main mechanisms of action of tDCS on suppressing tinnitus are discussed.

Methods: The study was performed in accordance with the PRISMA guidelines. The databases of the PubMed (1980–2018), Embase (1980–2018), PsycINFO (1850–2018), CINAHL, Web of Science, BIOSIS Previews (1990–2018), Cambridge Scientific Abstracts (1990–2018), and google scholar (1980–2018) using the set search terms. The date of the most recent search was 20 May, 2018. The randomized controlled trials that have assessed at least one therapeutic outcome measured before and after tDCS intervention were included in the final analysis.

Results: Different tDCS protocols were used for tinnitus ranging single to repeated sessions (up to 10) consisting of daily single session of 15 to 20-min and current intensities ranging 1–2 mA. Dorsolateral prefrontal cortex (DLPFC) and auditory cortex are the main targets of stimulation. Both single and repeated sessions showed moderate to significant treatment effects on tinnitus symptoms. In addition to improvements in tinnitus symptoms, the tDCS interventions particularly bifrontal DLPFC showed beneficial outcomes on depression and anxiety comorbid with tinnitus. Heterogeneities in the type of tinnitus, tDCS devices, protocols, and site of stimulation made the systematic reviews of the literature difficult. However, the current evidence shows that tDCS can be developed as an adjunct or complementary treatment for intractable tinnitus. TDCS may be a safe and cost-effective treatment for tinnitus in the short-term application.

Conclusions: The current literature shows moderate to significant therapeutic efficacy of tDCS on tinnitus symptoms. Further randomized placebo-controlled double-blind trials with large sample sizes are needed to reach a definitive conclusion on the efficacy of tDCS for tinnitus. Future studies should further focus on developing efficient disease- and patient-specific protocols.

Keywords: Transcranial direct current stimulation, Tinnitus, Treatment, Clinical efficacy

*Correspondence: Yadollahpour.a@gmail.com
[3] Department of Medical Physics, School of Medicine, Ahvaz Jundishapur University of Medical Sciences, Golestan Blvd, Ahvaz 61357-33118, Iran
Full list of author information is available at the end of the article

Background

Tinnitus is the perception of sound, in the ear or in the head, in the absence of any external acoustic stimulation which affects 10–15% of the adult population worldwide [1, 2]. The main risk factors of tinnitus include hearing loss, trauma to the auditory periphery such as a lesion to auditory nerve, abnormal plastic changes in auditory network, ototoxic medications, head injury, and depression [3]. Hearing loss is not necessarily a precondition of tinnitus; however, some studies have shown that different forms of hearing loss may have correlation with tinnitus [2, 4]. This disorder is usually accompanied by different mild to severe comorbidities such as depression, anxiety, and sleep disturbances that make it a debilitating condition [1, 2, 5].

Neuroimaging, neuroelectrophysiologic, and neuroanatomic studies have shown that maladaptive plastic changes in different auditory and non-auditory cerebral regions and abnormal neural activities of specific cortical regions might be the main etiology of tinnitus [6–10]. Tinnitus perception is an integrated output of a large and complicated brain network comprising of different subnetworks with overlapping functions [2, 11]. In this impaired network, each subnetwork represents a clinical aspect of tinnitus such as distress, loudness, and laterality [11–13]. Neurobiological and neuroimaging findings have shown that abnormal activities of the non-auditory regions associated with cognitive and attentional functions as well as limbic processes probably contribute to the unpleasant and distressing aspects of tinnitus [11, 14]. Structural and functional abnormalities in dorsolateral prefrontal cortex (DLPFC) [10, 15–17] and auditory cortex (AC) [2, 3, 18, 19] are associated with tinnitus. The DLPFC is a multifunction region that plays important roles in auditory processing and perception, auditory attention, top-down modulation of auditory processing, and modulating the input to primary AC [20–22]. Moreover, DLPFC is involved in regulating different cognitive functions. Therefore, in development of any treatment modality for tinnitus, this disorder should be considered as a complex and heterogamous condition involving a large network consisting of multiple overlapping brain networks. Considering the engagements of AC and DLPFC in the tinnitus perception, these regions may be good targets for any therapeutic intervention for tinnitus.

Several pharmacologic agents have been developed for tinnitus treatment; however, a large portion of the patients are resistant to the treatment [1]. In addition, most of the pharmacologic drugs are associated with different side effects that adversely influence the individual's daily and quality of life. So far, no definitive treatment has been proposed for tinnitus and several common causes of tinnitus remain elusive. In this regard, studies are ongoing to develop new efficient therapeutic modalities for tinnitus in two avenues including pharmacologic agents and non-pharmacologic modalities.

During the recent decades, several non-pharmacological modalities such as cognitive behavioral therapies [23], noise-masking modality [24], and neurofeedback [25] have been proposed for treatment of tinnitus; however, they have limited treatment efficacy and each of them have their own drawbacks.

Applications of brain stimulation and modulation techniques have been dramatically developed during the recent decade for treatment and management of neuropsychiatric disorders [26–31]. These modalities including repetitive transcranial magnetic stimulation (rTMS), deep brain stimulation, and electrical stimulation have shown promising outcomes in the disorders in which the abnormal neural activities and impaired neural interfaces are the main characteristics [26–30]. This significant contribution of neural stimulation and modulation modalities is mostly because of mutual interactions between the endogenous and exogenous electrical and magnetic fields. The therapeutic values of electric and magnetic fields have been reported in different disorders that support the above claim [32–35].

RTMS has shown therapeutic effects in tinnitus through eliminating the tinnitus symptoms and also improving the cognitive impairments comorbid with tinnitus [36–38]. However, this technique is relatively expensive and associated with side effects with lower mobility.

Transcranial direct current stimulation (tDCS) is a form of neuromodulation in which a low intensity direct current passes the brain tissues through a pair of electrodes placed on the scalp. The tDCS is a noninvasive, safe, cost-effective, and user friendly modality which has shown promising outcomes in treatment of different neuropsychiatric disorders as well as in improving cognitive functions in healthy individuals [39–43].

Tinnitus is associated by abnormal neural activities in different brain regions and also maladaptive neuroplasticity of specific regions. Therefore, tDCS applied over specific brain regions with appropriate anodal/cathodal placement has been expected to have beneficial effects for this disorder. Anodal and cathodal tDCS respectively increases (depolarizes) and reduces (hyperpolarizes) the cortical excitability of the exposed regions [44].

Several preclinical and clinical studies have been conducted on tinnitus and the initial findings were promising though controversial [45–48]. Studies are ongoing to reach a definitive answer on the clinical efficacy of tDCS in tinnitus.

Studies are ongoing to develop effective clinical protocols and to understand the mechanisms of action.

The present study aims to review the recent advances in applications of tDCS for tinnitus treatment. In addition, the clinical efficacy and the main mechanisms of action of the technique are discussed.

Methods

The databases of the PubMed (1980–2018), Embase (1980–2018), PsycINFO (1850 –2018), CINAHL, Web of Science, BIOSIS Previews (1990–2018), Cambridge Scientific Abstracts (1990–2018), and google scholar (1980–2018) using the set search terms. The study procedures were performed according to the guidelines of the PRISMA. The search terms were "transcranial direct current stimulation" OR "tDCS" AND "tinnitus" AND "treatment". The date of the most recent search was 20 May 2018. Bibliographies of the retrieved records and review articles were manually reviewed to identify the records that may have been missed in the initial search. The titles, abstracts, and keywords of all retrieved records were reviewed and the eligible records were entered in the final review based on the inclusion and exclusion criteria. Only published, peer-reviewed studies on human subjects available in English were considered for this review. The studies that investigated the treatment of different types of tinnitus with different tDCS devices and in different protocols against sham condition were included in the review. Studies of randomized controlled trials were included.

The studies should have assessed at least one therapeutic outcome measured before and after an intervention. The studies that assessed only cognitive measures, studies on animal and healthy subjects were also excluded. Clinical trials without a randomized controlled design, conference abstracts, narrative reviews, and editorials were excluded from the review.

Results

A total of 85 studies were identified at the screening step. In the identification phase, total of 33 records were excluded from the further assessment and 53 records were entered into the screening phase in which 8 conference abstracts, 1 book, 2 case reports and 4 editorials were excluded from the review. In the eligibility stage, 31 records remained in the study and 3 records from the additional records were added into the study where total of 34 studies were included for detailed review. Due to the heterogeneities in the patients and the tDCS devices and protocols as well as the target sides, the authors decided to comprehensively review the studies. The review focuses on the advances in applications of tDCS for treatment of tinnitus and the important factors in the resulting outcomes. In addition, the mechanisms of

actions of the tDCS in tinnitus treatment are discussed (Fig. 1).

Discussion

Tinnitus is a heterogeneous disorder in which several regions are involved in the tinnitus-related anomalies ranging primary and secondary auditory systems as well as non-auditory brain areas.

The general hypothesis in application of tDCS for treatment of tinnitus like other neuropsychiatric disorders is that anodal tDCS increases the neural excitability, whereas cathodal tDCS decreases it. As a result: anodal tDCS with excitatory effect can be applied on the regions with hypo-activity associated with an impairment to reach beneficial outcome. Similarly, cathodal tDCS that induces inhibitory effect can be applied over the regions with disease specific hyper-activities to reach beneficial effects.

The main approach in choosing the target site and electrode placement in tDCS applications in different neuropsychiatric disorders is modulating the impaired region(s) of the brain to alter the activities or functions of the region(s) towards normal conditions. In this regard, for tinnitus, the main objective is modulating either the tinnitus percept or its affective aspects like distress through disrupting the underlying pathological neural activities. The general hypothesis is that anodal tDCS increases the neural excitability, whereas cathodal tDCS decreases it [44, 49–51]. As a result: anodal tDCS with excitatory effect can be applied on the regions with hypo-activity associated with an impairment to reach beneficial outcome [52]. Similarly, cathodal tDCS that induces inhibitory effect can be applied over the regions with disease specific hyper-activities to reach beneficial effects [52].

Considering the tinnitus features and the associations between tinnitus and the structural and functional abnormalities in DLPFC [10, 15–17] and AC [2, 3, 18, 19], these two sites were the main targets in the previous tDCS studies in tinnitus. Initial tDCS studies have targeted the AC for tinnitus treatment and the findings were promising though controversial [53–55]. Moreover, modulating DLPFC activity using tDCS has been shown to enhance different cognitive functions in healthy individual and to improve different neuropsychiatric disorders, including tinnitus [17, 39, 40, 56–58].

The two main sites targeted in the previous studies for treatment of tinnitus were DLPFC [13, 59, 60] and AC [45, 54, 61]. Fregni et al. conducted the first study investigating tDCS in tinnitus in which they compared the effects of cathodal tDCS, anodal tDCS, and 10-Hz rTMS against sham stimulation over two sites of mesial parietal cortex and left temporoparietal area (LTA)

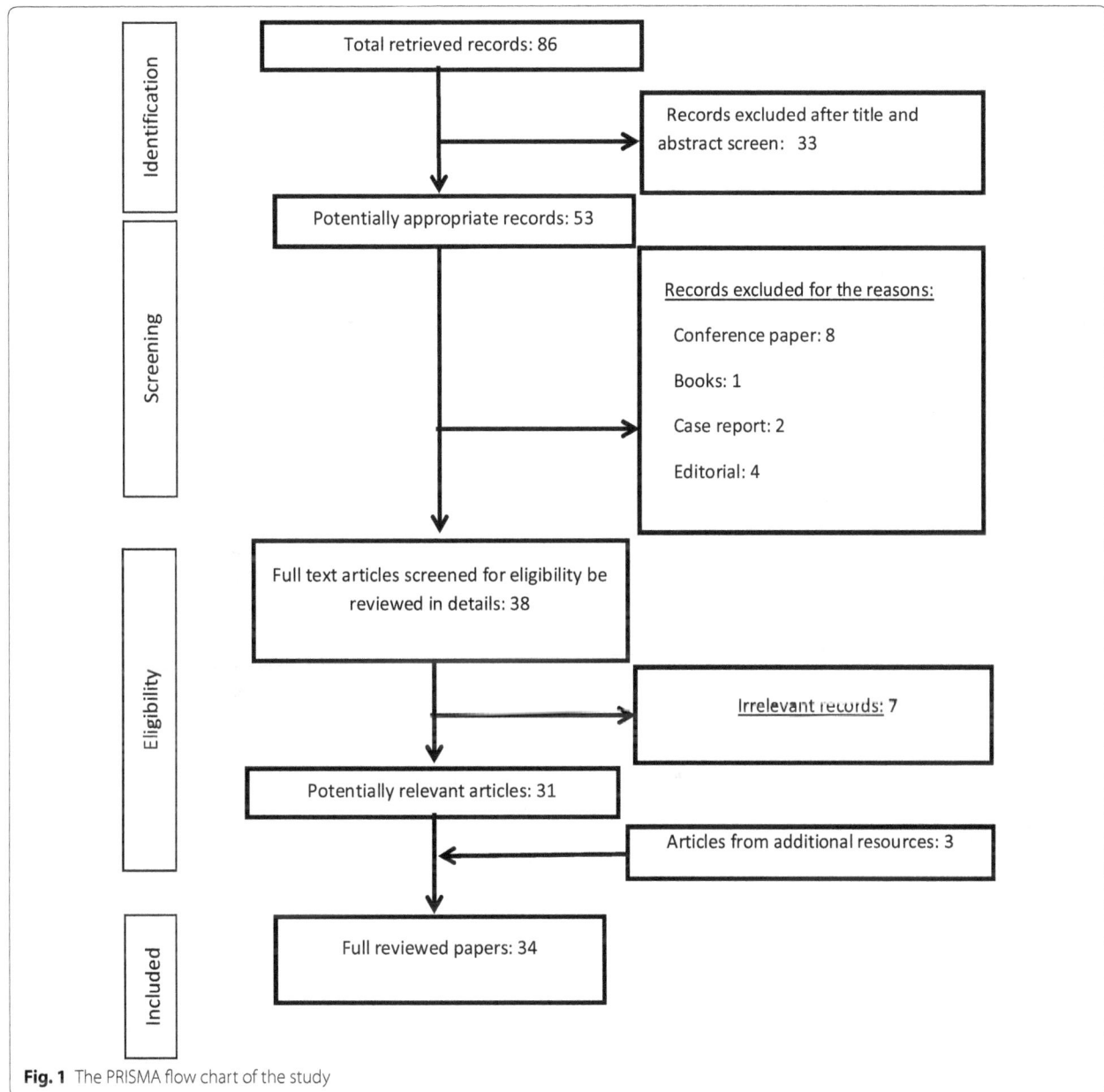

Fig. 1 The PRISMA flow chart of the study

on tinnitus symptoms [45]. They reported that 10 Hz rTMS and anodal tDCS of LTA significantly reduced the tinnitus symptoms; however, the effect was transient and short lasting. After this study, several clinical trials have been conducted to evaluate and develop the therapeutic efficacy of tDCS for treatment of tinnitus. Garin et al. investigated the outcomes of tDCS applied over LTA and reported significant improvements in tinnitus symptoms and interestingly they reported the beneficial effects lasted for several days in some patients [62]. Both Fregni et al. and Garin et al. reported that cathodal tDCS over the LTA with the

anode on the contralateral supraorbital area did not improve tinnitus symptoms.

Following these initial studies, other researchers have investigated the tDCS in single and repeated sessions over LTA and AC and reported controversial findings [54, 63, 64]. It seems that cathodal tDCS in single session is not effective on tinnitus treatment since cathodal tDCS is not strong enough to disturb or modulate the ongoing tinnitus-related abnormal cortical activities [65]. In this regard, repeated sessions of cathodal tDCS may have therapeutic effects on tinnitus based on the theoretical and experimental results. Therefore, repeated sessions of tDCS, longer period of each session and higher intensities have been designed to investigate the effects of cathodal tDCS in tinnitus [54, 60, 66, 67].

Following the initial studies focusing on temporoparietal area (TA) and AC, several studies have targeted prefrontal cortex (PFC), particularly DLPFC for tinnitus treatment. In these studies, the main target site was DLPFC and the most frequent electrode montage was bifrontal [13, 46, 59, 68]. Vanneste et al. were the first group reported the effects of bifrontal tDCS on tinnitus symptoms [13]. They investigated the effects of bifrontal tDCS over DLPFC (n = 478) in an open label study. They applied bifrontal tDCS (2 mA, each session 20 min) in two montages (anode right/cathode left (n = 448) and anode left/cathode right (n = 30) DLPFC) for 20 min. They reported no tinnitus-suppressing effect in the anode left/cathode right DLPFC tDCS. However, anode right/cathode left tDCS significantly reduced the tinnitus intensity or distress in 29.9% of the patients. In addition, they observed an interaction between the amount of distress reduction and the tinnitus laterality. However, they did not observe such interaction for the tinnitus intensity [13]. Vanneste et al. concluded that bifrontal tDCS could modulate the emotional aspects of tinnitus experienced by the patients [13].

The next studies conducted on bifrontal tDCS have reported that this montage both in anode left/cathode right or vice versa could improve the tinnitus-related depression and anxiety, respectively [47]. These effects could be attributed the roles of PFC and particularly DLPFC in modulating different non-auditory structures and networks involved in perception of the auditory and distress aspects of tinnitus as well as emotional functions.

To improve the tDCS protocol in targeting the optimal stimulation site for tinnitus treatment, De Ridder and Vanneste (n = 675) compared the efficacy of EEG-driven tDCS versus standard bifrontal tDCS [61]. They used source localized resting-state electrical activity to determine gamma-band functional connectivity as an index of the tinnitus network. On the one hand, the authors reported that standard bifrontal tDCS, with the anode right/cathode left DLPFC, significantly reduced tinnitus symptoms in 30% of the patients [61]. Moreover, the EEG-driven tDCS approach did not significantly improve the symptoms. The authors also tried to identify the mechanism of action of tDCS in suppressing the tinnitus symptoms through comparing the pre- and post-intervention of the source-localized resting-state electrical activity of the patients. They concluded that the tDCS induced changes are probably occurred through modulations of a large network consisting of pregenual anterior cingulate cortex, parahippocampal area, and right primary AC in resting-state

spontaneous brain activity. This study demonstrated that tDCS impacts both the direct target under the electrodes (DLPFC) and distant regions with functional connections with the exposed target [61]. This finding along with neuroimaging studies encourage further studies on the therapeutic outcomes of tDCS applied over non-auditory regions in tinnitus.

In line with the optimization of tDCS protocol for tinnitus, Shekhawat and Vanneste designed a trial to optimize the parameters of bifrontal tDCS over DLPFC for tinnitus suppression with the primary outcome of tinnitus loudness [68]. They designed a dose–response trial (n = 111) to optimize the current intensity (1.5 and 2 mA), stimulation duration (20 and 30 min), and number of tDCS sessions (2, 4, 6, 8, and 10 with 3–4 day washout period between each session). The patients received a minimum of 2 sessions during 1 week or maximum of 10 sessions during 5 weeks. Their findings showed a significant reduction in tinnitus loudness after DLPFC tDCS. The intensity and duration of each session did not show significant interaction with the outcome. In addition, they reported that increasing the number of sessions increases the amount of outcome, but after 6 sessions no further increase was observed and the amount of outcome reached a plateau trend [68].

Few studies have used different electrode montages than the previous studies triggering LTA or AC and DLPFC. For instance Pal et al. in a randomized, parallel, double-blind, sham-controlled study investigated the treatment efficacy and safety of cathodal tDCS to the AC with anode over the PFC [69]. They applied a 5-session tDCS over five consecutive days and assessed the tinnitus handicap inventory (THI) score as the primary outcome of tinnitus after the last session on day 5, and at 1 and 3 months post stimulation. They reported no beneficial effects of tDCS on the neither primary nor secondary outcome measures. Their findings showed that tDCS of the auditory and prefrontal cortices does not improve tinnitus but it is relatively safe protocol [69].

A line of studies have focused on combinations of tDCS with other treatment modalities including pharmacological and non-pharmacological modalities [63, 70]. Shekhawat et al. in a 7-month long double-blind randomized clinical trial investigated the effects of multisession anodal tDCS over LTA combined with the hearing aid sound therapy in patients with chronic tinnitus (n = 40). They applied anodal tDCS (2 mA intensity; 20-min duration) for 5 consecutive sessions with 24-h gap over the LTA, and then applied a hearing aid treatment for 6 months. Their findings showed a significant improvement in the overall Tinnitus Functional Index score as well as the tinnitus loudness and distress scores. They reported that after 3 months of hearing aid use, significant improvements were observed in tinnitus that were sustained at 6 months of use [63].

Teismann et al. investigated the effects of combined tailor-made notched music training (TMNMT) with tDCS on tinnitus symptoms. They applied TMNMT for 10 subsequent days (daily single session of 2.5 h). During the initial 30-min of the first 5 days of the TMNMT sessions, they concurrently applied tDCS (intensity: 2 mA) in anodal, cathodal, and sham groups. The active electrode was over the head surface over left AC; the reference electrode was put over right supraorbital cortex [70]. They observed a significant reduction in tinnitus handicap inventory (THI) score that reached its maximum value after the 5 days of treatment. The treatment effect remained significant for 31 days following the termination of the treatment. They also reported no significant difference between the anodal, cathodal, or sham tDCS groups.

It seems that tDCS over TA or AC may have greater therapeutic effects when combined with other non-medication modalities.

So far, most of the tDCS trials for tinnitus treatment have investigated the effects of single session tDCS on tinnitus symptoms. However, few studies have assessed the treatment effects of repeated sessions of tDCS on tinnitus symptoms. In these studies the number of total sessions ranged three to ten sessions consisting daily one session and current intensity ranging 1–2 mA and each session lasting 15 to 30 min. The main target sites in the tDCS applications in tinnitus treatment were temporal or temporoparietal (auditory) cortex [48, 54, 71, 72] and DLPFC [47, 55, 73]. The findings of these studies are promising though heterogeneous which encourage conducting further placebo-controlled randomized trials to shed more light on the clinical efficacy of the technique and mechanism of action involved in the effects. One important factor that should be further assessed in future studies is assessing the treatment outcomes for longer follow up periods since most of the previous studies have investigated the transient effects of tDCS and in few cases the after effect assessments were not beyond some hours.

Neuroimaging and neurobiological studies have demonstrated that the main features of tinnitus are hyperactivity and maladaptive plasticity in AC [2, 6, 9]. In tinnitus there are specific neural changes that start at the cochlear nucleus and project to the AC and non-auditory brain regions. The main cause of these neural anomalies is maladaptive neural plasticity. This maladaptive plasticity increases spontaneous firing rates of and synchrony among neurons in primary and secondary auditory systems that may generate the phantom percept. In addition to the abnormal neural activities and maladaptive plasticity present in the primary and secondary

ACs, disturbances in non-auditory brain structures and networks such as the insula, anterior cingulate cortex, and the DLPFC have been proposed as other possible pathologies of tinnitus [6, 8–10, 13, 18, 74, 75]. The perception of tinnitus has been reportedly as an integrated output of a complex tinnitus network consisting of different regions and subnetworks. It is assumed that each subnetwork of this network represents a clinical aspect of tinnitus such as distress, loudness, laterality, etc.

There are different hypotheses proposed to explain the therapeutic outcomes of tDCS in tinnitus symptoms. The first hypothesis is based on the disturbing theory of an ongoing neural activity associated with tinnitus. It is hypothesized that tDCS disturbs the abnormal ongoing neural activity induced by tinnitus. The second hypothesis is changing the maladaptive plasticity of tinnitus through repeated sessions of tDCS. Previous studies have shown that repeated sessions of tDCS depending on the polarity of the electrode could reduce or increase the neural excitability of the exposed regions and the resulting changes persist beyond the tDCS intervention [44, 76]. This altered excitability can lead to neuroplasticity with therapeutic effects for tinnitus [52]. Therefore, in the treatment of tinnitus with tDCS, the main idea is modulating the abnormal excitability in the auditory pathways and maladaptive plasticity in auditory and limbic cortexes through applying single or repeated sessions of tDCS. The clinical trials conducted so far have shown that single and repeated sessions of tDCS applied over DLPFC or AC may induce transient and long lasting therapeutic effects in tinnitus patients. The early studies have investigated the effects of single session tDCS and reported transient beneficial effect, but the effects did not last more than some hours.

Some evidence showed that the tDCS effects on tinnitus symptoms are probably induced through modulations of a large neural network comprising of pregenual anterior cingulate cortex, parahippocampal area, and right primary AC in resting-state spontaneous brain activity [61]. According to this hypothesis, the tDCS influences both the direct target under the electrodes and distant regions with functional connections with the direct target [61].

Most of the previous studies have investigated the physical parameters of tDCS to develop effective treatment protocols for tinnitus and also in other neuropsychiatric disorders including the electrode size, polarity, electrode placement and configuration, current amplitude and density, treatment duration, number of sessions and total dose. Findings of the recent studies as well as neuroimaging and neuroelectrophysiologic studies showed that tinnitus is a heterogeneous disease with different disease-specific features. It seems that in addition to the physical parameters of tDCS, the patient- and disease-specific factors including gender, audiometric variables, severity of tinnitus, tinnitus laterality and type, illness duration, and audiometric features of the patients might be important in exerting and/or the amount of therapeutic effects [47, 59, 60]. Therefore, at least one line of the future tDCS studies for treatment of tinnitus should focus on developing disease specific of tDCS protocols.

Conclusions

This study reviewed the advances in using tDCS for treatment of tinnitus and discussed the therapeutic efficacy of the technique and the main mechanisms of action in treatment of tinnitus symptoms and therapeutic effects. Reviewing the current clinical trials showed that tDCS has moderate and promising treatment outcomes in the treatment of tinnitus. In addition, tDCS has shown beneficial effects on different cognitive impairments comorbid with tinnitus including anxiety and depression. However, so far there is no standard tDCS protocol for tinnitus treatment for clinical applications.

The main limitations of the conducted trials are small sample size, heterogeneities in patients and treatment protocols, poor methodology design, as well as the heterogeneous nature of tinnitus.

To develop efficient tDCS protocols for tinnitus, the roles of specific features of patient and tinnitus such as audiometric features of the patients, tinnitus laterality, tinnitus type, and tinnitus duration should be evaluated as well as the effects of the stimulation parameters. Further prospective, randomized, placebo-controlled, double-blind studies with large sample sizes are needed to reach a definitive conclusion on the efficacy of tDCS for tinnitus patients. Future studies should focus on developing efficient disease- and patient-specific protocols.

Abbreviations

AC: auditory cortex; LTA: left temporoparietal area; PFC: prefrontal cortex; PRISMA: preferred reporting items for systematic reviews and meta-analyses; rTMS: repetitive transcranial magnetic stimulation; TA: temporoparietal area; tDCS: transcranial direct current stimulation; THI: tinnitus handicap inventory; TMNMT: tailor-made notched music training.

Authors' contributions

Conceptualization and design, TY and AY JS-R and DR-C and RO-P; Data acquisition, TY and AY and JS-R and DR-C and RO-P; Analysis and interpretation, TY and AY and JS-R and DR-C and RO-P; Writing-Original draft preparation, TY and DR-C and RO-P; Writing-Review & editing, AY and JS-R; Approval of manuscript, TY and AY and JS-R and DR-C and RO-P. All authors read and approved the final manuscript.

Author details

[1] Shanghai Key Laboratory of Psychotic Disorders, Shanghai Mental Health Center, Shanghai Jiao Tong University School of Medicine, Shanghai, China. [2] Co-innovation Center of Neuroregeneration, Nantong University, Nantong, Jiangsu, China. [3] Department of Medical Physics, School of Medicine, Ahvaz Jundishapur University of Medical Sciences, Golestan Blvd, Ahvaz 61357-33118, Iran. [4] Biomedical Engineering Department, Polytechnic University of Pachuca, Zempoala, Mexico. [5] Graduate and Research Department, Polytechnic University of Pachuca, Zempoala, Mexico.

Acknowledgements

Not applicable.

Competing interests

Ali Yadollahpour and Tifei Yuan are members of the editorial board for BMC Neuroscience. There is no other competing interest declared by authors.

Funding

Authors received no fund for this study.

References

1. Langguth B, Kreuzer PM, Kleinjung T, De Ridder D. Tinnitus: causes and clinical management. Lancet Neurol. 2013;12:920–30.
2. Baguley D, McFerran D, Hall D. Tinnitus. Lancet Lond Engl. 2013;382:1600–7. https://doi.org/10.1016/S0140-6736(13)60142-7.
3. Muhlnickel W, Elbert T, Taub E, Flor H. Reorganization of auditory cortex in tinnitus. Proc Natl Acad Sci USA. 1998;95:10340–3.
4. Husain FT, Schmidt SA. Using resting state functional connectivity to unravel networks of tinnitus. Hear Res. 2014;307:153–62.
5. Sindhusake D, Mitchell P, Newall P, Golding M, Rochtchina E, Rubin G. Prevalence and characteristics of tinnitus in older adults: the blue mountains hearing study: prevalencia y características del acúfeno en adultos mayores: el Estudio de audición blue mountains. Int J Audiol. 2003;42:289–94.
6. Schlee W, Hartmann T, Langguth B, Weisz N. Abnormal resting-state cortical coupling in chronic tinnitus. BMC Neurosci. 2009;10:11.
7. De Ridder D, Elgoyhen AB, Romo R, Langguth B. Phantom percepts: tinnitus and pain as persisting aversive memory networks. Proc Natl Acad Sci. 2011;108:8075–80.
8. Van Der Loo E, Congedo M, Vanneste S, Van De Heyning P, De Ridder D. Insular lateralization in tinnitus distress. Auton Neurosci. 2011;165:191–4.
9. Vanneste S, Van de Heyning P, De Ridder D. The neural network of phantom sound changes over time: a comparison between recent-onset and chronic tinnitus patients. Eur J Neurosci. 2011;34:718–31.
10. De Ridder D, Fransen H, Francois O, Sunaert S, Kovacs S, Van De Heyning P. Amygdalohippocampal involvement in tinnitus and auditory memory. Acta Otolaryngol. 2006;126:50–3.
11. Vanneste S, Plazier M, Van Der Loo E, Van de Heyning P, Congedo M, De Ridder D. The neural correlates of tinnitus-related distress. Neuroimage. 2010;52:470–80.
12. De Ridder D, Vanneste S, Congedo M. The distressed brain: a group blind source separation analysis on tinnitus. PLoS One. 2011;6:e24273.
13. Vanneste S, Plazier M, Ost J, van der Loo E, Van de Heyning P, De Ridder D. Bilateral dorsolateral prefrontal cortex modulation for tinnitus by transcranial direct current stimulation: a preliminary clinical study. Exp Brain Res. 2010;202:779–85.
14. Eggermont JJ. The neuroscience of tinnitus. Oxford: Oxford University Press; 2012.

15. Fitzgerald PB, Oxley TJ, Laird AR, Kulkarni J, Egan GF, Daskalakis ZJ. An analysis of functional neuroimaging studies of dorsolateral prefrontal cortical activity in depression. Psychiatry Res Neuroimaging. 2006;148:33–45.

16. Bodner M, Kroger J, Fuster JM. Auditory memory cells in dorsolateral prefrontal cortex. Neuroreport. 1996;7:1905–8.

17. Shekhawat GS, Stinear CM, Searchfield GD. Modulation of perception or emotion? a scoping review of tinnitus neuromodulation using transcranial direct current stimulation. Neurorehabil Neural Repair. 2015;29:837–46. https://doi.org/10.1177/1545968314567152.

18. Rauschecker JP, Leaver AM, Mühlau M. Tuning out the noise: limbic-auditory interactions in tinnitus. Neuron. 2010;66:819–26.

19. Schlee W, Schecklmann M, Lehner A, Kreuzer PM, Vielsmeier V, Poeppl TB, et al. Reduced variability of auditory alpha activity in chronic tinnitus. Neural Plast. 2014. https://doi.org/10.1155/2014/436146.

20. Lewis JW, Beauchamp MS, DeYoe EA. A comparison of visual and auditory motion processing in human cerebral cortex. Cereb Cortex. 2000;10:873–88.

21. Mitchell TV, Morey RA, Inan S, Belger A. Functional magnetic resonance imaging measure of automatic and controlled auditory processing. Neuroreport. 2005;16:457.

22. Voisin J, Bidet-Caulet A, Bertrand O, Fonlupt P. Listening in silence activates auditory areas: a functional magnetic resonance imaging study. J Neurosci. 2006;26:273–8.

23. Bruder GE, Stewart JW, Mercier MA, Agosti V, Leite P, Donovan S, et al. Outcome of cognitive–behavioral therapy for depression: relation to hemispheric dominance for verbal processing. J Abnorm Psychol. 1997;106:138.

24. Shekhawat GS, Kobayashi K, Searchfield GD. Methodology for studying the transient effects of transcranial direct current stimulation combined with auditory residual inhibition on tinnitus. J Neurosci Methods. 2015;239:28–33.

25. Khoramzadeh S, Saki N, Davoodi I, Nosratabadi M, Yadollahpour A. Investigating the therapeutic efficacy of neurofeedback treatment on the severity of symptoms and quality of life in patients with tinnitus. Int J Ment Health Addict. 2016;14:982–92. https://doi.org/10.1007/s11469-016-9670-6.

26. Paulus W. Transcranial electrical stimulation (tES—tDCS; tRNS, tACS) methods. Neuropsychol Rehabil. 2011;21:602–17.

27. George MS, Wassermann EM, Williams WA, Callahan A, Ketter TA, Basser P, Hallett M, Post RM. Daily repetitive transcranial magnetic stimulation (rTMS) improves mood in depression. Neuroreport. 1995;6:1853–6.

28. Yadollahpour A, Rashidi S, Kunwar PS. Repetitive transcranial magnetic stimulation in psychiatric disorders: a review of clinical advances. Asian J Pharm. 2017;11:S242–50. https://www.scopus.com/inward/record.uri?eid=2-s2.0-85026263088&partnerID=40&md5=d1da8a4d7df6be4b49b98f6620ead12c. Accessed 11 June 2018.

29. Yadollahpour A, Jalilifar M, Rashidi S. Transcranial direct current stimulation for the treatment of depression: a comprehensive review of the recent advances. Int J Ment Health Addict. 2017;15:434–43. https://doi.org/10.1007/s11469-017-9741-3.

30. Lisanby SH. Electroconvulsive therapy for depression. N Engl J Med. 2007;357:1939–45.

31. Lisanby S. Noninvasive brain stimulation for depression—the devil is in the dosing. N Engl J Med. 2017;376:2593–4.

32. Yadollahpour A, Jalilifar M, Rashidi S. Antimicrobial effects of electromagnetic fields: a review of current techniques and mechanisms of action. J Pure Appl Microbiol. 2014;8:4031–43. https://www.scopus.com/inward/record.uri?eid=2-s2.0-84923860983&partnerID=40&md5=4c6811a94a88290721c46a3a7d6c0c46. Accessed 11 June 2018.

33. Athanasiou A, Karkambounas S, Batistatou A, Lykoudis E, Katsaraki A, Kartsiouni T, et al. The effect of pulsed electromagnetic fields on secondary skin wound healing: an experimental study. Bioelectromagnetics. 2007;28:362–8.

34. McLeod KJ, Rubin CT, Donahue HJ. Electromagnetic fields in bone repair and adaptation. Radio Sci. 1995;30:233–44.

35. Yadollahpour A, Rashidi S. A review of electromagnetic field based treatments for different bone fractures. Biosci Biotechnol Res Asia. 2014;11:611–20. https://doi.org/10.13005/bbra/1313.

36. Kreuzer PM, Landgrebe M, Schecklmann M, Poeppl TB, Vielsmeier V, Hajak G, et al. Can temporal repetitive transcranial magnetic stimulation be enhanced by targeting affective components of tinnitus with frontal rTMS? A randomized controlled pilot trial. Front Syst Neurosci. 2011;5:88.

37. Lefaucheur JP, Brugières P, Guimont F, Iglesias S, Franco-Rodrigues A, Liégeois-Chauvel C, et al. Navigated rTMS for the treatment of tinnitus: a pilot study with assessment by fMRI and AEPs. Neurophysiol Clin. 2012;42:95–109.

38. Langguth B, Eichhammer P, Zowe M, Marienhagen J, Kleinjung T, Jacob P, et al. Low frequency repetitive transcranial magnetic stimulation (rTMS) for the treatment of chronic tinnitus–are there long-term effects? Psychiatr Prax. 2004;31:S52–4.

39. Yadollahpour A, Asl HM, Rashidi S. Transcranial direct current stimulation as a non-medication modality for attention enhancement: a review of the literature. Res J Pharm Technol. 2017;10:311–6. https://doi.org/10.5958/0974-360X.2017.00064.6.

40. Yadollahpour A, Jalilifar M, Rashidi S. Transcranial direct current stimulation for the treatment of depression: a comprehensive review of the recent advances. Int J Ment Health Addict. 2017. https://doi.org/10.1007/s11469-017-9741-3.

41. Baeken C, Brunelin J, Duprat R, Vanderhasselt M-A. The application of tDCS in psychiatric disorders: a brain imaging view. Socioaffective Neurosci Psychol. 2016;6:29588. https://doi.org/10.3402/SNP.V6.29588.

42. Trumbo M. Effect of transcranial direct current stimulation on the attention network task (ANT). University of New Mexico. 2012. https://digitalrepository.unm.edu/psy_etds/139/. Accessed 10 June 2018

43. Lefaucheur J-P, Antal A, Ayache SS, Benninger DH, Brunelin J, Cogiamanian F, et al. Evidence-based guidelines on the therapeutic use of transcranial direct current stimulation (tDCS). Clin Neurophysiol. 2017. https://doi.org/10.1016/j.clinph.2016.10.087.

44. Nitsche MA, Paulus W. Excitability changes induced in the human motor cortex by weak transcranial direct current stimulation. J Physiol. 2000;527:633–9.

45. Fregni F, Marcondes R, Boggio PS, Marcolin MA, Rigonatti SP, Sanchez TG, et al. Transient tinnitus suppression induced by repetitive transcranial magnetic stimulation and transcranial direct current stimulation. Eur J Neurol. 2006;13:996–1001.

46. Vanneste S, Langguth B, De Ridder D. Do tDCS and TMS influence tinnitus transiently via a direct cortical and indirect somatosensory modulating effect? a combined TMS-tDCS and TENS study. Brain Stimul. 2011;4:242–52. https://doi.org/10.1016/j.brs.2010.12.001.

47. Faber M, Vanneste S, Fregni F, De Ridder D. Top down prefrontal affective modulation of tinnitus with multiple sessions of tDCS of dorsolateral prefrontal cortex. Brain Stimul. 2012;5:492–8.

48. Shekhawat GS, Stinear CM, Searchfield GD. Transcranial direct current stimulation intensity and duration effects on tinnitus suppression. Neurorehabil Neural Repair. 2013;27:164–72. https://doi.org/10.1177/1545968312459908.

49. Romero Lauro LJ, Rosanova M, Mattavelli G, Convento S, Pisoni A, Opitz A, et al. TDCS increases cortical excitability: direct evidence from TMS–EEG. Cortex. 2014;58:99–111. https://doi.org/10.1016/j.cortex.2014.05.003.

50. Varoli E, Pisoni A, Mattavelli GC, Vergallito A, Gallucci A, Mauro LD, et al. Tracking the effect of cathodal transcranial direct current stimulation on cortical excitability and connectivity by means of TMS-EEG. Front Neurosci. 2018;12:319. https://doi.org/10.3389/fnins.2018.00319.

51. Pellicciari MC, Brignani D, Miniussi C. Excitability modulation of the motor system induced by transcranial direct current stimulation: a multimodal approach. Neuroimage. 2013;83:569–80. https://doi.org/10.1016/j.neuroimage.2013.06.076.

52. Roche N, Geiger M, Bussel B. Mechanisms underlying transcranial direct current stimulation in rehabilitation. Ann Phys Rehabil Med. 2015;58:214–9. https://doi.org/10.1016/J.REHAB.2015.04.009.

53. Shekhawat GS, Stinear CM, Searchfield GD. Transcranial direct current stimulation intensity and duration effects on tinnitus suppression. Neurorehabil Neural Repair. 2013;27:164–72. https://doi.org/10.1177/1545968312459908.

54. Forogh B, Mirshaki Z, Raissi GR, Shirazi A, Mansoori K, Ahadi T. Repeated sessions of transcranial direct current stimulation for treatment of chronic subjective tinnitus: a pilot randomized controlled trial. Neurol Sci. 2016;37:253–9. https://doi.org/10.1007/s10072-015-2393-9.

55. Shekhawat GS, Sundram F, Bikson M, Truong D, De Ridder D, Stinear CM, et al. Intensity, duration, and location of high-definition transcranial

direct current stimulation for tinnitus relief. Neurorehabil Neural Repair. 2016;30:349–59. https://doi.org/10.1177/1545968315595286.

56. Wang Y, Shen Y, Cao X, Shan C, Pan J, He H, et al. Transcranial direct current stimulation of the frontal-parietal-temporal area attenuates cue-induced craving for heroin. J Psychiatr Res. 2016;79:1–3. https://doi.org/10.1016/j.jpsychires.2016.04.001.

57. Baker JM, Rorden C, Fridriksson J. Using transcranial direct-current stimulation to treat stroke patients with aphasia. Stroke. 2010;41:1229–36.

58. Fröhlich F, Burrello TN, Mellin JM, Cordle AL, Lustenberger CM, Gilmore JH, et al. Exploratory study of once-daily transcranial direct current stimulation (tDCS) as a treatment for auditory hallucinations in schizophrenia. Eur Psychiatry. 2016;33:54–60. https://doi.org/10.1016/j.eurpsy.2015.11.005.

59. Vanneste S, De Ridder D. Bifrontal transcranial direct current stimulation modulates tinnitus intensity and tinnitus-distress-related brain activity. Eur J Neurosci. 2011;34:605–14.

60. Frank E, Schecklmann M, Landgrebe M, Burger J, Kreuzer P, Poeppl TB, et al. Treatment of chronic tinnitus with repeated sessions of prefrontal transcranial direct current stimulation: outcomes from an open-label pilot study. J Neurol. 2012;259:327–33.

61. De Ridder D, Vanneste S. EEG driven tDCS versus bifrontal tDCS for tinnitus. Front Psychiatry. 2012;3:84.

62. Garin P, Gilain C, Van Damme JP, de Fays K, Jamart J, Ossemann M, et al. Short- and long-lasting tinnitus relief induced by transcranial direct current stimulation. J Neurol. 2011;258:1940–8. https://doi.org/10.1007/s00415-011-6037-6.

63. Shekhawat GS, Searchfield GD, Stinear CM. Randomized trial of transcranial direct current stimulation and hearing aids for tinnitus management. Neurorehabil Neural Repair. 2014;28:410–9. https://doi.org/10.1177/1545968313508655.

64. Mori T, Takeuchi N, Suzuki S, Miki M, Kawase T, Izumi S-I. Anodal transcranial direct current stimulation over the auditory cortex improved hearing impairment in a patient with brainstem encephalitis. J Int Med Res. 2016;44:760–4. https://doi.org/10.1177/0300060516630843.

65. Vanneste S, De Ridder D. Noninvasive and invasive neuromodulation for the treatment of tinnitus: an overview. Neuromodulation Technol Neural Interface. 2012;15:350–60. https://doi.org/10.1111/j.1525-1403.2012.00447.x.

66. Yadollahpour A, Bayat A, Rashidi S, Saki N, Karimi M. Dataset of acute repeated sessions of bifrontal transcranial direct current stimulation for treatment of intractable tinnitus: a randomized controlled trial. Data Br. 2017;15:40–6.

67. Bayat A, Mayo M, Rashidi S, Saki N, Yadollahpour A. Repeated sessions of bilateral transcranial direct current stimulation on intractable tinnitus: a study protocol for a double-blind randomized controlled trial. F1000Research. 2018;7:317. https://doi.org/10.12688/f1000research.13558.1.

68. Shekhawat GS, Vanneste S. Optimization of transcranial direct current stimulation of dorsolateral prefrontal cortex for tinnitus: a non-linear dose-response effect. Sci Rep. 2018;8:8311. https://doi.org/10.1038/s41598-018-26665-1.

69. Pal N, Maire R, Stephan MA, Herrmann FR, Benninger DH. Transcranial direct current stimulation for the treatment of chronic tinnitus: a randomized controlled study. Brain Stimul. 2015;8:1101–7. https://doi.org/10.1016/j.brs.2015.06.014.

70. Teismann H, Wollbrink A, Okamoto H, Schlaug G, Rudack C, Pantev C. Combining transcranial direct current stimulation and tailor-made notched music training to decrease tinnitus-related distress—a pilot study. PLoS One. 2014;9:e89904. https://doi.org/10.1371/journal.pone.0089904.

71. Kreuzer PM, Lehner A, Schlee W, Vielsmeier V, Schecklmann M, Poeppl TB, et al. Combined rTMS treatment targeting the anterior cingulate and the temporal cortex for the treatment of chronic tinnitus. Sci Rep. 2015;5:18028.

72. Joos K, De Ridder D, Van de Heyning P, Vanneste S. Polarity specific suppression effects of transcranial direct current stimulation for tinnitus. Neural Plast. 2014;2014:1–8. https://doi.org/10.1155/2014/930860.

73. Vanneste S, De Ridder D. Bifrontal transcranial direct current stimulation modulates tinnitus intensity and tinnitus-distress-related brain activity. Eur J Neurosci. 2011;34:605–14. https://doi.org/10.1111/j.1460-9568.2011.07778.x.

74. Smits M, Kovacs S, De Ridder D, Peeters RR, Van Hecke P, Sunaert S. Lateralization of functional magnetic resonance imaging (fMRI) activation in the auditory pathway of patients with lateralized tinnitus. Neuroradiology. 2007;49:669–79.

75. Schlee W, Mueller N, Hartmann T, Keil J, Lorenz I, Weisz N. Mapping cortical hubs in tinnitus. BMC Biol. 2009;7:80.

76. Wagner BT. Non invasive brain stimulation : modeling and experimental analysis of transcranial magnetic stimulation and transcranial DC stimulation as a modality for neuropathology treatment technology. Cambridge: Harvard-MIT Division of Health Sciences And Tec; 2006.

10

Calcium currents in striatal fast-spiking interneurons: dopaminergic modulation of Ca_V1 channels

Ernesto Alberto Rendón-Ochoa, Teresa Hernández-Flores, Victor Hugo Avilés-Rosas, Verónica Alejandra Cáceres-Chávez, Mariana Duhne, Antonio Laville, Dagoberto Tapia, Elvira Galarraga and José Bargas* [iD]

Abstract

Background: Striatal fast-spiking interneurons (FSI) are a subset of GABAergic cells that express calcium-binding protein parvalbumin (PV). They provide feed-forward inhibition to striatal projection neurons (SPNs), receive cortical, thalamic and dopaminergic inputs and are coupled together by electrical and chemical synapses, being important components of the striatal circuitry. It is known that dopamine (DA) depolarizes FSI via D_1-class DA receptors, but no studies about the ionic mechanism of this action have been reported. Here we ask about the ion channels that are the effectors of DA actions. This work studies their Ca^{2+} currents.

Results: Whole-cell recordings in acutely dissociated and identified FSI from PV-Cre transgenic mice were used to show that FSI express an array of voltage gated Ca^{2+} channel classes: Ca_V1, $Ca_V2.1$, $Ca_V2.2$, $Ca_V2.3$ and Ca_V3. However, Ca_V1 Ca^{2+} channel carries most of the whole-cell Ca^{2+} current in FSI. Activation of D_1-like class of DA receptors by the D_1-receptor selective agonist SKF-81297 (SKF) enhances whole-cell Ca^{2+} currents through Ca_V1 channels modulation. A previous block of Ca_V1 channels with nicardipine occludes the action of the DA-agonist, suggesting that no other Ca^{2+} channel is modulated by D_1-receptor activation. Bath application of SKF in brain slices increases the firing rate and activity of FSI as measured with both whole-cell and Ca^{2+} imaging recordings. These actions are reduced by nicardipine.

Conclusions: The present work discloses one final effector of DA modulation in FSI. We conclude that the facilitatory action of DA in FSI is in part due to Ca_V1 Ca^{2+} channels positive modulation.

Keywords: Ca^{2+}-currents, Ca^{2+}-channels, Fast-spiking interneurons, Dopamine, D1-like dopamine receptors, Excitability

Background

Inhibitory GABAergic interneurons are part of striatal circuitry. They control striatal projection neurons output (SPNs), are a part of neuronal ensembles and participate in cognition, procedural learning and motor performance [1–8]. Among all striatal interneurons, parvalbumin-positive (PV+) fast spiking interneurons (FSI) are the most studied. They can fire at high frequencies with little adaptation and represent about 0.7% of the total neuronal population. Although the proportion of PV+ interneurons is small compared to spiny projection neurons (SPN), they have physiological relevance by providing feed forward perisomatic and dendritic inhibition to large numbers of SPNs [1, 2, 9]. FSI receive inputs from cortical and thalamic regions [3, 10, 11], are interconnected by gap junctions and GABAergic chemical synapses that may help to generate synchronized or correlated firing between them. Activation of FSI has widespread effects upon SPNs [12, 13].

*Correspondence: jbargas@ifc.unam.mx
División de Neurociencias, Instituto de Fisiología Celular, Universidad Nacional Autónoma de México, Circuito Exterior s/n Ciudad Universitaria, Col. Coyoacán, 04510 Ciudad de México, México

Striatal neurons receive massive dopaminergic innervation from the substantia nigra pars compacta (SNc) [14–16]. In vitro studies have shown that dopamine is an important modulator in the striatum which shapes excitability and circuitry management through, in part, the control of different receptors, ion channels, such as K^+, Ca^{2+} and synaptic channels, neurons and neuronal ensembles [17–19]. In FSI, DA binds to D5-type dopamine receptors, a member of the D1-class receptors [20, 21]. Activation of these receptors produces a depolarization accompanied by action-potential (AP) discharge in striatal FSI [20, 21], as well as in FSI from the prefrontal cortex [22, 23] and basolateral amygdala [24]. Although DA receptors expressed in striatal FSI are known, no description about their functional effectors has been made. In SPNs, dopamine modulates Ca^{2+} entry through somatic Ca_V1, $Ca_V2.1$ and $Ca_V2.2$ currents [25, 26] regulating firing frequency [25, 27]. In striatal cholinergic interneurons (CHI), dopamine modulates whole-cell Ca^{2+} current regulating firing properties, as well as the time course and shape of action potentials (AP) [28]. However, no study has been made to know whether calcium channels are involved on the depolarization produced by dopamine in FSI. Hence, this study was propose to find out: (1) the Ca^{2+} channel classes expressed in FSI, (2) if there is dopaminergic modulation of Ca^{2+} currents in FSI, and finally, (3) whether there are particular Ca^{2+} channels modulated by dopamine receptors. Accordingly, as a first approach, we use whole-cell recording in acutely dissociated striatal and identified FSI obtained from transgenic PV-cre mice in order to avoid indirect actions. Besides, whole cell current clamp recordings in slices as well as dynamic Ca^{2+} imaging with single cell resolution were performed. All techniques confirmed the hypothesis that D1-class receptor agonists enhance Ca^{2+} current carried by Ca_V1 channel leading to an increase in excitability of striatal FSI.

Methods
Experimental subjects and design
Experimental subjects, obtained from IFC bioterium were: B6; 12P2-$Pvalb^{tm1(cre)Arbr}$/J (PV-Cre; Silvia Arber, Friederich Miescher Institute; Jackson Labs, stock# 008069), called PV+ mice from now on. Experimental subjects were housed in acrilic cages (4–5 mice per cage; $19 \times 29 \times 12$ cm) with wood-based bedding and cardboard cylinders, kept on a 12:12 light/dark (light beginning at 8 am) period with a temperature maintained at 20–21 °C in IFC vivarium after surgery (see below) until used for experiments. All animals had standard rodent chow and water ad libitum. In order to identify isolated PV+ interneurons, PV-Cre transgenic mice at PD 21 (21 days, mean ± 4 days, 30 g mean ± 4, at 14–18 h),

were anesthetized i.p. with ketamine (Bayer 75 mg/kg) and xilazine (Bayer 10 mg/kg) and injected stereotaxically in a laminar flow hood (Telsar technologies. Model PV-30/60) in a dedicated, sterile room, with the following viral constructs (University of Pennsylvania Vector Core): AAV2/1.CAG.Flex.tdTomato.WPRE.bGH (Honguki Zeng) for whole cell recordings in isolated cells, AAV1.Syn.Flex.GCaMP6f.WPRE.SV40 [29], for calcium imaging recordings and AAV1.CAG.Flex.eGFP.WPRE. bGH (Allen institute) for some current clamp experiments in slices at the following coordinates relative to bregma (in mm): AP = 0.9, ML = ±1.2, DV = −3.2. The total virus volume injected was 0.8 µl over a period of 10 min (Fig. 1a). Animals were monitored for two weeks to ensure full recovery and fluorescent protein expression (Fig. 1b). A total of 45 infected PV-Cre mice were randomly assigned to 6 independent groups: for voltage clamp recordings of calcium currents (see next sections for details of the techniques) to observe contribution of Ca^{2+} channels classes (Fig. 2; n = 19 recordings from 18 different mice, below); effects of DA on Ca^{2+} currents (Fig. 3a, b; n = 8 recording from 8 different mice); SCH + SKF control group (Fig. 3c, d; n = 6 recordings from 4 different mice); nicardipine on DAergic actions (Fig. 4; n = 8 recordings from 6 different mice); current clamp recordings in slices (Fig. 5; n = 6 recordings from 6 different mice for SKF-nicardipine experiments and n = 4 for SKF-SCH experiments) and calcium imaging experiments (Fig. 6; n = 33; for imaging PV-cre identified FSI were extracted from 6 different experiments/slices from 3 different mice). The experimental units were single neuron recordings or changes in fluorescence ($\Delta F/F$ where ΔF = changes in fluorescence and F = basal fluorescence). Subject numbers were minimized to obtain statistical significance.

Preparation of dissociated neurons and slices
Brain slices and acutely dissociated neurons were obtained and described in previous work [30–34]. Briefly, infected PV-Cre mice were anesthetized (see above). The mice were decapitated, their brains were removed and submerged in iced saline solution containing (in mM): 126 NaCl, 3 KCl, 26 NaHCO$_3$, 2 CaCl$_2$, 1 MgCl$_2$, 11 glucose, 0.2 thiourea and 0.2 of ascorbic acid (25 °C; pH: 7.4 with HCl, 300 ± 5 mOsm/l with glucose; saturated with 95% O$_2$ and 5% CO$_2$). Using a vibratome (1000 Classic, Warner Instruments, Hamden, USA), sagittal brain slices of 300 µm thick were cut and placed in the same saline solution for 1 h at 34 °C. When recordings were done in slices, they were transferred to a submerged chamber and superfused at 5 ml/min with saline solution. When recordings were done in dissociated cells, the dorsal striatum was dissected from the slices and returned into the

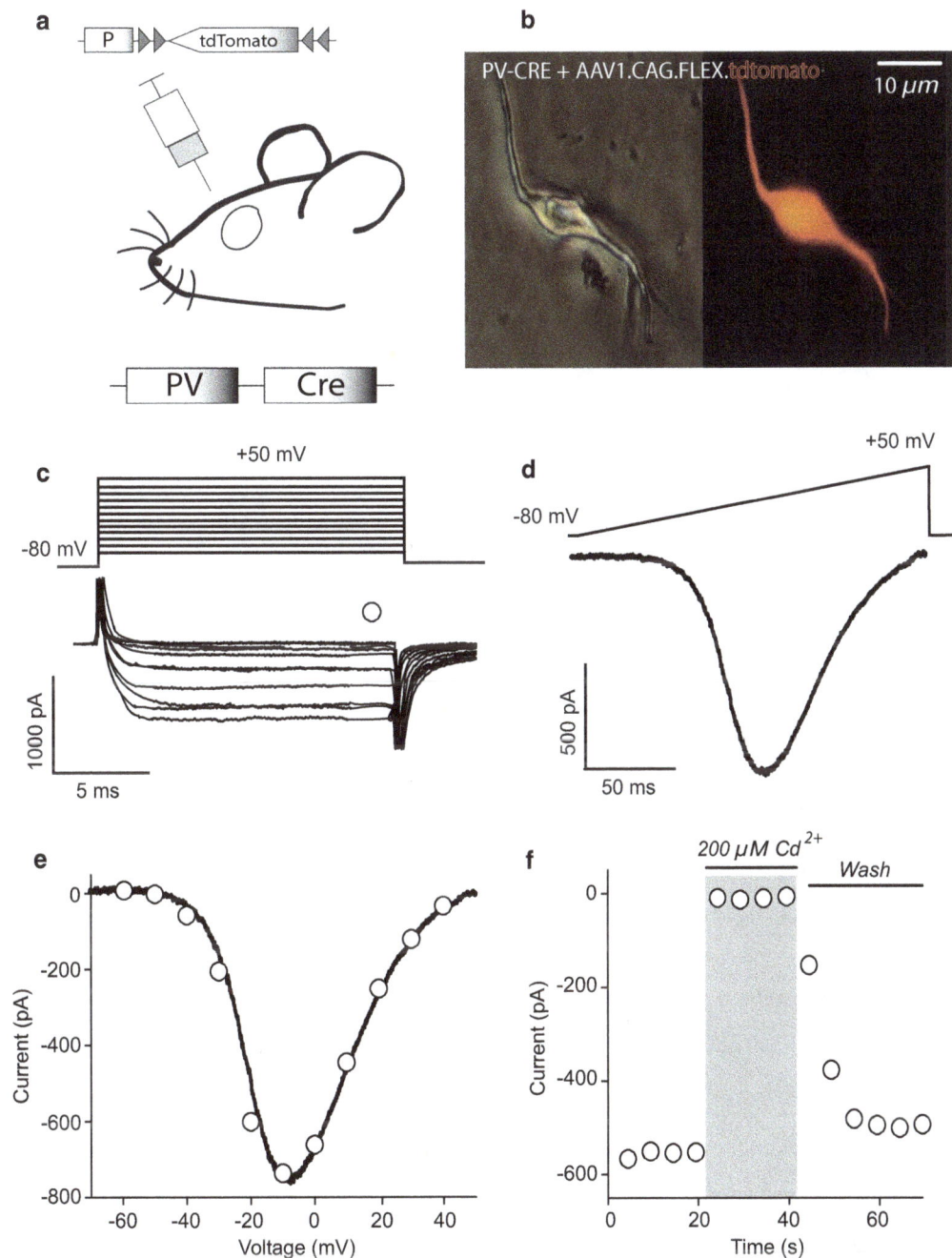

Fig. 1 Whole-cell Ca²⁺ currents in acutely dissociated FSI. **a** Schematic infection protocol in PV-cre mice with a viral construction containing tdTomato into the dorsal striatum. **b** Representative images of virally infected, acutely dissociated PV-cre FSI. Left: light microscopy; right: the same fluorescent tdTomato PV-cre cell. **c** Inward currents (bottom) elicited by rectangular voltage commands from − 80 to 50 mV (top) in 10 mV steps (tail currents are clipped). Empty circle shows where the amplitude current measurements were obtained. **d** Inward current in the same neuron elicited by a ramp command from − 80 to 50 mV (0.7 mV/ms). **e** Current–voltage relationship (I–V plot). Empty circles are measurements taken from currents elicited with voltage commands (as in **c**) and continuous line was the current obtained with the ramp command (as in **d**). Measurements using both protocols are superimposed. Note that measurements using the ramp command appear to "fit" measurements using the square commands suggesting good voltage control and space clamp. **f** Representative time course of Ca²⁺ current blockade during bath application of 200 μM Cd²⁺

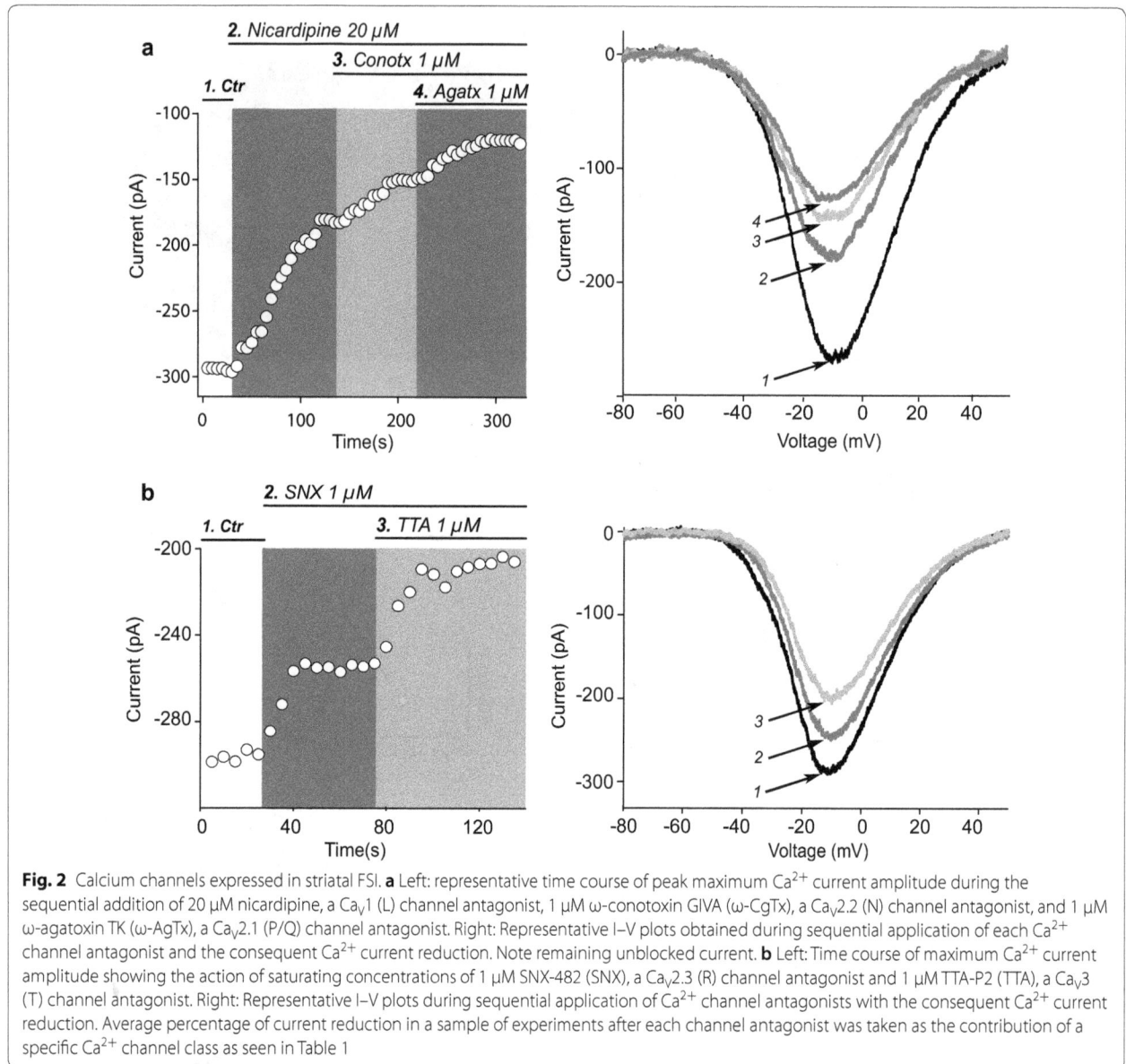

Fig. 2 Calcium channels expressed in striatal FSI. **a** Left: representative time course of peak maximum Ca²⁺ current amplitude during the sequential addition of 20 µM nicardipine, a Ca_V1 (L) channel antagonist, 1 µM ω-conotoxin GIVA (ω-CgTx), a $Ca_V2.2$ (N) channel antagonist, and 1 µM ω-agatoxin TK (ω-AgTx), a $Ca_V2.1$ (P/Q) channel antagonist. Right: Representative I–V plots obtained during sequential application of each Ca²⁺ channel antagonist and the consequent Ca²⁺ current reduction. Note remaining unblocked current. **b** Left: Time course of maximum Ca²⁺ current amplitude showing the action of saturating concentrations of 1 µM SNX-482 (SNX), a $Ca_V2.3$ (R) channel antagonist and 1 µM TTA-P2 (TTA), a Ca_V3 (T) channel antagonist. Right: Representative I–V plots during sequential application of Ca²⁺ channel antagonists with the consequent Ca²⁺ current reduction. Average percentage of current reduction in a sample of experiments after each channel antagonist was taken as the contribution of a specific Ca²⁺ channel class as seen in Table 1

saline solution containing 10 mM HEPES plus 0.5 mg/ml of papain (*Carica papaya*; Calbiochem, Cat# 5125. San Diego CA) at 34 °C. After 20–25 min of digestion, the striatum slices were transferred to a low Ca²⁺ (0.4 mM CaCl₂) saline solution. To obtain individual cells, the striatal slices were mechanical dissociated with a graded series of fire-polished Pasteur pipettes. The cell suspension (1 ml) was plated into a Petri dish mounted on the stage of an inverted microscope (Nikon Instruments, Melville, NY, 20 ×/0.4 NA). Cells were left for 10–15 min for neurons to adhere to the bottom of the dish. The dish contained 1 ml of the whole-cell recording saline solution (in mM): 0.001 tetrodotoxin (TTX), 140 NaCl, 3 KCl, 5

BaCl₂, 2 MgCl₂, 10 HEPES, and 10 glucose (pH: 7.4 with NaOH; 300 ± 5-mOsm/l with glucose). Thereafter, the cells were superfused at 1 ml/min with saline of the same composition at room temperature (approximate 25 °C). Tomato-positive neurons were visualized using a UV lamp (X-Cite; EXFO, Ontario, Canada; Fig. 1b). Dissociated neurons lack their distal dendrites and axon, so currents reported are somatic.

Voltage clamp recordings of calcium currents

Voltage-clamp recordings were performed on identified striatal PV+ interneurons with 12–15 µM soma diameter and whole-cell capacitance of 6–7 pF with short or

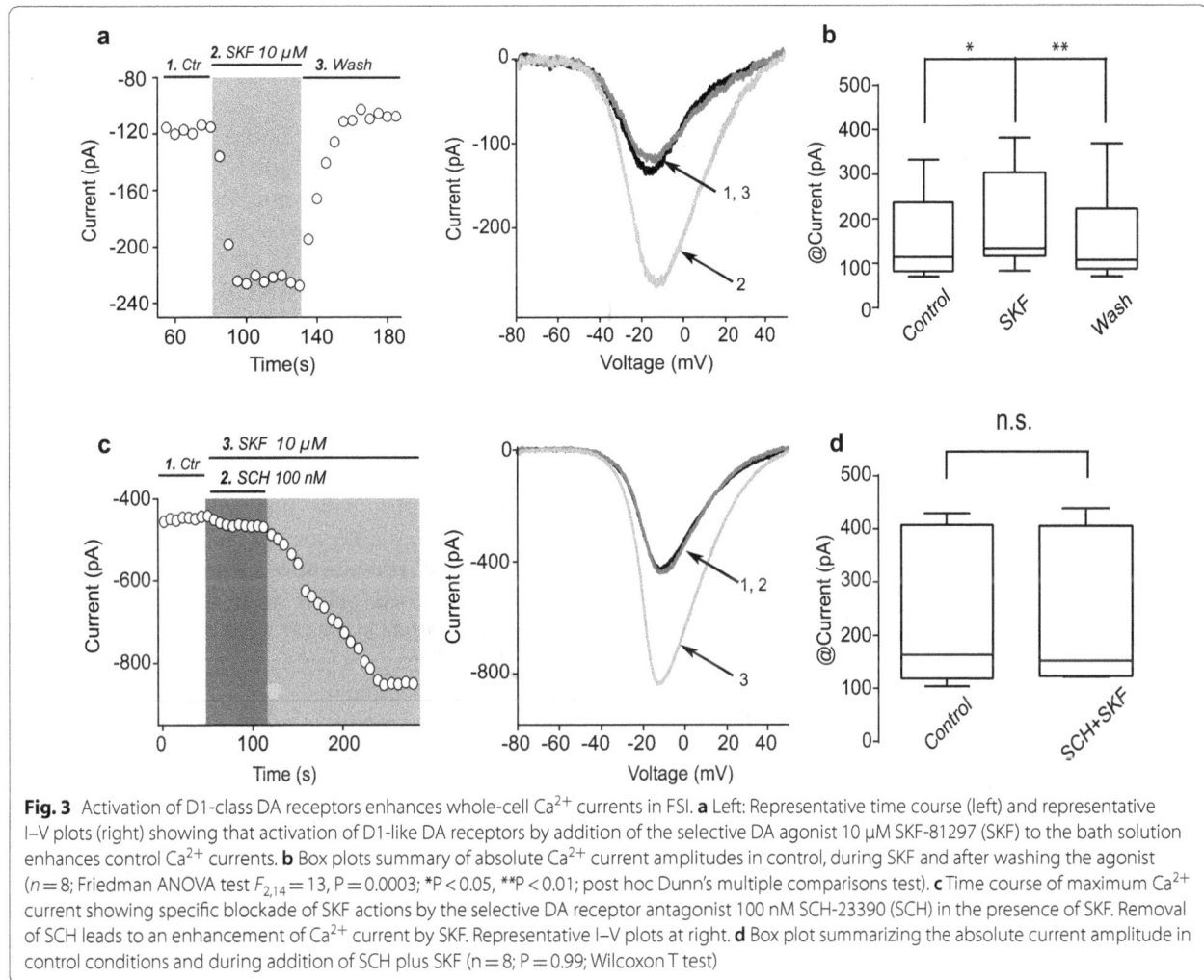

Fig. 3 Activation of D1-class DA receptors enhances whole-cell Ca^{2+} currents in FSI. **a** Left: Representative time course (left) and representative I–V plots (right) showing that activation of D1-like DA receptors by addition of the selective DA agonist 10 µM SKF-81297 (SKF) to the bath solution enhances control Ca^{2+} currents. **b** Box plots summary of absolute Ca^{2+} current amplitudes in control, during SKF and after washing the agonist ($n = 8$; Friedman ANOVA test $F_{2,14} = 13$, $P = 0.0003$; *$P < 0.05$, **$P < 0.01$; post hoc Dunn's multiple comparisons test). **c** Time course of maximum Ca^{2+} current showing specific blockade of SKF actions by the selective DA receptor antagonist 100 nM SCH-23390 (SCH) in the presence of SKF. Removal of SCH leads to an enhancement of Ca^{2+} current by SKF. Representative I–V plots at right. **d** Box plot summarizing the absolute current amplitude in control conditions and during addition of SCH plus SKF ($n = 8$; $P = 0.99$; Wilcoxon T test)

absent dendritic trunks [32, 34]. Patch pipettes of borosilicate glass (WPI, Sarasota, FL, USA) were pulled in a Flaming-Brown puller (Sutter Instrument Corporation, Novato, CA, USA) and fire polished prior to use. The internal saline solution contained (in mM): 180 N-methyl-D glucamine (NMDG), 40 HEPES, 10 EGTA, 4 $MgCl_2$, 2 ATP, 0.4 GTP and 0.1 leupeptin (pH = 7.2 with H_2SO_4; 280 ± 5 mOsm/l; room temperature around 25 °C). Whole-cell recordings used electrodes with D.C. resistance of 3–6 MΩ in the bath. Liquid junction potentials (5-10 mV) were corrected. Recordings of Ca^{2+} currents were obtained with an Axopatch 200B patch-clamp amplifier (Axon Instruments, Foster City, CA, USA) and controlled and monitored with pClamp (version 8.2, RRID: rid_000085) and a 125 kHz DMA interface (Axon Instruments, Foster City, CA, USA). We recorded currents passing through Ca^{2+} channels using Ba^{2+} as a charge carrier as shown in previous articles [31, 34, 35]. Ba^{2+} is a potent K^+ blocker. In addition, intracellular K^+

was replaced by 180 mM NMDG. Na^+ channels were blocked with 1 µM TTX. Currents isolated in this way were completely blocked by 200–400 µM Cd^{2+} (Fig. 1f) in this way, and for simplicity, we will refer to these currents as Ca^{2+} currents. Current–voltage relationships (I–V plots) were generated before and after drug application. Figure 1c shows representative Ca^{2+} currents evoked with 20 ms rectangular voltage commands from − 80 to 50 mV in 10 mV steps. Figure 1d shows a representative Ca^{2+} current in response to a voltage ramp command (0.7 mV/ms) from − 80 to 50 mV. When I–V plot from both methods coincide, space-clamp was considered acceptable (Fig. 1e). For clarity, most figures only show representative responses to voltage ramps.

Current clamp recordings in slices

Current clamp recordings were performed with the patch clamp technique in the whole cell configuration of PV+

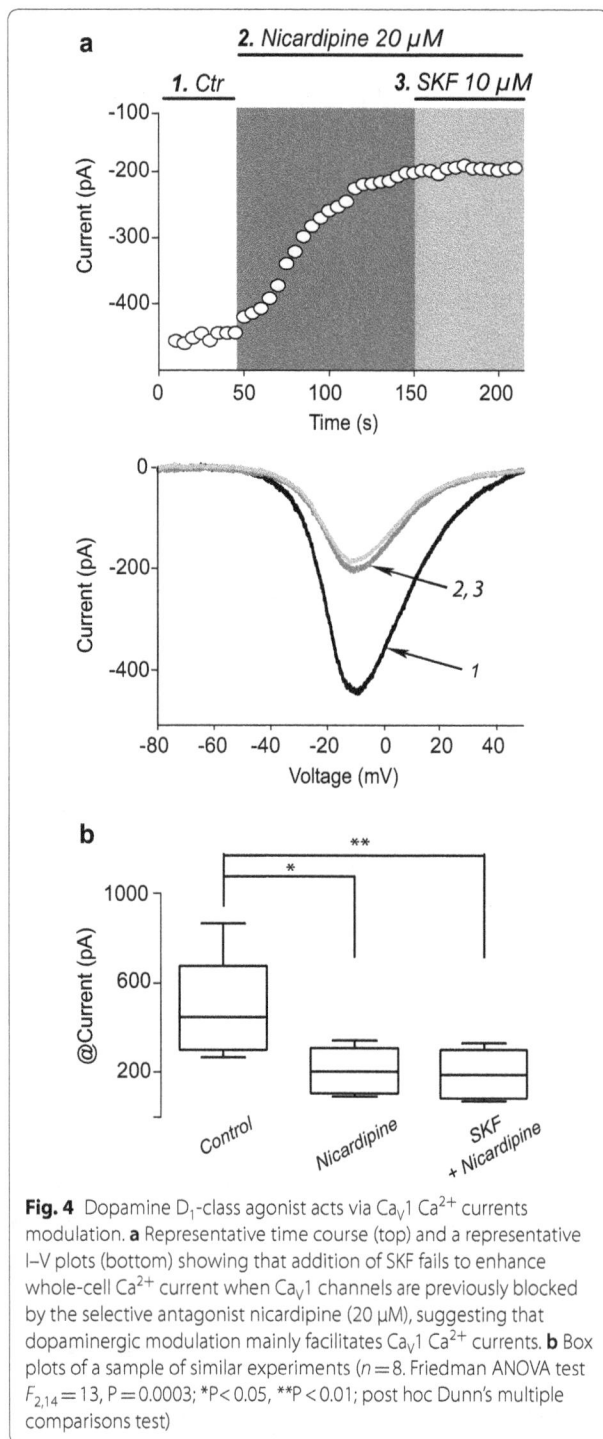

Fig. 4 Dopamine D$_1$-class agonist acts via Ca$_V$1 Ca^{2+} currents modulation. **a** Representative time course (top) and a representative I–V plots (bottom) showing that addition of SKF fails to enhance whole-cell Ca^{2+} current when Ca$_V$1 channels are previously blocked by the selective antagonist nicardipine (20 µM), suggesting that dopaminergic modulation mainly facilitates Ca$_V$1 Ca^{2+} currents. **b** Box plots of a sample of similar experiments ($n = 8$. Friedman ANOVA test $F_{2,14} = 13$, $P = 0.0003$; *$P < 0.05$, **$P < 0.01$; post hoc Dunn's multiple comparisons test)

were visualized with infrared differential interference contrast videomicroscopy and PV+ neurons were identified using epifluorescent illumination with a 40 × immersion objective (0.8 NA; Nikon Instruments, Melville, NY). Micropipettes were pulled (Sutter Instrument, Novato, CA) from borosilicate glass tubes (WPI, Sarasota, FL) to an outer diameter of 1.5-mm for a final D.C. resistance of 4–6 MΩ when filled with internal saline. The internal solution contained (in mM): 120 KSO$_3$CH$_4$, 10 NaCl, 10 EGTA, 10 HEPES, 0.5 CaCl$_2$, 2 MgCl$_2$, 2 ATP-Mg, and 0.3 GTP-Na (pH = 7.3, 290 mOsM/l). Recordings were made with an Axopatch 200A amplifier (Axon Instruments, Foster City, CA) and data were acquired with the Im-Patch© software designed in the Lab View environment (freely available for download at im-patch. com). Evoked firing responses at different depolarizing membrane potentials were obtained before and after a selective dopamine receptor agonist was administered. Current–voltage relationships made in current-clamp mode superimposed tightly with those performed in voltage-clamp mode at steady state, suggesting that neither bridge balance, nor series resistance, represented a problem in our recordings.

Digitalized electrophysiological data were imported and analyzed into Origin v8, Microcal (Northampton, MA), and MatLab (The Mathworks Inc. Natick, MA). Data are presented as the mean ± standard error (SEM). Firing rate plots were made by taking firing rate at rheobase in the different pharmacological conditions (Fig. 5c). Free-distribution statistical tests Wilcoxon's T test and Friedman, one-way ANOVA with post hoc Dunn's tests were used to assess statistical significance between paired or unpaired samples comparisons. Statistical significance was defined by P-values below 0.05.

Calcium imaging recordings

Calcium imaging recordings were obtained from PV+ neurons of mice infected with a Cre-dependent GCamp6f expression. Recordings were performed in saline solution containing (in mM): 126 NaCl, 2.5 KCl, 26 NaHCO$_3$, 1.2 NaHPO$_4$, 1 CaCl$_2$, 1.3 MgCl$_2$, 10 glucose, 0.2 thiourea and 0.2 of ascorbic acid (25 °C; pH: 7.4 with HCl, 300 ± 5 mOsm/l with glucose; saturated with 95% O$_2$ and 5% CO$_2$). For recordings, a microscope equipped with a 20 × 0.95 NA water-immersion objective (XLUMPlanFI, Olympus, Center Valley, PA) which has an image field of 750 × 750 µm, was used. To observe spontaneous changes in GCamp6f fluorescence intensity, light pulses at 488 nm (15–50 ms exposure) were delivered to the preparation with a Lambda LS illuminator (Sutter instruments, Petaluma, CA) connected to the microscope via optic fiber. Brief image sequences or movies (~ 180 s per epoch) were acquired with open access Im-Patch© software [6] at

neurons of infected mice ranging in age 28–60 days. Sagittal slices (250–300 µm thick) were cut using a vibratome (1000 Classic, Warner Instruments, Hamden, USA), transferred to a recording chamber and superfused continuously with oxygenated saline solution (5 ml/min) at room temperature (~ 25 °C). Neurons within the striatum

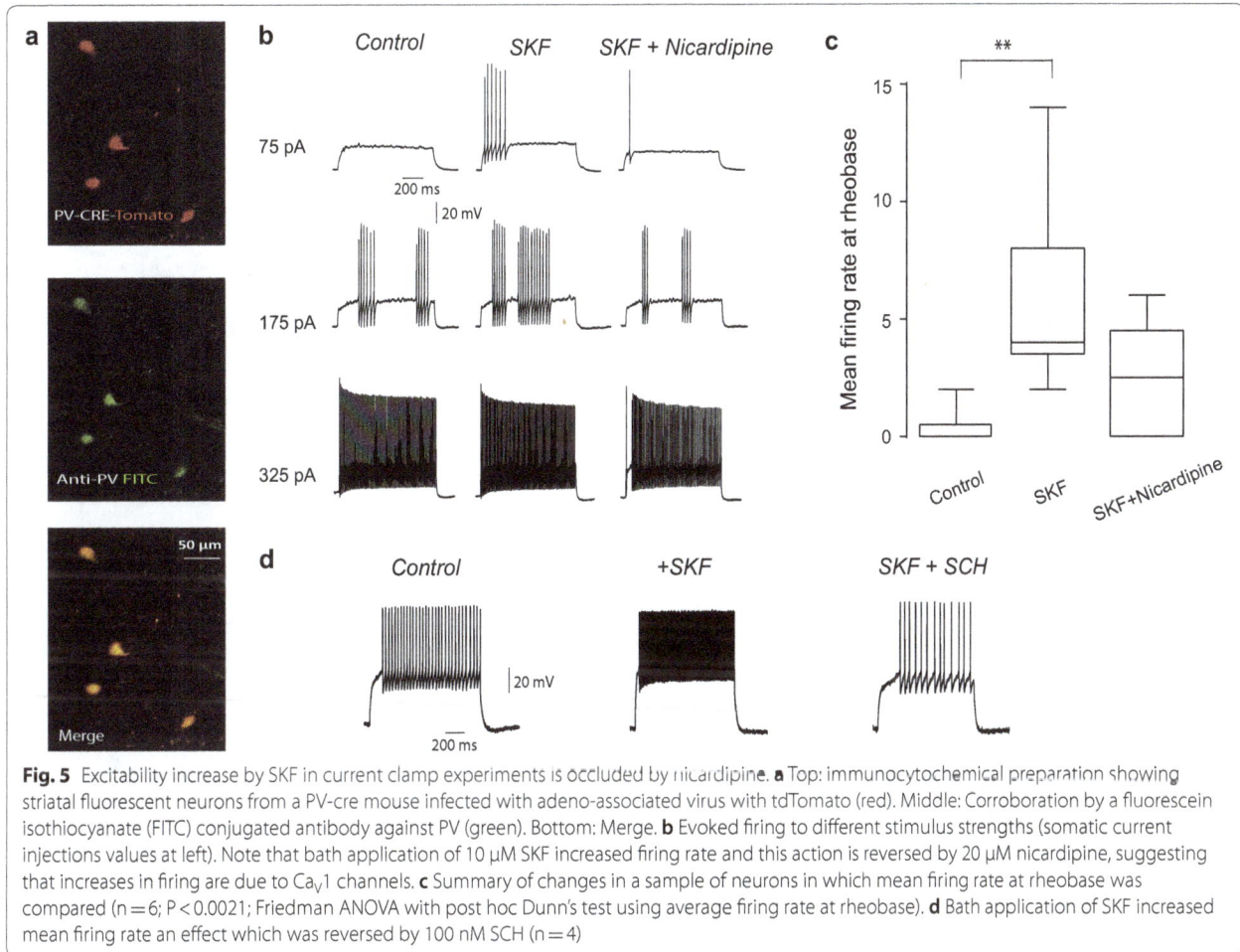

Fig. 5 Excitability increase by SKF in current clamp experiments is occluded by nicardipine. **a** Top: immunocytochemical preparation showing striatal fluorescent neurons from a PV-cre mouse infected with adeno-associated virus with tdTomato (red). Middle: Corroboration by a fluorescein isothiocyanate (FITC) conjugated antibody against PV (green). Bottom: Merge. **b** Evoked firing to different stimulus strengths (somatic current injections values at left). Note that bath application of 10 µM SKF increased firing rate and this action is reversed by 20 µM nicardipine, suggesting that increases in firing are due to Ca_V1 channels. **c** Summary of changes in a sample of neurons in which mean firing rate at rheobase was compared (n = 6; P < 0.0021; Friedman ANOVA with post hoc Dunn's test using average firing rate at rheobase). **d** Bath application of SKF increased mean firing rate an effect which was reversed by 100 nM SCH (n = 4)

time intervals of 5–10 min during ≥ 60 min with a cooled digital camera (CoolSnap K4, Photometrics, Tucson, AZ) and 100–250 ms/image frame. Ca^{2+} entry was seen as spontaneous neuronal intrasomatic Ca^{2+} transients in PV+ neurons whose first time derivative reflects the time of electrical activity [36]. Activity of each cell was illustrated as dots in a raster plot.

Inmunocytochemical procedures

PV-Cre mice were infected as described earlier. Mice were deeply anesthetized (see above) and perfused transcardially with a solution of 4% paraformaldehyde in PBS. Thereafter, animals were decapitated and their brains removed from the skull and fixed overnight with 4% paraformaldehyde in PBS. The brains were then cut on a vibratome into 40 µm slices that were incubated 30 min with 1% bovine albumina to block nonspecific binding sites and for 36 h with a rabbit polyclonal antibody against parvalbumin (anti PV 1:2000 Abcam dissolved in PBS containing 0.25% Triton-X). The slices were then rinsed thrice with PBS and incubated with a goat versus rabbit secondary antibody (1:200 Vector Laboratories, Burlingame, CA, dissolved in PBS containing 0.25% Triton-X) during 1 h. This antibody was conjugated with FITC (Vector Laboratories, Burlingame, CA). Samples were mounted with vectashield (Vector Laboratories, Burlingame, CA) and observed in a confocal microscope ZEISS LSM 700 (10 ×/1.0 NA) (n = 10).

Drugs

For dissociated cell recordings, drugs were applied with a gravity-fed system that positioned a glass capillary tube 100 µm from the recording cell in the direction of superfusion flow. Solution changes were performed with a D.C. controlled microvalve system (Lee; Essex, CT, USA). This method allowed reversible drug applications [26, 33]. For current clamp recordings drugs were administered into the bath saline. Substances used were the DA receptor D1-like selective agonist SKF 81297 (Cat# S143), DA receptor D1-like antagonist SCH 23390 (Cat# 125941-87-9), Ca^{2+} Ca_V1 antagonist nicardipine (Cat# N7510) all from Sigma-Aldrich-RBI (St Louis, MO, USA); Ca^{2+}

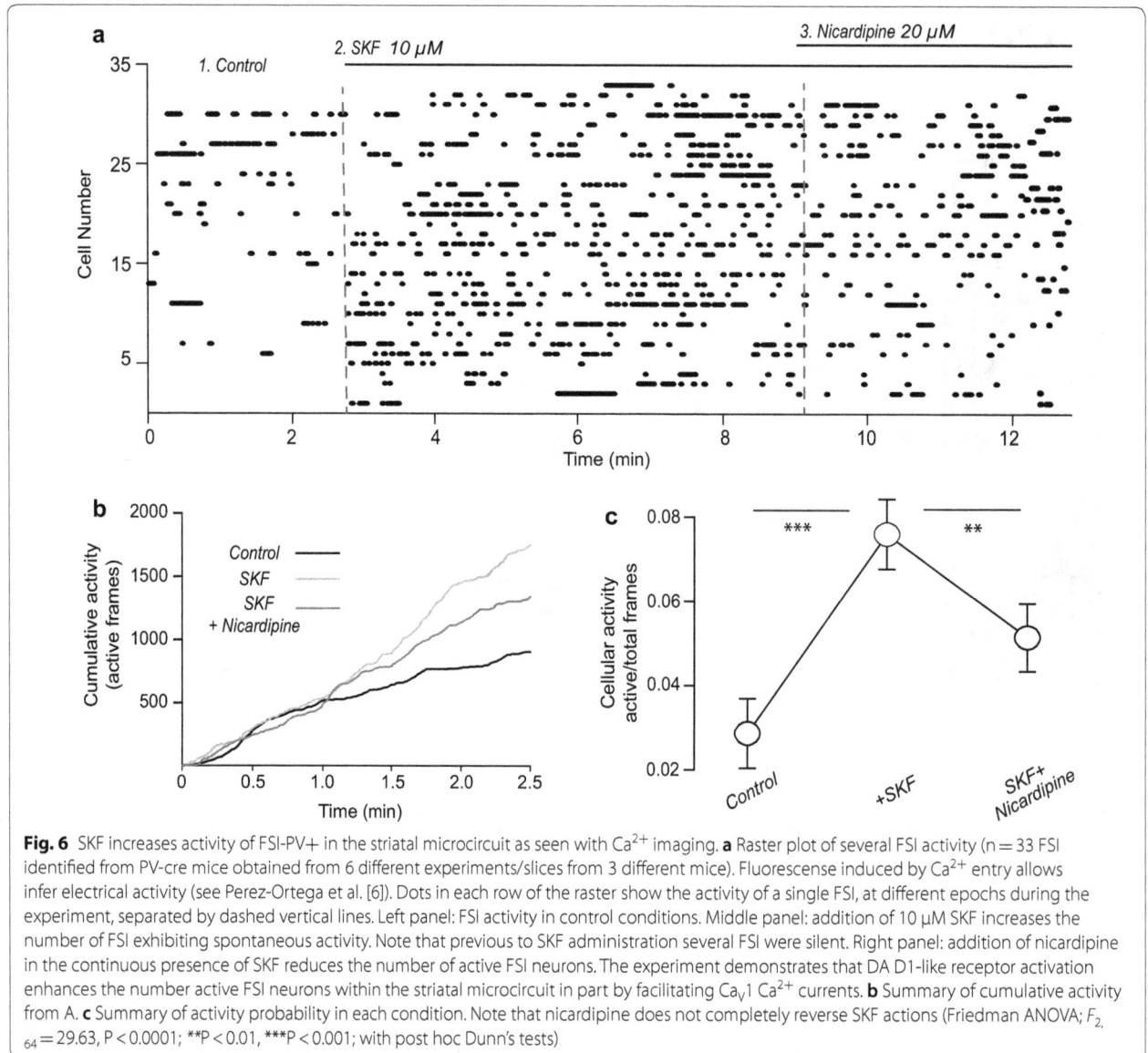

Fig. 6 SKF increases activity of FSI-PV+ in the striatal microcircuit as seen with Ca^{2+} imaging. **a** Raster plot of several FSI activity (n = 33 FSI identified from PV-cre mice obtained from 6 different experiments/slices from 3 different mice). Fluorescense induced by Ca^{2+} entry allows infer electrical activity (see Perez-Ortega et al. [6]). Dots in each row of the raster show the activity of a single FSI, at different epochs during the experiment, separated by dashed vertical lines. Left panel: FSI activity in control conditions. Middle panel: addition of 10 μM SKF increases the number of FSI exhibiting spontaneous activity. Note that previous to SKF administration several FSI were silent. Right panel: addition of nicardipine in the continuous presence of SKF reduces the number of active FSI neurons. The experiment demonstrates that DA D1-like receptor activation enhances the number active FSI neurons within the striatal microcircuit in part by facilitating Ca$_V$1 Ca^{2+} currents. **b** Summary of cumulative activity from A. **c** Summary of activity probability in each condition. Note that nicardipine does not completely reverse SKF actions (Friedman ANOVA; $F_{2, 64}$ = 29.63, P < 0.0001; **P < 0.01, ***P < 0.001; with post hoc Dunn's tests)

Ca$_V$2.2 blocker ω-conotoxin GVIA (Cat# C-300), Ca^{2+} Ca$_V$3 blocker TTA-P2 (Cat# T-155), Ca^{2+} Ca$_V$2.3 blocker SNX-482 (Cat# RTS-500), Na$^+$ blocker tetrodotoxin (TTX) (Cat# T-550) from Alomone Laboratories (Israel) and Ca^{2+} Ca$_V$2.1 blocker ω-agatoxin TK (Cat# 4294-s) from Peptides International (Louisville, KY).

Data analysis

Collected digitalized data were analyzed and plotted using commercial software (Origin v8, Microcal, Northampton, MA, USA; RIDD: rid_000069). We report mean ± SEM of peak Ca^{2+} currents changes for dissociated FSI recordings without assuming normal distributions. We also used the 5, 25, 50 (median), 75

and 95 percentile ranges of absolute current values represented as Tukey box plots. Friedman, Kruskal–Wallis or Wilcoxon test with post hoc Dunn for multiple comparisons tests were used (signaled in each Result). Friedman and Wilcoxon test were used when we compared the same samples in two or three different conditions (before, during and after application of a drug). P < 0.05 was used as significance threshold. Analysis was conducted by GraphPad Prism 6.01 (La Joya, CA). Here, Ba^{2+} currents are reported as Ca^{2+} currents and graphs summarizing sampling results are illustrated. For current clamp recordings, we report mean ± SEM of firing rate. For calcium imaging experiments, activity of each FSI was determined as the total number of active frames/total number of frames. Finally, to quantify the amount of activity on each experiment, a cumulative activity plot was built on each condition.

Contribution of each class of Ca^{2+} channel to the whole-cell Ca^{2+} current

The method to obtain the average contribution of a given class of Ca^{2+} channel to the whole cell Ca^{2+} current was described in previous work [37]. Briefly, to approximate the contribution of each class of Ca^{2+} channel, the amount of Ca^{2+} current blocked by a given antagonist: nicardipine, ω-conotoxin GVIA (ω-CgTx), ω-agatoxin TK (ω-AgTx), TTA-P2 (TTA) and SNX-482 (SNX) was obtained by subtraction in the same or different experiments. Hardly all antagonists could be tested in a single experiment, but the amount blocked by each antagonist was taken no matter the number or order of the antagonists tested. This amount of blocked current was defined as the contribution of that specific channel class to the whole-cell control Ca^{2+} current normalized to 100% without any antagonist. Thereafter the data was introduced in the following system of linear equations:

$$0_{X1} + N_{X2} + PQ_{X3} + T_{X4} + R_{X5} = A$$
$$L_{X1} + 0_{X2} + PQ_{X3} + T_{X4} + R_{X5} = B$$
$$L_{X1} + N_{X2} + 0_{X3} + T_{X4} + R_{X5} = C$$
$$L_{X1} + N_{X2} + PQ_{X3} + 0_{X4} + R_{X5} = D$$
$$L_{X1} + N_{X2} + PQ_{X3} + T_{X4} + 0_{X5} = E$$

where L, PQ, N, T and R are the contributions in percentage ($\pm$SEM) of each channel class: Ca_V1, $Ca_V2.2$, $Ca_V2.1$, Ca_V3 and $Ca_V2.3$ to the whole-cell Ca^{2+} current. For example, PQ refers to the current blockade by the selective P/Q type Ca^{2+} channel antagonist (ω-AgTx). Zero in the linear equation system means a blockade of a given Ca^{2+} channel class, thus, coefficients L, N, PQ, T or R were replaced by zero when the corresponding Ca^{2+} channel class was blocked. A, B, C, D or E stand for the mean percentage of Ca^{2+} current in the control (100%) with one channel class blocked (< 100%). Subscripts $X1$–$X5$ are the unknown variables, in other words, the values that multiply the coefficients L, N, PQ, T and R in order to determine percentage contribution of each channel to the whole-cell Ca^{2+} current.

Results

Striatal FSI express the Ca^{2+} binding protein PV [2, 38] and activation of the D5-type DA receptor from the D1-like class depolarizes FSI neurons to increase their action potentials (APs) firing rate [20, 21]. However, a final effector and whether DA enhances or decreases Ca^{2+} currents in FSI is unknown. With the help of PV-Cre transgenic mice we explored whether DA receptor actions in acutely dissociated striatal FSI modulate Ca^{2+} currents. In our experiments Na^+ and K^+ channels were blocked (Fig. 1c, d).

Ca^{2+} channels expressed in striatal FSI

FSI were identified using mice expressing Cre-recombinase under the control of the PV promoter (PV-Cre) and stereotaxic injections of an adeno-associated virus into the dorsal striatum allowed expression of a fluorescent protein (td-Tomato) only in striatal FSI. Acutely dissociated neurons were used in the first part of this study to avoid any indirect inputs from afferents, gap junctions, dendritic or axonal inputs. First, we estimated which Ca^{2+} channels are present in the soma and nearby dendrites of FSI and their percentage contribution to the overall whole cell Ca^{2+} current optimizing space clamp (Fig. 1e and current isolation; see Methods). Ca^{2+} entry through different calcium channels exert different and complex responses that vary in different cell types and localization within the cell body [37 for a review], therefore, one goal of this study was to determine the classes of voltage gated Ca^{2+} channels present in striatal FSI. Representative experiments with time courses of Ca^{2+} current amplitudes before and after application of specific channels antagonists is shown in Fig. 2a, b and percentage contribution of each Ca^{2+} channel class is summarized in Table 1. Antagonists were administered in different order or alone, and the current they reduced was compared with the whole cell Ca^{2+} current without any antagonist (see Methods). To determine whether Ca_V1 (L-type) contributed to the whole-cell current, application of nicardipine, a specific Ca_V1 Ca^{2+} channels antagonist was examined. As shown in Fig. 2a, nicardipine at saturating concentrations (20 μM) reduces whole-cell current amplitude by 38 $\pm$ 1.1%. This reduction was significant when whole cell current was normalized to 100% for the current without any antagonist in control conditions (n = 12; P = 0.0001; Kruskal–Wallis ANOVA with post hoc Dunn's test, used in this and next antagonists cases, percentages were obtained with the system of linear equations described in the Methods and compared to whole cell Ca^{2+} current without any drugs). This large amount of current flux through Ca_V1 Ca^{2+} channel might contribute to neuronal depolarization and AP generation after addition of D1-like agonist, since this current have a slow voltage-dependent inactivation [20, 25, 39, 40]; a main hypothesis tested below.

$Ca_V2.2$ (N) contribute to 23.4 $\pm$ 0.7% as revealed by 1 μM of ω-conotoxin GVIA (ω-CgTx) blockade, a specific $Ca_V2.2$ channel antagonist (Fig. 2a, Table 1; P = 0.0001; n = 14). Contribution of $Ca_V2.1$ (P/Q) was 11.1 $\pm$ 1.4% disclosed by ω-agatoxin TK (1 μM; Fig. 2a; Table 1; P = 0.0033). 1 μM SNX-482 revealed the presence of

Table 1 Contribution in percentage of the whole-cell Ca^{2+} current for each class of Ca^{2+} channel

Antagonist	Nicardipine	ω-conotoxin GVIA	ω-Agatoxin TK	SNX-482	TTA-P2
Concentration	20 µM	1 µM	1 µM	1 µM	1 µM
Ca^{2+} channel antagonist	Ca$_V$1	Ca$_V$2.2	Ca$_V$2.1	Ca$_V$2.3	Ca$_V$3
% of current blocked (mean ± S.E.M)	38 ± 1.1	23.4 ± 0.7	11.1 ± 1.4	20 ± 2	7.4 ± 2.3
n	12	14	14	6	13
p	0.0001	0.0001	0.0033	0.0009	0.0202

The first row (not counting the title) indicates the Ca^{2+} channel antagonist used. The second row contains saturating concentrations used. Third row stands for the specific Ca^{2+} channel class that was blocked. The fourth row displays the mean ± SEM of Ca^{2+} current blocked in percentage by each antagonist. Antagonists were tested alone or in sequence in different orders. Percentages were obtained from a system of linear equations that used data from all experiments (see Materials and methods). The fifth row shows samples size: the number of neurons tested with each antagonist. The sixth row indicates statistical significance or P-value of percentage blockade by each antagonist as compared to whole-cell current average before adding any antagonist (Kruskal–Wallis ANOVA with post hoc Dunn's test of each paired comparison against the control: whole-cell Ca^{2+} current)

Ca$_V$2.3 (R) Ca^{2+} channels: 20 ± 2% (Fig. 2b; Table 1; n = 6; P = 0.0009). Finally, Ca$_V$3 (T) Ca^{2+} channels contribute with 7.4 ± 2.3% (Fig. 2b; Table 1; n = 13; P = 0.0202). To conclude, representative components of high voltage gated (HVA) and low voltage gated (LVA) Ca^{2+} channels are present in FSI. The specific type and role of each of these channels is a matter of future studies out of the scope of the present work. We next concentrate on Ca$_V$1 Ca^{2+} channels which provide much of the whole cell Ca^{2+} current.

Activation of D1-class receptor enhances Ca^{2+} currents in acutely dissociated FSI

To know whether DA has effect on FSI Ca^{2+} currents, we performed whole-cell recordings in dissociated and identified FSI cells. Time course of peak current is shown in I–V plots of Fig. 3a before, during and after the administration of 10 µM of the DA receptor D1-like agonist SKF-81297 (SKF). SKF enhanced whole-cell Ca^{2+} currents in all FSI tested by an average of 34 ± 14% (Fig. 3a, b; n = 8. Friedman ANOVA test $F_{2,14} = 13$, P = 0.0003; *P < 0.05, **P < 0.01; with post hoc Dunn's test). Note that Ca^{2+} current returns to values similar to the control when the agonist is washed-off. Representative I–V plots (Fig. 3a right) are shown at different moments of the time course. Box plot in Fig. 3b summarizes the results from the previous sample of experiments showing that SKF actions were significant. The effect of the SKF was blocked by the presence of 100 nM of the DA receptor D1-like antagonist SCH 23390 (SCH; Fig. 3c). Removal of SCH leads to an increase in Ca^{2+} current in the presence of SKF showing that activation of D1-like DA receptors, most probably D5 [20, 21], enhances Ca^{2+} currents in FSI. No significant differences were found comparing controls and the combination SCH/SKF (Fig. 3d) (n = 8; Wilcoxon T test P > 0.9999). These results are consistent with the expression of D1-class DA receptors in FSI and show that DA enhances Ca^{2+} currents through the activation of these receptors.

D1-like receptors modulate Ca$_V$1 Ca^{2+} channel current

To further investigate the role of DA on Ca^{2+} currents we performed experiments blocking Ca^{2+} currents while activating DA receptors. Because Ca$_V$1 Ca^{2+} channels provide the most to the whole cell Ca^{2+} current we first blocked them [25]. Time course of peak current amplitude (top) and a representative I–V plots (bottom) are illustrated in Fig. 4a showing first, the action of 20 µM of the selective antagonist nicardipine on Ca$_V$1 currents. Then the action of subsequent application of the D1-like agonist SKF is shown. Nicardipine reduced Ca^{2+} current by 55.4 ± 7.8% in this sample (Fig. 4a, b; n = 8; Friedman ANOVA test $F_{2,14} = 13$, P = 0.0003; *P < 0.05, **P < 0.01 with post hoc Dunn's test). Note that in the presence of nicardipine subsequent addition of 10 µM SKF fail to elicit any change in the remaining Ca^{2+} current (P = 0.9999; Dunn's test). We conclude that the action of nicardipine occluded the action of SKF and therefore Ca$_V$1 Ca^{2+} channels are the final effectors of DA receptor modulation; without excluding other classes of channels (Na$^+$, K$^+$). This action is similar to that found in striatonigral projection neurons expressing D1-like receptors in both cell bodies and terminals [15, 41, 42]. It is also inferred that with respect to Ca^{2+} currents, there is no other effector for D1- receptor modulation in FSI.

D1-like receptors enhance FSI firing rate by modulating Ca$_V$1 Ca^{2+} channels

We then asked whether Ca$_V$1 Ca^{2+} channels modulation is robust enough to explain, in part, the increase in firing rate due to D1-like receptor modulation in FSI [20, 21]. Whole-cell current-clamp experiments on identified PV+ neurons in slices of transfected PV-Cre mice were performed. FSI in the dorsal striatum were identified based on adeno-associated virus containing td-Tomato

(Fig. 5a top left; see Methods) and corroborated with an antibody against PV conjugated to fluorescein isothiocyanate (FITC; Fig. 5a middle left). Merge is at the bottom in Fig. 5a. FSI were also identified by their electrophysiological phenotype: ability to fire at high firing rates with almost no frequency adaptation as well as stuttering (Fig. 5b). Representative recordings evoked by different intracellular current injections are shown in Fig. 5b: 10 μM SKF induced increases in mean firing rate at rheobase (n = 6; P < 0.0001; Friedman ANOVA with post hoc Dunn's test using average firing rate after 300 pA. Fig. 5c). Notably, subsequent administration of the Ca_V1 antagonist, nicardipine (20 μM), reversed in part the increase in firing rate induced by SKF. The same was true for a D1-receptor antagonist SCH (Fig. 5d; n = 4). Several seconds had to be taken between stimuli that evoke firing, before and after drugs administration, since in our hands, intensity-frequency plots exhibited hysteresis (adverse effect), a phenomenon that needs further investigation but out of the scope of the present report.

Activation of D1-class receptors enhances FSI activity in the dorsal striatal microcircuit

Finally, we asked whether activation of DA D1-class receptors can enhance the number of active FSI within the striatal microcircuit by enhancing Ca_V1 Ca^{2+} current. To test this hypothesis we performed calcium imaging experiments with single cell resolution [36] in slices from PV-Cre transgenic mice expressing GCaMP6f as a fluorophore. Using this technique we recorded spontaneous calcium transients of several PV+ neurons in different slices from three mice. The time derivative of these calcium transients indicates their firing time [36]. FSI may fire spontaneously in control conditions together with the firing of other striatal neurons. To avoid confounds we only graphed FSI activity using raster plots where dots in each row represent the moments of activity of single neurons (Methods). The firing of FSI from different slices (n = 6) are plotted together (Fig. 6a) as previously described [6, 36, 43]. Changes in fluorescence were obtained before, during and after application of SKF and SKF plus nicardipine. Raster plot of active FSI during a period of 13 min recording is shown in Fig. 6a (n = 33 identified FSI). The left panel in Fig. 6a shows the basal FSI activity in the striatal microcircuit without adding any excitatory drive or drug. Notice scarce FSI activity in control conditions. In contrast, administration of 10 μM SKF to the bath saline increased the number of active FSI (Fig. 6a middle panel). The subsequent addition of nicardipine in the presence of SKF reduced, but not completely reversed the enhanced activity. Figure 6b shows cumulative activity of all FSI neurons along time [43] and Fig. 6c shows activity probability under each

condition (mean ± SEM). To compare activity over time a cellular activity value for each neuron at each condition was calculated (frames with active neuron/total number of frames). In control conditions cellular activity was 0.03 ± 0.008, SKF raised activity to 0.07 ± 0.008 (Fig. 6b, c; Friedman ANOVA $F_{2, 64} = 29.63$, P < 0.0001; post hoc Dunn's test). This result indicates that DA increases the number of FSI firing within the striatal microcircuit in agreement with data from dissociated neurons and slice experiments. 20 μM nicardipine (Fig. 6a right panel) reduced FSI activity to 0.05 ± 0.008 (Fig. 6b, c; P < 0.001, Dunn's test).

Discussion

A summary of original data and findings of the present work follow: (1) all major classes of voltage gated Ca^{2+} channels are present in striatal FSI (Ca_V1, $C_V2.1-3$; Ca_V3). These results were obtained in voltage-clamp mode in identified dissociated FSI. Specific channel subtypes are still in need of investigation. (2) Contributions in percentage of each Ca^{2+} channel class are reported. Ca_V1 channels represent much of the whole cell Ca^{2+} current. (3) DA D_1-class receptors, probably D_5-type [21], up-modulate Ca_V1 carried current. (4) The Ca_V1 class is the only Ca^{2+} channel modulated by DA in FSI. This modulation is occluded by a previous administration of nicardipine or blocked by the antagonist SCH [20]. (5) Modulation of Ca_V1 Ca^{2+} channels is reflected in an increase in firing rate of FSI. These data were obtained in slices in current clamp mode. (6) Ca^{2+}-imaging recordings of several identified FSI obtained from different slices/animals showed that DA increases the number of FSI that are active in the striatal microcircuit. To our knowledge these are the first evidences of a molecular final effector for the DA-dependent modulation in striatal FSI, leading to a better understanding of the DA actions in the striatum.

Ca^{2+} channels expressed in FSI

Using pharmacological tools here we demonstrate that identified FSI from transgenic animals may be isolated in enough number to study the ion channels they express with whole-cell voltage clamp techniques in acutely dissociated preparations, thus eliminating indirect sources or confounds such as inputs from other neurons as well as gap junctions and chemical synapses between FSI themselves, this maneuver allows study specific Ca^{2+} currents [30, 33, 34, 37]. Striatal FSI seem to express all classes of voltage gated Ca^{2+} channels, HVA (Ca_V1, $Ca_V2.1$, $Ca_V2.2$ and $Ca_V2.3$) and LVA (Ca_V3), although, their contributions vary (Fig. 2a, b and Table 1). On average, Ca_V1 channels contribute the most to the whole cell Ca^{2+} current followed by $Ca_V2.2$ and $Ca_V2.3$ channels that altogether make up to more than 80% of the whole cell Ca^{2+} current. $Ca_V2.1$ and Ca_V3 make up the remaining current. Together with other ion channels [44–46], the studied Ca^{2+} channels shape the characteristic firing properties [28, 44–46] of FSI and may be orchestrated by signaling pathways as it occurs in striatal projection neurons (SPNs) [27, 30, 37, 40, 41]. Although it was not the goal of the present study to explore the role of each Ca^{2+} channel encountered, the variety found may imply that each channel has a specific role and ways to be modulated [6, 13, 14, 30, 35, 37, 40, 41]. Pathologies associated with striatal FSI, such as anxiety-like behaviors, schizophrenia or disorders such as Tourette's and Huntington's disease as well as some channelopathies [7, 47–51] may use this preparation to study associated changes.

Dopaminergic modulation of striatal FSI Ca^{2+} currents

A selective D1-class DA receptor agonist, SKF-81297, was used to investigate dopaminergic modulation. The DA receptor agonist enhanced Ca^{2+} currents specifically carried by Ca_V1 channels in FSI. A previous blockade of these channels with a dihydropyridine, nicardipine, completely occluded the action of the DA receptor agonist. Notably, this is similar to the dopaminergic modulation found in direct basal ganglia projection neurons (dSPNs) except that in the present case there was no need to block intracellular phosphatases [20].

Current through Ca_V1 channels has been associated with enhanced evoked depolarization and discharge facilitation [41, 52, 53]. Current clamp experiments in slices showed that this is also the case for striatal FSI as well as other neurons [37]. Ca_V1 also induces short-term synaptic depression and facilitates GABA release in SNr [53, 54]. Blockade of enhanced firing by nicardipine shows that Ca_V1 channels are in part responsible for these functions in striatal FSI. It would be interesting to know if FSI from other nuclei express this modulation or if it is particular for striatal FSI.

In addition, dynamic Ca^{2+} imaging of identified FSI with single cell resolution showed that the firing of these interneurons is enhanced in the striatal microcircuit by dopaminergic modulation. This action was partially blocked by nicardipine, lasted for several minutes without overt desensitization, suggesting that D1-class receptor activation, probably D5-type, increases feed-forward inhibition in the microcircuit [1, 55, 56]. Network analyses of this action in control and disease in vitro models [6] deserve further study. In addition, calcium recording was not performed in vivo, so the impact of excitatory drive from cortex and thalamus were not evaluated in the DAergic actions reported, although, in vitro studies have shown similar suprathreshold responses on thalamic and cortical stimuli, suggesting that both sources produces

similar feed-forward inhibition on SPN [11]. Given that the resonant frequency of FSI is within the gamma band [57], it may be logical to infer that DA modulation favors gamma (Piper) rhythms within neuronal circuits [4, 58–60]. On the other hand, aberrant or excessive gamma rhythms may be present during schizophrenia and L-DOPA induced dyskinesia [8, 18, 61].

However, the number of dopamine activated FSI within the striatal microcircuit does not return to control conditions after Ca_V1 Ca^{2+} channels are blocked. There could be various reasons for this behavior. One is that the DA receptor agonist not only affects FSI within the circuit, but turns on network activity in a way that does not return to control even after blocking Ca_V1 in FSI [19, 62]. Another explanation is that circuit activity or DA activates other ion channels in FSI [19]. Finally, FSI form networks of interconnected neurons both electrically and chemically [1, 2, 11]. This last property may correlate FSI firing making hard to study their individual cell responses in striatal brain slices.

Conclusion

To our knowledge this is the first demonstration that Ca_V1 channels are final effectors of DA modulation in FSI. In addition, we show the classes of Ca^{2+} channels that striatal FSI express and show evidence that Ca_V1 are the only ones modulated by D1-class receptors activation. Enhancement of Ca_V1 channels is a main cause for the increase in excitability of these interneurons due to DA receptors signaling, and collectively, this modulation increases the number of active FSI during striatal microcircuit operation. The demonstration that identified interneurons can be isolated for recording opens the pathway for future studies such as: to study other current classes (K^+, Na^+) and their modulation in interneurons in space clamp conditions, it also suggests comparisons between current phenotypes between FSIs from the striatum and other nucleus such as the cortex, and finally, quantitative single cell PCR may be used to prove whether different regions of the striatum possess different types of FSIs.

Abbreviations

FSI: fast spiking interneurons; PV: parvalbumin; HVA: high voltage activated; LVA: low voltage activated; SPN: spiny projection neurons; dSPN: striatonigral projection neurons; TTX: tetrodotoxin; SNc: sustantia nigra pars compacta; ChAT: giant cholinergic interneurons; DA: dopamine; HEPES: 4-(2-hydroxyethyl)-1-piperazineethanesulfonic acid; NMDG: N-methyl-D glucamine; eGFP: enhanced green fluorescent protein; iFr: instantaneous firing rate.

Authors' contributions

JB: conception of research. EAR-O, TH-F, VHA-R and JB: designed the isolated neurons and current clamp experiments. EAR-O, TH-F and VHA-R: performed isolated neuron electrophysiology experiments. MD and AL: performed, analyzed, interpreted and reported calcium imaging experiments. EAR-O, VAC-C: performed and analyzed current clamp experiments. AL: performed analytical code to obtain the contribution of Ca^{2+} channels. EAR-O, MD, VAC-C, VHA-R and TH-F: performed mice transfections. DT and EG: performed and analyzed inmunocytochemical experiments. EAR-O, VHA-R, VAC-C, AL, DT, EG and JB: interpreted and analyzed data. EAR-O and JB: wrote the manuscript. All authors participated actively with important experimental and intellectual content to the design, content, analysis, discussion and conclusions of the study. All authors read and approved the final manuscript.

Acknowledgements

Gabriela X Ayala and Ariadna Aparicio-Júarez for technical support and advice and to Dr. Claudia Rivera for animal care. A. Luna collaborated in some experiments.

Competing interests

The authors declare they have no competing interests.

Funding

This work was supported by Grants from Consejo Nacional de Ciencia y Tecnologia, Mexico (CONACyT, 251144 to EG and Frontera 57 to JB) and from Dirección General de Asuntos del Personal Académico, Universidad Nacional Autónoma de México (DGAPA-UNAM) IN201517 to EG and IN201417 to JB. After funding approval, funding institutions had no role in the design, collection, analyses, interpretation of data and writing of the manuscript. In addition, Ernesto Alberto Rendón-Ochoa had a CONACyT doctoral fellowship: 261720. Data in this work are part of his doctoral dissertation in the Programa de Maestría y Doctorado en Ciencias Bioquímicas, Facultad de Química, Universidad Nacional Autónoma de México.

References

1. Koós T, Tepper JM. Inhibitory control of neostriatal projection neurons by GABAergic interneurons. Nat Neurosci. 1999;2(5):467–72.

2. Koós T, Tepper JM. Dual cholinergic control of fast-spiking interneurons in the neostriatum. J Neurosci. 2002;22(2):529–35.

3. Ramanathan S, Hanley JJ, Deniau JM, Bolam JP. Synaptic convergence of motor and somatosensory cortical afferents onto GABAergic interneurons in the rat striatum. J Neurosci. 2002;22(18):8158–69.

4. Sohal VS, Zhang F, Yizhar O, Deisseroth K. Parvalbumin neurons and gamma rhythms enhance cortical circuit performance. Nature. 2009;459(7247):698–702.

5. Berke JD. Functional properties of striatal fast-spiking interneurons. Front Syst Neurosci. 2011;5(45):1–7.

6. Pérez-Ortega J, Duhne M, Lara-González E, Plata V, Gasca D, Galarraga E, Hernández-Cruz A, Bargas J. Pathophysiological signatures of functional connectomics in parkinsonian and dyskinetic striatal microcircuits. Neurobiol Dis. 2016;91:347–61.

7. Xu M, Li L, Pittenger C. Ablation of fast-spiking interneurons in the dorsal striatum, recapitulating abnormalities seen post-mortem in Tourette syndrome, produces anxiety and elevated grooming. Neuroscience. 2016;324:321–9.

8. Yamada H, Inokawa H, Hori Y, Pan X, Matsuzaki R, Nakamura K, Samejima K, Shisara M, Kimura M, Sakagami M, Minamimoto T. Characteristics of fast-spiking neurons in the striatum of behaving monkeys. Neurosci Res. 2016;105:2–18.

9. Tepper JM, Tecuapetla F, Koós T, Ibáñez-Sandoval O. Heterogeneity and diversity of striatal GABAergic interneurons. Front Neuroanat. 2010;4(150):1–18.

10. Reig R, Silberberg G. Multisensory integration in the mouse striatum. Neuron. 2014;83(5):1200–12.

11. Arias-García MA, Tapia D, Laville JA, Calderón VM, Ramiro-Cortés Y, Bargas J, Galarraga E. Functional comparison of corticostriatal and thalamostriatal postsynaptic responses in striatal neurons of the mouse. Brain Struct Funct. 2018;223(3):1229–53.

12. Gittis AH, Leventhal DK, Fensterheim BA, Pettibone JR, Berke JD, Kreitzer AC. Selective inhibition of striatal fast-spiking interneurons causes dyskinesias. J Neurosci. 2011;31(44):15727–31.

13. Damodaran S, Evans RC, Blackwell KT. Synchronized firing of fast-spiking interneurons is critical to maintain balanced firing between direct and indirect pathway neurons of the striatum. J Neurophysiol. 2014;111(4):836–48.

14. Surmeier DJ, Bargas J, Hemmings HC, Nairn AC, Greengard P. Modulation of calcium currents by a D1 dopaminergic protein kinase/phosphatase cascade in rat neostriatal neurons. Neuron. 1995;14:385–97.

15. Bolam JP, Hanley JJ, Booth PA, Bevan MD. Synaptic organization of the basal ganglia. J Anat. 2000;196:527–42.

16. Gerfen CR, Surmeier DJ. Modulation of striatal projection systems by dopamine. Annu Rev Neurosci. 2011;34:441–66.

17. Surmeier DJ, Carrillo-Reid L, Bargas J. Dopaminergic modulation of striatal neurons, circuits, and assemblies. Neuroscience. 2011;198:3–18.

18. Tritsch NX, Sabatini BL. Dopaminergic modulation of synaptic transmission in cortex and striatum. Neuron. 2012;76(1):33–50.

19. Carrillo-Reid L, Hernández-López S, Tapia D, Galarraga E, Bargas J. Dopaminergic modulation of the striatal microcircuit: receptor-specific configuration of cell assemblies. J Neurosci. 2011;31(42):14972–83.

20. Bracci E, Centonze D, Bernardi G, Calabresi P. Dopamine excites fast-spiking interneurons in the striatum. J Neurophysiol. 2002;87(4):2190–4.

21. Centonze D, Grande C, Usiello A, Gubellini P, Erbs E, Martin AB, Pisani A, Tognazzi N, Bernardi G, Moratalla R, Borrelli E, Calabresi P. Receptor subtypes involved in the presynaptic and postsynaptic actions of dopamine on striatal interneurons. J Neurosci. 2003;23(15):6245–54.

22. Gorelova N, Seamans JK, Yang CR. Mechanisms of dopamine activation of fast-spiking interneurons that exert inhibition in rat prefrontal cortex. J Neurophysiol. 2002;88(6):3150–66.

23. Kröner S, Krimer LS, Lewis DA, Barrionuevo G. Dopamine increases inhibition in the monkey dorsolateral prefrontal cortex through cell type-specific modulation of interneurons. Cereb Cortex. 2007;17(5):1020–32.

24. Kröner S, Rosenkranz JA, Grace AA, Barrionuevo G, Kro S. Dopamine modulates excitability of basolateral amygdala neurons in vitro dopamine. J Neurophysiol. 2005;93(3):1598–610.

25. Pérez-Garci E, Bargas J, Galarraga E. The role of Ca^{2+} channels in the repetitive firing of striatal projection neurons. NeuroReport. 2003;14(9):1253–6.

26. Perez-Rosello T, Figueroa A, Salgado H, Vilchis C, Tecuapetla F, Guzman JN, Galarraga E, Bargas J. Cholinergic control of firing pattern and neurotransmission in rat neostriatal projection neurons: role of $Ca_V2.1$ and $Ca_V2.2$ Ca^{2+} channels. J Neurophysiol. 2005;93(5):2507–19.

27. Bargas J, Ayala GX, Vilchis C, Pineda JC, Galarraga E. Ca^{2+}-activated outward currents in neostriatal neurons. Neuroscience. 1999;88(2):479–88.

28. Bennett BD, Callaway JC, Wilson CJ. Intrinsic membrane properties underlying spontaneous tonic firing in neostriatal cholinergic interneurons. J Neurosci. 2000;20(22):8493–503.

29. Chen TW, Wardill TJ, Sun Y, Pulver SR, Renninger SL, Baohan A, Schreiter ER, Kerr RA, Orger MB, Jayaraman V, Looger LL, Svoboda K, Kim DS. Ultrasensitive fluorescent proteins for imaging neuronal activity. Nature. 2013;499(7458):295–300.

30. Bargas J, Howe A, Eberwine J, Cao Y, Surmeier DJ. Cellular and molecular characterization of Ca^{2+} currents in acutely isolated, adult rat neostriatal neurons. J Neurosci. 1994;14(11):6667–86.

31. Perez-Burgos A, Perez-Rosello T, Salgado H, Flores-Barrera E, Prieto GA, Figueroa A, Galarraga E, Bargas J. Muscarinic M1 modulation of N and L types of calcium channels is mediated by protein kinase C in neostriatal neurons. Neuroscience. 2008;155(4):1079–97.

32. Perez-Burgos A, Prieto GA, Galarraga E, Bargas J. $Ca_V2.1$ channels are modulated by muscarinic M1 receptors through phosphoinositide hydrolysis in neostriatal neurons. Neuroscience. 2010;165(2):293–9.

33. Hernández-González O, Hernández-Flores T, Prieto GA, Pérez-Burgos A, Arias-García MA, Galarraga E, Bargas J. Modulation of Ca^{2+}-currents by sequential and simultaneous activation of adenosine A1 and A2A receptors in striatal projection neurons. Purinergic Signal. 2014;10(2):269–81.

34. Hernández-Flores T, Hernández-González O, Pérez-Ramírez MB, Lara-González E, Arias-García MA, Duhne M, Pérez-Burgos A, Prieto GA, Figueroa A, Galarraga E, Bargas J. Modulation of direct pathway striatal projection neurons by muscarinic M4-type receptors. Neuropharmacology. 2015;89:232–44.

35. Bargas J, Surmeier DJ, Kitai ST. High- and low-voltage activated calcium currents are expressed by neurons cultured from embryonic rat neostriatum. Brain Res. 1991;541(1):70–4.

36. Carrillo-Reid L, Tecuapetla F, Tapia D, Hernández-Cruz A, Galarraga E, Drucker-Colin R, Bargas J. Encoding network states by striatal cell assemblies. J Neurophysiol. 2008;99(3):1435–50.

37. Vilchis C, Bargas J, Pérez-Roselló T, Salgado H, Galarraga E. Somatostatin modulates Ca^{2+} currents in neostriatal neurons. Neuroscience. 2002;109(3):555–67.

38. Kawaguchi Y, Wilson CJ, Augood SJ, Emson PC. Striatal interneurones: chemical, physiological and morphological characterization. Trends Neurosci. 1995;18(12):527–35.

39. Catterall WA. Voltage-gated calcium channels. Cold Spring Harb Perspect Biol. 2011;3(8):1–23.

40. Hernandez-Lopez S, Tkatch T, Perez-Garci E, Galarraga E, Bargas J, Hamm H, Surmeier DJ. D2 dopamine receptors in striatal medium spiny neurons reduce L-type Ca^{2+} currents and excitability via a novel PLCb1-IP3-calcineurin-signaling cascade. J Neurosci. 2000;20(24):8987–95.

41. Hernandez-Lopez S, Bargas J, Surmeier DJ, Reyes A, Galarraga E. D1 receptor activation enhances evoked discharge in neostriatal medium spiny neurons by modulating an L-type Ca^{2+} conductance. J Neurosci. 1997;17(9):3334–42.

42. Guzmán JN, Hernández A, Galarraga E, Tapia D, Laville A, Vergara R, Aceves J, Bargas J. Dopaminergic modulation of axon collaterals interconnecting spiny neurons of the rat striatum. J Neurosci. 2003;23(26):8931–40.

43. Plata V, Duhne M, Pérez-Ortega JE, Barroso-Flores J, Galarraga E, Bargas J. Direct evaluation of L-DOPA actions on neuronal activity of parkinsonian tissue in vitro. Biomed Res Int. 2013;519184:1–7.

44. Rudy B, McBain CJ. Kv3 channels: voltage-gated K + channels designed for high-frequency repetitive firing. Trends Neurosci. 2001;24(9):517–26.

45. Erisir A, Lau D, Rudy B, Leonard CS. Function of specific K + channels in sustained high-frequency firing of fast-spiking neocortical interneurons. J Neurophysiol. 1999;82(5):2476–89.

46. Lenz S, Perney TM, Qin Y, Robbins E, Chesselet MF. GABA-ergic interneurons of the striatum express the Shaw-like potassium channel Kv3.1. Synapse. 1994;18(1):55–66.

47. Cepeda C, Galvan L, Holley SM, Rao SP, André VM, Botelho EP, Chen JY, Watson JB, Deisseroth K, Levine MS. Multiple sources of striatal inhibition are differentially affected in Huntington's disease mouse models. J Neurosci. 2013;33(17):7393–406.

48. Rossignol E, Kruglikov I, van den Maagdenberg AM, Rudy B, Fishell G. $Ca_V2.1$ ablation in cortical interneurons selectively impairs fast-spiking basket cells and causes generalized seizures. Ann Neurol. 2013;74(2):209–22.

49. Tottene A, Urbani A, Pietrobon D. Role of different voltage-gated Ca^{2+} channels in cortical spreading depression: specific requirement of P/Q-type Ca^{2+} channels. Channels. 2011;5(2):110–4.

50. Kataoka Y, Kalanithi PS, Grantz H, Schwartz ML, Saper C, Leckman JF, Vaccarino FM. Decreased number of parvalbumin and cholinergic interneurons in the striatum of individuals with Tourette syndrome. J Comp Neurol. 2010;518(3):277–91.

51. Kalanithi PS, Zheng W, Kataoka Y, DiFiglia M, Grantz H, Saper CB, Schwartz ML, Leckman JF, Vaccarino FM. Altered parvalbumin-positive neuron distribution in basal ganglia of individuals with Tourette syndrome. Proc Natl Acad Sci USA. 2005;102(37):13307–12.

52. Galarraga E, Hernández-López S, Reyes A, Barral J, Bargas J. Dopamine facilitates striatal EPSPs through an L-type Ca^{2+} conductance. NeuroReport. 1997;889(10):2183–6.

53. Tecuapetla F, Carrillo-Reid L, Bargas J, Galarraga E. Dopaminergic modulation of short-term synaptic plasticity at striatal inhibitory synapses. Proc Natl Acad Sci USA. 2007;104(24):10258–63.

54. Recillas-Morales S, Sanchez-Vega L, Ochoa-Sanchez N, Caballero-Floran I, Paz-Bermudez F, Silva I, Aceves J, Erlij D, Floran B. L-type Ca^{2+} channel activity determines modulation of GABA release by dopamine in the substantia nigra reticulata and the globus pallidus of the rat. Neuroscience. 2014;256:292–301.

55. Tepper JM, Wilson CJ, Koós T. Feedforward and feedback inhibition in neostriatal GABAergic spiny neurons. Brains Res Rev. 2008;58:272–81.

56. Wang W, Nitulescu I, Lewis JS, Lemos JC, Bamford IJ, Posielski NM, Storey GP, Phillips PE, Bamford NS. Overinhibition of corticostriatal activity following prenatal cocaine exposure. Ann Neurol. 2013;73:355–69.

57. Beatty JA, Song SC, Wilson CJ. Cell-type-specific resonances shape the responses of striatal neurons to synaptic input. J Neurophysiol. 2014;113(3):688–700.

58. Hu H, Gan J, Jonas P. Interneurons fast-spikin, parvalbumin + GABAergic interneurons: from cellular design to microcircuit function. Science. 2014;345(6196):1255263.

59. Siegle JH, Pritchett DL, Moore CI. Gamma-range synchronization of fast-spiking interneurons can enhance detection of tactile stimuli. Nat Neurosci. 2014;17(10):1371–9.

60. Brown P. Cortical drives to human muscle: the Piper and related rhythms. Prog Neurobiol. 2000;60(1):97–108.

61. McNally JM, McCarley RW. Gamma band oscillations: a key to understanding schizophrenia symptoms and neural circuit abnormalities. Curr Opin Psychiatry. 2016;29(3):202–10.

62. Tecuapetla F, Matias S, Dugue GP, Mainen ZF, Costa RM. Balanced activity in basal ganglia projection pathways is critical for contraversive movements. Nat Commun. 2014;5(4315):1–10.

11

Clinical features and risk factors of neurological involvement in Sjögren's syndrome

Wenjing Ye[1,2], Siyan Chen[3], Xinshi Huang[1], Wei Qin[1], Ting Zhang[1], Xiaofang Zhu[1], Xiaochun Zhu[1], Chongxiang Lin[4*] and Xiaobing Wang[1*]

Abstract

Background: To investigated distinct manifestations of Sjögren's syndrome (SS) patients with neurological complications and the potential risk factors associated with neurological complications in SS, and to produce a disease evaluation and neurological involvement prediction for SS.

Methods: 566 patients who fulfilled the 2002 classification criteria for SS from the Rheumatology Department of the First Affiliated Hospital of Wenzhou Medical University were included in the cross-sectional study. Clinical, immunological and histological characteristics were surveyed, and potential risk factors for neurological complications were examined by multivariate analysis.

Results: Among 566 SS patients, 184 (32.5%) patients had neurological involvement, with more than 10% got limbs pain, limbs numbness and cerebral infarction, respectively. Of these 184 SS patients with neurological complications, secondary SS (sSS) patients had a higher prevalence of peripheral nervous system (PNS) involvement than primary SS (pSS) patients (31.1 vs. 19%). And sSS patients showed higher total ESSPRI score and higher prevalence of xerostomia and low C3, C4 levels with more liver, articular involvement and saliva gland atrophy, and more severe lymphocyte infiltration in salivary glands than pSS patients. As for the specific factors associated with neurological involvement, low C3 level were found to be significant in pSS or sSS patients who were younger 50 year old, and ANA positivity, cardiac involvement, saliva gland atrophy were demonstrated to be associated in elder pSS patients. And xerophthalmia was found to be associated in sSS patients.

Conclusion: Low complement (C3) levels, xerophthalmia, ANA positive, cardiac involvement and labial salivary gland histological result were good ways to predict neurological complications in different subgroups of SS, which might provide insight into better clinical decision-making, especially at early stages of the disease.

Keywords: Sjögren's syndrome, Cross-sectional study, Neurological complication, Risk factor, Logistic model

Background

Sjögren's syndrome (SS) is a chronic autoimmune disease characterized by autoantibody secretion and lymphocytic infiltrates of exocrine glands leading to xerophthalmia and xerostomia [1]. Sjögren's syndrome is considered secondary (sSS) when it presents with associated autoimmune disorders, otherwise it's considered primary Sjögren's syndrome (pSS) [2]. It impacts 0.1–0.6% of the general adult population with a female to male ratio of 9:1 [3]. Besides dry eyes and dry mouth, pSS covers a broad spectrum of extraglandular clinical presentations, including vasculitis, arthralgia, renal tubular acidosis, pulmonary involvement, immunological abnormalities and neuropathy [4, 5].

Neurological disorders of SS including peripheral neuropathy and central neuropathy were investigated since

*Correspondence: 6785069@qq.com; gale820907@163.com
[1] Rheumatology Department, The First Affiliated Hospital of Wenzhou Medical University, Wenzhou, China
[4] Stomatological Department, The First Affiliated Hospital of Wenzhou Medical University, Wenzhou, China
Full list of author information is available at the end of the article

the 1980s [6], however, their prevalence are inconstant in different studies. It's documented that 10–20% of SS patients had peripheral nervous system (PNS) involvement [7]. However, the prevalence of central nervous system (CNS) manifestations of SS ranged from 2.5 to 60% [8], which may due to the lack of unified definition of CNS involvement in SS [9, 10]. Therefore, CNS and PNS complications are common but varied in SS. Furthermore, the association between clinical/serological manifestations and nervous system involvement remains unclear. To date no seroimmunological profiles had been shown as pathognomonic neither for neurological involvement in SS. The aim of this study was to evaluate the prevalence and symptoms of neurological complications in a population of patients with SS and to investigate the potential risk factors for neurological involvement to facilitate a comprehensive disease evaluation and prognosis prediction for Chinese SS patients.

Methods
Study population and clinical data
A total of 566 patients who fulfilled the 2002 classification criteria [8] for SS from the Rheumatology department of the First Affiliated Hospital of Wenzhou Medical University between January 1, 2013 and February 28, 2017 were enrolled in this study. The study was approved by the Ethical Committee of the First Affiliated Hospital of Wenzhou Medical University (approval # 16024). The study design conformed to current National Health and Family Planning Commission of China ethical standards, with written informed consent provided by all patients. sSS patients were diagnosed with systemic lupus erythematosus [11], systemic sclerosis [12], rheumatoid arthritis [13], inflammatory myopathies [14], mixed connective tissue disease [15], or primary biliary cirrhosis [16] according to existing classification criteria used in clinical practice. Clinical data as age of disease onset, age at diagnosis, the duration of the disease, oral and ocular dryness, constitutional symptoms, joints, skin, pulmonary, kidney, vasculitis, gastrointestinal tracts and endocrine involvement were collected.

Assessment of nervous system involvement
Peripheral neuropathy includes painful sensory neuropathy, sensory ataxic neuropathy, pure sensory trigeminal neuropathy, axonal sensorimotor polyneuropathy, mononeuritis multiplex, multiple cranial neuropathies, radiculoneuropathy and autonomic neuropathy. Involvement of peripheral nervous system was diagnosed by medical history, physical examination and electromyography. Involvement of central nervous system was confirmed

by case history brain computed tomography, cranial MRI, electromyography and psychiatric records. And the presentations we collect including headache, dizziness, physical pain, epilepsy, cognitive disorder, disturbance of consciousness, emotional problem, cerebral hemorrhage, cerebral infarction, demyelination, vascular stenosis and occlusion, aging brain, cerebral tumor, leukoaraiosis and nerve injury. Depression was diagnosed by psychiatrists.

Assessment of exocrine gland involvement and disease activity
All patients underwent a thorough review of medical history, physical examination and a series of assessments to evaluate the systemic condition. Xerostomia was diagnosed by testing timed whole unstimulated salivary flow and the histopathological result of labial salivary gland biopsy (LSGB). A lymphocytic focus score of ≥ 1 as a positive biopsy with more than 50 lymphocytes per 4 mm^2, based on the classification described previously [17]. Xerophthalmia was confirmed by an ophthalmologist by examining Schirmer's test [16], breakup time of tear film [18] and cornea fluorescent pigmentation [19].

Besides routine blood test, immunological tests including ANA, anti-Ro antibodies, anti-SSA antibodies, anti-SSB antibodies, rheumatoid factor, C3, C4, IgG, IgA, and IgM levels were performed using commercial techniques. Additionally, all patients were tested for acute inflammatory factors comprising erythrocyte sedimentation rate (ESR), and C-reactive protein (CRP) levels.

Disease manifestations were scored with the ESS-DAI summating the scores achieved per organ domain. The ESSDAI scores 12 organ domains on the severity of involvement, ranging from 0 to 3 points. And each patient was asked to assess the severity of dryness, fatigue, and pain over the preceding 2 weeks, each on a 10-point Likert scale. The average of the three items was regarded as ESSPRI value [20].

Statistical analysis
Continuous data were expressed as mean ± standard deviation, and counts and percentages were indicated for the categorical variables. Nonparametric Wilcoxon signed-rank test was used for paired comparison and Fisher's exact tests used for categorical data as appropriate. To examine correlations between risk factors and neuropathy, univariate analyses were used, firstly based on biological plausibility and literature review. Variables with a $P < 0.05$ in univariate analysis were then included in a multivariate analysis using logistic regression. Statistical significance was set at $P < 0.05$. All analyses were conducted using R v3.3.2 statistical software packages.

Results

The characteristics of Sjögren's syndrome patients with or without neurological involvement

The patient cohort comprised 566 individuals, with 415 pSS and 151 sSS patients. Demographic, clinical, histological, immunological, inflammatory features and outcome measures data collected from 415 pSS were presented in Table 1. The female to male ratio is 10:1. 290 (69.88%) pSS patients had no neurological involvements and 125 (30.12%) with neurological involvement. Most patients presented to the hospital in their 50s for the first interview, with an average disease course of approximate 4 years. Compared with pSS patients without neurological involvement, those with neurological involvement showed much higher total ESSDAI score with more

cardiac and constitutional domain involvements, but less glandular domain involvement. It is consistent with a lower prevalence of xerostomia in this subgroup. However, no significant difference in total ESSPRI scores was found between the two groups. pSS patients with neurological involvement showed a higher prevalence of ANA antibody and hypergammaglobulinemia, but reduced level of C3 ($P < 0.05$). No significant differences in Anti-SSA/SSB positive was found between the two subgroups ($P > 0.05$). Although pSS patients with neurological involvement seemed to use glucocorticoid more often with higher dose and longer duration, the differences didn't reach to the statistical significance ($P < 0.05$, Table 1). There are 92 (60.93%) sSS patients had no neurological involvements and 59 (39.07%) with neurological

Table 1 Demographic, clinical, histological, immunological, inflammatory features and outcome measures of Chinese primary Sjögren's syndrome patients with or without neurological involvement

	Without NP involvement 290	With NP involvement 125	P value
Age (years)	51.50 ± 13.73	52.81 ± 14.95	0.387
Sex, female, n (%)	28 (9.66%)	16 (12.80%)	0.34
Disease duration (months)	3.99 ± 6.01	4.30 ± 5.57	0.642
Hypertension, n (%)	57 (19.66%)	29 (23.20%)	0.414
Diabetes mellitus, n (%)	22 (7.59%)	12 (9.60%)	0.493
Hyperlipemia, n (%)	114 (39.31%)	37 (29.60%)	0.059
Xerostomia, n (%)	237 (81.72%)	88 (70.40%)	0.010
Xerophthalmia, n (%)	80 (27.59%)	44 (35.20%)	0.120
ESSDAI	6.60 ± 2.22	8.81 ± 3.45	< 0.001
ESSPRI	2.87 ± 1.51	2.97 ± 1.46	0.459
Constitutional domain involvement	65 (22.41%)	42 (33.60%)	0.017
Glandular domain involvement	189 (65.17%)	47 (37.60%)	< 0.001
Cardiac involvement, n (%)	133 (45.86%)	77 (61.60%)	0.003
LSGB, Lymphocytic focus ≥ 1	192 (66.21%)	76 (60.80%)	0.291
ANA positivity, n (%)	254 (87.59%)	120 (96.00%)	0.008
Anti-SSA/Ro60 positive, n (%)	214 (75.09%)	97 (78.23%)	0.494
Anti-Ro52 positive, n (%)	177 (62.11%)	79 (63.20%)	0.833
Anti-SSB positive, n (%)	134 (47.02%)	50 (40.00%)	0.188
Hypergammaglobulinemia (> 16 g/L), n	186 (64.14%)	120 (100.00%)	< 0.001
Low C3 level (< 0.9 g/L)	90 (31.03%)	54 (46.15%)	0.004
Low C4 level (< 0.1 g/L)	11 (4.17%)	6 (5.31%)	0.624
RF positive, n (%)	178 (61.38%)	59 (52.21%)	0.093
ESR (mm/h)	35.71 ± 23.84	32.43 ± 25.31	0.232
CRP (mg/L)	10.23 ± 21.68	12.76 ± 24.51	0.325
Glucocorticoid use	171 (58.97%)	81 (66.39%)	0.158
Moderate to high dose	46 (15.86%)	24 (19.20%)	0.405
Continuous use for > 1 year	81 (27.93%)	38 (30.40%)	0.610

Disease duration measured from the day diagnosed; moderate- to high-dose glucocorticoid: > 1 mg/kg/d prednisone; glucocorticoid use at any time for > 2 week

NP neurological, *ESSDAI* European League Against Rheumatism Sjögren's syndrome disease activity index, *ESSPRI* European League Against Rheumatism Sjögren's syndrome patient reported index, *ANA* antinuclear antibodies, *C3* complement component 3, *C4* complement component 4, *CRP* C-reactive protein, *ESR* erythrocyte sedimentation rate, *LSGB* labial salivary gland biopsy, *RF* rheumatoid factor

involvement. The comparison between with and without neurological involvement were not analyzed as sSS cases had different primary diseases with distinctive etiology and mechanism.

The characteristics of neurological involvement in Sjögren's syndrome patients

As shown in Table 2, the various manifestations of neurological involvements were categorized into five subgroups: PNS presentations, neuropsychiatric symptoms, unspecific neurological complaints, paroxysmal disease, and CNS radiological results. The prevalence of limbs pain, limbs numbness and cerebral infarction were all higher than 10%. Meanwhile, the occurrences of trigeminal neuralgia, epilepsy, cerebral hemorrhage, angiostegnosis, cerebral tumor and leukoaraiosis were comparatively low. Of note, there were 39 patients with neurological involvement had sleep problem as well.

Subtypes of neurological involvement in Sjögren's syndrome patients

Among 415 pSS patients, there were 125 of them had neurological involvement with 79 PNS involvement and 63 CNS involvement. 59 out of 151 sSS patients got neurological involvement. And sSS had a higher prevalence of PNS involvement than pSS (31.13 vs. 19.04%, $P < 0.05$), although no significant difference in CNS involvement (13.91 vs. 15.18%). Most of the sSS cases with neurological involvement were secondary to systemic lupus erythematosus (SLE) or rheumatoid arthritis (RA) (Table 3).

Table 3 Subtypes of neurological involvement in Sjögren's syndrome patients

	PNS involvement	CNS involvement
pSS (n = 125)	79	63
sSS (n = 59)	47	21
Rheumatoid arthritis	13	5
Systemic lupus erythematosus	28	13
Systemic sclerosis	1	0
Dermatomyositis/myositis	3	0
Primary biliary cirrhosis	0	3
Mixed connective tissue disease	1	1

Table 2 Features of neurological involvement in Sjögren's syndrome patients

Neurological involvement	Numbers	Percentage (%)
PNS presentations		
Limbs pain	35	0.190
Limbs numbness	25	0.136
Anaesthesia	8	0.043
Trigeminal neuralgia	1	0.005
Neuropsychiatric symptoms		
Depression	10	0.054
Cognitive dysfunction	4	0.022
Unspecific neurological complaints		
Headache	15	0.082
Dizziness	16	0.087
Muscular weakness	11	0.060
Paroxysmal disease		
Epilepsy	3	0.016
CNS radiological results		
Cerebral hemorrhage	2	0.011
Cerebral infarction	35	0.190
Demyelination	5	0.027
Angiostegnosis	3	0.016
Aging brain	11	0.060
Cerebral tumor	3	0.016
Leukoaraiosis	3	0.016

PNS peripheral nervous system, *CNS* central nervous system

Table 4 Analysis of multiple features of 184 Chinese Sjögren's syndrome patients with neurological involvement

	pSS 125	sSS 59	P value
Age (years)	52.81 ± 14.95	47.93 ± 16.22	0.084
Sex, female, n (%)	109 (87.20%)	56 (94.90%)	0.126
Disease duration (months)	51.57 ± 66.84	46.07 ± 68.73	0.955
Xerostomia, n (%)	88 (70.40%)	50 (84.70%)	0.036
Xerophthalmia, n (%)	44 (35.20%)	22 (37.30%)	0.783
ESSDAI	7.84 ± 2.83	8.81 ± 3.45	0.129
ESSPRI	2.77 ± 1.34	3.38 ± 1.63	0.038
Liver dysfunction, n (%)	41 (33.60%)	28 (49.10%)	0.047
Articular involvement, n (%)	46 (36.80%)	40 (67.80%)	<0.001
LSGB, lymphocytic focus ≥ 1	76 (60.80%)	50 (84.70%)	0.001
Saliva gland atrophy	78 (70.30%)	46 (86.80%)	0.021
Albumin levels (g/L)	37.35 ± 5.73	34.12 ± 5.94	<0.001
Low C3 level (< 0.9 g/L)	54 (46.20%)	36 (65.50%)	0.018
Low C4 level (< 0.1 g/L)	6 (5.30%)	11 (20.80%)	0.005
Antiphospholipid syndrome	0	6(10.17%)	<0.001

NP neurological, *ESSDAI* European League Against Rheumatism Sjögren's syndrome disease activity index, *ESSPRI* European League Against Rheumatism Sjögren's syndrome patient reported index, *ANA* antinuclear antibodies, *C3* complement component 3, *C4* complement component 4, *CRP* C-reactive protein, *ESR* erythrocyte sedimentation rate, *LSGB* labial salivary gland biopsy, *RF* rheumatoid factor

Features of Sjögren's syndrome patients with neurological involvement

As shown in Table 4, sSS showed higher total ESSPRI score and higher prevalence of xerostomia and low C3, C4 levels with more liver, articular involvement and saliva gland atrophy, while pSS had a higher level of albumin. And sSS showed more severe lymphocyte infiltration in salivary glands than pSS. There were 6 antiphospholipid syndrome cases were found in sSS but none in pSS.

Specific factors associated with neurological involvement in Sjögren's syndrome

A series of features commonly used in clinical practice were selected first by univariate analysis and then logistic regression analysis as potential risk factors for neurological involvement in SS. By univariate analysis a series of variables were found to be associated with neurological involvement, as shown in Table 5. And their independent risks for neurological involvement were further tested by multivariate analysis. As age is a key factor on neurological involvement, we did a stratification analysis

by separate the cohort into two subgroups. There were 248 patients younger than 50, and 318 were the opposite (including 50 years old). We found that male, low C3 level presented significant associations with neurological involvement in pSS patients who were younger than 50 year old, while ANA positivity, cardiac involvement, saliva gland atrophy were found significant in those older than 50 year old (Table 6). Xerophthalmia and low C3 level were demonstrated to be associated with neurological involvement in the younger subgroup of sSS patients, and xerophthalmia level also presented in the older subgroup (Table 6).

Discussion

This study is to investigate the neurological involvement in a Chinese SS cohort. The prevalence of peripheral and central nervous system are about 19 and 15.2% respectively in pSS, which lied in the wide ranges came from various studies [21, 22]. However, sSS seemed to complicate with more PNS manifestations (31.1%). Most of our sSS were secondary to SLE and RA. It's been reported the prevalence of neuropsychiatric syndromes in SLE at time of diagnosis with SLE were 28% [23], but the estimate incidence of neurological symptoms in RA were high up to 70% when mood disorders are included [24]. In our cohort, neuropsychiatric symptoms like depression is not uncommon, which should arouse more attention. Among various manifestations of neurological involvement, limbs pain, limbs numbness and cerebral infarction were most frequently seen in more than a third of the cohort which suggesting an ischemic mechanism and

Table 5 Univariate and multivariate analysis of factors associated with neurological involvement in primary and secondary Sjögren's syndrome

Independent variables	Univariate analysis OR (95% CI) P value	
	pSS	sSS
Age < 50		
Sex (male)	4.55 (1.27, 16.29) 0.020	–
ESSDAI	1.47 (1.26, 1.72) < 0.001	1.27 (1.05, 1.53) 0.0136
Xerophthalmia, n (%)		3.25 (1.03, 10.23) 0.0440
Low C3 level (< 0.9 g/L)	2.10 (1.06, 4.13) 0.032	3.83 (1.31, 11.24) 0.0143
Low C4 level (< 0.1 g/L)	–	3.50 (1.02, 12.00) 0.0463
RF positive, n (%)	–	0.32 (0.12, 0.87) 0.0251
ESR (mm/h)	0.98 (0.96, 1.00) 0.038	–
Age ≥ 50		
Constitutional domain involvement	1.96 (1.08, 3.55) 0.027	–
ESSDAI	1.52 (1.34, 1.72) < 0.001	1.44 (1.16, 1.80) 0.001
ANA positivity, n (%)	4.50 (1.02, 19.83) 0.047	–
Cardiac involvement, n (%)	2.28 (1.21, 4.31) 0.010	–
Xerophthalmia, n (%)	1.82 (1.02, 3.27) 0.044	4.82 (1.56, 14.95) 0.006
Low C3 level (< 0.9 g/L)	1.83 (1.01, 3.30) 0.046	–
Saliva gland atrophy	0.38 (0.19, 0.74) 0.004	–
ESR (mm/h)	–	0.98 (0.96, 1.00) 0.0336

NP neurological, ESSDAI European League Against Rheumatism Sjögren's syndrome disease activity index, ESSPRI European League Against Rheumatism Sjögren's syndrome patient reported index, ANA antinuclear antibodies, C3 complement component 3, C4 complement component 4, CRP C-reactive protein, ESR erythrocyte sedimentation rate, LSGB labial salivary gland biopsy, RF rheumatoid factor

Table 6 Multivariate analysis of factors associated with neurological involvement in primary and secondary Sjögren's syndrome

Independent variables	Multivariate analysis OR (95% CI) P value	
	pSS	sSS
Age < 50		
Sex (male)	4.56 (1.15, 20.01) 0.013	
Low C3 level (< 0.9 g/L)	2.21 (1.04, 4.82) 0.026	3.33 (1.92, 8.03) 0.021
Xerophthalmia, n (%)		3.03 (1.08, 7.45) 0.030
Age >= 50		
ANA positivity	5.52 (1.42, 37.28) 0.037	
Cardiac involvement	2.38 (1.18, 5.06) 0.013	
Saliva gland atrophy	0.28 (0.13, 0.59) 0.001	
Xerophthalmia, n (%)		4.07 (1.25, 14.35) 0.012

NP neurological, ESSDAI European League Against Rheumatism Sjögren's syndrome disease activity index, ESSPRI European League Against Rheumatism Sjögren's syndrome patient reported index, ANA antinuclear antibodies, C3 complement component 3, C4 complement component 4, CRP C-reactive protein, ESR erythrocyte sedimentation rate, LSGB labial salivary gland biopsy, RF rheumatoid factor

a vasculitis process in SS. Epilepsy had been described in pSS, but is not well characterized [7]. We also found 3 cases with epilepsy as their initial symptoms and were then diagnosed by neuropathists. When compare the differences between pSS and sSS, we found the later have higher frequencies of xerostomia, articular and saliva gland involvement and low complement prevalence. Given the wide involvement of neurological involvement in SS, tight control of neurological risk factors is needed for better prognosis.

For potential risk factors for neurological involvement, low C3 level was found to be associated in younger pSS patients, and ANA positivity, cardiac involvement, saliva gland atrophy were demonstrated to be associated in elder pSS patients. It revealed that cardiac event accumulates with age and plays a key role in neurological involvement. For example, a marked increase in the risk of stroke was found after acute myocardial infarction stroke revealed its strong association with high cardiovascular risk [25]. Saliva gland atrophy was confirmed by histology of LSGB. Significant lymphocytic in filtration in the LSGB, defined as a focus score (FS) ≥ 1, has a preponderant role in both AECG and ACR classifications and is a promising tool for prognosis [26]. It and has sensibility comparable to scintigraphy and sialography and could not be substituted by ultrasound for all patients [27]. However, the sensitivity and specificity of commonly seen saliva gland atrophy for SS remain unclear. Here, we reveal the potential relationship between saliva gland atrophy and neurological involvement in pSS, especially meaningful in the elder, while the pathogenesis to be further investigated. ANA positivity has been found to be associated with uveitis risk in Juvenile idiopathic arthritis [28] and is considered as a significant predictors of cardiovascular events and mortality in both those with and those without rheumatic diseases, which hints the its potential role in neurological involvement [29].

Furthermore, xerophthalmia were found to be associated with neurological involvement in both younger and older sSS patients, but low C3 level was only connected with those younger sSS patients. As is known, the complement system is a major component of the innate immune system, is becoming increasingly recognized as a critical participant in the acute inflammatory pathophysiology of acquired brain or spinal cord injury [30, 31]. C3 represents the central molecule of the complement cascade [32]. Low level of C3 in SS patients' serum which suggesting the excessive activation and consumption of complement system, was revealed to be an independent risk factor for neurological involvement both in pSS and sSS patients who were less than 50 years old. Our finding further supports the role of complement system in immunological associated neurological lesion. Also, the

different risk factors of neurological involvement in the two age subgroups suggested distinctive mechanisms of pathogenesis behind them.

The broad spectrums of clinical profiles, different classification criteria and ethnic diversity have posed challenges to a comprehensive and accurate appraisal of SS. In our study it's demonstrated that low C3 level is a good to predictor for neurological complications in younger SS, both in primary and secondary SS, which might provide insight into better clinical decision-making, especially at early stages of the disease.

However, limitation of this study should be considered, that we included a homogenous group of participants from one center, which might provide compelling results. As it is a cross-sectional study, is limited to correlation analysis and unable to support strong causal conclusions. And traditional risk factors like arteriosclerosis, age, hypertension, therapeutic side effects, were not adjusted in the present study, which might also play a key role in the development of the neurological complications in SS. Therefore, to further evaluate the role of complement neurological complications in SS, more data from heterogeneous SS patients with consecutive follow-up are highly recommended.

Conclusions

Low complement (C3) levels, xerophthalmia, ANA positive, cardiac involvement and labial salivary gland histological result were good ways to predict neurological complications in different subgroups of SS, which might provide insight into better clinical decision-making, especially at early stages of the disease.

Abbreviations

SS: Sjögren's syndrome; sSS: secondary Sjögren's syndrome; pSS: primary Sjögren's syndrome; PNS: peripheral nervous system; C3/C4: complement 3/ complement 4; CNS: central nervous system; LA: leukoaraiosis; LSGB: labial salivary gland biopsy; ESR: erythrocyte sedimentation rate; CRP: C-reactive protein; RF: rheumatoid factor; ANA: antinuclear antibodies; EULAR: European League Against Rheumatism; ESSDAI: European League Against Rheumatism Sjögren's syndrome disease activity index; ESSPRI: European League Against Rheumatism Sjögren's syndrome patient reported index.

Authors' contributions

XSH, WQ and TZ collected the clinical data of patients that enrolled in this study. XFZ and XCZ made substantial contributions to conception and design, and analyzed the patient data regarding the rheumatic disease. SYC assessed the nervous system involvement in SS patients and analyzed data regarding nervous system disease. CXL assessed the oral symptoms in SS patient. All authors involved in drafting the manuscript. WJY and XBW was the major contributor in revising the manuscript and given final approval of the version to be published. All authors agreed to be accountable for all aspects of the work in ensuring that questions related to the accuracy or integrity of any part of the work are appropriately investigated and resolved. All authors read and approved the final manuscript.

Author details

[1] Rheumatology Department, The First Affiliated Hospital of Wenzhou Medical University, Wenzhou, China. [2] Rheumatology Department, Ruian People's

Hospital, Wenzhou, China. [3] Neurology Department, The First Affiliated Hospital of Wenzhou Medical University, Wenzhou, China. [4] Stomatological Department, The First Affiliated Hospital of Wenzhou Medical University, Wenzhou, China.

Acknowledgements
We thank the patients for participating in this study. We also thank Professor Jianmin Li for providing expert advice on salivary gland pathology.

Competing interests
The authors declare that they have no competing interests.

Funding
No funding was obtained for this study.

References

1. Moreira I, Teixeira F, Silva AM, Vasconcelos C, Farinha F, Santos E. Frequent involvement of central nervous system in primary Sjögren syndrome. Rheumatol Int. 2015;35(2):289–94.
2. Vitali C, Bombardieri S, Moutsopoulos HM, Balestrieri G, Bencivelli W, Bernstein RM, Bjerrum KB, Braga S, Coll J, Vita SD. Preliminary criteria for the classification of Sjögren's syndrome. Results of a prospective concerted action supported by the European Community. Arthritis Rheum. 1993;36(3):340–7.
3. Mavragani CP, Moutsopoulos HM. The geoepidemiology of Sjögren's syndrome. Autoimmun Rev. 2010;9(5):A305–10.
4. Fox RI. Sjögren's syndrome. Lancet. 2005;366(9482):321–31.
5. Ramos Casals M, Brito Zerón P, Sisó Almirall A, Bosch Aparici FJ. Primary Sjogren syndrome. Br Med J. 2012;344:e3821.
6. Alexander EL, Provost TT, Stevens MB, Alexander GE. Neurologic complications of primary Sjögren's syndrome. Medicine (Baltimore). 1982;61(4):247–57.
7. Delalande S, de Seze J, Fauchais AL, Hachulla E, Stojkovic T, Ferriby D, Dubucquoi S, Pruvo JP, Vermersch P, Hatron PY. Neurologic manifestations in primary Sjogren syndrome: a study of 82 patients. Medicine (Baltimore). 2004;83(5):280–91.
8. Vitali C, Bombardieri S, Jonsson R, Moutsopoulos H, Alexander E, Carsons S, Daniels T, Fox P, Fox R, Kassan S. Classification criteria for Sjögren's syndrome: a revised version of the European criteria proposed by the American-European Consensus Group. Ann Rheum Dis. 2002;61(6):554–8.
9. Segal B, Carpenter A, Walk D. Involvement of nervous system pathways in primary Sjögren's syndrome. Rheum Dis Clin North Am. 2008;34(4):885–906, viii.
10. Le Guern V, Belin C, Henegar C, Moroni C, Maillet D, Lacau C, Dumas JL, Vigneron N, Guillevin L. Cognitive function and 99mTc-ECD brain SPECT are significantly correlated in patients with primary Sjogren syndrome: a case-control study. Ann Rheum Dis. 2010;69(1).132–7.
11. Tan EM, Cohen AS, Fries JF, Masi AT, Mcshane DJ, Rothfield NF, Schaller JG, Talal N, Winchester RJ. The 1982 revised criteria for the classification of systemic lupus erythematosus. Arthritis Rheum. 1982;25(11):1271–7.
12. Masi AT. Preliminary criteria for the classification of systemic sclerosis (scleroderma). Arthritis Rheum. 1980;23(5):581–90.
13. Aletaha D, Neogi T, Silman AJ, Funovits J, Felson DT, Bingham CO, Birnbaum NS, Burmester GR, Bykerk VP, Cohen MD. 2010 rheumatoid arthritis classification criteria: an American College of Rheumatology/European League Against Rheumatism collaborative initiative. Arthritis Rheum. 2010;62(9):2569–81.
14. Bohan A, Peter JB. Polymyositis and dermatomyositis. N Engl J Med. 1975;292(8):403–7.
15. Sharp GC, Anderson PC. Current concepts in the classification of connective tissue diseases: overlap syndromes and mixed connective tissue disease (MCTD). J Am Acad Dermatol. 1980;2(4):269–79.
16. Kaplan MM, Gershwin ME. Primary biliary cirrhosis. N Engl J Med. 2005;353(12):1261–73.
17. Guellec D, Cornec D, Jousse-Joulin S, Marhadour T, Marcorelles P, Pers J-O, Saraux A, Devauchelle-Pensec V. Diagnostic value of labial minor salivary gland biopsy for Sjögren's syndrome: a systematic review. Autoimmun Rev. 2013;12(3):416–20.
18. Goren MB, Goren SB. Diagnostic tests in patients with symptoms of keratoconjunctivitis sicca. Am J Ophthalmol. 1988;106(5):570–4.
19. Whitcher JP, Shiboski CH, Shiboski SC, Heidenreich AM, Kitagawa K, Zhang S, Hamann S, Larkin G, McNamara NA, Greenspan JS. A simplified quantitative method for assessing keratoconjunctivitis sicca from the Sjögren's Syndrome International Registry. Am J Ophthalmol. 2010;149(3):405–15.
20. Risselada AP, Kruize AA, Bijlsma JW. Clinical applicability of the EULAR Sjogren's syndrome disease activity index: a cumulative ESSDAI score adds in describing disease severity. Ann Rheum Dis. 2012;71(4):631.
21. Font J, Ramoscasals M, de la Red G, Pou A, Casanova A, García-Carrasco M, Cervera R, Molina JA, Valls J, Bové A, Ingelmo M, Graus F. Pure sensory neuropathy in primary Sjogren's syndrome. Longterm prospective followup and review of the literature. J Rheumatol. 2003;30(7):1552.
22. Bougea A, Anagnostou E, Konstantinos G, George P, Triantafyllou N, Kararizou E. A systematic review of peripheral and central nervous system involvement of rheumatoid arthritis, systemic lupus erythematosus, primary Sjögren's syndrome, and associated immunological profiles. Int J Chronic Dis. 2015;2015(6):1–11.
23. Muscal E, Brey RL. Neurological manifestations of systemic lupus erythematosus in children and adults. Neurol Clin. 2010;28(1):61–73.
24. Covic T, Cumming SR, Pallant JF, Manolios N, Emery P, Conaghan PG, Tennant A. Depression and anxiety in patients with rheumatoid arthritis: prevalence rates based on a comparison of the Depression, Anxiety and Stress Scale (DASS) and the hospital, Anxiety and Depression Scale (HADS). BMC Psychiatry. 2012;12:6.
25. Hachet O, Guenancia C, Stamboul K, Daubail B, Richard C, Bejot Y, Yameogo V, Gudjoncik A, Cottin Y, Giroud M, Lorgis L. Frequency and predictors of stroke after acute myocardial infarction: specific aspects of in-hospital and postdischarge events. Stroke. 2014;45(12):3514–20.
26. Milic VD, Petrovic RR, Boricic IV, Marinkovic-Eric J, Radunovic GL, Jeremic PD, Pejnovic NN, Damjanov NS. Diagnostic value of salivary gland ultrasonographic scoring system in primary Sjogren's syndrome: a comparison with scintigraphy and biopsy. J Rheumatol. 2009;36(7):1495–500.
27. Song GG, Lee YH. Diagnostic accuracies of sialography and salivary ultrasonography in Sjögren's syndrome patients: a meta-analysis. Clin Exp Rheumatol. 2014;32(4):516.
28. Heiligenhaus A, Heinz C, Edelsten C, Kotaniemi K, Minden K. Review for disease of the year: epidemiology of juvenile idiopathic arthritis and its associated uveitis: the probable risk factors. Ocul Immunol Inflamm. 2013;21(3):180–91.
29. Liang KP, Kremers HM, Crowson CS, Snyder MR, Therneau TM, Roger VL, Gabriel SE. Autoantibodies and the risk of cardiovascular events. J Rheumatol. 2009;36(11):2462–9.
30. Neher MD, Weckbach S, Flierl MA, Huber-Lang MS, Stahel PF. Molecular mechanisms of inflammation and tissue injury after major trauma—is complement the "bad guy"? J Biomed Sci. 2011;18:90.
31. Brennan FH, Anderson AJ, Taylor SM, Woodruff TM, Ruitenberg MJ. Complement activation in the injured central nervous system: another dual-edged sword? J Neuroinflammation. 2012;9:137.
32. Ricklin D, Hajishengallis G, Yang K, Lambris JD. Complement: a key system for immune surveillance and homeostasis. Nat Immunol. 2010;11(9):785–97.

12

PA28αβ overexpression enhances learning and memory of female mice without inducing 20S proteasome activity

Julia Adelöf[1,2], My Andersson[3], Michelle Porritt[2], Anne Petersen[1], Madeleine Zetterberg[1], John Wiseman[2] and Malin Hernebring[1,2*] (ID)

Abstract

Background: The proteasome system plays an important role in synaptic plasticity. Induction and maintenance of long term potentiation is directly dependent on selective targeting of proteins for proteasomal degradation. The 20S proteasome activator PA28αβ activates hydrolysis of small nonubiquitinated peptides and possesses protective functions upon oxidative stress and proteinopathy. The effect of PA28αβ activity on behavior and memory function is, however, not known. We generated a mouse model that overexpresses PA28α (PA28αOE) to understand PA28αβ function during healthy adult homeostasis via assessment of physiological and behavioral profiles, focusing on female mice.

Results: PA28α and PA28β protein levels were markedly increased in all PA28αOE tissues analyzed. PA28αOE displayed reduced depressive-like behavior in the forced swim test and improved memory/learning function assessed by intersession habituation in activity box and shuttle box passive avoidance test, with no significant differences in anxiety or general locomotor activity. Nor were there any differences found when compared to WT for body composition or immuno-profile. The cognitive effects of PA28αOE were female specific, but could not be explained by alterations in estrogen serum levels or hippocampal regulation of estrogen receptor β. Further, there were no differences in hippocampal protein expression of neuronal or synaptic markers between PA28αOE and WT. Biochemical analysis of hippocampal extracts demonstrated that PA28α overexpression did not increase PA28–20S peptidase activity or decrease K48-polyubiquitin levels. Instead, PA28αOE exhibited elevated efficiency in preventing aggregation in the hippocampus.

Conclusions: This study reveals, for the first time, a connection between PA28αβ and neuronal function. We found that PA28α overexpressing female mice displayed reduced depressive-like behavior and enhanced learning and memory. Since the positive effects of PA28α overexpression arose without an activation of 20S proteasome capacity, they are likely independent of PA28αβ's role as a 20S proteasome activator and instead depend on a recognized chaperone-like function. These findings suggest that proteostasis in synaptic plasticity is more diverse than previously reported, and demonstrates a novel function of PA28αβ in the brain.

Keywords: PA28αβ, Learning and memory, F2 hybrid transgenic mice, Behavioral phenotyping, 20S proteasome, Proteasome capacity, K48-linked protein ubiquitination

*Correspondence: malin.hernebring@gu.se
[1] Department of Clinical Neuroscience, Institute of Neuroscience
and Physiology, Sahlgrenska Academy at the University of Gothenburg,
Gothenburg, Sweden
Full list of author information is available at the end of the article

Background

The proteasome is a sophisticated multi-subunit protease comprising the 20S catalytic core and up to two proteasome activators that interact physically with 20S and control substrate entry to its inner proteolytic compartment. PA28αβ is a proteasome activator, which is produced upon interferon-γ stimulation [1] and oxidative stress [2]. Whilst involved in antigen processing and presentation by the major histocompatibility complex I (MHC-I) [3, 4], PA28αβ provides protective functions upon oxidative stress and proteinopathy as demonstrated in both animal and cell model studies [5–9].

Protective effects of PA28αβ have been found in mice, where an overexpression of PA28α specifically in cardiomyocytes lowered the myocardial infarct size upon ischemia/reperfusion (I/R) and preserved ventricular contractility after reperfusion [5]. Cardiomyocyte-specific overexpression of PA28α also prolonged lifespan of a desmin-related cardiomyopathy mouse model while reducing its associated proteinopathy [5]. Cultured rat cardiomyocytes overexpressing PA28α exhibit reduced apoptosis and protein oxidation upon hydrogen peroxide (H_2O_2) exposure [6]. Immortalized mouse embryonic fibroblasts (MEFs) exposed to a mild pre-treatment of H_2O_2 become less sensitive to a harsh H_2O_2 exposure compared to untreated cells. This H_2O_2 adaptation requires induction of PA28α [7, 8]. Furthermore, PA28α is essential for protein damage control during mouse ES cell differentiation [9].

The mechanism behind PA28αβ's protective effects is not known. In vitro studies using purified proteins have shown that PA28αβ can induce degradation of an oxidized protein substrate [7] and exhibit chaperone-like functions in collaboration with Hsp40, Hsp70 and Hsp90 [10].

It is well established that the proteasome system is important for the nervous system to function properly. Proteasome-dependent protein degradation is known to be critical for long-term potentiation (LTP) [11–16], a molecular mechanism central for learning and memory. Proteasome inhibition impairs murine memory and learning analyzed by one-trail inhibitory avoidance [15], taste aversion [16], auditory fear conditioning and context fear conditioning [17]. In addition, the proteasome system regulates synaptic transmission at both presynaptic and postsynaptic terminals in mammalian neurons [18–20]. However, the role of PA28αβ in neuronal function is an almost completely unexplored field. Protein expression patterns in the brain of healthy and disease subjects [21–24] suggest a role in neurodegenerative disease and traumatic brain injury, but no mechanistic studies have been performed.

We have generated a mouse model in which the gene encoding murine PA28α is overexpressed in all analyzed tissues (PA28αOE). The aim of this study is to characterize the behavior and physiology of female healthy adult mice to gain insight into the role of PA28αβ in normal physiological and cognitive functions.

Results

Generation and evaluation of the PA28αOE model

A targeting vector for PA28α overexpression (PA28αOE), which included the *CAG* promoter driving the expression of the coding region of *murine PA28α*, was targeted to the murine *Rosa26 locus* (see Fig. 1a). Correct integration in murine embryonic stem (ES) cells and murine splenocytes was confirmed by Targeted Locus Amplification (Cergentis).

Western blot analysis of male PA28αOE C57BL/6 mice ($n = 3$) confirmed that PA28α was overexpressed in heterozygous PA28αOE eye lens ($P = 0.0049$), left ventricle of the heart ($P < 1E-6$), mouse embryonic fibroblasts (MEFs; $P < 1E-5$) as well as in a mixed sample of frontal cortex and striatum of the brain ($P < 0.001$; Fig. 1b and Additional file 1). PA28α overexpression resulted in an upregulation of PA28β (the other PA28αβ subunit) in MEFs, frontal cortex and striatum from PA28αOE (detected in OE MEFs but below detection level in WT; Fig. 1b and Additional file 1), while PA28β mRNA levels were not affected (Fig. 1c and Additional file 1). This is in line with the previous finding in cardiomyocytes that PA28α overexpression stabilizes PA28β at the protein level [6]. Hence, all components of the PA28αβ complex are present in the tissues analyzed from the PA28αOE mouse model.

Female C57BL/6N × BALB/c F2 hybrid mice

Crosses between two inbred strains, hybrids, tend to be more genetically vigorous and less sensitive to adverse environmental conditions than inbred strains. To take advantage of these characteristics we generated C57BL/6N × BALB/c F2 hybrids for phenotypic profiling of the PA28αOE mouse model. We chose to analyze the mice at the age of 7–8 months, approximately corresponding to a human age of 32–34 years [25], to ensure focus on adult homeostasis. 10 wildtype (WT) and 6 PA28αOE heterozygous female F2 hybrid littermates were subjected to physiological and behavioral phenotypic profiling as outlined in Fig. 2a.

PA28αOE mice displayed no differences in body composition or immunological profile

PA28αOE mice appeared healthy and energetic, and were visually indistinguishable from WT with respect to appearance and behavior. There were no statistically

a

Wild-type allele   **R26 locus**

Targeting
vector

Targeted
allele

In vivo cre recombination

KI allele

b

c

Fig. 1 Generation and validation of the PA28αOE mouse model. **a** Structure of the targeting vector, targeted allele and KI allele (PA28αOE). **b** Representative western blots of PA28α in cultivated mouse embryonic fibroblasts (MEFs), frontal cortex and striatum (brain), eye lens and left ventricle of the heart and representative western blots of PA28β in MEFs and frontal cortex and striatum (brain) from litter mates of PA28αOE (OE) and wildtype (WT) C57BL/6 male mice (founder strain). Analysis demonstrated that PA28α is induced fivefold in MEFs ($P < 1E-5$; Student's *t* test), 3.2-fold in brain ($P < 0.001$), 15-fold in eye lens ($P = 0.0049$), and fourfold in heart ($P < 1E-6$), while PA28β is induced 2.7-fold in brain ($P = 0.0015$) (n = 3). The amount of PA28β was below detection level in WT MEFs, but detected in all OE MEFs (n = 3). **c** Relative levels of mRNA encoding PA28α and PA28β with 36b4 as a reference gene in a mixed sample of frontal cortex and striatum of the brain. Values are mean ± SEM normalized to mean WT-value ($P_{PA28\alpha} = 0.028$; n = 3). Two different splicing variants of the PA28β transcript were analyzed

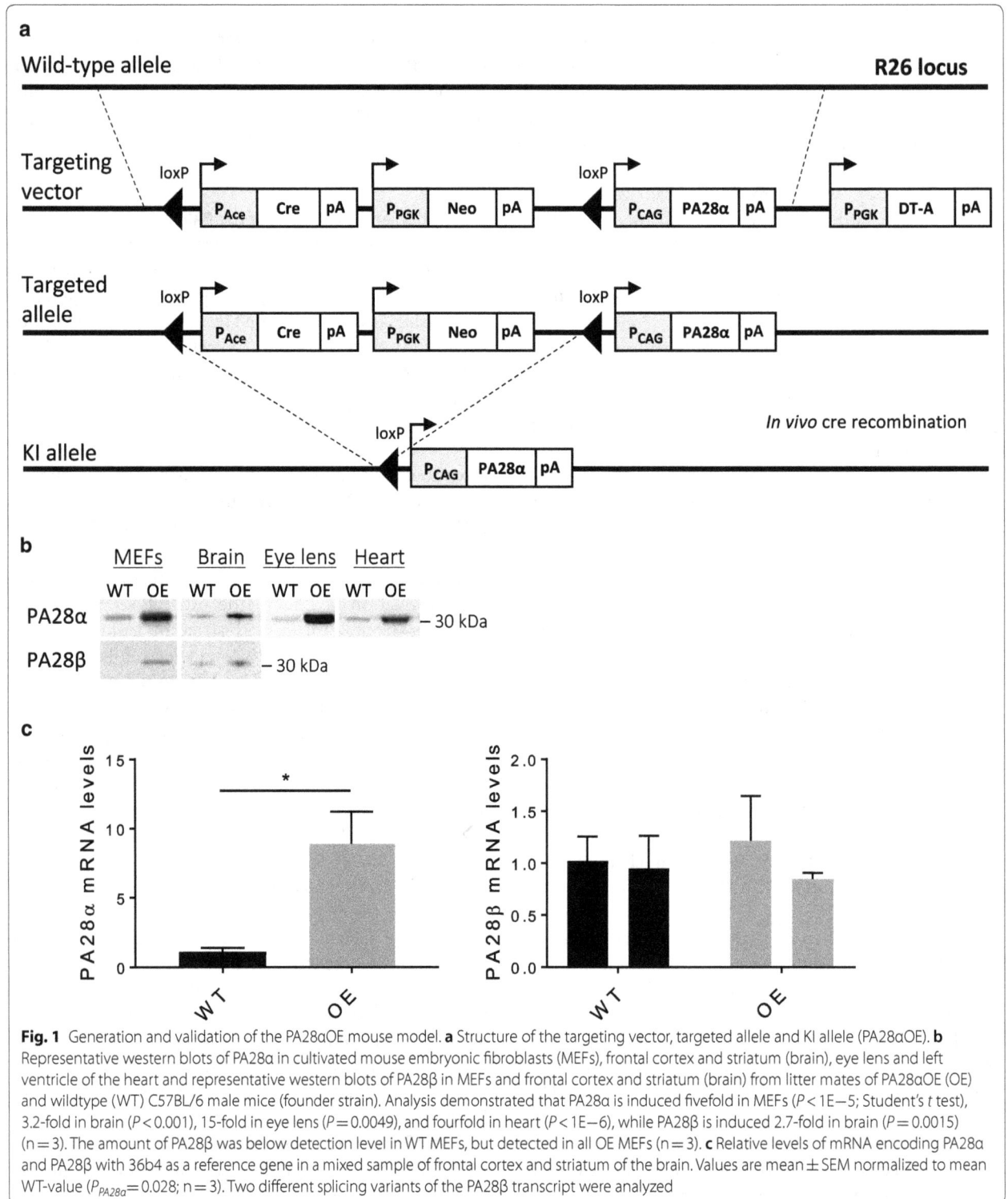

significant differences observed in the physiological parameters body temperature, body weight and length, fat mass, lean mass and bone density (Additional file 2). PA28αOE and WT mice had similar immunological

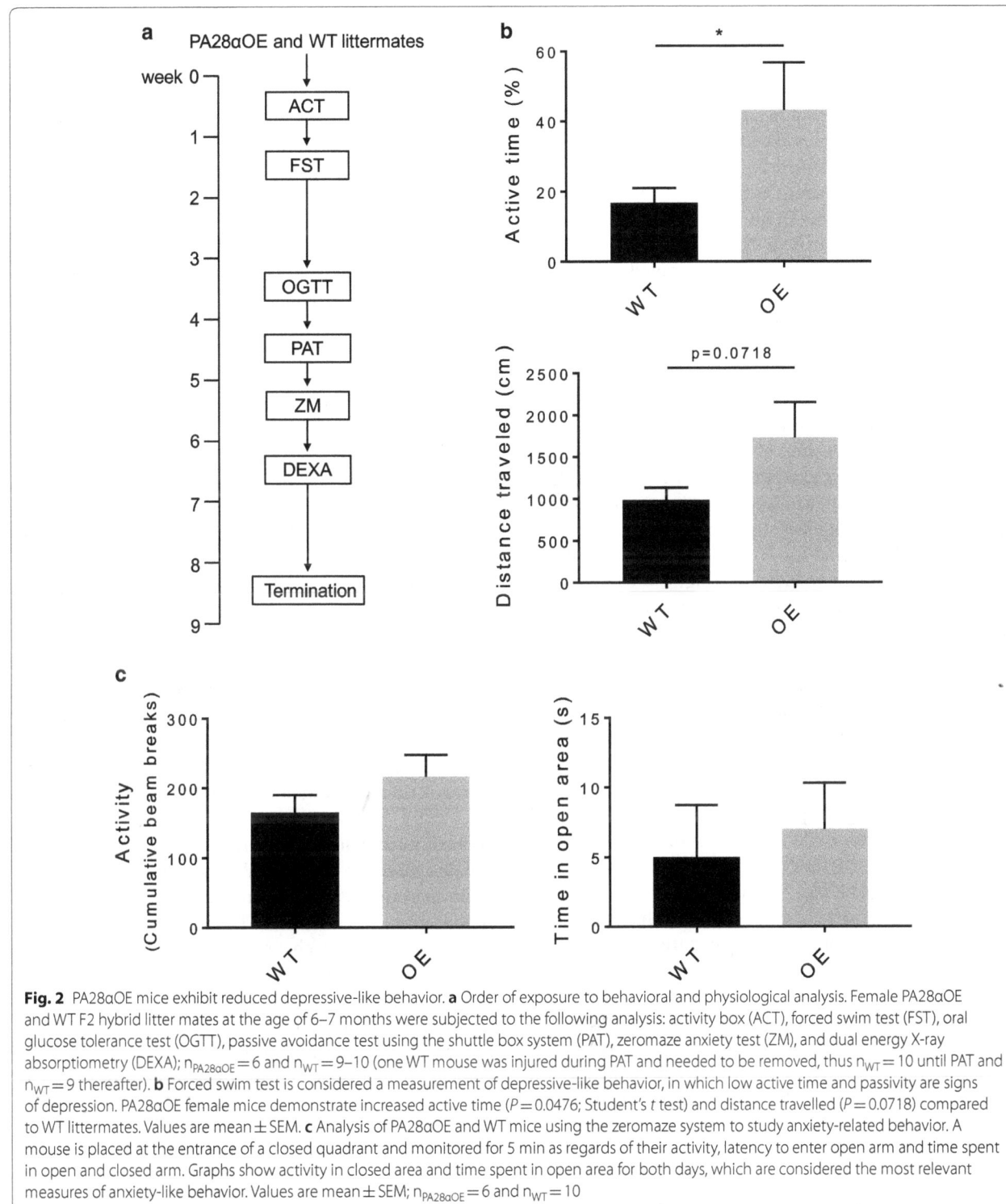

Fig. 2 PA28αOE mice exhibit reduced depressive-like behavior. **a** Order of exposure to behavioral and physiological analysis. Female PA28αOE and WT F2 hybrid litter mates at the age of 6–7 months were subjected to the following analysis: activity box (ACT), forced swim test (FST), oral glucose tolerance test (OGTT), passive avoidance test using the shuttle box system (PAT), zeromaze anxiety test (ZM), and dual energy X-ray absorptiometry (DEXA); $n_{PA28αOE} = 6$ and $n_{WT} = 9-10$ (one WT mouse was injured during PAT and needed to be removed, thus $n_{WT} = 10$ until PAT and $n_{WT} = 9$ thereafter). **b** Forced swim test is considered a measurement of depressive-like behavior, in which low active time and passivity are signs of depression. PA28αOE female mice demonstrate increased active time ($P = 0.0476$; Student's t test) and distance travelled ($P = 0.0718$) compared to WT littermates. Values are mean ± SEM. **c** Analysis of PA28αOE and WT mice using the zeromaze system to study anxiety-related behavior. A mouse is placed at the entrance of a closed quadrant and monitored for 5 min as regards of their activity, latency to enter open arm and time spent in open and closed arm. Graphs show activity in closed area and time spent in open area for both days, which are considered the most relevant measures of anxiety-like behavior. Values are mean ± SEM; $n_{PA28αOE} = 6$ and $n_{WT} = 10$

profiles with no differences in the levels of circulating granulocytes, monocytes, lymphocytes, NK cells, B cells, T cells, CD4 + T cells or CD8 + T cells (assayed at termination, Additional file 3), and displayed similar response in oral glucose tolerance test (OGTT, Additional file 4).

PA28αOE mice show decreased depressive-like behavior and increased learning

In the behavioral examinations, PA28αOE mice displayed a 400% increase in mean active time in the forced swim test (FST, Fig. 2b and Additional file 5; $P = 0.047$), indicating a reduction in depressive-like behavior compared to WT. This was not explained by a change between groups in terms of general anxiety or physical activity, as there were neither differences in anxiety levels, measured in the elevated zeromaze (Fig. 2c and Additional file 5), nor general physical activity as determined by activity box measurements (Locomotion, Fig. 3a and Additional file 6).

To determine if the decreased depressive like behavior displayed by the PA28αOE mice resulted in improved cognitive functions, we compared the time the animals spent in corners and the number of rearings (standing on hind legs, an indication of vigilance) during the first day of the activity box experiment (new environment) to the second day of trail (acquainted environment). On day 2, PA28αOE spent significantly more time in the corner (Fig. 3a and Additional file 6; $P = 0.034$) and exhibited a strong inclination to reduced rearing ($P = 0.065$), indicating enhanced intersessional habituation of PA28αOE compared to WT [26, 27]. A difference in learning capacity was apparent when the animals were exposed to the shuttle box passive avoidance test, all PA28αOE mice (6/6) stayed out of the dark compartment on day 2, where they experienced a mild electric shock the previous day, while only 2 out of 10 WT did the same (Fig. 3b and Additional file 6; $P = 0.0056$). This behavior did not result from a change in pain tolerance between WT and PA28αOE, determined by direct response in the shuttle box assay (see Methods section) and by the tail-flick method (Additional file 7). Taken together, PA28αOE mice display decreased depressive-like behavior and an increased capacity for learning compared to their WT littermates.

The cognitive effects of PA28αOE are female specific

As the previous experiments were performed with female mice, we wanted to determine whether these behavioral effects of PA28αOE were gender specific. To this end,

we subjected male C57BL/6N × BALB/c F2 hybrids (litter mates to the females analyzed) to the same cognitive behavioral tests. Male PA28αOE mice did not, however, display an increase in activity compared to WT when subjected to the forced swim test ($n \geq 5$; Additional file 8). Neither did they show any significant changes in learning compared to WT in the shuttle box passive avoidance, nor were there any indications of enhanced habituation in the male PA28αOE mice compared to WT in activity box measurements ($n \geq 5$; Additional file 8). Thus, we could not find any effect of PA28α overexpression in male mice on cognitive behavior in our behavioral tests suggesting that the effects of PA28αOE overexpression are female specific.

PA28αOE mice display no change in serum estrogen or hippocampal estrogen receptor regulation

As the declarative component of passive avoidance memory formation is formed in the hippocampus and fluctuating levels of estrogen directly affect hippocampal memory function [28], differences in estrogen levels between animal groups could explain the results obtained in our behavioral assays. To determine if this was the case, blood serum levels of estrogen was determined by ELISA, showing no differences in estrogen levels between PA28αOE and WT (Additional file 9), nor in the levels of S105-phosphorylated estrogen receptor β from hippocampal extracts (Additional file 9). This suggests that the resulting differences in behavior are neither a result of differences in serum levels of estrogen nor hippocampal regulation of estrogen receptor β.

PA28αOE mice exhibit no differences in hippocampal protein expression of neuronal or synaptic markers

As proteasome-dependent protein degradation is crucial for long-term potentiation (LTP) [11–16] we investigated if there were global changes in the amount of AMPA receptors and/or synaptic markers in the PA28αOE mice that could explain their increased learning capacity. Isolation of hippocampus (9 WT and 6 PA28αOE female F2 hybrids) and subsequent WB analysis revealed no differences in neuronal density of neurons, measured by

(See figure on next page.)

Fig. 3 PA28αOE mice exhibit improved learning/memory. **a** Activity box measurements of exploratory behavior; locomotion, rearing and corner time in novel (day 1) and acquainted (day 2) environment. On day 2, PA28αOE females spent longer time in the corners ($P = 0.034$; two-way ANOVA repeated measurements, followed by Sidak test, $F(1, 14) = 5498$), and exhibited a strong tendency of reduced rearing [$P = 0.065$; $F(1, 14) = 3992$], both of which are indicators of more proficient habituation. Locomotion on day 2 between PA28αOE and WT is not statistically different ($P = 0.19$). Values are mean ± SEM. **b** Shuttle box passive avoidance test assesses learning and memory capability. On day 1 ($P_{day1} = 0.194$, Mantel–Cox survival test) a small electric shock was given to PA28αOE female mice and their wildtype female littermates upon voluntarily entering a dark compartment. As shown, on day 2 there is a significant difference between PA28αOE and WT in re-entering the compartment ($P_{day2} = 0.0056$). Maximum assay time was 300 s (i.e. no entry = 300 s). Dashed lines correspond to 95% confidence interval

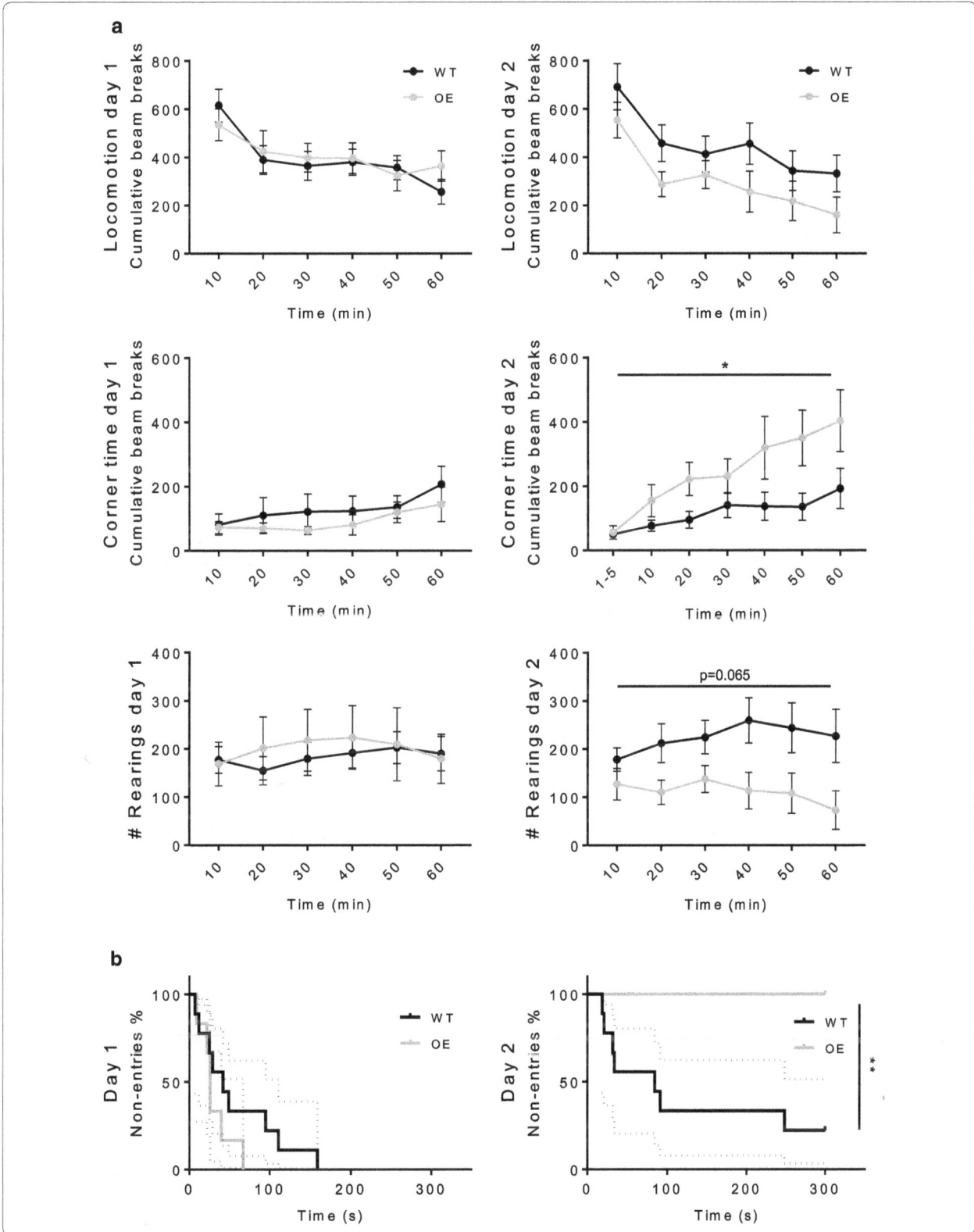

expression of the neuronal nuclear marker NeuN (Additional file 9) or synaptic density, measured as expression of adhesion molecule N-Cadherin, together with the presynaptic vesicle glycoprotein Synaptophysin and the excitatory postsynaptic density protein PSD-95 (Additional file 9). The AMPA receptor subunits GluA1 and GluA2 did not differ in expression between animal groups, nor the expression of Spinophilin, a postsynaptic density protein involved in spine formation (Additional file 9). However, expression of GluA2, Synaptophysin and GluA1 varied greatly but correlated to each other and to the level of S105-phosphorylated estrogen receptor β (Additional file 9; correlation coefficients: $CC_{GluA2-Synphys}$: 0.93; $CC_{GluA2-GluA1} = 0.92$; $CC_{GluA2-S105-ER\beta} = 0.72$; $CC_{Synphys-GluA1} = 0.83$; $CC_{Synphys-S105-ER\beta} = 0.61$; $CC_{GluA1-S105-ER\beta} = 0.84$).

LTP in the hippocampus is dependent on activation of calcium calmodulin kinase II [29] and is positively modulated by cAMP response element-binding protein [30] suggesting that increased activation of these could correlate to enhanced learning. We could, however, find no differences in phosphorylated CaMKII or phosphorylated CREB between PA28αOE and WT hippocampi (Additional file 9).

Hence, global expression levels of neuronal, synaptic or LTP markers cannot explain the cognitive differences observed between WT and PA28αOE female mice.

PA28αOE mice do not demonstrate induced proteasome activity

The prevailing view of PA28αβ's molecular function in the cell is activation of the 20S proteasome. We performed proteasome activity assays on hippocampal extracts from WT and PA28αOE female mice to investigate whether the cognitive effects observed upon PA28α overexpression are associated with such activation. The interactions between the 20S proteasome and its different

regulators are perturbed or compromised by mutually exclusive extraction conditions [31–33]. Thus, to detect PA28-dependent activation of 20S proteasome capacity (digestion of fluorogenic peptides in vitro), conditions specifically optimizing the interaction between 20S and PA28αβ need to be used [e.g. no salt; 31, 32].

We detected a threefold increase in PA28-dependent proteasome capacity upon IFN-γ treatment after using conditions optimizing PA28–20S interaction (MEFs, positive control, Fig. 4a and Additional file 10). However, in PA28αOE hippocampi there was no induction in PA28-dependent proteasome capacity compared to WT hippocampi (Fig. 4a and Additional file 10; n ≥ 3, animals used in the phenotypic profiling). This was unexpected since PA28α is capable of self-assembly in vitro into a heptamer ring [34, 35], which can activate 20S proteasome capacity [36]. To further analyze this, PA28-dependent proteasome capacities of PA28αOE and WT MEFs were determined, also demonstrating a lack of induction in PA28αOE (Additional file 11, 12).

Western analysis of hippocampal K48-linked polyubiquitinated proteins, generally targeted for proteasomal degradation, showed a clear trend of increased levels in PA28αOE (Fig. 4b and Additional file 13; $P = 0.051$), indicating reduced 26S proteasome activity and in line with PA28α overexpression being unable to activate proteasome activity. 20S proteasome capacity was not induced in PA28αOE hippocampi (Fig. 4c and Additional file 10) and hippocampal levels of proteasome related markers Rpt2 (19S subunit), β5 (20S) and β5i (20Si) did not differ between WT and PA28αOE (Fig. 4d and Additional file 13), while PA28α overexpression in PA28αOE hippocampi was verified (Fig. 4d).

For these reasons, we conclude that the improved cognitive functions observed upon PA28α overexpression arise without an increase in 20S proteasome activity,

(See figure on next page.)

Fig. 4 PA28α overexpression does not increase hippocampal PA28-dependent proteasome activity, but enhances aggregation prevention capacity in the hippocampus. **a** The PA28-dependent proteasome capacity determined by suc-LLVY-AMC digestion (i.e. β5/β5i chymotrypsin-like activity) under PA28–20S optimizing conditions, with interferon-γ treated MEFs serving as positive control (compare C – FNγ to C + IFNγ). Activity presented is activity inhibited by the proteasome-specific inhibitor epoxomicin (5 μM), which corresponded to 70–98% of total activity (see Methods). Values are mean ± SEM; $n_{PA28\alpha OE} = 3$ and $n_{WT} = 4$; differences are not statistically significant ($P = 0.72$). **b** Representative blot of K48-linked polyubiquitin western analysis and quantification of K48-linked polyubiquitinated protein signal from western analysis, $P = 0.051$; Student's t test). Values are mean ± SEM; $n_{PA28\alpha OE} = 6$ and $n_{WT} = 8$. **c** 20S proteasome capacity (in the presence of 0.02% SDS) in protein extracts made from PA28αOE and WT right hippocampus, values are mean ± SEM; $n_{PA28\alpha OE} = 3$ and $n_{WT} = 4$. **d** Western analysis of the proteasome related markers Rpt2 (19S subunit), β5 (20S) and β5i (20Si) in protein extracts made from PA28αOE and WT left hippocampus. PA28α is induced 13-fold in PA28αOE hippocampus ($P < 1E-12$; Student's t test). *Estimated kDa marker placement based on 20 kDa and 37 kDa marker bands. "n.d." = not included in assay due to limited amount of extract. **e** Aggregation prevention of heat-sensitive luciferase in the presence of hippocampal protein extracts at 42 °C. Luciferase aggregation prevention capacity was calculated as percentage of non-aggregated luciferase compared to samples without cell extracts. Boiled extracts served as negative control and did not prevent aggregation. Values are mean ± SEM; $n_{PA28\alpha OE} = 9$ and $n_{WT} = 10$ ($P = 0.036$; Student's t test). **f** A model of PA28αβ effects on cognitive functions through its role as a chaperone rather than a 20S proteasome activator

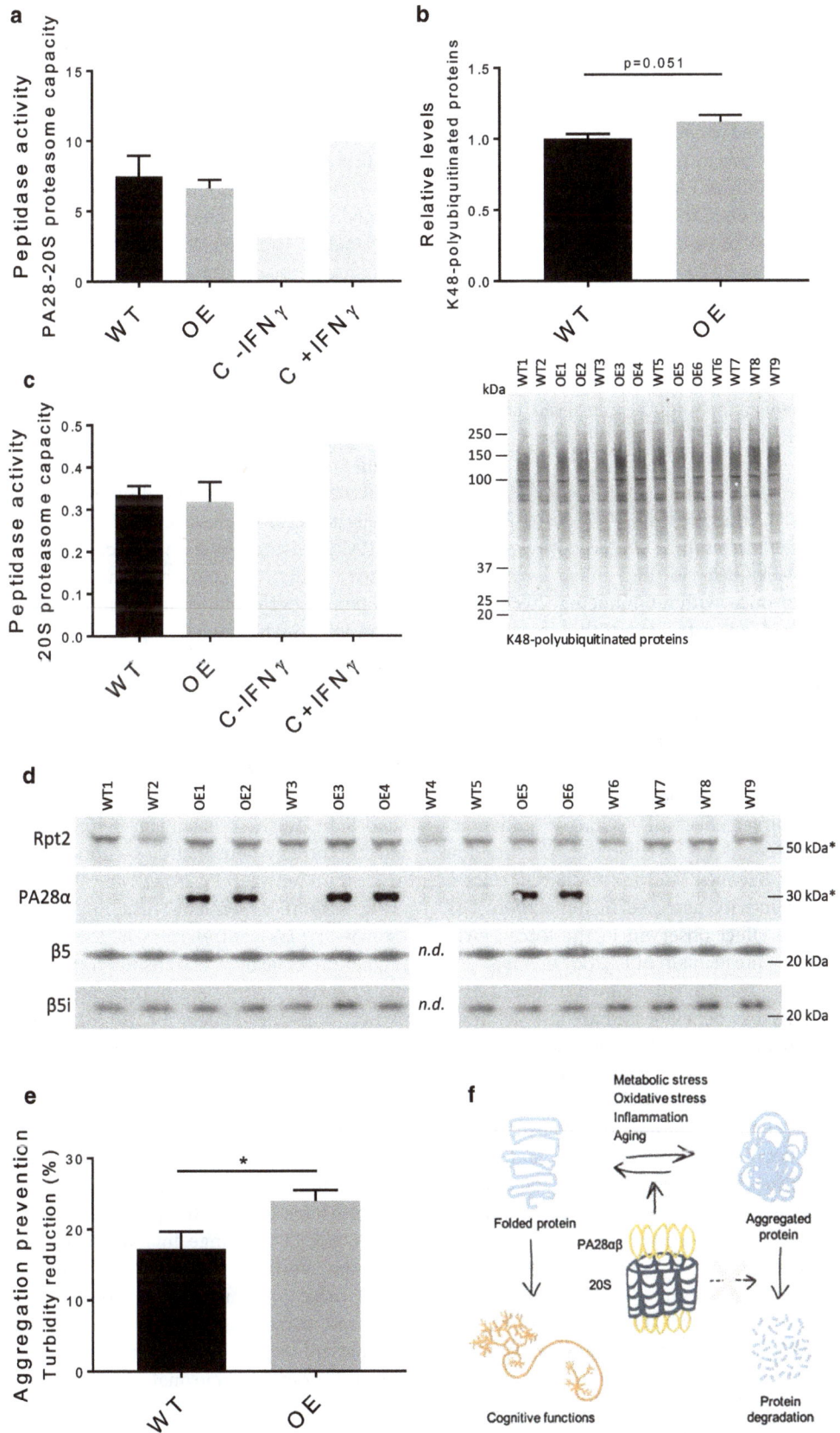

and are therefore likely not dependent on this molecular function of PA28αβ.

PA28αOE hippocampus extracts prevent aggregation more efficiently than WT

PA28αβ has a recognized chaperone-like activity not necessarily coupled to its role as a 20S proteasome activator [10, 37]. Therefore, WT and PA28αOE female hippocampal extracts were analyzed to determine their capacity to prevent aggregation of heat sensitive luciferase. Hippocampal extracts from PA28αOE were more efficient in preventing aggregation than WT hippocampal extracts (Fig. 4e and Additional file 13; $P = 0.036$). Thus, as depicted in Fig. 4f, chaperone-like functions of PA28αβ, rather than its role as a proteasome activator, are likely part of the mechanism behind the observed cognitive effects in PA28αOE.

Discussion

This study couples, for the first time, PA28αβ to neuronal function and demonstrates that PA28α overexpression reduces depressive-like behavior and enhances learning/memory in female mice without inducing 20S proteasome activity. Instead, our data suggest that the observed effects on cognitive capacity is exerted by PA28αβ chaperone-like functions.

The forced swim test is an established behavioral model to assess emotional state of rodents [38]. The increased activity time of PA28αOE mice compared to WT could point to an antidepressant action of overexpressing PA28α, though a direct effect of PA28α on enhancing locomotion activity could not be ruled out. We found no difference, however, between WT and PA28αOE mice in general locomotor activity, assessed in the activity box, supporting that the effect observed in the forced swim test is a stress coping mechanism of PA28αOE mice.

Open-field tests are traditionally known to assess emotionality and anxiety-like behavior and are also acknowledged to assay locomotion and exploratory behavior [39–41]. In a new environment, the innate behavior of mice is to explore, specifically the periphery, and avoid the open areas of the box. Habituation is considered the simplest form of learning and memory [26] and can be measured intrasessionally (within-session) which is proposed to primarily reflect adaptation [42] or intersessionally (between sessions) by repeated exposures, reflecting learning and memory [27].

We found no differences in the behavior between PA28αOE and WT during day 1 in the activity box. This indicates that there is no difference between WT and PA28αOE mice in general locomotor activity, adaptation (intrasessional habituation) or anxiety-like behavior; the latter confirmed by zeromaze anxiety analysis.

However, on day 2, PA28αOE mice changed their behavior and spent more time in the corner and tended to reduce their number of rearings. Increased corner time and reduced rearing are both indicators of anti-exploratory behavior signifying that PA28αOE mice habituate faster. The increased capacity for learning was further confirmed in the shuttle box passive avoidance test. On day 2, no PA28αOE female mice entered the avoidance-trained area in the shuttle box, in stark contrast to WT littermates. Thus, results from both activity box analysis and shuttle box passive avoidance test demonstrate an increased learning capacity of PA28αOE female mice.

Remarkably, none of the cognitive behavioral effects from PA28α overexpression were observed in male littermates, indicating that these effects are female specific. Results in the forced-swim test have been shown to be dependent on several factors, such as age of animals, strain and gender [38, 43]. A possible explanation for our results could be an innate difference between male and female mice in depressive-like behavior that is reversed by PA28α overexpression, which in females unleashes positive effects on cognitive functions. Comparing male and female performance in the forced swim test shows a trend for a higher baseline activity in males, though not statistically significant. As depressive-like behavior and function of the hippocampus are closely linked [44], the increased capacity for learning could point to a direct effect of PA28αβ in the hippocampus. Upon examination, we found no alterations in serum estrogen levels or hippocampal regulation of estrogen receptor β that could shed light on the mechanism behind the sex difference. Further, no key neuronal or synaptic markers differed in expression between PA28αOE and WT hippocampi.

Proteasome-dependent protein degradation is well known to play central roles in long term potentiation, regulation of synaptic transmission, and synaptic plasticity. However, this study presents data strongly indicating that the effects of PA28α overexpression on memory/learning are not dependent on PA28αβ as a proteasome activator. Analysis of hippocampi from WT and PA28αOE littermates revealed that PA28α overexpression did not increase PA28-dependent 20S peptidase activity or decrease K48-linked polyubiquitin levels. It is important to note that, even though data presented here demonstrates that proteolysis is not generally enhanced in PA28αOE, a change in individual peptides/proteins, although unlikely, cannot be excluded. In addition, an increase in neuronal proteasome activity has been observed in response to learning [15, 45] and it is possible that enhanced PA28αβ expression specifically modulates this complex neuronal activation state in a manner leading to improved memory, while baseline proteasome activity is unaltered.

Previous studies overexpressing PA28α have demonstrated a minor increase in proteasome activity [6, 46]. However, none of those experiments included a positive control (interferon-γ treated cells or purified $20S \pm PA28\alpha\beta$) and were either not conducted under PA28–20S optimizing conditions [6] or not negatively controlled [specific 20S proteasome inhibitor; 46]. In the in vivo study of cardiomyocyte PA28α overexpression [5], enhanced proteasome function was verified by expression of the reporter gene GFPdgn (GFP fused to degron CL1) [5, 47]. Degradation of GFPdgn is however not only dependent on the proteasome itself, but is also a reflection of the efficiency in recognition and unfolding of this particular substrate. The reduction in GFPdgn observed upon PA28α overexpression may thus instead be a result of PA28αβ chaperone functions.

As opposed to proteasome activation, our data suggest that the observed effects on cognition is exerted by PA28αβ chaperone-like functions, since hippocampal extracts from PA28αOE prevented protein aggregation more efficiently than hippocampal extracts from WT. PA28αβ has previously been shown to be able to collaborate with Hsp40, Hsp70 and Hsp90 to refold a denatured protein substrate [10]. In addition, PA28αβ can compensate for Hsp90 functions in major histocompatibility complex class I antigen processing [37].

As a chaperone, PA28αβ may play a direct role in neuron protein homeostasis and metabolism, affecting firing, signaling, action potential generation as well as vesicular transport and release. Improved learning in PA28αOE mice could be due to an elevated capacity for cellular memory formation, i.e. an enhanced probability for inducing LTP or an increase in the actual magnitude of LTP. Induction and expression of LTP is ultimately expressed as number of AMPA-receptors in the synapse [48] but whole-hippocampi analysis of GluA1 and A2 did not reveal any differences between WT and PA28αOE. A chaperone-like activity could be an explanation for this, as PA28αβ could exert its effect by increasing AMPA-receptor stability, rather than number, thus increasing availability of AMPA-receptors in the membrane and subsequently the likelihood of AMPA-recruitment to the synapse.

In addition, or alternatively, to a direct role in neuron function, PA28αβ chaperone-like activity could be part of the mechanism behind its protective effects against oxidative stress and proteinopathy, and thus the positive effects on cognitive capacity by PA28α overexpression could be a result of neuroprotection. Oxidative stress and proteinopathy are central for the progression and/or detrimental effects of many diseases that cause decline in cognitive functions, including neurodegenerative diseases and neuronal injury after stroke and head trauma

[49, 50]. Hence, PA28α overexpression may increase the fitness and exert effects protecting against these diseases, perhaps acting at the core of early aging events.

Conclusions

In this study, we demonstrate that overexpression of PA28α and concomitant upregulation of PA28β protein reduces depressive-like behavior and enhances learning and memory in female mice. The overexpression of PA28α does not increase PA28αβ-dependent proteasome activity but could still be linked to its protective functions upon oxidative stress and proteinopathy. The underlying mechanism to these protective effects may instead involve chaperone-like functions of PA28αβ.

Methods

Animal care, diets and termination

C57BL/6N (Charles River, Lyon, France), BALB/c (Harlan Laboratories, Horst, the Netherlands) and C57BL/6N × BALB/c F2 hybrid mice were housed in a temperature controlled room (21 °C) with a 12:12 h light–dark cycle (dawn: 5.30–6.00 am, dusk: 5.30–6 pm) and controlled humidity (45–55%). They were checked daily had free access to water and regular chow diet (R3; Lactamin, Kimstad Sweden) containing 12% fat, 62% carbohydrates, and 26% protein (energy percentage), with a total energy content of 3 kcal/g. At termination, mice were euthanized under 5% isoflurane anesthesia and decapitated. Blood samples for hematology were collected by intra-cardiac puncture, tissues were isolated, directly transferred to dry ice, and kept at − 80 °C until biochemical analyses.

Generation of PA28αOE mice

A knock-in strategy was used to target the murine *Rosa26* locus in order to generate mice carrying a murine PA28α overexpression cassette at this site. The targeting vector was built using homologous recombination in bacteria [51] and a C57 mouse BAC served as template for the extraction of *Rosa26* homology arms. The targeting vector contained the *CAG* promoter [52] driving the expression of the coding region of *murine PA28α* and a rabbit β-globin poly (A) signal (CAG-PA28α-pA) and a neomycin phosphotransferase (Neo) selectable marker cassette. The *PGK-gb2-neo* cassette with CAG-PA28α-pA was inserted into a *Rosa26* targeting vector comprised of a 1.5 kb 5′ and 5 kb 3′ homology arms of *Rosa26*, and a PGK-diphtheria toxin A (*DTA*) gene for negative selection (Fig. 1a). The Neo selectable marker cassette, which was flanked by *loxp* sites, was deleted in the germline of the chimeric mice generating the KI allele using a self-excising Neo strategy. After linearization, the targeting construct was electroporated into C57BL/6N mouse embryonic stem (ES) cells which were then grown in media containing G418 (200 µg/ml). Thus, the PA28αOE mouse line was established on a pure C57BL/6 genetic background. PCR screens and Targeted Locus Amplification (Cergentis, Utrecht, the Netherlands) analyses revealed clones that had undergone the desired homologous recombination event. Several of these clones were expanded and injected into Balb/cOlaHsd blastocysts to generate chimeric males which were then bred to C57BL/6JOlaHsd females and black-coated offspring were genotyped on both sides of the homology arms for correct integration into the *Rosa26* locus.

SDS–PAGE and Western blot analysis

MEFs, brain sample containing frontal cortex and striatum, left ventricle of the heart, and hippocampi were lysed with a modified RIPA buffer (50 mM Na_2HPO_4 pH 7.8; 150 mM NaCl; 1% Nonidet P-40; 0.5% deoxycholate; 0.1% SDS; 1 mM DTPA; 1 mM pefablock). Cell debris was removed by centrifugation at 5000 g for 10 min and protein concentration was determined using the Pierce™ BCA Protein Assay Kit (Thermo Fisher Scientific). Eye lenses were lysed by sonication (Branson Ultrasonic Corp., Danbury, CT, USA) in PBS [53]. Samples were prepared for SDS–PAGE as described [54], separated by sodium dodecyl sulfate (SDS)-polyacrylamide gel electrophoresis (PAGE), transferred onto a nitrocellulose membrane (Invitrogen, Bleiswjik, the Netherlands) and probed with rabbit mAb PA28α (#9643; Cell Signaling Technology, Inc., Leiden, the Netherlands), rabbit pAb PA28β (#2409), rabbit mAb GluA2 (#13607), rabbit pAb N-Cadherin (#4061), rabbit pAb GluA1 (#13185), rabbit pAb β5/PSMB5 (#11903), rabbit mAb Phospho-CaMKII Thr286 (#12716), rabbit mAb Phospho-CREB Ser133 (#9198), rabbit pAb polyubiquitin K48-linkage specific (ab190061; Abcam, Cambridge UK), goat pAb PSD-95 (ab12093), rabbit pAb GluA1 (ab31232), rabbit mAb Synaptophysin (ab32127), rabbit pAb Spinophilin (ab203275), rabbit mAb NeuN (ab177487), rabbit pAb Estrogen Receptor beta phospho S105 (ab62257), rabbit pAb Rpt2/S4 (ab3317), or rabbit pAb β5i/LMP7 (ab3329). IRDye 800CW-labelled goat anti-rabbit, 680CW-labelled goat anti-mouse, 800CW-labelled donkey anti-goat IgG antibodies (LI-COR Biosciences, Cambridge, UK) were used for detection and blots were analyzed with the Odyssey infrared imaging system and software (LI-COR Biosciences), except for lens samples for which HRP-conjugated secondary Ab was used and luminescence after ECL reaction was imaged using ImageQuant LAS 500 (GE Healthcare, Piscataway, NJ, USA). Blots were quantified using the ImageJ software. Equal total

protein present of each sample on the membrane was confirmed using the Novex reversible membrane protein stain (IB7710, Invitrogen) according to manufacturer's instructions.

RNA extraction and quantitative (qPCR) analysis

Total RNA was extracted using Stat60 (CS-502, Tel-Test Inc) as per manufacturer's recommendations. cDNA was synthesized on 1 µg total RNA using the High-Capacity cDNA Reverse Transcription Kit (#4368814 Applied Biosystems, Thermo Fisher Scientific) according to manufacturer's instructions. Synthesized cDNA was analyzed in triplicates by qPCR using iQTM SYBRH Green Supermix and the QuantStudio 7 Flex system (Applied Biosystems, Thermo Fisher Scientific). For primer sequences, see Additional file 14.

Study design of physiological and behavioral phenotypic profiling

10 Wildtype (WT) and 6 PA28αOE heterozygous female F2 hybrid littermates at the age of 6 months were subjected to a 2-month protocol of physiological and behavioral phenotypic profiling as outlined in Fig. 2a. The mice were housed 4 in each cage with 2 WT-cages, 1 PA28αOE-cage, and 1 mixed cage. The genotype was not indicated on the cage, and the animal number to genotype was not decoded until after data analysis. The animals were analyzed cage by cage in the following order: WT-cage 1, PA28αOE-cage, WT-cage 2, mixed cage. Shuttle box and zeromaze were performed in 3 rounds with 6 mice each round as follows: (1) 4 WT from WT-cage 1 and 2 PA28αOE from PA28αOE-cage, (2) 2 PA28αOE from PA28αOE-cage and 2 WT from WT-cage 2, (3) 2 WT from WT-cage 2 and 2 PA28αOE and 2 WT from mixed cage. Activity box was performed in 2 rounds with 8 mice each round as follows: (1) 4 WT from WT-cage 1 and 4 PA28αOE from PA28αOE-cage, (2) 4 WT from WT-cage 2 and 2 WT from WT-cage 2 and 2 PA28αOE and 2 WT from mixed cage. All animal experiments were carried out at 10–11 am, except activity box that was carried out at 10–12 am.

Activity box

Activity box is an open field activity-like test to study general activity, exploratory behavior, signs of anxiety, stress and depression [55]. The mice are three dimensionally recorded by infrared sensors built into the walls (8Lx8Bx8H) of a sound-proof opaque box (50 × 50 × 50 cm) with a low intensity lamp into the lid of the box (Kungsbacka mät och regler, Fjärrås, Sweden). The mice were placed in the middle of the box and recorded for 1 h in this novel environment. On the following day, they were recorded again in the—now considered—acquainted environment. The parameters recorded as events/5 min were horizontal activity, peripheral activity, rearing activity, peripheral rearing, rearing time, locomotion, and corner time.

Forced swim test

This test is performed to analyze mice for signs of depression [55, 56]. The assembly consists of a transparent plexiglas cylinder with 25 cm inner diameter and 60 cm in length with a grey, circular plastic platform hanging from wires on the outside of the cylinder, approximately 20 cm from the top (bespoke construction, AstraZeneca Gothenburg), and filled with room tempered (22 °C) water in level with the platform. A single mouse is placed on the water surface inside the cylinder and its behavior is monitored by a video camera placed directly above the cylinder for 6 min and 20 s, of which the last 4 min are used in calculation (MouseTracker analysis software).

Oral glucose tolerance test (OGTT)

Oral glucose tolerance test (OGTT) baseline measurements were obtained after 5 h of fasting, followed by oral glucose dosing (6.7 ml/kg). Insulin levels was measured with Ultra-sensitive mouse insulin ELISA kit (Crystal Chem, Zaandam, Netherlands) according to manufacturer's instructions and glucose levels by AccuChek mobile blood glucose meter (Roche Diagnostics Scandinavia, Solna, Sweden) at baseline and after 15, 30, 60, 120 min from dosing.

Shuttle box passive avoidance test

Passive avoidance testing was performed using the shuttle box system (Accuscan Instruments Inc., Columbus, OH, USA). This test is used to study memory performance in mice and is carried out over 2 days [55, 57, 58]. The system consists of a cage centrally divided by a wall into two compartments, one of which has transparent walls (the bright compartment) while the other is covered from all sides with opaque walls (the dark compartment). Both chambers are equipped with sensors that determine the location of the mouse and the central wall has a mechanical sliding door that can be programmed to open or close. The cage floor is made of stainless steel grid, which can deliver a mild electric shock to the mouse upon certain stimuli. On the first day, a mouse is released into the well-lit compartment and tends to migrate to the dark compartment when the central door opens (30 s after mouse entry). Upon entry to the dark compartment, the central door closes and the mouse is exposed to a mild electric shock (0.3 mA). Intensity of pain response was monitored. All mice responded to the electric shock

by a vocal response ("beep") and a jump, indicating similar strength of discomfort. On the second day, the mouse is released as before into the well-lit compartment and when the central door opens, may or may not enter the dark compartment. The time taken to enter the dark compartment is recorded on both days and a longer interval or no entry on the second day indicates memory response. Maximum assay time is 300 s each day.

Elevated zeromaze monitoring system

The elevated zeromaze system (Accuscan Instruments Inc.) was used to study anxiety-related behavior [55, 59, 60]. The maze is made up of a circular Perspex platform, elevated 75 cm above the floor, 5 cm wide and 40 cm inner diameter, equally divided into four quadrants, of which two quadrants on opposite sides of the platform are closed by 30 cm high Perspex transparent walls with photocell transceivers, while the other two quadrants are open and bordered by a Perspex lip (0.5 cm high), a security and tactile guide on the open quadrants. During testing, a mouse is placed at the entrance of a closed quadrant and monitored for 5 min. Activity in closed arm, latency to enter open arm, and time spent in open and closed arm are the parameters analyzed.

Body composition and core temperature

Core body temperature of the mice was obtained with a rectal probe thermometer (ELFA AB, Sweden). Under 2% isoflurane sedation the mice were analyzed by dual energy X-ray absorptiometry (DEXA) using Lunar PIXImus Densitometer (GE Medical Systems, Madison, WI, USA) to determine body fat (g), body fat (%), lean body mass (g), and total BMD (g/cm^2) [55].

Immunoprofiling of peripheral blood

Blood samples for hematology (in EDTA tubes, Microvette CB300, Sarstedt, Nürnbrecht, Germany) were collected from the left atrium of the heart under isoflurane anesthesia, prior to necropsy. Leucocytes and erythrocytes were isolated by centrifugation and stained with 1:50 dilutions of MS CD45 HRZN V500 mAb (#561487; BD Diagnostics, Stockholm, Sweden), MS F4/80 PE T45-2342 (#565410), MS CD4 PERCP mAb (#561090), MS CD19 APC mAb (#561738), CD8 APC-Cy7 mAb (#561967), NK1.1 FITC mAb (#553164), and CD3e conjugated to BD Horizon V450 (#560804). Erythrocytes were lysed with BD FACS lysis buffer and analyzed using flow cytometry (FACS Fortessa, BD Bioscience, Stockholm, Sweden) with appropriate filter settings, gating on live cells.

Blood serum preparation and β-estradiol detection

Blood samples for blood serum preparation were collected from the left atrium of the heart under isoflurane anesthesia, prior to necropsy, incubated at room temperature for 30–45 min, and coagulates were removed by centrifugation. Relative β-estradiol serum levels were detected by the Mouse/Rat Estradiol ELISA-Kit (SKU: ES180S-100, Calbiotech, Spring Valley, CA USA) according to manufacturer's instructions.

Cell culture and IFN-γ treatment of embryonic fibroblasts

MEFs from C57BL/6N females that had been mated with C57BL/6N PA28αOE heterozygote males, were isolated at E13.5 as described [61], with the following exceptions: embryos were isolated individually, heads were used for genotyping and the trypsin treatment was for 45 min in 0.05% trypsin–EDTA solution with 1% chicken serum (Gibco, Thermo Fisher Scientific, Gothenburg, Sweden) under gentle agitation. Cells were cultivated in DMEM (Dulbecco's modified Eagle's medium, Thermo Fisher Scientific) supplemented with 10% fetal bovine serum (FBS), 1% Penicillin/streptomycin and 1% non-essential amino acids at 37 °C under 5% CO_2 and ambient oxygen. For positive control in the analysis of PA28αβ-dependent proteasome capacity, 150 U/mL recombinant mouse IFN-γ (Thermo Fisher Scientific) was added to the culture media 24 h prior harvest.

Proteasome capacity assays

PA28–20S or 20S proteasome capacity was analyzed as previously described [32] with some modifications. Cells were lysed in 25 mM Tris/HCl (pH 8.3) by 4 cycles of high-speed centrifugation (20,000 g) and resuspension at 4 °C, cell debris was removed by centrifugation at 5000 g for 10 min and protein concentration was determined using the BCA Protein Assay kit (Pierce, Thermo Fisher Scientific). The chemotryptic activity was assayed by hydrolysis of the fluorogenic peptide succinyl-Leu-Leu-Val-Tyr-7-amino-4-methylcoumarin (suc-LLVY-AMC; Calbiochem Merck-Millipore, Darmstadt, Germany). 10 μg total protein was incubated with 200 μM suc-LLVY-AMC in 50 mM Tris/HCl (pH 8.3) and 0.5 mM DTT for PA28–20S activity or 50 mM Tris/HCl (pH 8.3), 0.5 mM DTT and 0.02% SDS for 20S activity in a total volume of 100 μL; fluorescence was monitored using 390 nm excitation and 460 nm emission filters with free AMC as standard (Molekula Ltd., Gillingham, UK) and activity was determined as the slope of fluorescence over time divided by total protein. Protein levels in the assay were determined by SDS–PAGE, InstantBlueTM (Expedeon Ltd., Cambridge UK) staining, and analysis using the Odyssey infrared

imaging system and software (LI-COR Biosciences). Activity upon proteasome inhibition with 5 μM epoxomicin (Sigma-Aldrich, Stockholm, Sweden) is considered non-specific/background activity. Epoxomicin inhibited the PA28–20S proteasome capacity to $70 \pm 9\%$ (mean $\pm$ SD) of WT, $77 \pm 10\%$ of PA28αOE, 98.3% of untreated MEFs and 99.8% of interferon-γ treated MEFs; and epoxomicin inhibited the 20S proteasome capacity to $94 \pm 3\%$ of WT, $95 \pm 3\%$ of PA28αOE, 85% of untreated MEFs and 81% of interferon-γ treated MEFs.

Luciferase aggregation prevention

Luciferase aggregation prevention capacity was analyzed as previously described [62] with some modifications. To increase the number of n in the analysis, hippocampi from females of similar age (5–6 months) of the C57BL/6N background, 6 WT and 6 PA28αOE, were included to the 4 WT and 3 PA28αOE hippocampi from the C57BL/6N × BALB/c F2 hybrids. Right hippocampi were lysed in extraction buffer (25 mM Tris/HCl, 100 mM NaCl, 5 mM $MgCl_2$, 1 mM ATP, and 5% glycerol, pH 7.4) by 4 cycles of high-speed centrifugation (20,000 g) and resuspension at 4 °C. Cell debris was removed by centrifugation at 5000 g for 10 min and 1 mM DTT was added after an aliquot was set aside for protein concentration determination with the BCA Protein Assay kit (Pierce, Thermo Fisher). Heat-sensitive luciferase (200 nM; L9506; Sigma-Aldrich) was heat-denatured at 42 °C in 50 mM Tris pH 7.6, 2 mM EDTA, in the presence of 4.5 μg protein extracts or corresponding volume of extraction buffer. Aggregation of luciferase was determined as light scattering at 340 nm at 42 °C. At around 80% of maximum, the increase in turbidity of the positive control (without protein extract) started to plateau, and the closest time point was chosen for analysis (40 min in the experiments on hybrid hippocampal extracts and 20 min at 42 °C in the experiments with C57). The turbidity of the positive control was considered maximum aggregation (100%). Turbidity of the negative control with no addition of heat-sensitive luciferase did not change over time and was considered background. Luciferase aggregation prevention capacity was calculated as percentage of non-aggregated luciferase. Extracts that had been incubated at 99 °C for 45 min served as negative control to the cell extract and did not prevent aggregation.

Statistical analysis

Comparisons between two groups were performed with unpaired t test assuming two-tailed distribution and equal variances and differences were considered significant at $P < 0.05$. Statistical analysis of the activity box corner time day 2 (Fig. 3a) by two-way ANOVA repeated measurements followed by Sidak multiple comparisons test and of the shuttle box PAT (Fig. 3b) was done by Mantel–Cox survival test; both in GraphPad Prism and the null hypothesis was rejected at the 0.05 level.

Additional files

Additional file 1. The raw data used to produce Fig. 1.

Additional file 2. Physiological parameters of WT and PA28αOE F2 C57BL/6NxBALB/c mice.

Additional file 3. The cellular immune profiles of PA28αOE and WT mice.

Additional file 4. Blood glucose and insulin response in oral glucose tolerance test (OGTT) of PA28αOE and WT mice.

Additional file 5. The raw data used to produce Fig. 2.

Additional file 6. The raw data used to produce Fig. 3.

Additional file 7. Tail-flick pain tolerance analysis of PA28αOE.

Additional file 8. Cognitive behavior of male PA28αOE.

Additional file 9. Hippocampal neuronal markers and serum estrogen levels of PA28αOE and WT mice.

Additional file 10. The raw data used to produce Fig. 4a and 4c.

Additional file 11. PA28-dependent proteasome activity of PA28αOE and WT MEFs.

Additional file 12. The raw data used to produce Additional file 11.

Additional file 13. The raw data used to produce Fig. 4b, 4d, 4e and Additional file 9.

Additional file 14. Sequences of primers used for real-time quantitative (qPCR) analysis.

Abbreviations
GFPdgn: GFP fused to degron CL1, reporter gene; H_2O_2: hydrogen peroxide; LTP: long-term potentiation; MHC-I: major histocompatibility complex I; MEFs: mouse embryonic fibroblasts; PA28αOE: PA28α overexpression mouse model; WT: wildtype.

Authors' contributions
JA, MA, MZ, JW and MH designed research; JA, AP, JW and MH performed research; JA, MA, MP and MH analyzed the data; JA, MA and MH wrote the manuscript; all authors critically revised the manuscript for important intellectual content. All authors read and approved the final manuscript.

Author details
[1] Department of Clinical Neuroscience, Institute of Neuroscience and Physiology, Sahlgrenska Academy at the University of Gothenburg, Gothenburg, Sweden. [2] IMED Biotech Unit, Discovery Biology, Discovery Sciences, AstraZeneca, Gothenburg, Sweden. [3] Department of Clinical Sciences, Epilepsy Centre, Lund University, Lund, Sweden.

Acknowledgements
We thank Viktor Verdier for performing MEF proteasome activity assays; Åsa Rensfeldt for PA28α and PA28β detection in MEFs and MEF isolation support; Johan K Johansson and Mikael Bjursell for the help of setting up the phenotyping analysis; Liselotte Andersson, Johan K Johansson, Anna Thorén and Seren Necla Sevim for technical assistance in sample harvesting; Sarah Dorbéus and Pernilla Eliasson for FACS analysis support; the Translational Genomics group at AstraZeneca for generation and validation of the PA28αOE mouse line; and Elin Blomberg for artistic input to the illustration in Fig. 4f.

Competing interests
The authors declare that they have no competing interests.

Funding
This Project is financially supported by the Swedish Foundation for Strategic Research (SSF), Herman Svensson Foundation, Ögonfonden, and by AstraZeneca AB. None of these organizations had any role in study design, collection, analysis of data, interpretation of data, or manuscript writing.

References
1. Joon Young A, Nobuyuki T, Kin-ya A, Hiroshi H, Chiseko N, Keiji T, et al. Primary structures of two homologous subunits of PA28, a γ-interferon-inducible protein activator of the 20S proteasome. FEBS Lett. 1995;366:37–42.
2. Pickering AM, Koop AL, Teoh CY, Ermak G, Grune T, Davies KJA. The immunoproteasome, the 20S proteasome, and the PA28αβ proteasome regulator are oxidative-stress-adaptive proteolytic complexes. Biochem J. 2010;432:585–94.
3. Cascio P. PA28αβ: the enigmatic magic ring of the proteasome? Biomolecules. 2014;4:566.
4. Vigneron N, Van den Eynde B. Proteasome subtypes and regulators in the processing of antigenic peptides presented by class I molecules of the major histocompatibility complex. Biomolecules. 2014;4:994.
5. Li J, Horak KM, Su H, Sanbe A, Robbins J, Wang X. Enhancement of proteasomal function protects against cardiac proteinopathy and ischemia/reperfusion injury in mice. J Clin Investig. 2011;121:3689–700.
6. Li J, Powell SR, Wang X. Enhancement of proteasome function by PA28α overexpression protects against oxidative stress. FASEB J. 2011;25:883–93.
7. Pickering AM, Davies KJA. Differential roles of proteasome and immunoproteasome regulators PA28αβ, PA28γ and PA200 in the degradation of oxidized proteins. Arch Biochem Biophys. 2012;523:181–90.
8. Pickering AM, Linder RA, Zhang H, Forman HJ, Davies KJA. Nrf2-dependent induction of proteasome and PA28αβ regulator are required for adaptation to oxidative stress. J Biol Chem. 2012;287:10021–31.
9. Hernebring M, Fredriksson Å, Liljevald M, Cvijovic M, Norrman K, Wiseman J, et al. Removal of damaged proteins during ES cell fate specification requires the proteasome activator PA28. Sci Rep. 2013;3:1381.
10. Minami Y, Kawasaki H, Minami M, Tanahashi N, Tanaka K, Yahara I. A critical role for the proteasome activator PA28 in the Hsp90-dependent protein refolding. J Biol Chem. 2000;275:9055–61.
11. Hegde AN, Goldberg AL, Schwartz JH. Regulatory subunits of cAMP-dependent protein kinases are degraded after conjugation to ubiquitin: a molecular mechanism underlying long-term synaptic plasticity. Proc Natl Acad Sci USA. 1993;90:7436–40.
12. Hegde AN, Inokuchi K, Pei W, Casadio A, Ghirardi M, Chain DG, et al. Ubiquitin C-terminal hydrolase is an immediate-early gene essential for long-term facilitation in Aplysia. Cell. 1997;89:115–26.
13. Fonseca R, Vabulas RM, Hartl FU, Bonhoeffer T, Nägerl UV. A balance of protein synthesis and proteasome-dependent degradation determines the maintenance of LTP. Neuron. 2006;52:239–45.
14. Karpova A, Mikhaylova M, Thomas U, Knöpfel T, Behnisch T. Involvement of protein synthesis and degradation in long-term potentiation of schaffer collateral CA1 synapses. J Neurosci. 2006;26:4949–55.
15. Lopez-Salon M, Alonso M, Vianna MRM, Viola H, Souza ETM, Izquierdo I, et al. The ubiquitin–proteasome cascade is required for mammalian long-term memory formation. Eur J Neurosci. 2001;14:1820–6.
16. Rodriguez-Ortiz CJ, Balderas I, Saucedo-Alquicira F, Cruz-Castañeda P, Bermudez-Rattoni F. Long-term aversive taste memory requires insular and amygdala protein degradation. Neurobiol Learn Mem. 2011;95:311–5.
17. Jarome TJ, Werner CT, Kwapis JL, Helmstetter FJ. Activity dependent protein degradation is critical for the formation and stability of fear memory in the Amygdala. PLoS ONE. 2011;6:24349.
18. Colledge M, Snyder EM, Crozier RA, Soderling JA, Jin Y, Langeberg LK, et al. Ubiquitination regulates PSD-95 degradation and AMPA receptor surface expression. Neuron. 2003;40:595–607.

19. Kato A, Rouach N, Nicoll RA, Bredt DS. Activity-dependent NMDA receptor degradation mediated by retrotranslocation and ubiquitination. Proc Natl Acad Sci USA. 2005;102:5600–5.

20. Yao I, Takagi H, Ageta H, Kahyo T, Sato S, Hatanaka K, et al. SCRAPPER-dependent ubiquitination of active zone protein RIM1 regulates synaptic vesicle release. Cell. 2007;130:943–57.

21. Braineac—The Brain eQTL Almanac. http://www.braineac.org/. Accessed 1 June 2018.

22. McNaught KSP, Jnobaptiste R, Jackson T, Jengelley T-A. The pattern of neuronal loss and survival may reflect differential expression of proteasome activators in Parkinson's disease. Synapse. 2010;64:241–50.

23. Yao X, Liu J, McCabe JT. Alterations of cerebral cortex and hippocampal proteasome subunit expression and function in a traumatic brain injury rat model. J Neurochem. 2008;104:353–63.

24. Matarin M, Salih Dervis A, Yasvoina M, Cummings Damian M, Guelfi S, Liu W, et al. A genome-wide gene-expression analysis and database in transgenic mice during development of amyloid or tau pathology. Cell Reports. 2015;10:633–44.

25. Flurkey KCJ, Harrison DE. The mouse in aging research. Burlington: American College Laboratory Animal Medicine (Elsevier); 2007.

26. Bolivar VJ. Intrasession and intersession habituation in mice: from inbred strain variability to linkage analysis. Neurobiol Learn Mem. 2009;92:206–14.

27. Fraley SM, Springer AD. Memory of simple learning in young, middle-aged, and aged C57/BL6 mice. Behav Neural Biol. 1981;31:1–7.

28. Liu F, Day M, Muñiz LC, Bitran D, Arias R, Revilla-Sanchez R, et al. Activation of estrogen receptor-beta regulates hippocampal synaptic plasticity and improves memory. Nat Neurosci. 2008;11(3):334–43.

29. Herring BE, Nicoll RA. Long-term potentiation: from CaMKII to AMPA receptor trafficking. Annu Rev Physiol. 2016;78:351–65.

30. Kim J, Kwon JT, Kim HS, Han JH. CREB and neuronal selection for memory trace. Front Neural Circ. 2013;7:44.

31. Rivett AJ, Bose S, Pemberton AJ, Brooks P, Onion D, Shirley D, et al. Assays of proteasome activity in relation to aging. Exp Gerontol. 2002;37:1217–22.

32. Hernebring M. 26S and PA28–20S proteasome activity in cytosolic extracts from embryonic stem cells. In: Turksen K, editor. Embryonic stem cell protocols. New York: Springer; 2016. p. 359–67.

33. Bose S, Brooks P, Mason GG, Rivett AJ. γ-Interferon decreases the level of 26 S proteasomes and changes the pattern of phosphorylation. Biochem J. 2001;353:291–7.

34. Zhang Z, Clawson A, Rechsteiner M. The proteasome activator 11 S regulator or PA28: contribution by Both α and β Subunits to proteasome activation. J Biol Chem. 1998;273:30660–8.

35. Knowlton JRJS, Whitby FG, Realini C, Zhang Z, Rechsteiner M, Hill CP. Structure of the proteasome activator REGalpha (PA28alpha). Nature. 1997;390:639–43.

36. Yao Y, Huang L, Krutchinsky A, Wong M-L, Standing KG, Burlingame AL, Wang CC. Structural and functional characterizations of the proteasome-activating protein PA26 from trypanosoma brucei. J Biol Chem. 1999;274:33921–30.

37. Yamano T, Murata S, Shimbara N, Tanaka N, Chiba T, Tanaka K, et al. Two distinct pathways mediated by PA28 and hsp90 in major histocompatibility complex class I antigen processing. J Exp Med. 2002;196:185–96.

38. Petit-Demouliere B, Chenu F, Bourin M. Forced swimming test in mice: a review of antidepressant activity. Psychopharmacology. 2005;177(3):245–55.

39. Walsh RN, Cummins RA. The open-field test: a critical review. Psychol Bull. 1976;83:482–504.

40. Crawley JN. Exploratory behavior models of anxiety in mice. Neurosci Biobehav Rev. 1985;9:37–44.

41. Carter M, Shieh J. Guide to research techniques in neuroscience. 2nd ed. San Diego: Academic; 2015.

42. Muller U, Cristina N, Li ZW, Wolfer DP, Lipp HP, Rulicke T, et al. Behavioral and anatomical deficits in mice homozygous for a modified beta-amyloid precursor protein gene. Cell. 1994;79:755–65.

43. Võikar V, Kõks S, Vasar E, Rauvala H. Strain and gender differences in the behavior of mouse lines commonly used in transgenic studies. Physiol Behav. 2001;72(1–2):271–81.

44. Campbell S, MacQueen G. The role of the hippocampus in the pathophysiology of major depression. J Psychiatry Neurosci. 2004;29(6):417–26.

45. Jarome TJ, Kwapis JL, Ruenzel WL, Helmstetter FJ. CaMKII, but not protein kinase A, regulates Rpt6phosphorylation and proteasome activity during the formation of long-term memories. Front Behav Neurosci. 2013;7:115.

46. Seo H, Sonntag KC, Isacson O. Generalized brain and skin proteasome inhibition in Huntington's disease. Ann Neurol. 2004;56:319–28.

47. Kumarapeli ARK, Horak KM, Glasford JW, Li J, Chen Q, Liu J, et al. A novel transgenic mouse model reveals deregulation of the ubiquitin-proteasome system in the heart by doxorubicin. FASEB J. 2005;19:2051–3.

48. Henley JM, Wilkinson KA. Synaptic AMPA receptor composition in development, plasticity and disease. Nat Rev Neurosci. 2016;17:337–50.

49. Noor JI, Ikeda T, Mishima K, Aoo N, Ohta S, Egashira N, et al. Short-term administration of a new free radical scavenger, Edaravone, is more effective than its long-term administration for the treatment of neonatal hypoxic-ischemic encephalopathy. Stroke. 2005;36:2468–74.

50. Otani H, Togashi H, Jesmin S, Sakuma I, Yamaguchi T, Matsumoto M, et al. Temporal effects of edaravone, a free radical scavenger, on transient ischemia-induced neuronal dysfunction in the rat hippocampus. Eur J Pharmacol. 2005;512:129–37.

51. Datsenko KA, Wanner BL. One-step inactivation of chromosomal genes in Escherichia coli K-12 using PCR products. PNAS. 2000;97:6640–5.

52. Hitoshi N, Ken-ichi Y, Jun-ichi M. Efficient selection for high-expression transfectants with a novel eukaryotic vector. Gene. 1991;108:193–9.

53. Petersen A, Zetterberg M. The immunoproteasome in human lens epithelial cells during oxidative stress. Invest Ophthalmol Vis Sci. 2016;57(11):5038–45.

54. Ballesteros M, Fredriksson Å, Henriksson J, Nyström T. Bacterial senescence: protein oxidation in non-proliferating cells is dictated by the accuracy of the ribosomes. EMBO J. 2001;20:5280–9.

55. Gerdin AK, Surve VV, Jönsson M, Bjursell M, Björkman M, Edenro A, et al. Phenotypic screening of hepatocyte nuclear factor (HNF) 4-γ receptor knockout mice. Biochem Biophys Res Commun. 2006;349:825–32.

56. Porsolt RD, Le Pichon M, Jalfre M. Depression: a new animal model sensitive to antidepressant treatments. Nature. 1977;266:730–2.

57. Bammer G. Pharmacological investigations of neurotransmitter involvement in passive avoidance responding: a review and some new results. Neurosci Biobehav Rev. 1982;6:247–96.

58. Misane I, Ogren SO. Selective 5-HT1A antagonists WAY 100635 and NAD-299 attenuate the impairment of passive avoidance caused by scopolamine in the rat. Neuropsychopharmacology. 2003;28:253–64.

59. Shepherd JK, Grewal SS, Fletcher A, Bill DJ, Dourish CT. Behavioural and pharmacological characterisation of the elevated "zero-maze" as an animal model of anxiety. Psychopharmacology. 1994;116:56–64.

60. Tang X, Sanford LD. Home cage activity and activity-based measures of anxiety in 129P3/J, 129X1/SvJ and C57BL/6J mice. Physiol Behav. 2005;84:105–15.

61. Jozefczuk J, Drews K, Adjaye J. Preparation of mouse embryonic fibroblast cells suitable for culturing human embryonic and induced pluripotent stem cells. J Vis Exp. 2012;64:3854.

62. Fredriksson Å, Johansson Krogh E, Hernebring M, Pettersson E, Javadi A, Almstedt A, et al. Effects of aging and reproduction on protein quality control in soma and gametes of Drosophila melanogaster. Aging Cell. 2012;11:634–43.

13

Blue light induces a neuroprotective gene expression program in *Drosophila* photoreceptors

Hana Hall[1†], Jingqun Ma[1,2†], Sudhanshu Shekhar[3], Walter D. Leon-Salas[4] and Vikki M. Weake[1,5*] [ID]

Abstract

Background: Light exposure induces oxidative stress, which contributes to ocular diseases of aging. Blue light provides a model for light-induced oxidative stress, lipid peroxidation and retinal degeneration in *Drosophila melanogaster*. In contrast to mature adults, which undergo retinal degeneration when exposed to prolonged blue light, newly-eclosed flies are resistant to blue light-induced retinal degeneration. Here, we sought to characterize the gene expression programs induced by blue light in flies of different ages to identify neuroprotective pathways utilized by photoreceptors to cope with light-induced oxidative stress.

Results: To identify gene expression changes induced by blue light exposure, we profiled the nuclear transcriptome of *Drosophila* photoreceptors from one- and six-day-old flies exposed to blue light and compared these with dark controls. Flies were exposed to 3 h blue light, which increases levels of reactive oxygen species but does not cause retinal degeneration. We identified substantial gene expression changes in response to blue light only in six-day-old flies. In six-day-old flies, blue light induced a neuroprotective gene expression program that included upregulation of stress response pathways and downregulation of genes involved in light response, calcium influx and ion transport. An intact phototransduction pathway and calcium influx were required for upregulation, but not downregulation, of genes in response to blue light, suggesting that distinct pathways mediate the blue light-associated transcriptional response.

Conclusion: Our data demonstrate that under phototoxic conditions, *Drosophila* photoreceptors upregulate stress response pathways and simultaneously, downregulate expression of phototransduction components, ion transporters, and calcium channels. Together, this gene expression program both counteracts the calcium influx resulting from prolonged light exposure, and ameliorates the oxidative stress resulting from this calcium influx. Thus, six-day-old flies can withstand up to 3 h blue light exposure without undergoing retinal degeneration. Developmental transitions during the first week of adult *Drosophila* life lead to an altered gene expression program in photoreceptors that includes reduced expression of genes that maintain redox and calcium homeostasis, reducing the capacity of six-day-old flies to cope with longer periods (8 h) of light exposure. Together, these data provide insight into the neuroprotective gene regulatory mechanisms that enable photoreceptors to withstand light-induced oxidative stress.

Keywords: *Drosophila*, Blue light, Retinal degeneration, Transcriptome, Photoreceptor, RNA-seq

*Correspondence: vweake@purdue.edu
†Hana Hall and Jingqun Ma have contributed equally to this work
[1] Department of Biochemistry, Purdue University, West Lafayette, IN 47907, USA
Full list of author information is available at the end of the article

Background

Light itself, although essential for vision, poses a stress to the visual system through photogeneration of reactive oxygen species [1]. Oxidative stress has been linked to the onset of human retinal degeneration [1]. The specialized nature and composition of photoreceptor neurons may increase their sensitivity to oxidative damage due to the energy demands of vision, the high concentration of peroxidation-sensitive polyunsaturated fatty acids, and exposure to light [2, 3]. In particular, lipid peroxidation, the oxidation of membrane lipids, is an emerging hallmark of both neurodegenerative and age-associated ocular disease [3, 4]. Lipid peroxidation, once initiated, induces a cycle of oxidative damage that harms cellular membranes and eventually culminates in cell death [5]. Cells possess endogenous protective mechanisms to withstand lipid peroxidation and maintain redox homeostasis including gene regulatory mechanisms [6]. However, the neuroprotective mechanisms utilized by photoreceptors to withstand the oxidative stress generated as a normal part of light exposure are not fully understood.

In *Drosophila*, as in other organisms, blue light wavelengths induce retinal degeneration [7–9]. Blue light ($\lambda = 480$ nm) activates the G-protein coupled receptor Rhodopsin 1 (Rh1) within the rhabdomere, the light sensing organelle, of R1–R6 photoreceptors [10]. Upon blue illumination, Rh1 is activated to metarhodopsin initiating the phototransduction cascade [10]. In flies, metarhodopsin can be converted back to Rh1 by orange light ($\lambda = 580$ nm) [10–12]. Persistent production of metarhodopsin in the presence of blue light leads to its endocytosis and prolonged calcium influx, both of which can induce cell death [13–18]. The prolonged calcium influx resulting from blue light exposure increases levels of reactive oxygen species in the eye including hydrogen peroxide and lipid peroxidation [19]. We previously showed that lipid peroxidation is a major contributor to blue light-induced retinal degeneration because feeding flies lipophilic antioxidants, or overexpressing Cytochrome-b5, suppressed lipid peroxidation and enhanced photoreceptor survival [19]. Thus, blue light exposure in flies provides a model for light-induced oxidative stress and lipid peroxidation, hallmarks of age-associated ocular and neurodegenerative disease [3, 4].

Although blue light induces retinal degeneration in mature flies, our previous results showed that very young flies are resilient to longer periods of blue light (Fig. 1a). Newly-eclosed flies, that have recently emerged from the pupal case and are less than one day old, did not undergo retinal degeneration in response to prolonged blue light [19]. In contrast, mature flies that are only six days old, underwent severe retinal degeneration when exposed to the same level of blue light [19]. Blue light-induced retinal degeneration required an intact phototransduction pathway and calcium influx, mediated by the transient receptor potential (*trp*) calcium channel [19]. Since blue light provides a model for light-induced lipid peroxidation in the eye, we sought to identify the gene regulatory mechanisms utilized by *Drosophila* photoreceptors to cope with the oxidative stress resulting from blue light exposure. Here, we profiled the transcriptome of *Drosophila* photoreceptors following short blue light exposure at different ages to gain insight into neuroprotective pathways that enable photoreceptors to withstand light-induced oxidative stress.

Results

Blue light induces neuroprotective gene expression changes in photoreceptors

To identify gene regulatory mechanisms involved in the response of photoreceptors to blue light-induced oxidative stress, we profiled the transcriptome of photoreceptor cells in flies that were exposed to blue light relative to dark control. Here, we exposed flies to 3 h blue light, which we previously showed was sufficient to increase levels of reactive oxygen species in the eye of six-day-old flies, but not in one-day-old flies [19]. This shorter 3 h blue light exposure resulted in less than 1% rhabdomere loss at both ages (Additional file 1: Figure S1), enabling us to isolate intact photoreceptor nuclei for RNA-seq analysis. To isolate photoreceptor nuclear RNA, we used previously developed methods to affinity-purify *Rh1-Gal4 > KASH-GFP* tagged nuclei from R1–R6 cells in adult heads [20, 21]. Since white-eyed flies are sensitized to blue light [9], we depleted eye pigments from *Rh1-Gal4 > KASH-GFP* flies, which have red eyes due to the presence of the *mini-white* transgene marker, by introducing homozygous mutations for *cn* and *bw* [22, 23]. We then exposed one- or six-day-old flies to 3 h of blue light and isolated photoreceptor nuclear RNA for RNA-seq analysis (Fig. 1b).

To test the enrichment of photoreceptor transcripts using our affinity-isolation procedure, we compared the transcriptome of the whole head homogenate (pre-isolation) and post-isolation sample from the control dark treated day one flies. Consistent with previous results using this affinity-isolation approach [20], the post-isolation samples differed substantially from the pre-isolation samples based on the principal component analysis (Additional file 1: Figure S2A). We identified 521 genes, including GFP, as significantly enriched using edgeR analysis (False Discovery Rate, FDR < 0.05, Fold change, FC > 2) in the post-isolation samples relative to the pre-isolation samples (Additional file 1: Figure S2B, Additional file 2: Table S1). These genes were

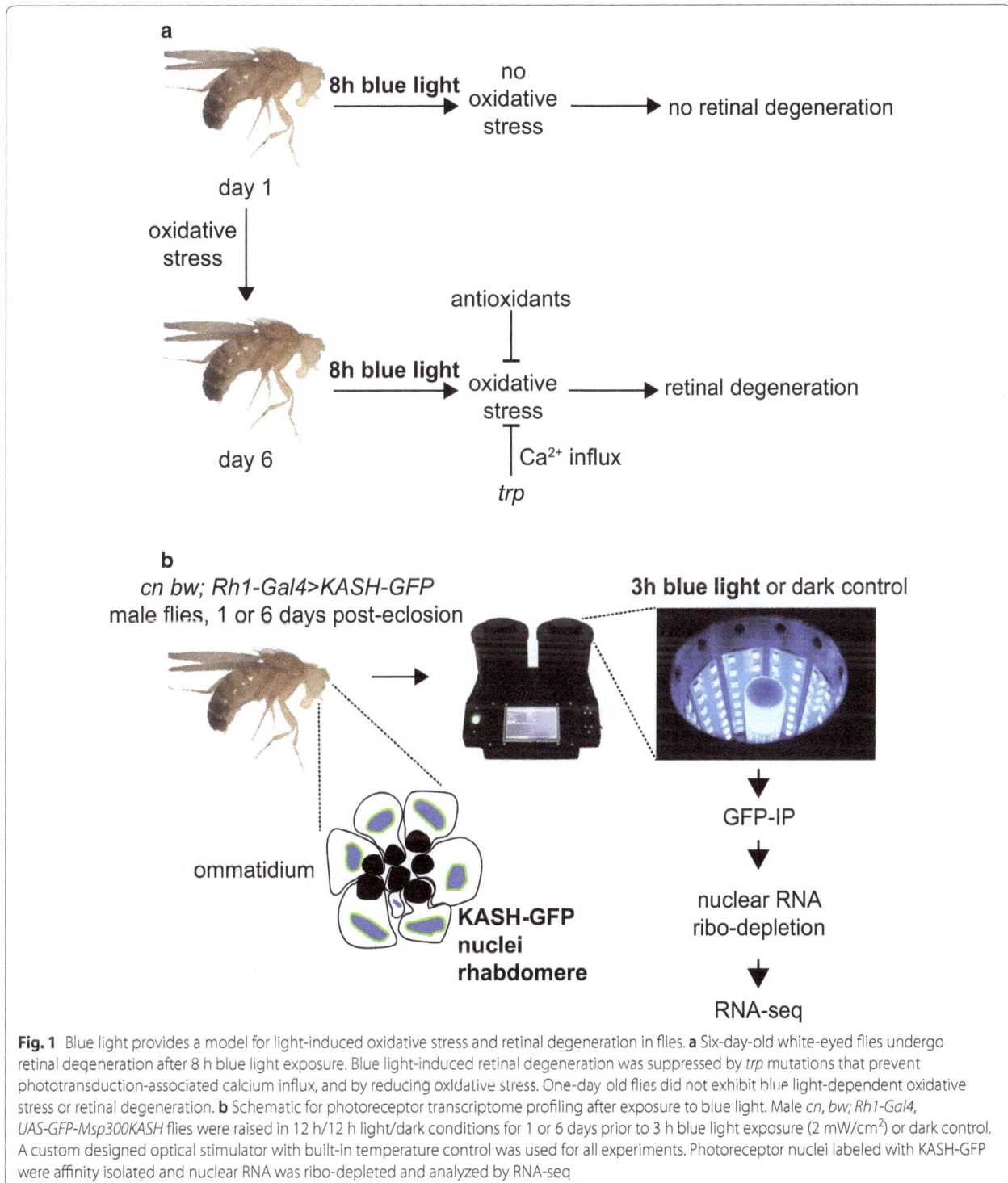

Fig. 1 Blue light provides a model for light-induced oxidative stress and retinal degeneration in flies. **a** Six-day-old white-eyed flies undergo retinal degeneration after 8 h blue light exposure. Blue light-induced retinal degeneration was suppressed by *trp* mutations that prevent phototransduction-associated calcium influx, and by reducing oxidative stress. One-day old flies did not exhibit blue light-dependent oxidative stress or retinal degeneration. **b** Schematic for photoreceptor transcriptome profiling after exposure to blue light. Male *cn, bw; Rh1-Gal4, UAS-GFP-Msp300KASH* flies were raised in 12 h/12 h light/dark conditions for 1 or 6 days prior to 3 h blue light exposure (2 mW/cm^2) or dark control. A custom designed optical stimulator with built-in temperature control was used for all experiments. Photoreceptor nuclei labeled with KASH-GFP were affinity isolated and nuclear RNA was ribo-depleted and analyzed by RNA-seq

enriched for Gene Ontology (GO) terms associated with photoreceptor development and function (Additional file 3: Table S2). Thus, we conclude that our post-isolation samples are enriched for photoreceptor-expressed transcripts.

Next, we compared the photoreceptor-enriched transcriptome of day one and day six flies that had been exposed to blue light or the dark control. Multidimensional scaling plots revealed that both age and light treatment influenced the variation in gene expression between

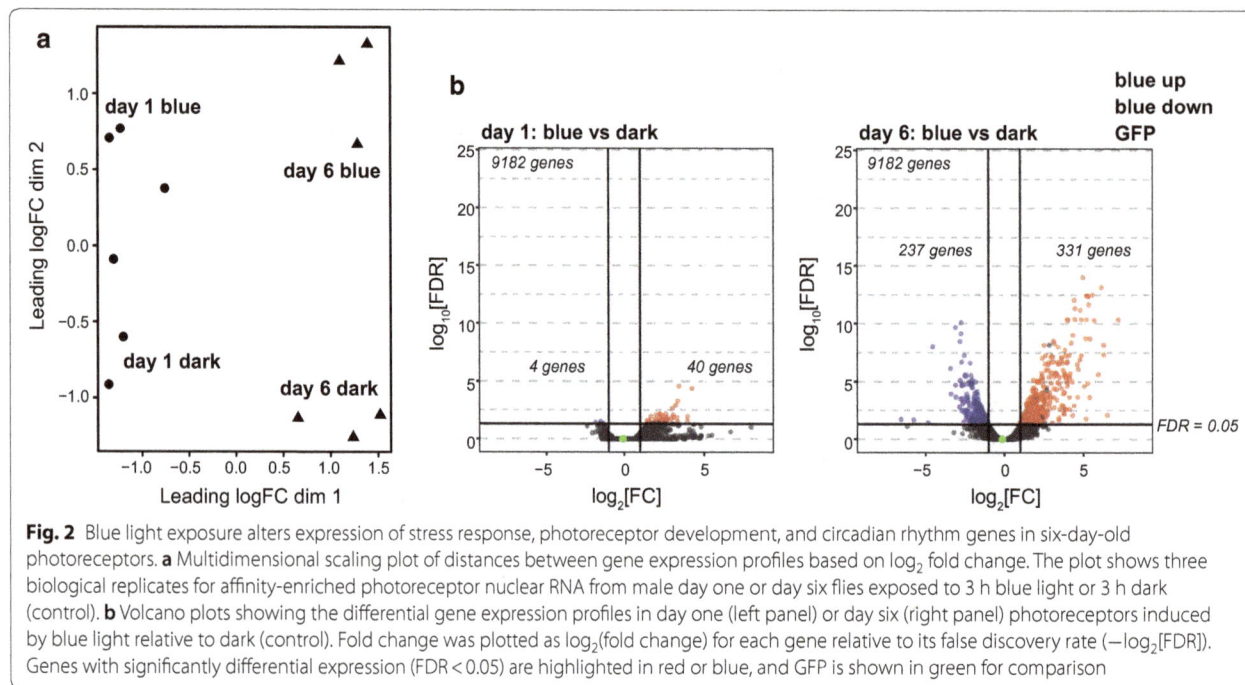

Fig. 2 Blue light exposure alters expression of stress response, photoreceptor development, and circadian rhythm genes in six-day-old photoreceptors. **a** Multidimensional scaling plot of distances between gene expression profiles based on $\log_2$ fold change. The plot shows three biological replicates for affinity-enriched photoreceptor nuclear RNA from male day one or day six flies exposed to 3 h blue light or 3 h dark (control). **b** Volcano plots showing the differential gene expression profiles in day one (left panel) or day six (right panel) photoreceptors induced by blue light relative to dark (control). Fold change was plotted as $\log_2$(fold change) for each gene relative to its false discovery rate ($-\log_2$[FDR]). Genes with significantly differential expression (FDR < 0.05) are highlighted in red or blue, and GFP is shown in green for comparison

the samples, with the three biological replicates for each treatment and age grouping together (Fig. 2a). To identify genes that showed altered expression profiles upon blue light treatment, we used edgeR analysis to identify differentially expressed genes in blue versus dark treated samples from day one or day six flies. Only 40 and four genes were significantly up- or downregulated (FDR < 0.05), respectively, in day one photoreceptors upon blue light stress (Fig. 2b). In contrast, 331 and 237 genes were significantly up- or downregulated, respectively, in day six photoreceptors upon blue light stress (Fig. 2b). Only six genes were uniquely regulated in response to blue light in day one photoreceptors, and most of these genes also showed strong, albeit not significant, fold changes in gene expression in day six flies (Additional file 1: Fig. S3). These data indicate that six-day-old flies exhibit substantial gene expression changes in photoreceptors in response to blue light, whereas these gene expression changes are largely absent in newly-eclosed flies. We previously observed that in contrast to six-day-old flies, one-day-old flies did not show increased levels of reactive oxygen species upon blue light exposure [19]. Together, these observations suggest that one-day-old flies experience much lower levels of blue light-induced oxidative stress than mature, six-day-old flies.

Next, we asked if the gene expression changes that we observed in response to blue light in day six flies could be neuroprotective since 3 h blue light exposure increased oxidative stress levels in the eye but did not cause retinal

degeneration (Additional file 1: Fig. S1). GO term enrichment analysis revealed that pathways associated with the response to unfolded proteins, environmental stresses such as heat, ion transport and protein translation were upregulated in response to blue light exposure in six-day-old flies (Table 1, Additional file 3: Table S2). The blue light-upregulated genes included many heat shock protein genes such as *Hsc70-2*, *Hsc70-3*, *Hsc70-5*, *Hsp68*, *Hsp70Aa* and *Hsp70Bc* that are part of the Heat Shock Protein 70 superfamily of chaperones. These chaperones are upregulated in response to chemical and thermal stress, resolve misfolded and aggregated proteins, and are implicated in having a protective role in neurodegenerative disease [24]. In addition, several genes encoding proteins involved in ion transport were upregulated in response to blue light. These genes include mitochondrial transporters such as *Thiamine pyrophosphate carrier protein 1* (*Tpc1*) and *CG5646*, several putative organic cation transporters such as *CG14855*, *CG14856* and *SLC22A*, and the gap junction protein *Innexin 7* (*Inx7*), which together might restore calcium and energy homeostasis within photoreceptors following blue light exposure. Several genes associated with protein translation were also upregulated in response to blue light including several cytoplasmic aminoacyl-tRNA synthetases (e.g. *GluProRS/Aats-glupro*, *GlyRS/Aats-gly*, *TrpRS/Aats-trp*). Specialized translation is associated with the stress response [25], but increased translation following blue light might also be required to restore Rh1 levels, which

Table 1 Enriched biological process GO terms identified for day 6 blue versus dark upregulated genes

GO term	Description	p value	FDR	Enrichment	Genes
GO:0006418	tRNA aminoacylation for protein translation	4.50E−06	0.00646	6.82	Aats-glupro, CG10802, Aats-thr, Aats-gly, Aats-cys, CG33123, Aats-trp, CG17259, Aats-asp
GO:0006399	tRNA metabolic process	0.000895	0.292	3.06	Aats-glupro, CG10802, CG6353, Aats-thr, Aats-gly, CG33123, Aats-cys, Aats-trp, CG17259, CG18596, Aats-asp
GO:0006820	Anion transport	0.000111	0.0532	3.05	CG14857, CG14856, CG5535, CG7589, CG14855, CG5802, CG13646, CG5646, Jhl-21, CG9864, CG42575, w, MFS3, Tpc1, CG7442
GO:0015695	Organic cation transport	0.000128	0.0574	13.47	CG5646, CG3476, CG7442, Tpc1
GO:0015696	Ammonium transport	0.000465	0.167	10.1	CG5646, w, CG3476, CG7442
GO:0009631	Cold acclimation	0.000338	0.143	18.18	Hsp23, Hsp26, Hsp83
GO:0006457	Protein folding	0.00042	0.159	3.13	Hsp68, Hsp23, CG14894, Hsp70Bc, Hsp26, Hsc70-3, Hsc70-5, Hsp70Aa, Hsc70-2, Hsp83, wbl, CG5525
GO:0042026	Protein refolding	2.37E−08	0.00017	14.26	Hsp68, Hsp23, Hsp26, Hsp70Bc, Hsc70-3, Hsc70-5, Hsc70-2, Hsp70Aa
GO:0061077	Chaperone-mediated protein folding	8.51E−06	0.00555	6.34	Hsp68, Hsp23, Hsp26, Hsp70Bc, Hsc70-3, Hsc70-5, Hsc70-2, Hsp70Aa, CG5525
GO:0009408	Response to heat	0.000101	0.0516	4.27	Hsp68, Hsp23, Nup98-96, Hsp26, Hsp70Bc, Hsc70-3, Hsc70-5, Hsc70-2, Hsp70Aa, Hsp83
GO:0006986	Response to unfolded protein	7.39E−06	0.00589	11.36	Hsp68, Hsp70Bc, Hsc70-3, Hsc70-5, Hsc70-2, Hsp70Aa
GO:0006458	'de novo' protein folding	1.13E−05	0.00626	8.48	Hsp68, Hsp70Bc, Hsc70-3, Hsc70-5, Hsc70-2, Hsp70Aa, CG5525
GO:0051085	Chaperone cofactor dependent protein refolding	2.93E−06	0.00525	12.99	Hsp68, Hsp70Bc, Hsc70-3, Hsp70Aa, Hsc70-2, Hsc70-5
GO:0034605	Cellular response to heat	8.56E−06	0.00511	7.35	Hsp68, Nup98-96, Hsp70Bc, Hsc70-3, Hsc70-5, Hsc70-2, Hsp70Aa, Hsp83
GO:0035080	Heat shock-mediated polytene chromosome puffing	0.000338	0.135	18.18	Nup98-96, Hsp70Bc, Hsp70Aa

are depleted due to endocytosis of activated metarhodopsin [14, 16]. Although DNA repair was not identified in the GO term enrichment analysis, several genes associated with repair of DNA damage were upregulated in response to blue light including *DNA ligase III* (*lig3*), *mutagen-sensitive 205* (*mus205*), *Replication Protein A 70* (*RpA-70*), *Inverted repeat-binding protein* (*Irbp*), *Inverted repeat binding protein 18 kDa* (*Irbp18*), *Replication factor C subunit 4* (*RfC4*), *Xrp1*, *nbs*, and *CG3448*. Thus, blue light exposure initiates a transcriptional stress response in photoreceptors that induces repair mechanisms to combat protein misfolding and DNA damage, and to restore Rh1 levels and ion homeostasis.

In addition to the genes that were upregulated in response to blue light, a similar number of genes were downregulated in response to blue light exposure in day six, but not day one, flies. Intriguingly, these blue light-downregulated genes were enriched for GO terms related to photoreceptor function and phototransduction including regulation of membrane potential, rhodopsin metabolism, and response to light stimulus (Table 2, Additional file 3: Table S2). Several genes involved in regulating

membrane potential were downregulated in response to blue light including potassium and chloride channels and their regulators such as *Chloride channel-a* (*ClC-a*), *Slowpoke* (*slo*), *Shaker* (*Sh*), *small conductance calcium-activated potassium channel* (*SK*), *ether a go–go* (*eag*), *Slip1*, Na^+-*driven anion exchanger 1* (*Ndae1*) and *Hyperkinetic* (*Hk*). In addition, factors involved in post-translational modification and maturation of rhodopsin such as *Hexosaminidase 1* (*Hexo1*), *alpha-Mannosidase class II b* (*alpha-Man-IIb*), and *fused lobes* (*fdl*) were downregulated in response to blue light. Most strikingly, several genes with well-characterized roles in phototransduction were significantly downregulated in day six flies upon blue light exposure. These genes include components of the phototransduction machinery such as *retinal degeneration A* (*rdgA*), *retinal degeneration C* (*rdgC*), *Histidine decarboxylase* (*Hdc*), *Calcium, integrin binding family member 2* (*Cib2*), and the calcium channel *trp*. Several other genes involved in voltage-gated calcium influx into photoreceptors were also downregulated in response to blue light including Ca^{2+}-*channel protein alpha¹ subunit D* (*Ca-alpha1D*), Ca^{2+}-*channel-protein-beta-subunit*

Table 2 Enriched biological process GO terms identified for day 6 blue versus dark downregulated genes

GO term	Description	p value	FDR	Enrichment	Genes
GO:0009886	Post-embryonic animal morphogenesis	0.000318	0.127	2.49	*app, ewg, mirr, ara, oc, so, dlg1, sd, Cbl, jumu, CG30456, psq, RhoGEF2, Exn, mthl1, CG33275, zfh2, CG13366*
GO:0009653	Anatomical structure morphogenesis	0.00041	0.134	1.77	*app, kek4, ewg, oc, vri, dlg1, dnt, ric8a, Cbl, jumu, csw, RhoGEF2, Prosap, mthl1, Moe, CG13366, zfh2, Hr39, slik, CHES-1-like, Shroom, fru, mirr, CG13188, caup, ara, so, gl, sd, psq, CG30456, Crg-1, fred, pyd, Exn, CG33275*
GO:0042693	Muscle cell fate commitment	0.000539	0.133	42.96	*caup, ara*
GO:0006357	Regulation of transcription by RNA polymerase II	0.000989	0.177	1.97	*CHES-1-like, mirr, ewg, Mef2, fru, caup, ara, oc, dlg1, gl, so, sd, onecut, psq, Eip74EF, Crg-1, Nfl, csw, jing, tim, jigr1, Camta, Hr39, Elp3*
GO:0006355	Regulation of transcription, DNA-templated	3.00E—04	0.154	1.8	*CTCF, ewg, Kdm4B, tinc, oc, vri, dlg1, jumu, onecut, Eip74EF, csw, Nfl, tim, zfh2, Hr39, Elp3, Pdp1, CHES-1-like, fru, Mef2, mirr, CG13188, caup, ara, Hmt4-20, Hmx, gl, so, sd, psq, Crg-1, jing, jigr1, Camta, wts, thoc5*
GO:0030001	Metal ion transport	0.000378	0.135	3.67	*eag, Hk, Ca-alpha1D, Ndae1, Ca-beta, Sh, SK, trp, olf186-F, slo*
GO:0042391	Regulation of membrane potential	2.52E—05	0.0903	5.05	*eag, inaF-D, Ca-alpha1D, Prosap, Sh, inaF-C, SK, Slob, Moe, slo*
GO:0007619	Courtship behavior	0.000837	0.162	9.04	*eag, rut, Sh, gb*
GO:0048150	Behavioral response to ether	0.000539	0.138	42.96	*eag, Sh*
GO:0007617	Mating behavior	5.54E—05	0.0993	4.62	*eag, tim, rut, fru, Sh, gb, dlg1, Moe, Hr39, slo*
GO:0007275	Multicellular organism development	0.000177	0.141	3.25	*ewg, fru, Mef2, mirr, CG2681, oc, vri, dlg1, dnt, cdi, Elp3, Pdp1, Sema-1b*
GO:0046154	Rhodopsin metabolic process	4.33E—05	0.104	11.93	*fdl, rdgA, alpha-Man-IIb, trp, Hexo1*
GO:0001745	Compound eye morphogenesis	0.000177	0.127	4.44	*fred, mirr, caup, ara, pyd, oc, so, gl, sd*
GO:0008049	Male courtship behavior	0.000892	0.168	5.26	*fru, gb, dlg1, Moe, Hr39, slo*
GO:0045433	Male courtship behavior, veined wing generated song production	0.000837	0.167	9.04	*fru, Moe, Hr39, slo*
GO:0045938	Positive regulation of circadian sleep/wake cycle, sleep	0.000122	0.124	14.32	*Hk, homer, Sh, mld*
GO:0045187	Regulation of circadian sleep/wake cycle, sleep	0.000344	0.13	7.95	*Hk, tim, homer, mld, Sh*
GO:0042752	Regulation of circadian rhythm	0.000248	0.148	4.77	*Hk, tim, homer, mld, Sh, CG33275, gl, so*
GO:0007623	Circadian rhythm	0.000404	0.138	3.99	*Hk, tim, Mef2, dlg1, vri, so, gl, Pdp1, slo*
GO:0016057	Regulation of membrane potential in photoreceptor cell	0.000638	0.147	16.11	*inaF-D, SK, Moe*
GO:1902680	Positive regulation of RNA biosynthetic process	0.000803	0.175	2.37	*Mef2, mirr, caup, ara, oc, gl, so, sd, jumu, onecut, Eip74EF, Nfl, jing, Camta, thoc5, Hr39, Pdp1*
GO:0035120	Post-embryonic appendage morphogenesis	0.000543	0.13	3.26	*mirr, ara, Exn, mthl1, CG33275, sd, zfh2,, Cbl, jumu, CG30456, psq*
GO:0045317	Equator specification	0.000236	0.154	21.48	*mirr, caup, ara*
GO:0009887	Animal organ morphogenesis	0.000159	0.143	2.72	*mirr, ewg, CG13188, caup, ara, oc, gl, so, vri, sd, dnt, fred, pyd, Prosap, mthl1, CG13366, Hr39*
GO:0045935	Positive regulation of nucleobase-containing compound metabolic process	0.00072	0.161	2.32	*mirr, Mef2, caup, ara, oc, gl, so, sd, jumu, tankyrase, onecut, Eip74EF, Nfl, jing, Camta, thoc5, Hr39, Pdp1*
GO:0007635	Chemosensory behavior	8.68E—05	0.124	4.38	*mura, smi35A, gish, rut, Sh, gb, nord, Moe, trp, psq*
GO:0007610	Behavior	2.40E—05	0.172	2.36	*nord, oc, dlg1, vri, hppy, CG13192, eag, smi35A, gish, tim, Sh, Prosap, mld, Moe, Elp3, Hr39, Hk, Mef2, fru, gb, trp, psq, slo, mura, t, homer, rut*
GO:0035025	Positive regulation of Rho protein signal transduction	0.000317	0.134	11.45	*RhoGEF2, Exn, CG33275, CG30456*
GO:0009314	Response to radiation	5.00E—04	0.138	3.09	*smi35A, tim, CG30118, rdgA, CG9236, Sh, Camta, dlg1, wts, gl, Hdc, trp*
GO:0009416	Response to light stimulus	0.000275	0.152	3.53	*smi35A, tim, rdgA, CG30118, CG9236, Sh, Camta, dlg1, gl, Hdc, trp*

(*Ca-beta*), and *olf186-F*, which encodes a subunit of the store-operated calcium entry channel. Previously, we showed that blue light-induced retinal degeneration required an intact phototransduction pathway and Trp-mediated calcium influx [19]. Here, our data suggest that under phototoxic conditions, photoreceptors downregulate expression of phototransduction components and calcium channels, potentially as part of a neuroprotective response to mitigate the calcium influx resulting from light exposure.

Blue light-induced changes in gene expression show different temporal profiles

Exposure to moderate levels of stress protects photoreceptors against retinal degeneration [26]. To test if exposure to light stress would increase basal expression levels of stress response genes, we asked if the changes in gene expression that occurred in photoreceptors in response to blue light returned to pre-treatment levels after different intervals of dark exposure, post light-treatment. To do this, we exposed male six-day-old *cn bw; Rh1-Gal4 > KASH-GFP* flies to 3 h blue light or dark control, and then incubated flies for 0, 3, 6 or 24 h in the dark. We then dissected eyes and examined expression of several blue light-regulated genes using qPCR. We normalized expression of each gene to the pre-treatment control, and compared relative expression levels between the blue and dark samples for each time point. We examined four blue light-induced genes, *branchless* (*bnl*), *Heat shock protein 26* (*Hsp26*), *RpA-70* and *Xrp1* and two blue light-repressed genes, *Checkpoint suppressor 1-like* (*CHES-1-like*) and *trp* (Fig. 3). The four upregulated genes all showed different expression

profiles following exposure to 3 h blue light: *Xrp1* and *RpA-70* showed significantly increased expression in blue light versus dark control at 0, 3 and 6 h post-treatment, but returned to basal levels by 24 h post-treatment. In contrast, *bnl* and *Hsp26* levels remained high 24 h after blue light exposure. The two downregulated genes, *CHES-1-like* and *trp*, showed significantly decreased expression levels immediately post-treatment (0 h) but returned to basal levels by 3 h post-treatment. These data indicate that blue light-repression of genes is transient and might require continual exposure to the light source. In contrast, exposure to blue light increases expression of stress response genes, some of which remain at relatively high levels up to 1 day after flies are removed from the source of light stress.

An intact phototransduction pathway and calcium influx are required for blue light-induced upregulation of stress response genes, but not downregulation of visual function genes

Phototransduction in R1–R6 photoreceptors initiates with the light-sensing G-protein coupled receptor, Rhodopsin 1 (Rh1 encoded by *ninaE*), and culminates in calcium influx, largely mediated by the Trp channel [11]. We previously showed that blue light-induced retinal degeneration requires both phototransduction and calcium influx because rhabdomere loss was suppressed by mutations that reduce Rh1 protein levels to ~ 1% of wild-type levels (*ninaE*[7]) [27] or reduce Trp expression (*trp*[9]) [19]. To test if phototransduction and calcium influx were necessary for blue light-regulated gene expression changes, we examined expression of blue light-regulated genes in eyes from *ninaE*[7] or *trp*[9] flies. We compared gene

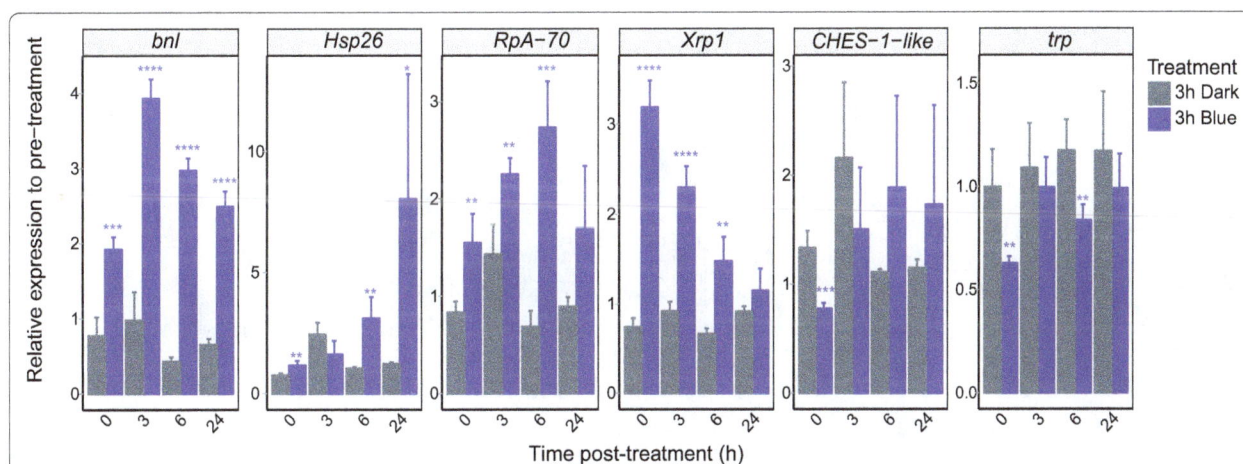

Fig. 3 Blue light-induced changes in gene expression are transient. Six-day-old male *cn, bw; Rh1-Gal4, UAS-GFP-Msp300KASH* flies were exposed to 3 h blue light exposure or dark control, and gene expression was analyzed in dissected eyes at 0, 3, 6 or 24 h following treatment by qPCR. Expression is shown relative to the geometric mean of *RpL32* and *elF1A* and is normalized to the pre-treatment sample, which is set to one. *p* values, *t* test between blue treatment and dark control at the same time post-treatment (*p < 0.05; **p < 0.01; ***p < 0.001; ****p < 0.0001; n = 4)

expression to white-eyed w^{1118} flies, which lack eye pigment but have otherwise normal phototransduction. We exposed six-day-old male flies of each genotype to 3 h blue light and examined gene expression relative to the dark control at either 0 or 3 h post-treatment by qPCR in dissected eyes (Fig. 4). We examined four blue light-upregulated genes, *bnl*, *Heat shock protein 83* (*Hsp83*), *RpA-70* and *Xrp1*, and three downregulated genes, *retinal degeneration A* (*rdgA*), *retinal degeneration C* (*rdgC*) and *Shaker* (*Sh*). Blue light exposure resulted in increased expression of *bnl*, *Hsp83*, *RpA-70* and *Xrp1* either at 0 or 3 h post-treatment in w^{1118} flies, and mutations in *ninaE* and *trp* suppressed this increase (Fig. 4). In contrast, *ninaE and trp* mutations did not suppress the downregulation of *rdgA*, *rdgC* or *Sh* upon blue light exposure. We did not observe significant differences in basal levels of expression of any of the seven blue-light regulated genes tested between w^{1118}, *ninaE* and *trp* flies in the dark controls relative to the pre-treatment samples (data not shown). We note that while *trp* expression was significantly reduced in *ninaE* flies, calcium influx is already suppressed in *ninaE* mutants because Rh1 functions upstream of the Trp channel in the phototransduction cascade. Together, these data indicate that the blue light-induced and repressed genes are regulated via distinct pathways. Blue light-upregulated genes require an intact phototransduction cascade and calcium influx, whereas blue light-repressed genes do not. Instead, blue light-downregulated genes are repressed only immediately after light exposure, suggesting that light itself might be involved in the transient repression of these genes.

Developmental transitions in photoreceptor gene expression correlate with the differential susceptibility to blue light between day one and six

Since we did not observe substantial changes in gene expression upon blue light exposure in day one flies, we next wondered if underlying changes in gene expression between day one and day six photoreceptors could account for the differential susceptibility to blue light. Supporting this hypothesis, day one flies have lower basal levels of hydrogen peroxide than day six flies, even prior to blue light exposures [19]. Principal component analysis of the blue and dark treated RNA-seq samples revealed that both light treatment and age contributed to differences in the gene expression profile (Fig. 2a). Indeed, we identified 106 and 496 genes that were significantly up- or downregulated, respectively, between day one and day six in photoreceptors in the absence of blue light exposure (Fig. 5a). Importantly, we did not observe differences in GFP expression between day one and day six samples (Fig. 5a). Further, we did not observe any differences in enrichment of GFP in day one versus day six affinity purifications based on qPCR (data not shown). Thus, affinity-enrichment of photoreceptor nuclear RNA was not affected by differences in age.

Next, we asked if the changes in gene expression between day one and day six resembled those gene expression changes observed in aging photoreceptors. We compared the gene expression changes observed between day one and day six in *cn bw; Rh1-Gal4 > KASH-GFP* flies with those observed between day 10 and 40 in pigmented male *Rh1-Gal4 > KASH-GFP* flies [20]. To do this, we performed gene set enrichment analysis to

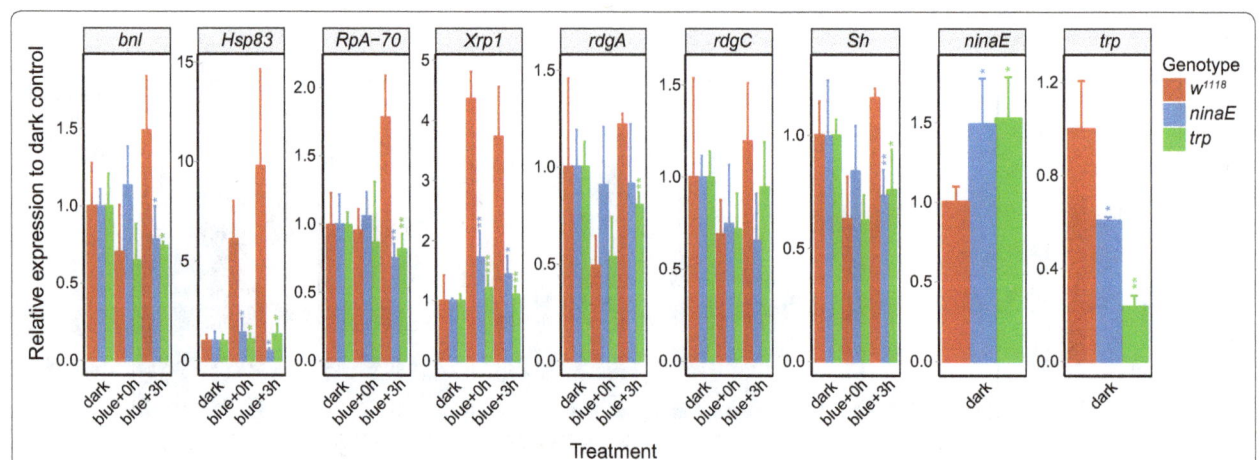

Fig. 4 An intact phototransduction pathway and calcium influx are required for blue light-induced upregulation of stress response genes, but not downregulation of visual function genes. Six-day-old male w^{1118}, $ninaE^7$ and trp^9 flies were exposed to 3 h blue light or dark control, and gene expression was analyzed in dissected eyes at 0 or 3 h following treatment by qPCR. Expression is shown relative to the geometric mean of *RpL32* and *elF1A* and is normalized to the dark control for each genotype, which is set to one. *p* values, *t* test between $ninaE^7$ or trp^9 and w^{1118} at the same time post-treatment (*p < 0.05; **p < 0.01, ***p < 0.001; n = 3)

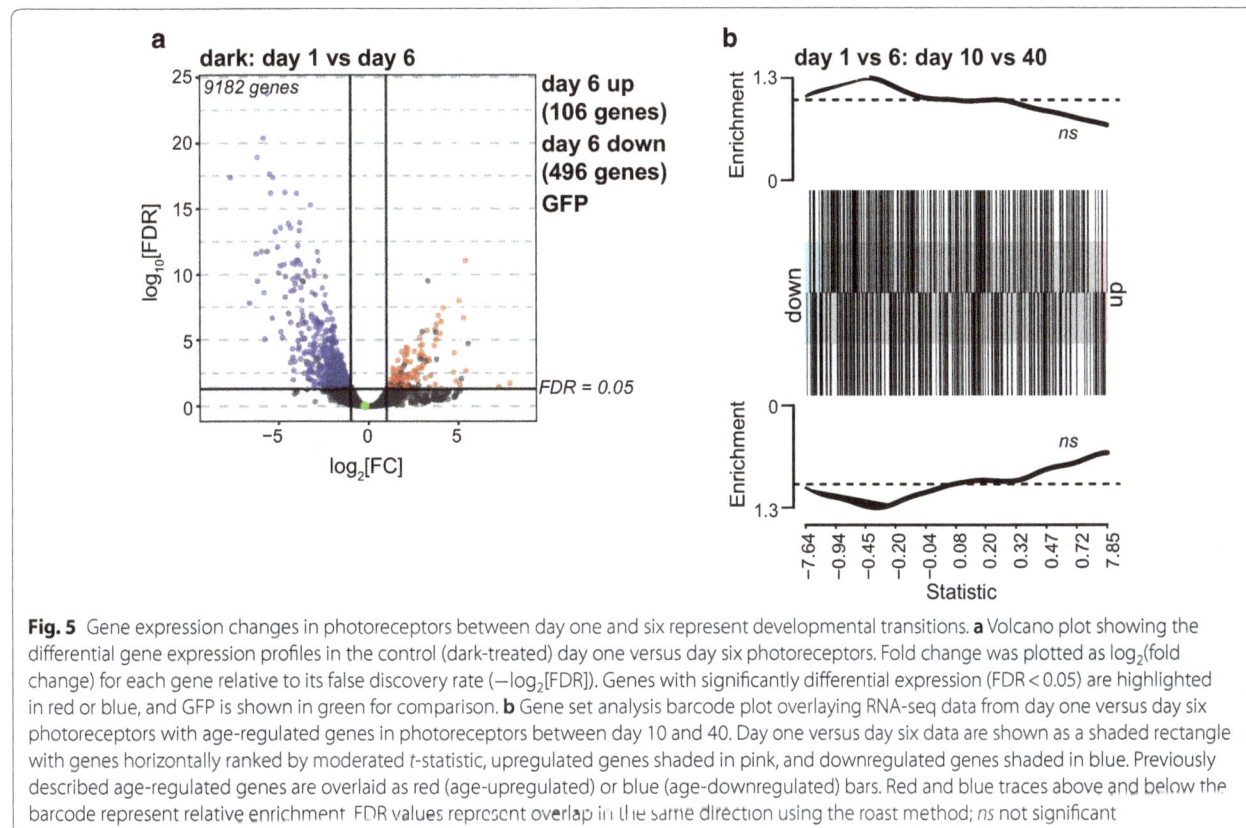

Fig. 5 Gene expression changes in photoreceptors between day one and six represent developmental transitions. **a** Volcano plot showing the differential gene expression profiles in the control (dark-treated) day one versus day six photoreceptors. Fold change was plotted as $\log_2$(fold change) for each gene relative to its false discovery rate ($-\log_2$[FDR]). Genes with significantly differential expression (FDR < 0.05) are highlighted in red or blue, and GFP is shown in green for comparison. **b** Gene set analysis barcode plot overlaying RNA-seq data from day one versus day six photoreceptors with age-regulated genes in photoreceptors between day 10 and 40. Day one versus day six data are shown as a shaded rectangle with genes horizontally ranked by moderated t-statistic, upregulated genes shaded in pink, and downregulated genes shaded in blue. Previously described age-regulated genes are overlaid as red (age-upregulated) or blue (age-downregulated) bars. Red and blue traces above and below the barcode represent relative enrichment. FDR values represent overlap in the same direction using the roast method; *ns* not significant

compare the gene expression changes between day one and six with day 10 and 40, and asked if these expression changes showed significant enrichment in either direction. We did not observe any significant enrichment of either up- or downregulated genes between day one and six, and day 10 and 40 (Fig. 5b). Thus, the gene expression changes that occur between day one and six in photoreceptors differ from those observed during later stages of the aging process in photoreceptors, suggesting that these gene expression changes between day one and six do not reflect aging. Consistent with these observations, white-eyed flies show peak reproductive capacity between 3 and 6 days post-eclosion [28]. Moreover, the fly strains used in our experiments show maximum life spans of up to 80 days under our growth conditions at 25 °C [20]. Together, these data suggest that the changes in gene expression between early post-eclosion at day one and day six do not represent aging.

Instead, we wondered if the changes in gene expression between day one and day six represented developmental transitions between newly-eclosed flies and mature, young adults. Strikingly, almost five times as many genes were downregulated between day one and day six as compared with upregulated genes. Whereas the genes that are upregulated between day one and day

six were enriched for several stress-related pathways including response to hypoxia, defense response, and heat response (Table 3), the downregulated genes were enriched for pathways associated with photoreceptor and/or eye development (Table 4). We observed reduced expression of genes involved in Notch signaling such as *Notch* (*N*), *Delta* (*Dl*), *Serrate* (*Ser*) and *fringe* (*fng*). Notch signaling plays an important role during eye development and specification of photoreceptor fate [29, 30], and our data suggest that newly-eclosed flies still show some activity of this pathway, but that this rapidly declines over the first few days post-eclosion. We next asked if some of these changes in gene expression could reduce the ability of day six flies to withstand blue light exposure. Indeed, some of the genes that were downregulated in the first week of life could account for the increased susceptibility of older flies to blue light. For example, day six flies showed reduced expression of *Calphotin* (*Cpn*), encoding an immobile calcium buffer required for rhabdomere development [31]. *Cpn* hypomorph flies develop light-induced retinal degeneration [13], suggesting that reductions in *Cpn* expression could reduce the ability of six-day-old flies to buffer the increased calcium levels that are necessary for blue light-induced retinal degeneration [19]. In addition, day six flies showed reduced

Table 3 Enriched biological process GO terms identified for day 6 versus day 1 upregulated genes

GO term	Description	p value	FDR	Enrichment	Genes
GO:0055093	Response to hyperoxia	0.000213	0.0899	24.23	*AttA, AttB, DptB*
GO:0050830	Defense response to Gram-positive bacterium	6.04E−05	0.0394	11.69	*AttA, Dro, AttB, TotM, DptB*
GO:0009617	Response to bacterium	1.38E−05	0.0142	5.42	*AttA, Dro, Lectin-galC1, cathD, TotM, AttB, DptB, TotX, TotA, TotC*
GO:0051704	Multi-organism process	5.45E−07	0.000977	4.36	*AttA, DrsI4, Dro, cathD, TotM, AttB, TotX, TotC, jumu, Est-6, Npl4, Lectin-galC1, CG34215, DptB, DrsI5, TotA*
GO:0051707	Response to other organism	1.02E−07	0.000732	5.31	*AttA, DrsI4, Dro, cathD, TotM, AttB, TotX, TotC, jumu, Npl4, Lectin-galC1, CG34215, DptB, DrsI5, TotA*
GO:0019731	Antibacterial humoral response	2.85E−06	0.00408	21.15	*AttA, Lectin-galC1, Dro, AttB, DptB*
GO:0098542	Defense response to other organism	1.05E−05	0.0125	5.01	*AttA, Lectin-galC1, Dro, DrsI4, cathD, AttB, TotM, CG34215, DrsI5, DptB, jumu*
GO:0030431	Sleep	4.99E−05	0.0397	6.02	*bgm, AttA, Cyp6g1, CG8435, CG8329, Iris, Amy-p, CG16926*
GO:0006952	Defense response	5.33E−05	0.0382	3.88	*CG10433, AttA, Lectin-galC1, Dro, DrsI4, cathD, AttB, TotM, CG34215, DrsI5, DptB, jumu*
GO:0009605	Response to external stimulus	2.34E−05	0.021	2.97	*CG6188, AttA, DrsI4, Dro, cathD, AttB, TotM, TotX, Slob, TotC, jumu, Npl4, Lectin-galC1, CG9236, CG34215, DptB, DrsI5, TotA*
GO:1901607	Alpha-amino acid biosynthetic process	0.000826	0.296	9.35	*CG6188, CG5840, CG10184, CG1315*
GO:0009109	Coenzyme catabolic process	0.000125	0.0749	88.84	*CG6188, CG8665*
GO:0006805	Xenobiotic metabolic process	0.000156	0.0747	26.65	*Cyp6g1, St1, CG17322*
GO:0046689	Response to mercury ion	0.000125	0.0691	88.84	*Cyp6g1, TotA*
GO:0034605	Cellular response to heat	0.000478	0.19	10.77	*TotM, TotX, TotA, TotC*

expression of several genes with important roles in maintaining cellular redox homeostasis including *Peroxidase* (*Pxd*), which converts hydrogen peroxide to water. Moreover, 10 of the 96 annotated Cytochrome P450 genes (*Cyp28d1, Cyp317a1, Cyp4c3, Cyp4e1, Cyp4e3, Cyp4s3, Cyp6a20, Cyp6a8, Cyp6a9,* and *Cyp9b1*) were downregulated between day one and day six. The upregulation of stress-related pathways between day one and six suggests that photoreceptors experience considerable stress as a normal part of their early life, potentially resulting from exposure to white light. In addition, the downregulation of many genes involved in signaling and developmental processes supports the idea that major developmental transitions occur in photoreceptors between the late pupal/newly-eclosed adult and mature-young adult stage. We propose that these collective changes in gene expression in the first week of adult life diminish the capacity of photoreceptors to maintain homeostasis under phototoxic conditions, resulting in their susceptibility to blue light-induced retinal degeneration.

Transcription factor-binding motifs are enriched in the promoters of blue light-regulated genes

What factors mediate the blue light-induced changes in gene expression in photoreceptors? Our qPCR analysis indicated that there were different pathways associated with blue light-upregulated and downregulated changes

in gene expression. An intact phototransduction pathway and calcium influx were only required for upregulation, but not downregulation, of genes in response to blue light. Thus, these data suggest that light-induced calcium influx activates the blue light-upregulated genes, whereas the blue light-downregulated genes are repressed, perhaps transiently, by exposure to light itself. To identify potential transcription factors that could mediate blue light-induced changes in gene expression, we examined the promoters of blue light up- or downregulated genes for enriched sequence motifs using hypergeometric optimization of motif enrichment (HOMER) [32]. Using this approach, we identified different sets of significantly enriched promoter motifs for blue light up- and downregulated genes (Additional file 1: Fig. S4, Fig. S5). These promoter motifs corresponded to potential binding sites for different transcription factors (Additional file 4: Table S3). Four of the promoter motifs identified for the blue light-upregulated genes contained potential binding sites for Heat shock factor (Hsf), a key mediator of the stress response [33]. In addition, a potential binding site for the AP-1 transcription factor, composed of Jun-related antigen (Jra) and Kayak (Kay) in flies, was present in one of the promoter motifs identified for the blue light-upregulated genes. Interestingly, a transcription co-activator that is important for redox-sensing by AP-1, *multiprotein bridging factor 1* (*mbf1*), was upregulated

Table 4 Enriched biological process GO terms identified for day 6 versus day 1 downregulated genes

GO term	Description	p value	FDR	Enrichment	Genes
GO:0032502	Developmental process	6.95E−12	6.23E−C9	1.65	5-HT2, Inx2, CG9634, e, CG17211, Mdr65, sas, fz, Mmp1, dlp, Cht5, uif, cv-2, rpr, Acp65Aa, W, aret, fng, N, Sb, pk, spz5, Cry, vkg, l(3)mbn, Phk-3, scb, Aph-4, Cpr66D, knk, RhoGAP15B, Cpr100A, Cpr49Ac, Pkg21D, ETHR, Cpr49Ah, Cpr49Af, ec, Cpr49Ae, how, ds, Sema-5c, LanB1, Fas2, dnd, grh, stl, out, TwdlT, Cad74A, esg, Cpr47Ea, miple2, blot, melt, DAAM, Cg25C, fj, Ccp84Ad, drd, Ccp84Ab, bnb, CG31475, spz3, TwdlE, Ccp84Aa, Cpr62Bc, Cpr62B0, kkv, Cpr73D, DI, qsm, aay, prc, Cht2, pio, ple, d, dp, CG10348, fw, Pxd, pot, Duox, wdp, Gp150, serp, verm, pbl, Ser, Gasp, Sobp, Tie, mys, scaf, laccase2, Cpr97Ea, Cpr76Bd, Cpr97Eb, Sox14, Cpr50Cb, Cad99C, trn, slow, moody, Ptp10D, aos, Cpr64Aa, Cpr47Ef, CG10641, CG15515, Cpr64Ac, sv, cue, CG10702, Pvr, ken, CG9509, resilin, lz, vn, rdo, CG34375, CG9850, pip, CG17111, Cpr92F, hbs, Cht7, Pu, CG34461, Irk2, Fas3, Cpr11A, CG16857, CG13183, CG13188, conv, CG16884, Ets98B, M6, Sesn, obst-A, Tsp, Cad96Ca, ft, nrv2
GO:0032501	Multicellular organismal process	2.43E−06	0.000693	1.52	bmm, Inx2, e, NLaz, Mdr65, CG10226, sas, fz, Mmp1, dlp, Cht5, cv-2, Oamb, aret, W, N, fng, CG34371, pk, Cry, Phk-3, CG30427, scb, Aph-4, knk, CG4221, Cht6, CG10936, Cpr49Ac, CG10407, ec, how, ds, ogre, CG5541, Sema-5c, CG14457, Fas2, grh, esg, miple2, ltd, CG5867, CG8483, Cg25C, fj, drd, Ccp84Ad, bnb, Obp56e, Jhe, kkv, Cpr73D, DI, aay, CG12344, pio, ple, Cht2, dp, pot, Swim, verm, CG10383, Oatp58Dc, CG42326, pbl, Ser, Tie, mys, Sox14, slow, moody, Ptp10D, CG14259, aos, Obp83g, ImpL2, cue, CG12121, Pvr, CG10702, ken, lz, vn, CG34375, CG15117, pip, GlyP, Cht7, Pu, Fas3, Peritrophin-A, cv, CG2650, Sesn, CG17974, Tsp, Cad96Ca, ft, CG31189, nrv2, CG11852
GO:0044550	Secondary metabolite biosynthetic process	5.67E−05	0.0107	5.6	bond, yellow-h, yellow-e, yellow-d2, ltd, yellow-c, CG31121
GO:0000003	Reproduction	4.59E−05	0.00889	3.11	Ccp84Ad, NLaz, Peritrophin-A, CG2650, Aph-4, CG14259, Obp56e, CG42326, CG14457, CG15117, CG17974, CG31189, CG10407, CG8483, CG5867, CG11852
GO:0007185	Transmembrane receptor protein tyrosine phosphatase signaling pathway	0.000412	0.0462	15.76	CG13183, CG13188, Gp150
GO:1901071	Glucosamine-containing compound metabolic process	1.75E−14	2.09E−11	7.58	CG13643, CG13183, CG8192, Cda4, CG13188, CG13676, CG14304, Peritrophin-A, serp, obst-B, verm, CG14608, obst-A, Cda5, knk, Cht5, Cht6, kkv, Gasp, CG7714, Cht7, Cht2
GO:0006030	Chitin metabolic process	8.39E−16	2.01E−12	8.56	CG13643, CG13183, CG8192, Cda4, CG13676, CG13188, CG14304, Peritrophin-A, serp, obst-B, verm, CG14608, obst-A, Cda5, knk, Cht5, Cht6, kkv, Gasp, CG7714, Cht7, Cht2
GO:0017144	Drug metabolic process	7.05E−09	3.61E−06	3.35	CG13643, CG8192, Cda4, e, Duox, obst-B, serp, verm, CG14608, Cda5, Cht5, Gasp, Cht7, Pu, CG13183, CG13676, CG13188, CG14304, CG7059, Peritrophin-A, Ahcy89E, obst-A, knk, Cht6, kkv, CG7714, su(f), Cht2, ple
GO:0006022	Aminoglycan metabolic process	1.10E−12	1.13E−09	6.04	CG3038, CG13643, CG13183, CG8192, Cda4, CG13676, CG13188, CG14304, Peritrophin-A, serp, obst-B, verm, CG14608, obst-A, Cda5, knk, Cht5, Cht6, kkv, Gasp, CG7714, Cht2

Table 4 (continued)

GO term	Description	p value	FDR	Enrichment	Genes
GO:0048856	Anatomical structure development	3.95E−15	7.08E−12	1.99	CG9634, Mdr65, fz, sas, Mmp1, dlp, Cht5, Acp65Aa, aret, W, N, fng, Sb, spz5, Cry, vkg, l(3)mbn, Phk-3, scb, Aph-4, Cpr66D, knk, Cpr100A, Pkg21D, Cpr49Ac, Cpr49Ah, Cpr49Af, Cpr49Ae, how, Sema-5c, LanB1, Fas2, grh, TwdlT, stl, out, esg, Cpr47Ea, melt, DAAM, cg25C, drd, Ccp84Ad, Ccp84Ab, bnb, spz3, TwdlE, Ccp84Aa, Cpr62Bc, Cpr62Bb, kkv, Cpr73D, Dl, aay, prc, pio, Cht2, ple, d, dp, CG10348, fw, pot, Duox, wdp, Gp150, serp, verm, pbl, Ser, Gasp, Sobp, Tie, mys, laccase2, Cpr97Ea, Cpr76Bd, Sox14, Cpr97Eb, Cpr50Cb, slow, moody, Ptp10D, Cpr64Aa, aos, Cpr47Ef, Cpr64Ac, CG15515, CG10641, sv, cue, Pvr, CG10702, ken, CG9509, resilin, lz, vn, CG34375, rdo, CG9850, pip, Cpr92F, Cht7, Pu, lrk2, CG34461, CG16857, Cpr11A, Fas3, conv, CG16884, M6, obst-A, Sesn, Tsp, Cad96Ca, ft, nrv2
GO:0009611	Response to wounding	0.000369	0.0427	3.35	Cht5, kkv, Spn28Dc, Cad96Ca, scb, Cht7, CG11089, Mmp1, lz, Cht2, ple
GO:0006032	Chitin catabolic process	7.01E−07	0.000239	9.34	Cht6, Cht5, Cda4, serp, verm, Cht7, Cda5, Cht2
GO:0042737	Drug catabolic process	0.000365	0.0429	3.94	Cht6, Cht5, Cda4, serp, verm, su(t), Cht7, Cda5, Cht2
GO:0022404	Molting cycle process	4.33E−06	0.00107	7.64	Cht6, Cht5, dp, pot, e, Cht7, Cht2, pio
GO:0009886	Post-embryonic animal morphogenesis	0.000163	0.0212	2.03	d, dp, how, fw, pot, ds, Duox, fz, Mmp1, dlp, vn, Ser, Fas2, cv-2, rpr, scaf, mys, Cg25C, W, fng, N, fj, pk, trn, aos, RhoGAP15B, Pvr, Dl, ft, pio
GO:0046667	Compound eye retinal cell programmed cell death	0.000843	0.0851	8.41	Dl, W, N, ec
GO:0060541	Respiratory system development	3.22E−05	0.00641	3.2	dp, conv, serp, Ptp10D, verm, Mmp1, knk, kkv, grh, esg, Dl, nrv2, DAAM, W, N, pio
GO:0007475	Apposition of dorsal and ventral imaginal disc-derived wing surfaces	0.000178	0.0224	6.64	dp, how, pot, Dl, mys, pio
GO:0048731	System development	0.000398	0.0453	2.08	dp, ken, serp, verm, Mmp1, pbl, vn, grh, esg, mys, melt, DAAM, W, N, spz5, conv, spz3, Aph-4, Ptp10D, knk, kkv, Dl, aay, nrv2, pio
GO:0008362	Chitin-based embryonic cuticle biosynthetic process	3.77E−08	1.42E−05	10.51	dp, kkv, pot, Gasp, grh, obst-A, knk, Cht2, pio
GO:0042335	Cuticle development	1.35E−30	4.83E−27	8.56	dp, pot, Duox, resilin, Cht5, Gasp, grh, TwdlT, Cpr92F, Cpr47Ea, Acp65Aa, Cht7, Pu, laccase2, Cpr97Ea, Ccp84Ad, drd, CG34461, Cpr768d, Cpr97Eb, Cpr11A, Ccp84Ab, Cpr50Cb, l(3)mbn, TwdlE, Cpr64Aa, Cpr66D, Cpr62Bc, Ccp84Aa, Cpr47Ef, obst-A, Cpr64Ac, CG15515, knk, Cpr62Bb, kkv, Cpr100A, Cpr73D, Cpr49Ac, Cpr49Ah, Cpr49Af, Cpr49Ae, Cht2, pio
GO:0040005	Chitin-based cuticle attachment to epithelium	0.000107	0.0167	21.02	dp, pot, pio
GO:0016339	Calcium-dependent cell–cell adhesion via plasma membrane cell adhesion molecules	1.16E−06	0.000379	8.85	ds, Cad99C, Cad87A, Cad74A, Cad96Ca, ft, mys, scb
GO:0044331	Cell-cell adhesion mediated by cadherin	0.000333	0.0398	7.51	ds, Cad99C, Cad87A, Cad74A, ft
GO:0007156	Homophilic cell adhesion via plasma membrane adhesion molecules	7.02E−09	3.87E−06	8.14	Fas2, CG16857, Fas3, fw, ds, Cad99C, Cad96Ca, Cad87A, Cad74A, ft, fz, hbs
GO:0035112	Genitalia morphogenesis	0.000178	0.0228	6.64	Fas2, Pvr, rpr, scaf, mys, N
GO:0007157	Heterophilic cell–cell adhesion via plasma membrane cell adhesion molecules	0.000119	0.0178	5.88	Fas3, ds, ft, scb, mys, hbs, N
GO:0042067	Establishment of ommatidial planar polarity	2.53E−08	1.01E−05	8.26	fj, d, pk, fw, ds, Dl, ft, fz, hbs, aos, N

Table 4 (continued)

GO term	Description	p value	FDR	Enrichment	Genes
GO:0090066	Regulation of anatomical structure size	0.000323	0.0393	2.23	fj, dp, ds, Cad99C, conv, slow, fz, serp, verm, Mmp1, knk, obst-A, pbl, Fas2, kkv, grh, Gasp, Cad96Ca, ft, nrv2, DAAM, aret
GO:0035150	Regulation of tube size	7.28E−09	3.48E−06	6.18	fj, ds, conv, fz, serp, verm, Mmp1, knk, obst-A, Fas2, kkv, Gasp, grh, ft, nrv2
GO:0035159	Regulation of tube length, open tracheal system	7.94E−10	5.18E−07	8.54	fj, ds, conv, serp, fz, verm, Mmp1, knk, Fas2, kkv, grh, ft, nrv2
GO:0035152	Regulation of tube architecture, open tracheal system	1.29E−08	5.42E−06	4.91	fj, ds, conv, serp, fz, verm, Mmp1, obst-A, knk, Fas2, kkv, uif, Gasp, grh, ft, mys, nrv2, DAAM
GO:0098742	Cell–cell adhesion via plasma-membrane adhesion molecules	9.80E−09	4.39E−06	6.06	fw, CG16857, Fas3, ds, Cad99C, fz, scb, Fas2, Cad96Ca, Cad74A, Cad87A, ft, mys, hbs, N
GO:0098609	Cell–cell adhesion	2.59E−06	0.000714	4.09	fw, Fas3, CG16857, ds, Cad99C, fz, scb, Fas2, Cad87A, Cad74A, Cad96Ca, ft, mys, hbs, N
GO:0007155	Cell adhesion	4.01E−11	3.19E−08	4.26	fw, how, ds, Swim, fz, Mmp1, sprt, LanB1, Fas2, Cad74A, mys, hbs, N, Fas3, CG16857, zye, Cad99C, trn, scb, CG15080, ImpL2, Tsp, Cad87A, Cad96Ca, ft, Dl, nrv2, prc
GO:0090099	Negative regulation of decapentaplegic signaling pathway	0.000995	0.0964	12.61	Irk2, Fs, scaf
GO:0006031	Chitin biosynthetic process	7.01E−05	0.0129	14.01	kkv, CG13183, CG13188, knk
GO:0060439	Trachea morphogenesis	0.000157	0.0209	12.01	kkv, CG13183, CG13188, verm
GO:0048085	Adult chitin-containing cuticle pigmentation	0.000722	0.0773	5.25	kkv, e, Duox, CG10625, CG9134, ple
GO:0001838	Embryonic epithelial tube formation	0.000995	0.0977	12.61	kkv, Mmp1, knk
GO:0048585	Negative regulation of response to stimulus	0.00095	0.0946	1.87	nimA, slif, wdp, fz, dlp, pbl, l(2)34Fc, Fas2, Ser, uif, Coop, Tie, scaf, GlyP, fng, N, Irk2, pk, Spn28Dc, aos, Sesn, ImpL2, CG4096, Fs, Cad96Ca, CG10702, Pvr, ft
GO:0023057	Negative regulation of signaling	0.000788	0.0819	1.92	nimA, wdp, fz, dlp, pbl, Fas2, Ser, uif, Coop, Tie, scaf, fng, N, ImpL2, CG4096, Fs, Cad96Ca, CG10702, Pvr, ft, egr, CG12344
GO:0048067	Cuticle pigmentation	1.84E−07	6.59E−05	7.01	Pu, kkv, yellow-h, yellow-e, e, Duox, yellow-d2, CG10625, CG9134, yellow-c, ple
GO:0043473	Pigmentation	2.65E−06	0.000705	5.04	Pu, kkv, yellow-h, yellow-e, e, Duox, yellow-d2, ltd, CG10625, CG9134, yellow-c, ple
GO:0046148	Pigment biosynthetic process	0.000283	0.035	3.45	Pu, se, santa-maria, yellow-h, yellow-e, e, yellow-d2, ltd, yellow-c, DhpD, CG31121
GO:0007508	Larval heart development	0.000107	0.0163	21.02	scb, mys, prc
GO:0035001	Dorsal trunk growth, open tracheal system	0.000157	0.0213	12.01	scb, mys, verm, Mmp1
GO:0035161	Imaginal disc lineage restriction	0.000843	0.0863	8.41	Ser, Dl, fng, N
GO:0007451	Dorsal/ventral lineage restriction, imaginal disc	7.01E−05	0.012	14.01	Ser, Dl, N, fng
GO:0035170	Lymph gland crystal cell differentiation	0.000412	0.0455	15.76	Ser, lz, N
GO:0042438	Melanin biosynthetic process	1.18E−05	0.00282	13.14	yellow-h, yellow-e, e, yellow-d2, yellow-c

in response to blue light [34]. Surprisingly, while expression of the unfolded protein response mediator *Inositol-requiring enzyme-1* (*Ire1*) was upregulated in response to blue light, we only identified one potential binding site for the Ire1-activated transcription factor, X box binding protein-1 (Xbp1), in the blue light-downregulated genes. One attractive candidate for a transcription factor that could mediate the light and calcium-dependent changes in gene expression is the Calmodulin-binding transcription activator (Camta) that activates expression of genes that are involved in deactivation of rhodopsin signaling [35]. *Camta* expression was reduced upon blue light exposure, and a potential Camta binding site (CGCG motif, motif 28) was present in the promoters of blue light-upregulated genes (Additional file 1: Fig. S4). However, canonical Camta-target genes such as *F box and leucine-rich-repeat gene 4* (*Fbxl4*) and CG7227 were not differentially expressed in response to blue light, suggesting that these Camta-regulated genes do not respond to blue light under the conditions used for our experiment.

Discussion

The eye is susceptible to light-induced oxidative stress, which has been implicated in photoreceptor damage in a variety of eye diseases [36, 37]. To characterize the light stress response in *Drosophila* photoreceptors, we profiled the transcriptome of photoreceptors exposed to high intensities of blue light. Although longer durations of blue light induce severe retinal degeneration in white-eyed flies [19, 38], shorter exposures to blue light induced major gene expression changes in photoreceptors but did not cause retinal degeneration. Instead, blue light induced expression of a broad range of genes involved in stress response, together with a concomitant reduction in expression of genes required for the light response including voltage-gated calcium, potassium and chloride ion channels. We expect that these transcriptional changes would result in altered protein levels; however, this has not been tested in this study. Previous studies showed that very young flies (1 day post-eclosion) were resistant to blue light-induced retinal degeneration, and our work revealed that the blue light-induced transcriptional changes differed according to the age of the fly; mature flies (6 days post-eclosion) showed substantially more differentially expressed genes in response to blue light exposure than very young flies (1 day post-eclosion). The increase in susceptibility to blue light between day one and six correlated with developmental transitions in photoreceptor gene expression, which included reduced expression of genes that function in redox and calcium homeostasis (Fig. 6a). Together, our data support a model in which mature adult flies upregulate stress response pathways in an effort to deal with light-induced oxidative

stress, and concomitantly quench the light response to diminish phototransduction-associated calcium influx (Fig. 6b). Newly-eclosed flies might be able to withstand blue light exposure better because of an increased capacity to buffer the calcium influx and oxidative stress resulting from prolonged phototransduction. Indeed, relatively young, yet mature, flies (day six) can withstand moderate blue light exposure without significant retinal degeneration but lose the ability to resist longer durations of light exposure. Recent work demonstrated that white-eyed flies (w^{1118}), but not their pigmented counterparts, undergo age-associated retinal degeneration under normal light/dark cycles by 30 days [39]. Thus, the acute blue light paradigm used in our study may reveal insight into mechanisms associated with age-associated retinal degeneration.

The transient, blue light-dependent downregulation of the calcium channel gene, *trp*, in day six flies corresponds well with our previous observations that mutations in *trp* suppress blue light-induced retinal degeneration. However, many voltage-gated potassium and chloride channels were also downregulated in response to blue light. Could decreasing activity of potassium or chloride channels ameliorate phototoxicity in flies? Excessive calcium influx is associated with brain ischemia-induced neuronal death, and potassium channel blockers reduced hypoxia-induced neuronal apoptosis in rodent models of ischemia [40]. However, eye-specific knockdown of *ATPα*, a subunit of a sodium/potassium channel, using the *longGMR-Gal4* driver caused age-dependent retinal degeneration in flies [41]. It is currently unclear whether transient repression of other voltage-gated ion channels in photoreceptors could attenuate retinal degeneration under phototoxic conditions.

How could exposure to blue light downregulate expression of genes, independent of phototransduction or calcium influx? In *Drosophila*, the blue light receptor cryptochrome (*cry*) entrains circadian rhythms to light–dark cycles via light-activated degradation of the clock protein Timeless (*tim*) [42]. Fly photoreceptors possess a functional circadian clock and express *PAR-domain protein 1* (*Pdp1*), *tim*, and *cry* [43–45]. We observed an enrichment of genes involved in circadian rhythm among the blue light-downregulated genes (Table 2). Regulators of the circadian clock including *tim*, *Pdp1*, and *vrille* (*vri*) were downregulated in response to blue light in day six, but not day one flies (Additional file 2: Table S1). When we compared the blue light-regulated genes in six-day-old flies with genes showing rhythmic expression patterns in fly heads [46], we found that 14 and 24 of the blue light up- and downregulated genes respectively (including *trp*) overlapped with the 331 genes showing rhythmic expression profiles in heads. While in flies Cry is thought to

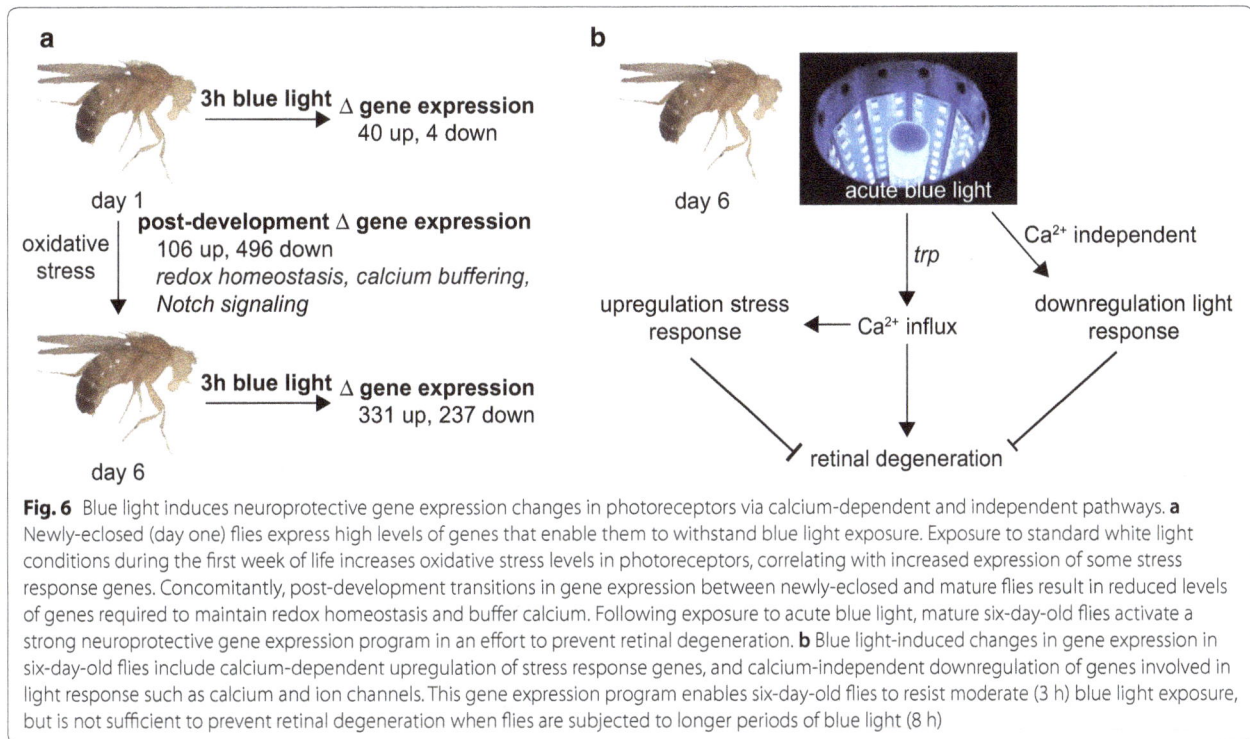

Fig. 6 Blue light induces neuroprotective gene expression changes in photoreceptors via calcium-dependent and independent pathways. **a** Newly-eclosed (day one) flies express high levels of genes that enable them to withstand blue light exposure. Exposure to standard white light conditions during the first week of life increases oxidative stress levels in photoreceptors, correlating with increased expression of some stress response genes. Concomitantly, post-development transitions in gene expression between newly-eclosed and mature flies result in reduced levels of genes required to maintain redox homeostasis and buffer calcium. Following exposure to acute blue light, mature six-day-old flies activate a strong neuroprotective gene expression program in an effort to prevent retinal degeneration. **b** Blue light-induced changes in gene expression in six-day-old flies include calcium-dependent upregulation of stress response genes, and calcium-independent downregulation of genes involved in light response such as calcium and ion channels. This gene expression program enables six-day-old flies to resist moderate (3 h) blue light exposure, but is not sufficient to prevent retinal degeneration when flies are subjected to longer periods of blue light (8 h)

mainly function by mediating light-dependent degradation of Timeless, some data suggest that Cry also acts as a transcriptional repressor in peripheral circadian clocks because loss of *cry* and *period (per)* in the eye leads to ectopic expression of *tim* [47]. However, we would expect to observe increased, rather than decreased, *tim* levels following blue light exposure if Cry-mediated transcriptional repression was involved because blue light causes degradation of Cry [42]. Thus, we propose that some unknown part of the circadian gene regulatory machinery regulates a light-dependent gene expression program in photoreceptors that attenuates the light response under strong illumination. Other transcription factors such as Kayak, which has a promoter motif in the blue light-upregulated genes, have been shown to affect expression of circadian-regulated genes in pacemaker neurons [48]. We note that the design of our study presents some difficulty in teasing out a potential role for circadian pathway components because we cannot readily distinguish between gene expression changes that occur in response to blue light and expression changes that occur in response to dark incubation, which we used as a control for these experiments. Our data suggest that the dark incubation does not itself cause major changes in gene expression because day one flies showed very few gene expression changes in response to blue light relative to dark control. Further, the subsets of genes tested by qPCR in dissected eyes showed similar directions of change to the RNA-seq analysis when normalized to a pre-treatment sample (Fig. 3). Thus, we speculate that some components of the circadian machinery are coopted in *Drosophila* photoreceptors to repress the expression of light response pathway genes in response to strong illumination.

Conclusions

Although light is essential for vision, it also poses a stress to photoreceptor cells within the eye. Young flies at 6 days post-eclosion undergo retinal degeneration when exposed to prolonged blue light exposure. Here, we show that exposure to blue light induces substantial gene expression changes in photoreceptors from six-day-old flies. In these flies, blue light upregulates stress response pathways and downregulates light response genes to mitigate oxidative stress, and quench the light response. Newly-eclosed flies, which are resilient to blue light-induced retinal degeneration, show no such changes in gene expression. Our data suggest that newly-eclosed flies express higher levels of genes that help withstand light stress because of their recent transition from the developing pupal to early adult stage. Together, the results from this study provide insight into neuroprotective pathways utilized by photoreceptors to resist light-induced oxidative stress.

Methods

Stocks, genetics, and blue light treatment

All genotypes used in this study are described in Additional file 3: Table S4. Mated male flies were used for all experiments. Flies were cultured on standard cornmeal food at 25 °C with 12 h/12 h light/dark cycle except for $ninaE^7$ and trp^9 flies, which together with the w^{1118} controls for those experiments, were raised in the dark prior to blue light treatment to prevent light-dependent retinal degeneration [49]. Flies homozygous for KASH-GFP, $P\{w^{+mC}=UAS\text{-}GFP\text{-}Msp300KASH\}attP2$, under the control of Rh1-Gal4 ($P\{ry^{+t7.2}=rh1\text{-}GAL4\}3$, ry^{506} [BL8691] were crossed to cn bw to deplete eye pigments [22]. For aging experiments, 400 male flies were collected from 0 to 8 h post-eclosion and aged for 12 h (day one; 12–19 h) or 6 days. Flies were exposed to 3 h of blue light ($\lambda = 465$ nm) at 8000 lx (2 mW/cm^2) using a custom designed optical stimulator with temperature control (23–25 °C) [38].

Immunostaining and confocal microscopy

Adult fly retinas were dissected and stained with phalloidin (A22287, 1:100, Thermo Fisher Scientific) as described previously [20]. Laser scanning confocal imaging was performed using a Nikon A1R inverted confocal microscope under a 60X/1.30 NA oil immersion Nikon Plan Fluor objective. Confocal images were collected either as single planes or 1.0 μm z-stacks using NIS-Elements software. Retinal cell degeneration was quantified by assessing rhabdomere loss (presence/absence phalloidin-positive rhabdomere) for R1–R6 cells per ommatidium using stacked images. Rhabdomere loss was quantified in five independent male flies (single eye/fly) for four independent light exposures (paired blue light versus dark controls).

RNA isolation, RNA-seq, and qPCR analysis

RNA-seq analysis: Heads were collected from ~400 male flies of the indicated treatments and ages and GFP-labeled photoreceptor nuclei were affinity purified as previously described [20, 21]. Total nuclear RNA was extracted using Trizol reagent (Life Technologies), followed by Direct-zol RNA Micro-prep kit (R2062, Zymo Research) including DNase treatment. RNA (35 ng) was used to generate uniquely barcoded, strand-specific and rRNA depleted library using NuGen Ovation RNA seq Systems 1-16 for Model Organism (0350, Nugen). All samples were added to a single pool that was clustered in two lanes of a HiSeq 2500 single-end rapid flowcell to generate 50 base reads per cluster. Quantitative PCR (qPCR) analysis: RNA was isolated from dissected eyes using Trizol (Invitrogen) and qPCR analysis was performed on cDNA generated from 100 ng RNA using random hexamers relative to a standard curve of serially diluted cDNA. Relative expression for each gene was normalized to the geometric mean of two reference genes (*eukaryotic translation initiation factor 1A, eIF1A* and *Ribosomal protein L32, RpL32*). Primers are listed in Additional file 4: Table S5.

RNA-seq data analysis

Three biological samples were analyzed for each of the following ages and treatments: day one 3 h dark (pre-isolation, whole head homogenate), day one 3 h dark (post-isolation), day one 3 h blue (post-isolation), day six 3 h dark (post-isolation), day six 3 h blue (post-isolation). Reads were trimmed using Trimmomatic (v0.36) and mapped against the bowtie2 (v2.3.2) [50] indexed *D. melanogaster* genome (Drosophila_melanogaster.BDGP6.89) using Tophat (v 2.1.1) [51]. The raw counts matrix was generated by Htseq-count (v0.7.0) applying strand-specific assay (fr-secondstrand), union mode, and default parameters [52]. Differential expression analysis was performed on genes with greater than one count per million (CPM) in at least three samples. Differentially expressed genes were detected using *glmTreat* generalized linear model analysis in edgeR (v3.18.1) [53] with a FDR of < 0.05. A FC of 2 was applied to *glmTreat* analysis of the pre versus post samples only. Gene set enrichment analysis between age-regulated genes (day 10 vs day 40) [20] and differentially expressed genes between day one and day six (dark controls) was performed using *mroast* and visualized using *barcode plot* in edgeR. All plots were generated in R (v3.4.1) using custom scripts.

GO term analysis

GO term enrichment analysis was performed using GOrilla [54] relative to the background gene set of all expressed genes with CPM >1 in at least three of the samples. Only GO terms with non-redundant gene members are shown in Tables 1 and 2. Complete GO term enrichment analyses and parameters used for GOrilla are described in Additional file 3: Table S2.

Motif analysis

Significantly-enriched promoter motifs were identified using HOMER (v4.9, Hypergeometric Optimization of Motif EnRichment) [32] as previously described [20]. The background gene set of all expressed genes with CPM > 1 in at least three of the samples was used for enrichment analysis.

Additional files

Additional file 1: Fig. S1. The blue light treatment conditions used for RNA-seq analysis do not induce retinal degeneration. **Fig. S2.** Affinity-enrichment of photoreceptor nuclear RNA from day one dark-treated flies. **Fig. S3.** Newly-eclosed flies do not show any unique blue light-induced gene expression changes. **Fig. S4.** Promoter motifs enriched at blue light-regulated genes. **Fig. S5.** Distribution of promoter motifs in blue light-regulated genes.

Additional file 2: Table 1. Significantly differentially expressed genes identified under each comparison.

Additional file 3: Table 2. GO term analysis of differentially regulated genes.

Additional file 4: Table 3. Transcription factors matches for all motifs identified for blue light-regulated genes.

Additional file 5: Table 4. Fly stocks used in this study.

Additional file 6: Table 5. Primers used in this study.

Abbreviations

CPM: counts per million; FDR: false discovery rate; FC: fold change; GFP: green fluorescent protein; GEO: gene expression omnibus; GO: gene ontology; h: hour; HOMER: hypergeometric optimization of motif enrichment; KASH: Klarsicht, Anc-1, Syn3-1 homology; qPCR: quantitative polymerase chain reaction; Rh1: rhodopsin 1; Trp: transient receptor potential.

Authors' contributions

JM performed the RNA-seq studies, HH and SS performed qPCR analysis, and WL constructed and supported the optical stimulator. JM and VW analyzed the data. JM, HH and VW wrote the manuscript in consultation with the other authors. All authors read and approved the final manuscript.

Author details

[1] Department of Biochemistry, Purdue University, West Lafayette, IN 47907, USA. [2] Present Address: Janelia Research Campus, Ashburn, VA 20147, USA. [3] Interdisciplinary Life Science (PULSe), Purdue University, West Lafayette, IN 47907, USA. [4] Purdue Polytechnic Institute, Purdue University, West Lafayette, IN 47907, USA. [5] Purdue University Center for Cancer Research, Purdue University, West Lafayette 47907, USA.

Acknowledgements

We thank the Bloomington Drosophila Stock Center (NIH P40OD018537) for flies. We thank Donald F. Ready for discussions regarding the blue light stress model and Yong Zhang for his comments on the manuscript.

Competing interests

The authors declare that they have no competing interests.

Funding

The authors thank the Ralph W. and Grace M. Showalter Research Trust, National Institutes of Health R01EY024905 to VW, Purdue University Center for Cancer Research (American Cancer Society Institutional Research Grant, IRG #58-006-53; NIH P30 CA023168) for funding to support this work. The content is solely the responsibility of the authors and does not necessarily represent the official views of the NIH.

References

1. Jarrett SG, Boulton ME. Consequences of oxidative stress in age-related macular degeneration. Mol Aspects Med. 2012;33(4):399–417.
2. Winkler BS, Boulton ME, Gottsch JD, Sternberg P. Oxidative damage and age-related macular degeneration. Mol Vis. 1999;5:32.
3. Handa JT, Cano M, Wang L, Datta S, Liu T. Lipids, oxidized lipids, oxidation-specific epitopes, and Age-related macular degeneration. Biochim Biophys Acta. 2017;1862(4):430–40.
4. Gaschler MM, Stockwell BR. Lipid peroxidation in cell death. Biochem Biophys Res Commun. 2017;482(3):419–25.
5. Niki E. Lipid peroxidation: physiological levels and dual biological effects. Free Radic Biol Med. 2009;47(5):469–84.
6. Burnside SW, Hardingham GE. Transcriptional regulators of redox balance and other homeostatic processes with the potential to alter neurodegenerative disease trajectory. Biochem Soc Trans. 2017;45(6):1295–303.
7. Kim GH, Kim HI, Paik SS, Jung SW, Kang S, Kim IB. Functional and morphological evaluation of blue light-emitting diode-induced retinal degeneration in mice. Graefes Arch Clin Exp Ophthalmol. 2016;254(4):705–16.
8. Jaadane I, Boulenguez P, Chahory S, Carre S, Savoldelli M, Jonet L, Behar-Cohen F, Martinsons C, Torriglia A. Retinal damage induced by commercial light emitting diodes (LEDs). Free Radic Biol Med. 2015;84:373–84.
9. Stark WS, Carlson SD. Blue and ultraviolet light induced damage to the Drosophila retina: ultrastructure. Curr Eye Res. 1984;3(12):1441–54.
10. Katz B, Minke B. Drosophila photoreceptors and signaling mechanisms. Front Cell Neurosci. 2009;3:2.
11. Hardie RC, Juusola M. Phototransduction in Drosophila. Curr Opin Neurobiol. 2015;34:37–45.
12. Montell C. Drosophila visual transduction. Trends Neurosci. 2012;35(6):356–63.
13. Weiss S, Minke B. A new genetic model for calcium induced autophagy and ER-stress in Drosophila photoreceptor cells. Channels (Austin). 2015;9(1):14–20.
14. Kiselev A, Socolich M, Vinos J, Hardy RW, Zuker CS, Ranganathan R. A molecular pathway for light-dependent photoreceptor apoptosis in Drosophila. Neuron. 2000;28(1):139–52.
15. Satoh AK, Ready DF. Arrestin1 mediates light-dependent rhodopsin endocytosis and cell survival. Curr Biol. 2005;15(19):1722–33.
16. Alloway PG, Howard L, Dolph PJ. The formation of stable rhodopsin-arrestin complexes induces apoptosis and photoreceptor cell degeneration. Neuron. 2000;28(1):129–38.
17. Weiss S, Kohn E, Dadon D, Katz B, Peters M, Lebendiker M, Kosloff M, Colley NJ, Minke B. Compartmentalization and Ca^{2+} buffering are essential for prevention of light-induced retinal degeneration. J Neurosci. 2012;32(42):14696–708.
18. Wang T, Xu H, Oberwinkler J, Gu Y, Hardie RC, Montell C. Light activation, adaptation, and cell survival functions of the Na^+/Ca^{2+} exchanger CalX. Neuron. 2005;45(3):367–78.
19. Chen X, Hall H, Simpson JP, Leon-Salas WD, Ready DF, Weake VM. Cytochrome b5 protects photoreceptors from light stress-induced lipid peroxidation and retinal degeneration. NPJ Aging Mech Dis. 2017;3:18.
20. Hall H, Medina P, Cooper DA, Escobedo SE, Rounds J, Brennan KJ, Vincent C, Miura P, Doerge R, Weake VM. Transcriptome profiling of aging Drosophila photoreceptors reveals gene expression trends that correlate with visual senescence. BMC Genom. 2017;18(1):894.
21. Ma J, Weake VM. Affinity-based isolation of tagged nuclei from Drosophila tissues for gene expression analysis. J Vis Exp. 2014. https://doi.org/10.3791/51418.
22. Tearle R. Tissue specific effects of ommochrome pathway mutations in Drosophila melanogaster. Genet Res. 1991;57(3):257–66.
23. Yoshihara Y, Mizuno T, Nakahira M, Kawasaki M, Watanabe Y, Kagamiyama H, Jishage K, Ueda O, Suzuki H, Tabuchi K, et al. A genetic approach to visualization of multisynaptic neural pathways using plant lectin transgene. Neuron. 1999;22(1):33–41.

24. Brehme M, Voisine C, Rolland T, Wachi S, Soper JH, Zhu Y, Orton K, Villella A, Garza D, Vidal M, et al. A chaperome subnetwork safeguards proteostasis in aging and neurodegenerative disease. Cell Rep. 2014;9(3):1135–50.

25. de Nadal E, Ammerer G, Posas F. Controlling gene expression in response to stress. Nat Rev Genet. 2011;12(12):833–45.

26. Mendes CS, Levet C, Chatelain G, Dourlen P, Fouillet A, Dichtel-Danjoy ML, Gambis A, Ryoo HD, Steller H, Mollereau B. ER stress protects from retinal degeneration. EMBO J. 2009;28(9):1296–307.

27. Washburn T, O'Tousa JE. Molecular defects in Drosophila rhodopsin mutants. J Biol Chem. 1989;264(26):15464–6.

28. Hanson FB, Ferris FR. Quantitative study of fecundity in Drosophila melanogaster. J Exp Zool. 1929;54(3):485–506.

29. Tomlinson A, Struhl G. Delta/Notch and Boss/Sevenless signals act combinatorially to specify the Drosophila R7 photoreceptor. Mol Cell. 2001;7(3):487–95.

30. Cagan RL, Ready DF. Notch is required for successive cell decisions in the developing Drosophila retina. Genes Dev. 1989;3(8):1099–112.

31. Yang Y, Ballinger D. Mutations in calphotin, the gene encoding a Drosophila photoreceptor cell-specific calcium-binding protein, reveal roles in cellular morphogenesis and survival. Genetics. 1994;138(2):413–21.

32. Heinz S, Benner C, Spann N, Bertolino E, Lin YC, Laslo P, Cheng JX, Murre C, Singh H, Glass CK. Simple combinations of lineage-determining transcription factors prime cis-regulatory elements required for macrophage and B cell identities. Mol Cell. 2010;38(4):576–89.

33. Gomez-Pastor R, Burchfiel ET, Thiele DJ. Regulation of heat shock transcription factors and their roles in physiology and disease. Nat Rev Mol Cell Biol. 2018;19(1):4–19.

34. Jindra M, Gaziova I, Uhlirova M, Okabe M, Hiromi Y, Hirose S. Coactivator MBF1 preserves the redox-dependent AP-1 activity during oxidative stress in Drosophila. EMBO J. 2004;23(17):3538–47.

35. Han J, Gong P, Reddig K, Mitra M, Guo P, Li HS. The fly CAMTA transcription factor potentiates deactivation of rhodopsin, a G protein-coupled light receptor. Cell. 2006;127(4):847–58.

36. Organisciak DT, Vaughan DK. Retinal light damage: mechanisms and protection. Prog Retin Eye Res. 2010;29(2):113–34.

37. Beatty S, Koh H, Phil M, Henson D, Boulton M. The role of oxidative stress in the pathogenesis of age-related macular degeneration. Surv Ophthalmol. 2000;45(2):115–34.

38. Chen X, Leon-Salas WD, Zigon T, Ready DF, Weake VM. A programmable optical stimulator for the Drosophila eye. HardwareX. 2017;2:13–33.

39. Ferreiro MJ, Perez C, Marchesano M, Ruiz S, Caputi A, Aguilera P, Barrio R, Cantera R. Drosophila melanogaster white mutant w(1118) undergo retinal degeneration. Front Neurosci. 2017;11:732.

40. Wei L, Yu SP, Gottron F, Snider BJ, Zipfel GJ, Choi DW. Potassium channel blockers attenuate hypoxia- and ischemia-induced neuronal death in vitro and in vivo. Stroke. 2003;34(5):1281–6.

41. Luan Z, Reddig K, Li HS. Loss of Na(+)/K(+)-ATPase in Drosophila photoreceptors leads to blindness and age-dependent neurodegeneration. Exp Neurol. 2014;261:791–801.

42. Michael AK, Fribourgh JL, Van Gelder RN, Partch CL. Animal cryptochromes: divergent roles in light perception, circadian timekeeping and beyond. Photochem Photobiol. 2017;93(1):128–40.

43. Cyran SA, Buchsbaum AM, Reddy KL, Lin MC, Glossop NR, Hardin PE, Young MW, Storti RV, Blau J. vrille, Pdp1, and dClock form a second feedback loop in the Drosophila circadian clock. Cell. 2003;112(3):329–41.

44. Stanewsky R, Kaneko M, Emery P, Beretta B, Wager-Smith K, Kay SA, Rosbash M, Hall JC. The cryb mutation identifies cryptochrome as a circadian photoreceptor in Drosophila. Cell. 1998;95(5):681–92.

45. Yoshii T, Todo T, Wulbeck C, Stanewsky R, Helfrich-Forster C. Cryptochrome is present in the compound eyes and a subset of Drosophila's clock neurons. J Comp Neurol. 2008;508(6):952–66.

46. Rodriguez J, Tang CH, Khodor YL, Vodala S, Menet JS, Rosbash M. Nascent-Seq analysis of Drosophila cycling gene expression. Proc Natl Acad Sci U S A. 2013;110(4):E275–84.

47. Collins B, Mazzoni EO, Stanewsky R, Blau J. Drosophila CRYPTOCHROME is a circadian transcriptional repressor. Curr Biol. 2006;16(5):441–9.

48. Ling J, Dubruille R, Emery P. KAYAK-alpha modulates circadian transcriptional feedback loops in Drosophila pacemaker neurons. J Neurosci. 2012;32(47):16959–70.

49. Sengupta S, Barber TR, Xia H, Ready DF, Hardie RC. Depletion of PtdIns(4,5)P(2) underlies retinal degeneration in Drosophila trp mutants. J Cell Sci. 2013;126(Pt 5):1247–59.

50. Langmead B, Salzberg SL. Fast gapped-read alignment with Bowtie 2. Nat Methods. 2012;9(4):357–9.

51. Trapnell C, Pachter L, Salzberg SL. TopHat: discovering splice junctions with RNA-Seq. Bioinformatics. 2009;25(9):1105–11.

52. Anders S, Huber W. Differential expression analysis for sequence count data. Genome Biol. 2010;11(10):R106.

53. Robinson MD, McCarthy DJ, Smyth GK. edgeR: a Bioconductor package for differential expression analysis of digital gene expression data. Bioinformatics. 2010;26(1):139–40.

54. Eden E, Navon R, Steinfeld I, Lipson D, Yakhini Z. GOrilla: a tool for discovery and visualization of enriched GO terms in ranked gene lists. BMC Bioinformatics. 2009;10:48.

14

Zinc and linoleic acid pre-treatment attenuates biochemical and histological changes in the midbrain of rats with rotenone-induced Parkinsonism

Ngala Elvis Mbiydzenyuy[1,3] (iD), Herbert Izo Ninsiima[1], Miriela Betancourt Valladares[2] and Constant Anatole Pieme[3]*

Abstract

Background: Studies have suggested the supplementation of Zinc and Linoleic acid in the management of neurodegenerative disorders but none has investigated the combined effects. Little is known about the neuroprotective effects of either Zinc or Linoleic acid or their combination against development of Parkinsonism. This study was designed to investigate the neuroprotective effects of Zinc and Linoleic acid in rotenone-induced Parkinsonism in rats.

Methods: Thirty-six young adult female rats weighing 100–150 g divided into six groups were used. Rats were induced with Parkinsonism by subcutaneous administration of rotenone (2.5 mg/kg) once a day for seven consecutive days. The rats received dimethyl sulfoxide (DMSO)/Olive oil or rotenone dissolved in DMSO/Olive oil. Groups III and IV received Zinc (30 mg/kg) or Linoleic acid (150 µl/kg) while group V received a combination of both, 2 weeks prior to rotenone injection. Groups II and VI served as negative (rotenone group) and positive (Levodopa groups) controls respectively. Oxidative stress levels were assessed by estimating Lipid peroxidation (MDA), total antioxidant capacity, Superoxide dismutase, reduced Glutathione (GSH), glutathione peroxidase and catalase in the midbrain. Histological examination was done to assess structural changes in the midbrain.

Results: There was a significant prevention in lipid peroxidation and decrease in the antioxidant status in intervention-treated groups as compared to the rotenone treated group. In addition, histological examination revealed that Parkinsonian rat brains exhibited neuronal damage. Cell death and reduction in neuron size induced by rotenone was prevented by treatment with zinc, linoleic acid and their combination.

Conclusion: These results suggest that zinc and linoleic acid and their combination showed significant neuroprotective activity most likely due to the antioxidant effect.

Keywords: Neuroprotection, Antioxidant, Brain, Nutrition, Ageing

*Correspondence: apieme@yahoo.fr
[3] Department of Biochemistry and Physiological Sciences, Faculty of Medicine and Biomedical Sciences, University of Yaounde I, Yaounde, Cameroon
Full list of author information is available at the end of the article

Background

Parkinsonism is a general term that refers to neurological disorder that causes movement disorders. These disorders include supranuclear palsy, vascular Parkinsonism, dementia with Lewy bodies, corticobasal degeneration and drug induced-Parkinsonism [44]. The pathophysiology of the latter is related to drug-induced changes in the basal ganglia motor circuit secondary to dopaminergic neuron destruction [21]. The consequence of nigrostriatal fibre degeneration is a loss of nerve endings in the striatum which contain tyrosine hydroxylase, and thus a reduced production of dopamine in the striatum. This produces tremor bradykinesia, rigidity and postural instability [18].

The aetiology of PD is considered to be associated with environmental exposures to various factors and genetic mutations [10]. Suggested environmental factors related to the aetiology of PD include exposure to herbicides and pesticides, intake of contaminated well-water and neurotoxins for example rotenone. Oxidative stress has been suggested as the common underlying mechanism in both sporadic and genetic cases of PD. This leads to cellular dysfunction [19]. The oxidative stress brings about death of dopaminergic neurons in the substantia nigra pars compacta. The initiators of these cascade of processes associated with generation of oxidative stress in the nigral dopaminergic neurons are thought to be the reactive oxygen species (ROS) produced during inflammation of the neurons, dysfunction of the mitochondria and metabolism of dopamine [22]. Micronutrients and trace elements have been described as key components in the combat against these ROS and hence the onset and progression of neurodegenerative disorders [5].

Current treatment of Parkinson's disease (PD) is based on dopamine replacement therapy, but chronic administration may cause motor fluctuations and dyskinesias, increased free radical formation, accelerating neuronal degeneration in some PD patients. Studies in rodents showed that levodopa/carbidopa do not offer neuroprotection as well. Several agents have been investigated for neuroprotection against development of Parkinson disease or for slowing down the degeneration dopaminergic neurons, yet none has successfully offered neuroprotection.

Zinc homeostasis has been implicated in several processes related to brain aging and the onset and development of age-related neurodegenerative disorders. Serum Zinc did not significantly correlate with age of onset and duration of the disease in a study of Zinc status in PD patients [56] suggesting that Zinc does not play any role. Studies have found that Zinc deficiency accompanies many cases of PD as shown by significant low levels of Zinc in the cerebrospinal fluid (CSF) of PD patients.

Zinc has been shown to play an important role in protecting dopaminergic neurons against free radicals and toxins from the environment by stimulating metallothionein production [26]. Another micronutrient essential for influencing signal transduction, neurochemistry, enzymes, membrane proteins and gene expression is the omega-6 polyunsaturated fatty acids of which Linoleic acid is the major long chain PUFA [7]. Omega-6 PUFAs also modulates transmission in cholinergic, serotoninergic and dopaminergic systems. Dopamine storage vesicle formation have been shown to significantly reduce in prolonged omega-6 PUFA deficiency [58]. Omega-6 PUFA is involved in inflammation, neurotrophic support, and oxidative stress through modulation of expression of genes responsible for that. Despite all these, the neuroprotective effects of omega-6 PUFA in PD are yet to be investigated elaborately [30].

There is therefore the need to investigate the potentials of micronutrients and trace elements offering protective effects in the brain or slowing down the degeneration processes that occur in toxin-induced neurodegeneration.

Using the hypothesis that mitochondrial dysfunction and oxidative injury underlie neurodegeneration in PD; the inclusion of metabolic modifiers may provide an alternative and early intervention approach. In order to investigate this we used a toxin-induced model of Parkinsonism to assess the protective effects of the trace element Zinc and micronutrient Linoleic acid. These agents may provide a potential neuroprotective therapy aimed for use as a prophylaxis to delay the onset or halt the progressive nature of Parkinsonism.

Methods

Chemicals and drugs

Rotenone (Sigma-Aldrich, St Louis, SA) was dissolved in 1:1 (v/v) dimethylsulfoxide (DMSO, Sigma-Aldrich, St Louis, SA). Zinc dust (10 g) (Sigma-Aldrich, St Louis, SA) was dissolved in distilled water; Linoleic acid (Sigma-Aldrich, St Louis, SA). All other chemicals and reagents were obtained from the Biochemistry and Physiology laboratories of the University of Yaounde 1 Cameroon and were of analytical grade.

Animals

Female wistar rats were used in the present study. Their weight ranged between 100 and 150 g. Rats were housed in groups of six in stainless steel cages under hygienic laboratory conditions (temperature of 25 °C and reversed 12/12 h light/dark cycle). Water and food pellets were given ad libitum. All the experimental protocols were approved by the Institutional Animal Care and Ethics Committees at the Kampala International University

Western Campus and Faculty of Medicine and Biomedical Sciences, University of Yaounde 1, Cameroon under the reference number No 2017/01/699/CE/CNERSH/SP.

Experimental design

Thirty-six young adult female rats aged 8–12 weeks and weighing 100–150 g, obtained from the animal house, Department of Physiological Sciences and Biochemistry University of Yaounde I, Cameroon and acclimated in a room at temperature of 25 ± 1 °C were used. Rotenone (2.5 mg/kg dose, s.c.) was employed to induce experimental Parkinsonism [52]. Rotenone was prepared to be injected in a volume of 1 ml/kg body weight. The rotenone solution was first prepared as a 50X stock in 100% dimethylsulfoxide (DMSO) by dissolving 125 mg of rotenone in 1 ml of DMSO. 40 µl of the stock solution was then diluted in 1960 µl of olive oil. The solution was vortexed to create an emulsion of the DMSO containing rotenone and Olive oil. Fresh solution was prepared every 2–3 times in a week. Rotenone is sensitive to light, so it was stored in small vials and protected from light by wrapping the vials with foil papers and kept in refrigerator. Before administering the Rotenone solution to rats, the vials were inverted several times or vortexed to obtain a uniform mixture with the DMSO/Olive oil. Each rat received a volume of 1 ml/kg of Rotenone and control animals received the vehicle only (Olive oil/DMSO).

Group I (normal control) received the vehicle Olive oil/DMSO once a day through the study period of 3 weeks; Group II (negative control) as described by Fujikawa et al. [13] and Ojha et al. [33] received 2.5 mg/kg of rotenone subcutaneously once a day consecutively for the last 7 days of the experiment. Group III received Zn (30 mg/kg b.w.) according to Partyka et al. [36] and Anna Partyka et al. [37] orally for 3 weeks in drinking water once per day and rotenone (2.5 mg/kg) once a day for the last seven consecutive days. Group IV received a daily dose of Linoleic acid (150 µg/kg) subcutaneously for 3 weeks once per day and rotenone (2.5 mg/kg) once a day for the last seven consecutive days. Group V received both Zinc (30 mg/kg) and Linoleic acid (150 µg/kg) orally and subcutaneously once per day for 3 weeks respectively and rotenone (2.5 mg/kg) once a day for the last seven consecutive days. Group VI served as a positive control and received Levodopa (6 mg/kg) orally once per day with rotenone (2.5 mg/kg) once a day consecutively for 7 days.

Brain tissue processing

At the end of the experiment, the rats were fasted overnight and humanely sacrificed by cervical dislocation without anaesthesia. The whole brain of each rat was rapidly dissected, removed and rinsed in ice-cold isotonic saline. The whole brain was weighed and immediately the midbrain region was isolated and this isolated brain section was used for further investigations. Portions of the midbrain were removed to use for histological assessments. The remainder midbrain tissues were homogenized with ice-cold 0.1 M phosphate buffer saline (pH 7.4). Tissue homogenate (10% w/v) was prepared in 50 mM phosphate buffer saline (pH 7.4) using a Symphony type Eperndorff homogenizer. The brain homogenate was centrifuged at 2000g for 10 min at 4 °C. The pellet which contained debris and nuclei was discarded. The supernatant was then again centrifuged at 12,000g for 20 min to obtain post mitochondrial supernatant. The supernatant was kept at -80 °C until determination of the levels and activity of oxidative stress markers [25].

Brain oxidative stress marker assessments
Brain lipid peroxidation

The method described by Stocks et al. [47] was used to measure lipid peroxidation. A coloured complex called thiobarbituric acid reactive substance is formed from a reaction of malondialdehyde and thiobarbituric acid. The complex was assayed spectrophotometrically at 532 nm and expressed in micro moles.

Brain total antioxidant capacity

The Ferric Reducing Antioxidant Power (FRAP) was used as a method of measuring the total antioxidant capacity of the homogenate [4]. This method determines the capacity of the homogenate to reduce ferric iron to ferrous iron at a pH of 3.6. A deep blue coloured compound of ferrous tripyridyltriazine (TPTZ-Fe-2+) is formed as a result of the reduction of ferric tripyridyltriazide (TPTZ-Fe3+). The absorbance was measured at 593 nm and the results were expressed in micromolar.

Brain reduced glutathione

The method of Boyne and Ellman [6] was used to estimate the level of reduced GSH in the brain homogenate. To precipitate the tissue proteins in the homogenate, it was mixed with 0.1 M phosphate buffer (pH 7.4) and then added to equal volume of 20% trichloroacetic acid containing 1 mM EDTA. The mixture stood for 5 min before it was centrifuged for 10 min at 2000 rpm. The supernatant was then transferred to a new set of test tubes, to which was added 1.8 ml of the Ellman's reagent (5,5′-dithio bis-2-nitrobenzoic acid). The reaction mixture was measured at 412 nm against blank.

Brain superoxide dismutase activity

The method of Misra and Fridovich [32] was used to assay the activity of superoxide dismutase. The method is based on the principle that super oxide inhibits the oxidation of adrenaline to adrenochrome. Each 3-ml of the reaction mixture contained 0.1-ml tissue homogenate, 2.8 ml of Potassium phosphate buffer (0.1 M, pH 7.4), and 0.1-ml pyrogallol solution (2.6 mM in 10 mM HCl). The pink product formed, adenochrome was detected in a spectrophotometer at 480 nm. The results were expressed as units/mg protein.

Brain catalase activity

The method of Sinha [45] was used to assay catalase activity. A volume of 0.5 ml of the homogenate was added to the reaction mixture which contained 1 ml of 0.01 M phosphate buffer (pH 7.0), 0.5 ml of 0.2 M H_2O_2, and 0.4 ml H_2O. The tubes were all heated at 95 °C for 10 min. To terminate the reaction, 2 ml of dichromate/acetic acid mixture was added to it. To the control, the homogenate was added after the addition of acid reagent. The absorbance was read at 570 nm, the enzyme activity was expressed as micromoles of H_2O_2/min/mg of protein.

Brain glutathione peroxidase

A colorimetric assay kit was used to assay the activity of glutathione peroxidase (GPx) (Sigma-Aldrich, Germany). This test is based on the principle that reduction of organic peroxide by glutathione peroxidase produces oxidized glutathione which is immediately converted to its reduced form (GSH) at the same time oxidizing NADPH to NADP+. The oxidation of NADPH was monitored spectrophotometrically using as a decrease in absorbance at 340 nm [14].

Total brain protein

Quantitative estimation of brain homogenate total protein was carried out according to the Biuret method Gornall et al. [17]. This was done in order to quantify the concentration of proteins in the samples.

Light microscopic examination

Small sections of each midbrain from the normal control and the various treated animals were fixed on 10% paraformaldehyde to assess for histological changes. Thin frozen brain sections of 30 μm from were obtained using microtome. The tissues were dehydrated in ascending grades of alcohol following fixation, and were then embedded in wax. Approximately 5–7 μm thick paraffin sections were cut and then subjected to hematoxylin–eosin staining as described by Fischer et al. [11]. Appearances of necrosis, apoptosis, size and quantity of cells were observed. The prepared slides were sent to the histopathology Department of the University of Yaounde, 1 Teaching Hospital for specialist observation and interpretation.

Statistical analysis

Results were collected, tabulated and expressed as mean ± S.E.M. Measurements were analyzed using one-way analysis of variance, ANOVA, followed by Tukey's multiple comparisons test. All statistical tests were done employing Graph Pad Prism version 6. Differences were considered significant at $p \leq 0.05$.

Results

In this present study, subcutaneous administration of rotenone (2.5 mg/kg) to rats consecutively for 7 days produced biochemical alterations accompanied by histological changes in the neurons in the midbrain.

Percentage survival

Repeated treatment of rats in this study with rotenone resulted in morbidity and mortality in rats. Death began occurring from the 4th day of administration of rotenone. The percentage survival of rats at the end of the experiment was found to reach 83% (5 out of 6). Death of rats occurred in the rotenone (01), zinc and Linoleic (01) and levodopa group (01). The survival of rats was not improved by treatment with Zinc and Linoleic acid as compared to rotenone group. From day 3, some animals showed severe weakness, apparent weight loss and locomotive inability. Rats that died during the course of the experiment were excluded from statistical analysis.

Biochemical measurements

Lipid peroxidation by MDA measurement

In the estimation of MDA levels, all animals in each group showed variable levels of MDA (Fig. 1 and Table 1). There was significant increase in levels of MDA in rotenone treated animals ($p < 0.0001$), when compared with normal control animals (0.03 ± 0.01 to 0.44 ± 0.06). There was significant decrease in MDA levels in Zinc treated animals (0.44 ± 0.06 to 0.03 ± 0.01; $p < 0.0001$), Linoleic acid (0.44 ± 0.06 to 0.02 ± 0.00; $p < 0.0001$), and a combination of both (0.44 ± 0.06 to 0.07 ± 0.03; $p < 0.0001$) when compared with rotenone treated animals. The effect of the zinc, Linoleic acid and the combination was significantly greater when compared to the Levodopa group ($p < 0.0001$ Table 1). There was however no significant difference in MDA levels of the combination when compared with individual treatments. Zinc lowered the MDA levels to normal control group levels (0.03 ± 0.01 to 0.03 ± 0.01), while Linoleic acid and the combination groups lowered to near normal control levels (0.03 ± 0.01 to 0.02 ± 0.00 and 0.03 ± 0.01 to 0.07 ± 0.03) respectively.

Table 1 Effect of zinc and linoleic acid and their combination on LPO and the antioxidant system enzymes in mid brain of rotenone treated rats

Groups	MDA (µmoles/mg protein) Mean ± SEM	TAC (µmoles/mg protein)	GSH (µmoles/mg protein)	SOD (UI/mg protein)	CAT (µmole H$_2$O$_2$/min/mg protein)	GPx (UI/ml enzymes)	TP (mg protein)
Vehicle (n = 6)	0.03 ± 0.01	699.2 ± 3.473	4.44 ± 0.43	6.68 ± 1	0.64 ± 0.01	0.0200 ± 0.003536	10.67 ± 1.052
Rotenone (n = 5)	0.44 ± 0.06[a]	554.6 ± 8.921[a]	0.57 ± 0.18[a]	1.42 ± 0.63[a]	0.22 ± 0.03[a]	0.0062 ± 0.002131	9.370 ± 0.3590
Zinc (n = 6)	0.03 ± 0.01*,c	686.7 ± 8.559*	3.91 ± 0.31*	5.16 ± 0.24[b]	0.74 ± 0.03*,d	0.0358 ± 0.006778[b]	10.41 ± 0.06512
Linoleic acid (n = 6)	0.02 ± 0.00*,c	702.1 ± 4.699*	3.76 ± 0.49*	5.34 ± 1.04[b]	0.74 ± 0.04*,d	0.0752 ± 0.004758*,c	10.95 ± 0.2067
Zinc + linoleic acid (n = 5)	0.07 ± 0.03*,c	630.2 ± 33.28[b]	3.62 ± 0.34*	7.11 ± 0.73[b]	0.68 ± 0.05*	0.0812 ± 0.007716*,c	11.30 ± 0.6652
Levodopa (n = 5)	0.43 ± 0.04	692.7 ± 3.239*	3.69 ± 0.23*	5.09 ± 0.55[b]	0.50 ± 0.08[b]	0.0170 ± 0.0030	11.28 ± 0.3937

Total protein and antioxidant biomarker activity and concentration in the midbrain of the experimental groups. Results are expressed as mean ± SEM

LPO lipid peroxidation

[a] p ≤ 0.0001 compared to vehicle group; [b]p ≤ 0.05 compared to rotenone group; [c]p ≤ 0.0001 compared to levodopa group, [d]p ≤ 0.05 compared to levodopa group

*p ≤ 0.0001 compared to rotenone group

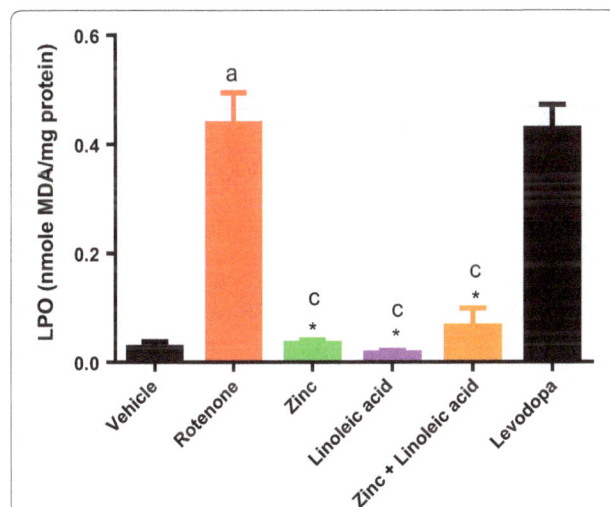

Fig. 1 Lipid peroxidation (MDA) levels in the midbrain of experimental groups. [a]p ≤ 0.0001 compared to vehicle group, [c]p ≤ 0.0001 compared to levodopa group, *p ≤ 0.0001 compared to rotenone group

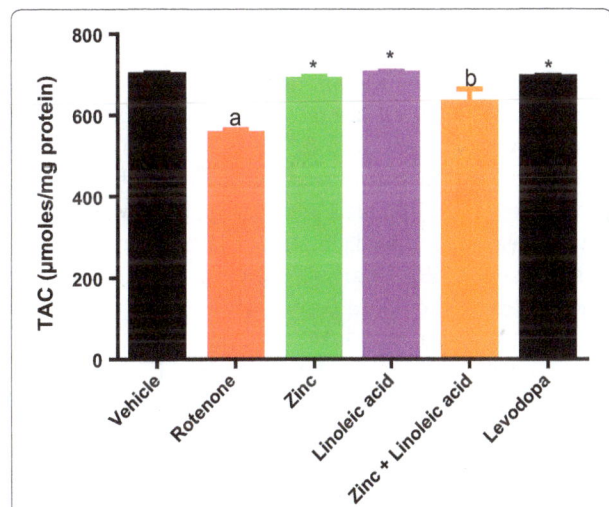

Fig. 2 Total antioxidant capacity (TAC) levels in the midbrain of experimental groups. [a]p ≤ 0.0001 compared to vehicle group, [b]p ≤ 0.05 compared to rotenone group, *p ≤ 0.0001 compared to rotenone group

Levodopa did not significantly reduce the MDA levels (0.44 ± 0.06 to 0.43 ± 0.04, p > 0.05, Table 1). The effect of linoleic acid and the combination was significant when compared to levodopa (p < 0.0001).

Total antioxidant capacity

The total antioxidant capacity in rotenone-treated rats presented in the Fig. 2 and Table 1 was found to significantly (p ≤ 0.05) decrease compared to vehicle-treated rats (699.2 ± 3.473 to 554.6 ± 8.921). The zinc and linoleic acid groups had significantly prevented the decrease in total antioxidant capacity (TAC) caused by rotenone administration (554.6 ± 8.921 to 686.7 ± 8.559; 554.6 ± 8.921 to 702.1 ± 4.699 respectively) (p < 0.0001); their combination also prevented this decrease in TAC caused by rotenone administration (554.6 ± 8.921 to 630.2 ± 33.28) (p ≤ 0.05, Fig. 2). The effect of the combination was not significant when compared to single treatments (p > 0.05, Fig. 2). Zinc, linoleic acid, the combination and levodopa all increased TAC to near normal control levels.

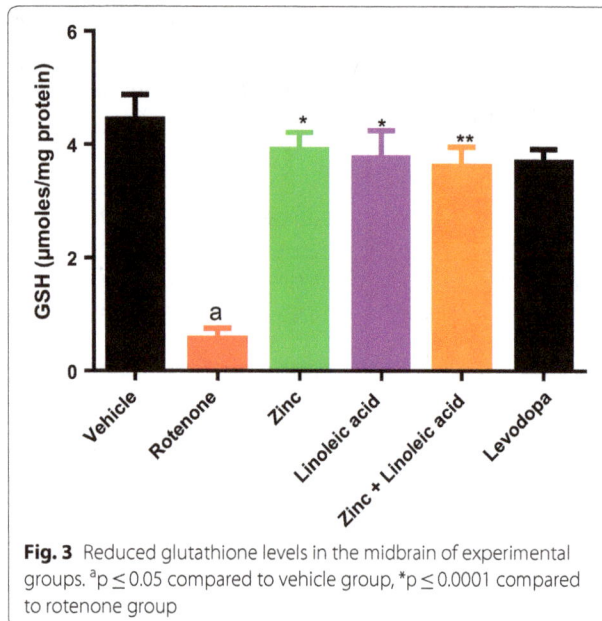

Fig. 3 Reduced glutathione levels in the midbrain of experimental groups. ^{a}p ≤ 0.05 compared to vehicle group, *p ≤ 0.0001 compared to rotenone group

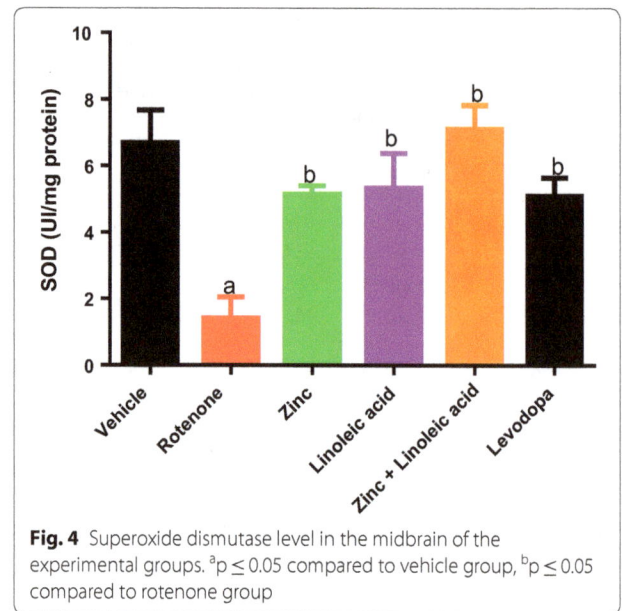

Fig. 4 Superoxide dismutase level in the midbrain of the experimental groups. ^{a}p ≤ 0.05 compared to vehicle group, ^{b}p ≤ 0.05 compared to rotenone group

Reduced glutathione concentration

There was significant decrease of reduced glutathione (GsH) level (4.44 ± 0.43 to 0.57 ± 0.18) in brain content in rotenone treated groups as compared to the vehicle group (p ≤ 0.0001) (Table 1 and Fig. 3). There was significant increase in reduced glutathione levels in zinc treated animals i.e. 0.57 ± 0.18 to 3.91 ± 0.31 (p < 0.0001), linoleic acid 0.57 ± 0.18 to 3.76 ± 0.49 (p < 0.0001), and a combination of both i.e. 0.57 ± 0.18 to 3.62 ± 0.34 (p < 0.0001) when compared with rotenone treated animals i.e. 0.57 ± 0.18. The combination of zinc and linoleic acid did not significantly increase GSH levels when compared to individual treatment (p > 0.05, Table 1, Fig. 3). Levodopa significantly increased brain GSH levels compared to the rotenone group (0.57 ± 0.18 to 3.69 ± 0.23). The effect of zinc, linoleic acid, their combination and levodopa was not significant compared to the normal control group.

Superoxide dismutase

There was a significant decrease in SOD activity in rotenone-treated rats as compared to vehicle-treated rats (6.68 ± 1 to 1.42 ± 0.63; p ≤ 0.05, Fig. 4 and Table 1). The zinc group had a significant increase in SOD activity as compared to rotenone group (1.42 ± 0.63 to 5.16 ± 0.24, p < 0.05). The linoleic acid group showed a similar effect (1.42 ± 0.63 to 5.34 ± 1.04, p < 0.05), as did their combination enhanced SOD activity as compared to rotenone group (1.42 ± 0.63 to 7.11 ± 0.73, p ≤ 0.05, Fig. 4). The combination of zinc and linoleic acid also significantly increased SOD activity when compared to individual treatment (p < 0.05, Fig. 4). The effect of zinc, linoleic

acid, their combination and levodopa was not significant when compared to the normal control group. Also the effect of zinc, linoleic acid and their combination was not significant when compared to levodopa (p > 0.05).

Glutathione peroxidase

The glutathione peroxidase activity was not significantly decreased in rotenone-treated rats as compared to vehicle-treated rats (0.0200 ± 0.003536 to 0.0062 ± 0.002131 p > 0.05, Fig. 5 and Table 1). The linoleic acid and the combination group had significant increase in GPx activity as compared to rotenone group (0.0062 ± 0.002131 to 0.0752 ± 0.004758 and 0.0062 ± 0.002131 to 0.0812 ± 0.007716 respectively, p < 0.0001, Table 1); the zinc group also showed a significant effect (0.0062 ± 0.002131 to 0.0358 ± 0.006778, p ≤ 0.05, Fig. 5). The effects of zinc and linoleic acid on increasing GPx activity were significant in comparison to the normal control group (0.0200 ± 0.003536 to 0.0358 ± 0.006778 and 0.0200 ± 0.003536 to 0.0752 ± 0.004758 respectively, p < 0.0001). The effects of linoleic acid and the combination was significant when compared to levodopa (p < 0.0001) while zinc effect was not significant (p > 0.05).

Catalase

Catalase activity in the vehicle treated group was found to be 0.64 ± 0.01 µM of H_2O_2 used/min/mg protein (Fig. 6). Rotenone treatment resulted in a significant decrease in CAT level in the midbrain as compared to the vehicle-treated group (0.64 ± 0.01 to 0.22 ± 0.03, p < 0.0001). The zinc group (0.22 ± 0.03 to 0.74 ± 0.03), linoleic acid group (0.22 ± 0.03 to 0.74 ± 0.04) and their combination

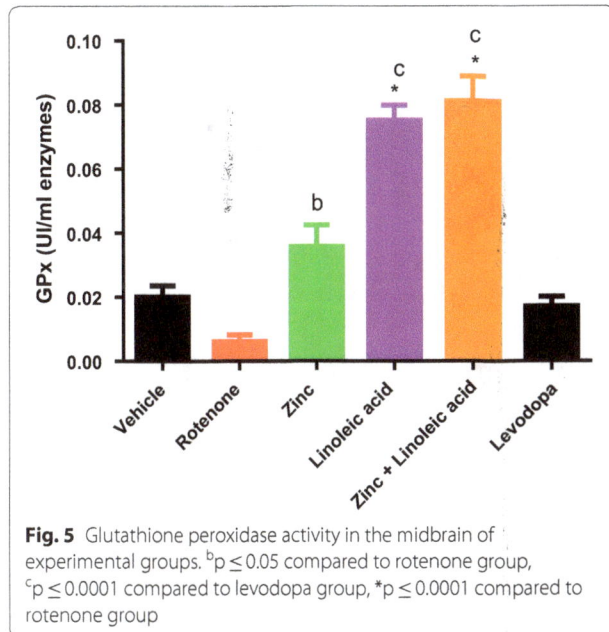

Fig. 5 Glutathione peroxidase activity in the midbrain of experimental groups. [b]$p \leq 0.05$ compared to rotenone group, [c]$p \leq 0.0001$ compared to levodopa group, *$p \leq 0.0001$ compared to rotenone group

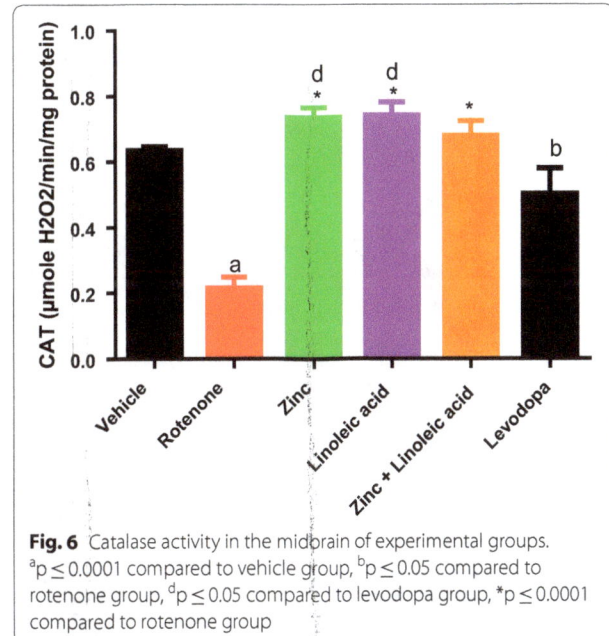

Fig. 6 Catalase activity in the midbrain of experimental groups. [a]$p \leq 0.0001$ compared to vehicle group, [b]$p \leq 0.05$ compared to rotenone group, [d]$p \leq 0.05$ compared to levodopa group, *$p \leq 0.0001$ compared to rotenone group

$(0.22 \pm 0.03$ to $0.68 \pm 0.05)$ had a significant increase in CAT activity as compared to rotenone group; $(p \leq 0.0001,$ Fig. 6). The combination of zinc and linoleic acid however did not significantly increase catalase activity when compared to individual treatment $(p > 0.05,$ Table 1, Fig. 6). The CAT activity increasing effects of zinc, Linoleic acid and their combination was not significant when compared to the normal control and levodopa groups.

Histopathology

The vehicle-treated group animals showed normal neuronal density and normal cellularity of neurons with no atypical cells, no visible cell death (Fig. 7). In rotenone treated group there was neuronal cell death, slight structural damage to the midbrain. The zinc group showed midbrain structure with slight hyperplasia of cells, presence of micro vacuolization and augmented number of cells reflecting cellular injury however with small blood vessels. There was no visible cell death in the linoleic acid group. The combination group showed normal neuron cell population, with some cells appearing multinucleated. The levodopa group showed slight cellularity of the midbrain region with multinucleated cells. There was no apparent cell death.

Discussion

The present study was done to evaluate the role of Zinc and Linoleic acid and their combination, as neuroprotective agents against rotenone-induced parkinsonism. As shown previously [2] intraperitoneal injection of rotenone over 7 days precipitates biochemical and histological deficits in the midbrain of rats. Interestingly, pretreatment of rats with Zinc or Linoleic acid prevented the decrease in total brain antioxidant capacity and activities of antioxidant enzymes.

In animal model studies, Rotenone (an alkaloidal pesticide), a specific inhibitor of complex I is employed to increase oxidative stress-mediated neuropathology [50]. More specifically, it is used to generate toxin-based rodent models of Parkinson's disease [43]. Because of its mechanism of action involving oxidative stress, exposure of rodents to Rotenone provides a valuable model for studying both mechanisms of oxidative stress and neuroprotection by antioxidant agents [39]. Pathologically, Rotenone induces the degeneration of the nigrostriatal dopaminergic pathway which is one of the cardinal pathological markers of Parkinson's disease [2, 50].

A number of studies have shown that the dopaminergic neurons in PD exists in a state of constant oxidative stress, due in part largely to the generation of H_2O_2 [24]. Lipid peroxidation measured by MDA levels was observed to be elevated in rotenone treated animals than controls. This agrees with other studies which suggest that oxidative damage is involved in the neuronal abnormalities in PD [28, 53]. However, treatment with zinc and linoleic acid or their combination reduced MDA levels and therefore lipid peroxidation and brought it to control levels. The reduction of MDA levels and thus lipid peroxidation by zinc is in line with the study of Ozturk et al. [34] who investigated the effects of zinc deficiency and supplementation on malondialdehyde and glutathione levels in blood and tissues of

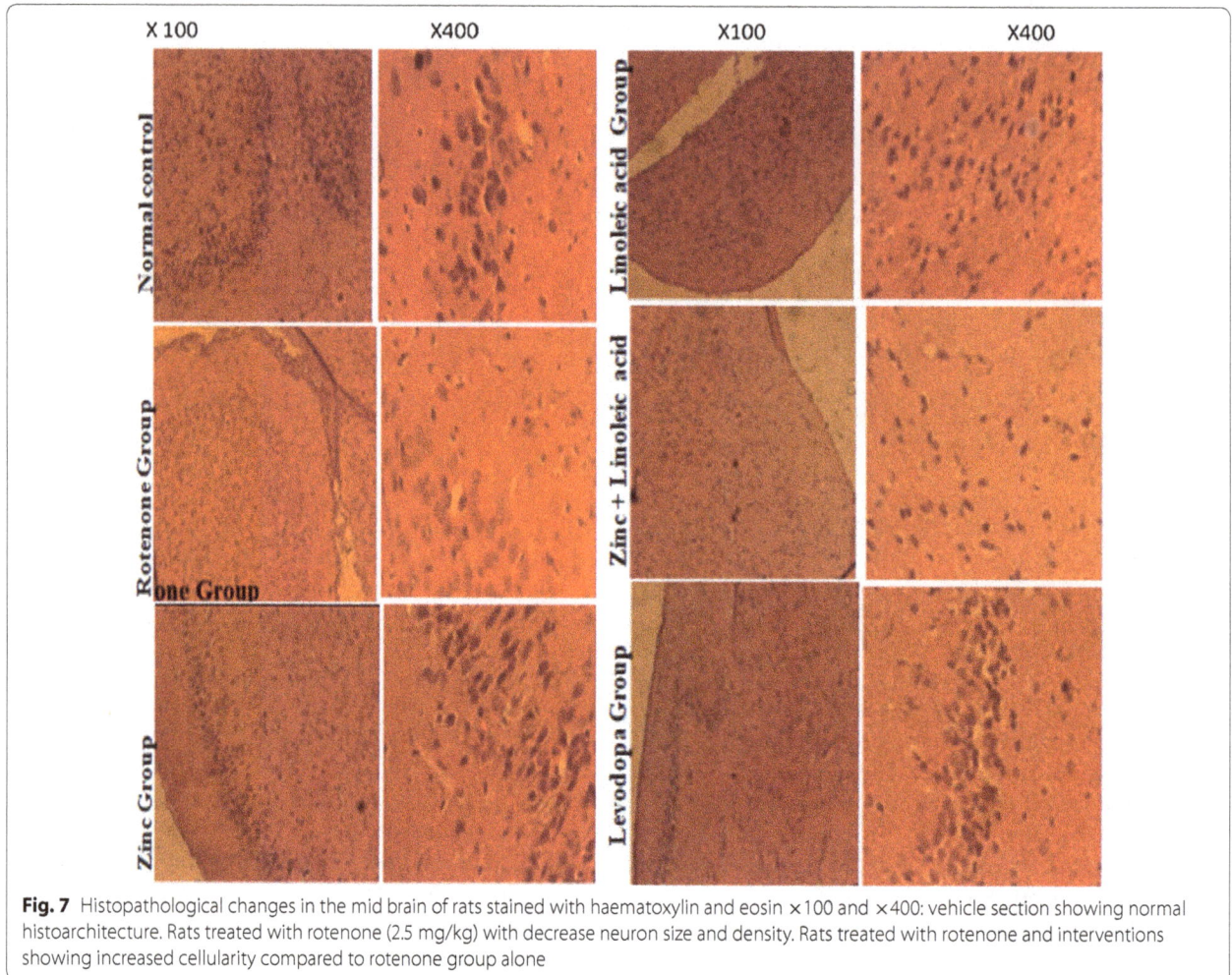

Fig. 7 Histopathological changes in the mid brain of rats stained with haematoxylin and eosin ×100 and ×400: vehicle section showing normal histoarchitecture. Rats treated with rotenone (2.5 mg/kg) with decrease neuron size and density. Rats treated with rotenone and interventions showing increased cellularity compared to rotenone group alone

rats performing swimming exercise, and showed that zinc supplemented rats had increased reduced glutathione and decreased MDA levels. The lowered MDA levels due to linoleic acid corroborates with the studies of Yang and colleagues who showed reduced MDA levels in the hippocampus of diabetic rats on administration of omega-3 PUFA [55]. The mechanism involved in lowering lipid peroxidation by linoleic acid appears to involve detoxification of peroxy radicals and other ROS species [16].

Decreased levels of GSH might play an important role in inducing oxidative stress in brain [57]. Such levels have been detected in remaining neurons and in SNpc of PD patients as compared to controls of similar age [49]. In this present study, GSH levels were lower in rotenone treated animals. Studies have shown decreased levels of GSH leads to oxidative damage to DNA, protein and lipids in PD [8, 48, 54]. Oral administration of zinc and subcutaneous administration of Linoleic acid increased GSH levels. Zinc has been suggested to exert this GSH-increased level effect through the actions of

metallothionein [40]. On the other hand the GSH activity-increasing effect of linoleic acid corroborates with the study of Ahmad and Beg [1], who evaluated the therapeutic effect of omega-6 linoleic acid and thymoquinone enriched extracts from Nigella sativa oil in the mitigation of lipidemic oxidative stress in rats. The effects of linoleic acid on GSH may be due to their direct antioxidant effects or the prevention of GSH oxidation.

The rotenone treated group showed a significant decrease in glutathione peroxidase activity. This agrees with the studies of Testa et al. [51]. Zinc pre-treatment was able to increase glutathione peroxidase activity. This corroborates with the study of the effect of zinc supplementation on glutathione peroxidase activity and selenium concentration in the serum, liver and kidney of rats chronically exposed to cadmium by Gałażyn-Sidorczuk et al. [14], showed that zinc significantly increased glutathione peroxidase levels. Linoleic acid in the study of Ahmad and Beg [1] also protected glutathione peroxidase activity by 90%.

SOD activity in the group treated with rotenone was found to be reduced. Complex-I of the mitochondrial respiratory chain is a major source of superoxide free radicals. The loss in SOD activity might contribute to increase in oxidative stress in rotenone treated animals [12, 27]. A lowered SOD activity would be detrimental in cases when superoxide radical production is increased. The decrease in SOD activity following rotenone treatment might be due to inactivation of SOD by ROS [12]. Administration of zinc was beneficial in restoring the SOD activity. This agrees with the studies of Paz Matias et al. [38] who investigated the effect of zinc supplementation on superoxide dismutase activity in patients with ulcerative rectocolitis. In the study of Ahmad and Beg [1], omega-6 linoleic acid supplementation also increased SOD activity.

The present study showed reduced CAT activity in rotenone-treated rats as compared to vehicle-treated rats. This agrees with the studies of Liu et al. [26], Prema et al. [41] and Soczynska et al. [46]. A study by Sharma and Bafna [42] showed a non-significant increase in the activity of CAT in rotenone treated rats compared to vehicle-treated rats. Zinc and linoleic acid increased the activity of CAT compared to the rotenone treated group. Zinc effect on Catalase activity agrees on the study of [35] who investigated the effect of zinc supplementation on antioxidant status and immune response in buffalo calves and showed that zinc supplementation increased Catalase activity. The protective effects of linoleic acid might reflect its ability to improve energy metabolism and repair damaged layers of lipids, hence suppressing the exudation of free electrons from the mitochondrial electron transport system, which is a prerequisite reaction to generate free radicals [29].

The antioxidant effect of Zinc has been suggested to work via metallothionein by regulating the secretion of pro-inflammatory cytokines and these metallothionein's are strong scavengers of free radicals [20, 31]. Linoleic acid with efficient free radical scavenging capacity could be involved in lowering MDA and slowing the degradation of the antioxidant enzymes CAT, SOD and GPx on its administration [9, 23], thus improving the total antioxidant capacity. The combination of zinc and linoleic acid showed remarkable antioxidant effect by lowering MDA levels and increasing GSH, SOD above the levels of individual interventions. Zinc and Linoleic acid antioxidant activity from the combination group did not show additive effect, supporting cited literature that Zinc and Linoleic acid act through independent pathways. We however suggest that either of the two facilitate the activity of the other.

The Levodopa treated group showed a significant increase in the total antioxidant capacity, levels and activity of antioxidant markers (Table 1) compared to the rotenone treated group. This corroborates with previous studies of Testa et al. [51], who evaluated the Levodopa and carbidopa antioxidant activity in normal lymphocytes in vitro, examining their implication for oxidative stress in Parkinson's disease. Their studies showed that Levodopa protected DNA from damage, scavenged free radicals and modulated the expression of genes involved in cellular oxidative metabolism.

In histopathological findings visible neuronal cell loss in the midbrain was identified that indicates the damage of neurons at this region in rotenone treated animals. Findings from earlier studies have shown that the substantia nigra is more vulnerable to damage by rotenone [26]. This may be attributed to higher susceptibility of the neurons in this region to free radicals. Histological findings in the midbrain were more correlated with impaired motor coordination responses along with biochemical evidences [51]. This may indicate that the midbrain area responds highly to oxidative stress caused by rotenone. This vulnerability of the midbrain to rotenone-induced oxidative stress has also been demonstrated in other studies [43]. Zinc and linoleic acid and their combination improved the neuronal loss in the midbrain caused by rotenone administration. The decreases in necrotic cells observed in the zinc treated group agrees with the studies of Galvão et al. [15] who also observed a decrease in the number of necrotic cells in hippocampus as well as cortex of zinc supplemented group for both male and female pups, in a study investigating the effect of "Prenatal zinc in adult rat offspring exposed to lipopolysaccharide during gestation". Linoleic acid effect on the midbrain corroborates with the studies of Beltz et al. [3], who investigated the effect of Linoleic acid on hippocampal neurogenesis. They advanced suggestions that linoleic acid plays this role via increasing expression of brain derived neurotrophic factor. The group treated with Levodopa were protected from neuronal loss in the midbrain region.

Limitations

Even though the study did not set out to investigate sex difference or confounding role of female sex hormones, the use of female rats in this study was a matter of choice motivated by the limited studies conducted on the effect of these micronutrients and trace elements on female rats. It is worth noting that the impact of the differences in estrous cycles of the rats could not be accounted for. It has been shown that estrous cycle variation, a consequence of variation in the levels of reproductive hormones, also influence the expression of genes responsible for production of antioxidants [32].

Our experimental design did not consider the impact of this variation on the results.

Conclusion

In the present study, repeated systemic administration of rotenone (2.5 mg/kg doses, s.c.) in rats produced increased midbrain lipid peroxidation and impaired antioxidant status, accompanied by histological changes. Zinc, Linoleic acid and their combination prevented the increase in MDA levels and decrease in brain antioxidant status induced by rotenone treatment. Cell death and reduction in neuron size induced by rotenone was prevented by treatment with zinc, linoleic acid and their combination. However further studies are needed to explore the possible mechanisms involved in this behavioral effect.

Abbreviations

CAT: Catalase; DMSO: Dimethylsulfoxide; DAergic: Dopaminergic; G-Px: Glutathione peroxidase; MDA: Malondialdehyde; PD: Parkinson's disease; ROS: Reactive oxygen species; PBS: Phosphate-buffered saline; PUFAs: Poly-unsaturated fatty acids; GSH: Reduced glutathione; SNpc: Substantia nigra pars compacta; SOD: Superoxide dismutase.

Authors' contributions

All authors contributed extensively to the work presented in this paper. NEM and HIN conceived the work, NEM, HIN, MBV and CAP designed the work. NEM and CAP collected and analyzed the data. NEM, HIN, MBV and CAP interpreted the data. NEM drafted the article and HIN, MBV, CAP did a critical revision of the manuscript. All authors read and approved the final manuscript.

Author details

[1] Department of Physiology, Faculty of Biomedical Sciences, Kampala International University, Western Campus, Ishaka, Uganda. [2] Department of Human Physiology, University of Medical Sciences, Camagüey, Cuba. [3] Department of Biochemistry and Physiological Sciences, Faculty of Medicine and Biomedical Sciences, University of Yaounde I, Yaounde, Cameroon.

Acknowledgements

The authors greatly acknowledge the cooperation of the staff of the animal house, University of Yaounde 1, Cameroon for technical support and space for the study. The authors thanks the facilitator of the IBRO-ARC fourth scientific writing workshop for guidance for writing the manuscript.

Competing interests

The authors declare that they have no competing interests.

Funding

The authors declare no funding whatsoever was obtained for this study.

References

1. Ahmad S, Beg ZH. Evaluation of therapeutic effect of omega-6 linoleic acid and thymoquinone enriched extracts from Nigella sativa oil in the mitigation of lipidemic oxidative stress in rats. Nutrition. 2016;32(6):649–55. https://doi.org/10.1016/j.nut.2015.12.003.
2. Alam M, Schmidt WJ. Rotenone destroys dopaminergic neurons and induces parkinsonian symptoms in rats. Behav Brain Res. 2002;136(1):317–24. https://doi.org/10.1016/S0166-4328(02)00180-8.
3. Beltz BS, Tlusty MF, Benton JL, Sandeman DC. Omega-3 fatty acids upregulate adult neurogenesis. Neurosci Lett. 2007;415(2):154–8. https://doi.org/10.1016/j.neulet.2007.01.010.
4. Benzie I, Strain J. The ferric reducing ability of plasma (FRAP) as a measure of "antioxidant power": the FRAP assay. Anal Biochem. 1996. https://doi.org/10.1006/abio.1996.0292.
5. Blesa J, Trigo-Damas I, Quiroga-Varela A, Jackson-Lewis VR. Oxidative stress and Parkinson's disease. Front Neuroanat. 2015;9(July):91. https://doi.org/10.3389/fnana.2015.00091.
6. Boyne AF, Ellman GL. A methodology for analysis of tissue sulfhydryl components. Anal Biochem. 1972;46(2):639–53. https://doi.org/10.1016/0003-2697(72)90335-1.
7. Calon F, Cole G. Neuroprotective action of omega-3 polyunsaturated fatty acids against neurodegenerative diseases: evidence from animal studies. Prostaglandins Leukot Essent Fat Acids. 2007;77(5–6):287–93. https://doi.org/10.1016/j.plefa.2007.10.019.
8. Chinta SJ, Andersen JK. Redox imbalance in Parkinson's disease. Biochim Biophys Acta Gen Subj. 2008. https://doi.org/10.1016/j.bbagen.2008.02.005.
9. Eckert GP, Lipka U, Muller WE. Omega-3 fatty acids in neurodegenerative diseases: focus on mitochondria. Prostaglandins Leukot Essent Fat Acids. 2013;88(1):105–14. https://doi.org/10.1016/j.plefa.2012.05.006.
10. Elbaz A, Tranchant C. Epidemiologic studies of environmental exposures in Parkinson's disease. J Neurol Sci. 2007;262(1–2):37–44. https://doi.org/10.1016/j.jns.2007.06.024.
11. Fischer AH, Jacobson KA, Rose J, Zeller R. Hematoxylin and eosin (H & E) staining. CSH Protoc. 2005;2008(4):pdb.prot4986. https://doi.org/10.1016/0016-5085(95)23032-7.
12. Fridovich I. Superoxide radical and superoxide dismutases. Ann Rev Biochem. 1995;64(1):97–112. https://doi.org/10.1146/annurev.biochem.64.1.97.
13. Fujikawa T, Kanada N, Shimada A, Ogata M, Suzuki I, Hayashi I, Nakashima K. Effect of sesamin in Acanthopanax senticosus HARMS on behavioral dysfunction in rotenone-induced parkinsonian rats. Biol Pharm Bull. 2005;28(1):169–72. https://doi.org/10.1248/bpb.28.169.
14. Galazyn-Sidorczuk M, Brzóska MM, Rogalska J, Roszczenko A, Jurczuk M. Effect of zinc supplementation on glutathione peroxidase activity and selenium concentration in the serum, liver and kidney of rats chronically exposed to cadmium. J Trace Elem Med Biol. 2012;26(1):46–52. https://doi.org/10.1016/j.jtemb.2011.10.002.
15. Galvão MC, Chaves-Kirsten GP, Queiroz-Hazarbassanov N, Carvalho VM, Bernardi MM, Kirsten TB. Prenatal zinc reduces stress response in adult rat offspring exposed to lipopolysaccharide during gestation. Life Sci. 2015;120:54–60. https://doi.org/10.1016/j.lfs.2014.10.019.
16. Gladine C, Newman JW, Durand T, Pedersen TL, Galano JM, Demougeot C, Comte B. Lipid profiling following intake of the omega 3 fatty acid DHA identifies the peroxidized metabolites F4-neuroprostanes as the best predictors of atherosclerosis prevention. PLoS ONE. 2014. https://doi.org/10.1371/journal.pone.0089393.
17. Gornall AG, Bardawill CJ, David MM. Determination of serum proteins by means of the biuret reaction. J Biol Chem. 1949;177(2):751–66.
18. Hallett M. Tremor: pathophysiology. Parkinsonism Relat Disord. 2014. https://doi.org/10.1016/S1353-8020(13)70029-4.
19. Henchcliffe C, Beal MF. Mitochondrial biology and oxidative stress in Parkinson disease pathogenesis. Nat Clin Pract Neurol. 2008;4(11):600–9. https://doi.org/10.1038/ncpneuro0924.
20. Hijova E. Metallothioneins and zinc: their functions and interactions. Bratisl Lekarske Listy. 2004;105(5–6):230–4.
21. Hirose G. Drug induced parkinsonism. J Neurol. 2006;253(S3):iii22–4. https://doi.org/10.1007/s00415-006-3004-8.

22. Hwang O. Role of oxidative stress in Parkinson's disease. Exp Neurobiol. 2013;22(1):11–7. https://doi.org/10.5607/en.2013.22.1.11.

23. Innis SM. Dietary omega 3 fatty acids and the developing brain. Brain Res. 2008. https://doi.org/10.1016/j.brainres.2008.08.078.

24. Jenner P, Olanow CW. Oxidative stress and the pathogenesis of Parkinson's disease. Neurology. 1996;47(6 Suppl 3):S161–70. https://doi.org/10.1212/WNL.47.6_Suppl_3.161S.

25. Kaur H, Chauhan S, Sandhir R. Protective effect of lycopene on oxidative stress and cognitive decline in rotenone induced model of Parkinson's disease. Neurochem Res. 2011;36(8):1435–43. https://doi.org/10.1007/s11064-011-0469-3.

26. Lehto SM, Ruusunen A, Tolmunen T, Voutilainen S, Tuomainen TP, Kauhanen J. Dietary zinc intake and the risk of depression in middle-aged men: a 20-year prospective follow-up study. J Affect Disord. 2013;150(2):682–5. https://doi.org/10.1016/j.jad.2013.03.027.

27. Liochev SI, Fridovich I. The effects of superoxide dismutase on H_2O_2 formation. Free Radic Biol Med. 2007;42(10):1465–9. https://doi.org/10.1016/j.freeradbiomed.2007.02.015.

28. Liu CB, Wang R, Pan HB, Ding QF, Lu FB. Effect of lycopene on oxidative stress and behavioral deficits in rotenone induced model of Parkinson's disease. Zhongguo Ying Yong Sheng Li Xue Za Zhi. 2013;29(4):380–4.

29. Liu J, Killilea DW, Ames BN. Age-associated mitochondrial oxidative decay: improvement of carnitine acetyltransferase substrate-binding affinity and activity in brain by feeding old rats acetyl-L-carnitine and/or R-alpha-lipoic acid. Proc Natl Acad Sci USA. 2002;99(4):1876–81. https://doi.org/10.1073/pnas.261709098.

30. Luchtman DW, Meng Q, Song C. Ethyl-eicosapentaenoate (E-EPA) attenuates motor impairments and inflammation in the MPTP-probenecid mouse model of Parkinson's disease. Behav Brain Res. 2012;226(2):386–96. https://doi.org/10.1016/j.bbr.2011.09.033.

31. Maret W. Zinc and human disease. Metal Ions Life Sci. 2013;13:389–414. https://doi.org/10.1007/978-94-007-7500-8-12.

32. Misra HP, Fridovich I. The role of superoxide anion in the autoxidation of epinephrine and a simple assay for superoxide dismutase. J Biol Chem. 1972;247(10):3170–5.

33. Ojha S, Javed H, Azimullah S, Khair SBA, Haque ME. Neuroprotective potential of ferulic acid in the rotenone model of Parkinson's disease. Drug Des Dev Ther. 2015;9:5499–510. https://doi.org/10.2147/DDDT.S90616.

34. Ozturk A, Baltaci AK, Mogulkoc R, Oztekin E, Sivrikaya A, Kurtoglu E, Kul A. Effects of zinc deficiency and supplementation on malondialdehyde and glutathione levels in blood and tissues of rats performing swimming exercise. Biol Trace Elem Res. 2003;94(2):157–66. https://doi.org/10.1385/BTER:94:2:157.

35. Parashuramulu S, Nagalakshmi D, Rao DS, Kumar MK, Swain PS. Effect of zinc supplementation on antioxidant status and immune response in buffalo calves. Anim Nutr Feed Technol. 2015;15(2):179–88. https://doi.org/10.5958/0974-181X.2015.00020.7.

36. Partyka A, Jastrzebska-Wiesek M, Nowak G. Evaluation of anxiolytic-like activity of zinc. In: 17th international congress of the polish pharmacological society Krynica Zdroj Poland; 2010. vol. 62, pp. 57–58.

37. Partyka A, Jastrzębska-Więsek M, Szewczyk B, Stachowicz K, Sałwińska A, Poleszak E, Nowak G. Anxiolytic-like activity of zinc in rodent tests. Pharmacol Rep. 2011;63(4):1050–5. https://doi.org/10.1016/S1734-1140(11)70621-1.

38. Paz Matias J, Costa e Silva DM, Climaco Cruz KJ, Gomes da Silva K, Monte Feitosa M, Oliveira Medeiros LG, do Nascimento Nogueira N. Effect of zinc supplementation on superoxide dismutase activity in patients with ulcerative rectocolitis. Nutr Hosp. 2015;31(3):1434–7. https://doi.org/10.3305/nh.2015.31.3.8402.

39. Perfeito R, Cunha-Oliveira T, Rego AC. Revisiting oxidative stress and mitochondrial dysfunction in the pathogenesis of Parkinson disease–resemblance to the effect of amphetamine drugs of abuse. Free Radic Biol Med. 2012;53(9):1791–806. https://doi.org/10.1016/j.freeradbiomed.2012.08.569.

40. Prasad AS. Zinc: an antioxidant and anti-inflammatory agent: role of zinc in degenerative disorders of aging. J Trace Elem Med Biol. 2014. https://doi.org/10.1016/j.jtemb.2014.07.019.

41. Prema A, Janakiraman U, Manivasagam T, Arokiasamy JT. Neuroprotective effect of lycopene against MPTP induced experimental Parkinson's disease in mice. Neurosci Lett. 2015;599:12–9. https://doi.org/10.1016/j.neulet.2015.05.024.

42. Sharma N, Bafna P. Effect of Cynodon dactylon on rotenone induced Parkinson's disease. Orient Pharm Exp Med. 2012;12(3):167–75. https://doi.org/10.1007/s13596-012-0075-1.

43. Sherer TB, Betarbet R, Testa CM, Seo BB, Richardson JR, Kim JH, Greenamyre JT. Mechanism of toxicity in rotenone models of Parkinson's disease. J Neurosci. 2003;23(34):10756–64.

44. Shin HW, Chung SJ. Drug-Induced parkinsonism. J Clin Neurol (Korea). 2012;8(1):15–21. https://doi.org/10.3988/jcn.2012.8.1.15.

45. Sinha AK. Colorimetric assay of catalase. Anal Biochem. 1972;47(2):389–94. https://doi.org/10.1016/0003-2697(72)90132-7.

46. Soczynska JK, Kennedy SH, Chow CS, Woldeyohannes HO, Konarski JZ, McIntyre RS. Acetyl-L-carnitine and α-lipoic acid: possible neurotherapeutic agents for mood disorders? Expert Opin Investig Drugs. 2008;17(6):827–43. https://doi.org/10.1517/13543784.17.6.827.

47. Stocks J, Gutteridge JMC, Sharp RJ, Dormandy TL. The inhibition of lipid autoxidation by human serum and its relation to serum proteins and α to copherol. Clin Sci Mol Med. 1974;47(3):223–33.

48. Surapaneni K, Venkataramana G. Status of lipid peroxidation, glutathione, ascorbic acid, vitamin E and antioxidant enzymes in patients with osteoarthritis. Indian J Med Sci. 2007. https://doi.org/10.4103/0019-5359.29592.

49. Tamilselvam K, Braidy N, Manivasagam T, Essa MM, Prasad NR, Karthikeyan S, Guillemin GJ. Neuroprotective effects of hesperidin, a plant flavanone, on rotenone-induced oxidative stress and apoptosis in a cellular model for Parkinson's disease. Oxidative Med Cell Longev. 2013. https://doi.org/10.1155/2013/102741.

50. Tanner et al. Rotenone, paraquat, and Parkinson's disease. Environ Health Perspect. 2011;119(6):866–72. http://www.sertox.com.ar/modules.php?name=News&file=article&sid=3681.

51. Testa CM, Sherer TB, Greenamyre JT. Rotenone induces oxidative stress and dopaminergic neuron damage in organotypic substantia nigra cultures. Mol Brain Res. 2005;134(1):109–18. https://doi.org/10.1016/j.molbrainres.2004.11.007.

52. Thiffault C, Langston JW, Di Monte DA. Increased striatal dopamine turnover following acute administration of rotenone to mice. Brain Res. 2000;885(2):283–8. https://doi.org/10.1016/S0006-8993(00)02960-7.

53. Tsang AHK, Chung KKK. Oxidative and nitrosative stress in Parkinson's disease. Biochem Biophys Acta. 2009;1792(7):643–50. https://doi.org/10.1016/j.bbadis.2008.12.006.

54. Vinish M, Anand A, Prabhakar S. Altered oxidative stress levels in Indian Parkinson's disease patients with PARK2 mutations. Acta Biochim Pol. 2011;58(2):165–9.

55. Yang R-H, Wang F, Hou X-H, Cao Z-P, Wang B, Xu X-N, Hu S-J. Dietary ω-3 polyunsaturated fatty acids improves learning performance of diabetic rats by regulating the neuron excitability. Neuroscience. 2012;212:93–103. https://doi.org/10.1016/j.neuroscience.2012.04.005.

56. Zawada WM, Banninger GP, Thornton J, Marriott B, Cantu D, Rachubinski AL, Jones SM. Generation of reactive oxygen species in 1-methyl-4-phenylpyridinium (MPP+) treated dopaminergic neurons occurs as an NADPH oxidase-dependent two-wave cascade. J Neuroinflammation. 2011;8(1):129. https://doi.org/10.1186/1742-2094-8-129.

57. Zeevalk GD, Razmpour R, Bernard LP. Glutathione and Parkinson's disease: is this the elephant in the room? Biomed Pharmacother. 2008;62(4):236–49. https://doi.org/10.1016/j.biopha.2008.01.017.

58. Zimmer L, Delpal S, Guilloteau D, Aïoun J, Durand G, Chalon S. Chronic n-3 polyunsaturated fatty acid deficiency alters dopamine vesicle density in the rat frontal cortex. Neurosci Lett. 2000;284(1–2):25–8. https://doi.org/10.1016/S0304-3940(00)00950-2.

Transcranial focused ultrasound stimulation of motor cortical areas in freely-moving awake rats

Wonhye Lee[†], Phillip Croce[†], Ryan W. Margolin, Amanda Cammalleri, Kyungho Yoon and Seung-Schik Yoo[*] [iD]

Abstract

Background: Low-intensity transcranial focused ultrasound (tFUS) has emerged as a new non-invasive modality of brain stimulation with the potential for high spatial selectivity and penetration depth. Anesthesia is typically applied in animal-based tFUS brain stimulation models; however, the type and depth of anesthesia are known to introduce variability in responsiveness to the stimulation. Therefore, the ability to conduct sonication experiments on awake small animals, such as rats, is warranted to avoid confounding effects of anesthesia.

Results: We developed a miniature tFUS headgear, operating at 600 kHz, which can be attached to the skull of Sprague–Dawley rats through an implanted pedestal, allowing the ultrasound to be transcranially delivered to motor cortical areas of unanesthetized freely-moving rats. Video recordings were obtained to monitor physical responses from the rat during acoustic brain stimulation. The stimulation elicited body movements from various areas, such as the tail, limbs, and whiskers. Movement of the head, including chewing behavior, was also observed. When compared to the light ketamine/xylazine and isoflurane anesthetic conditions, the response rate increased while the latency to stimulation decreased in the awake condition. The individual variability in response rates was smaller during the awake condition compared to the anesthetic conditions. Our analysis of latency distribution of responses also suggested possible presence of acoustic startle responses mixed with stimulation-related physical movement. Post-tFUS monitoring of animal behaviors and histological analysis performed on the brain did not reveal any abnormalities after the repeated tFUS sessions.

Conclusions: The wearable miniature tFUS configuration allowed for the stimulation of motor cortical areas in rats and elicited sonication-related movements under both awake and anesthetized conditions. The awake condition yielded diverse physical responses compared to those reported in existing literatures. The ability to conduct an experiment in freely-moving awake animals can be gainfully used to investigate the effects of acoustic neuromodulation free from the confounding effects of anesthesia, thus, may serve as a translational platform to large animals and humans.

Keywords: Transcranial focused ultrasound, FUS, Brain stimulation, Motor cortex, Wearable headgear, Awake rat, Ketamine/xylazine, Isoflurane

*Correspondence: yoo@bwh.harvard.edu
[†]Wonhye Lee and Phillip Croce have contributed equally to this work
Department of Radiology, Brigham and Women's Hospital, Harvard
Medical School, 75 Francis Street, Boston, MA 02115, USA

Background

Over the past few decades, various brain stimulation techniques have significantly contributed to enhancing our current understanding of neural/neuronal function and offered non-pharmacological options for the treatment of neurological and neuropsychiatry diseases [1–3]. Approaches, such as deep brain stimulation (DBS) or epidural cortical stimulation (EpCS) [3], allow for stimulating brain regions with excellent spatial specificity, but require invasive surgical procedures. Transcranial direct current stimulation (tDCS) and transcranial magnetic stimulation (TMS) provide non-invasive alternatives to the surgical procedures, but may not reach deep brain areas with a centimeter-scale area for stimulation, limiting spatial specificity [1, 2]. Optogenetic techniques are capable of modulating cellular level activity of the brain [4]; however, the necessary genetic modification of neurons to gain light-sensitivity and limited transcranial penetration of stimulatory light may obstruct its translational application in humans.

Focused ultrasound (FUS) technique allows for the non-invasive, focal delivery of mechanical pressure waves to regional biological tissues [5–7], measuring a few millimeters in diameter and length. The advances in FUS techniques have further enabled the transcranial delivery of acoustic energy to specific regions of the brain [8–10]. This transcranial FUS (tFUS) technique has been utilized for non-invasive functional neurosurgery by thermally ablating localized deep brain structures, whereby the ultrasound waves are delivered at high acoustic intensities [11, 12]. tFUS has also been applied to temporarily open the blood-brain barrier (BBB) when combined with intravascular administration of microbubbles (detailed review can be found in [13]). In addition to these therapeutic potentials, tFUS, given in a train of pulses at a low-intensity (under the threshold for heat generation), has been shown to reversibly modulate regional brain excitability [14–17]. Taking advantage of the exquisite ability to transcranially reach deep brain areas [18, 19] as well as cortical areas [20–25] with high spatial selectivity, low-intensity tFUS has rapidly gained momentum as a new mode of non-invasive brain stimulation [26, 27].

FUS has shown to modulate excitability in motor/visual cortical areas in rabbits [17], stimulated various motor cortices in mice [16, 28–32], suppressed epileptic seizure electroencephalographic (EEG) activities [33], and altered the extracellular neurotransmitter level [34, 35] and anesthesia time in rats [36]. Investigations have also been conducted to study the effect of varying acoustic parameters [37] and spatial profile of neuromodulation using a rat model [38, 39]. Additionally, tFUS has stimulated the motor and visual cortices in sheep and elicited corresponding electrophysiological

responses [24]. The majority of these studies, conducted on anesthetized animals, showed a degree of variability in response to the stimulation, depending on the types and depths of anesthesia [24, 28, 31, 37, 40]. To examine the behavioral responses to FUS, without the confounding effects from anesthesia, experimentations in an awake setting are desired, and several recent studies on non-human primates and human subjects started to demonstrate the feasibility of tFUS in brain stimulation without the use of anesthesia [18, 20–23, 25, 41, 42].

We were motivated to develop a technique that will allow tFUS to be applied among unanesthetized, freely-moving small animals. Typically, a FUS transducer, much larger in size than the animal's head, is maneuvered with optional image/visual-guidance for its stereotactic application during anesthesia [17, 24, 28, 30, 31, 37, 43]. To enable the experimentation in freely-moving small animals, one critical technical element is to make the transducer wearable. Accordingly, we developed a miniaturized, light-weight FUS transducer that can be worn (and detachable) by Sprague–Dawley rats (anesthetized) and demonstrated that FUS can be delivered to their primary somatosensory areas, with possibility for inducing long-term neuromodulatory effects [44]. A 3D-printed applicator that is designed to adjust the position of the transducer was attached to a pedestal, which was implanted onto the rat skull. The design enabled the individual adjustment of location/depth/orientation of the sonication focus. Recently, Li et al. [45] developed a dual-channel miniature FUS system that can stimulate two separate regions of the mice brain, and observed stimulation-mediated behaviors and extracellular neural action potentials. In their study, the transducers were surgically-fixed to the skull, which granted the use of the system among freely-moving mice. In the present study, we applied our wearable tFUS platform to stimulate motor cortical areas of freely-moving awake rats, and examined sonication-related behavioral responses from three different experimental conditions—(1) freely-moving awake status, (2) ketamine/xylazine anesthesia, and (3) isoflurane anesthesia. The response rates and latencies to the sonication were compared. After the completion of the sonication sessions, histological analysis was conducted on the rat brains to assess the presence of any undesirable tissue damage.

Methods

Ethical statement

All animal experiments were conducted under the approval of the local Institutional Animal Care and Use Committee.

Preparation of the miniature FUS transducer/headgear

A small (16 mm in diameter, 12 mm in height) and light (~6 g in weight) FUS transducer was built in-house (Fig. 1a) [44]. A disc-shape zirconate titanate (PbZr$_x$Ti$_{(1-x)}$O$_3$; PZT) ceramic (American Piezo Ceramics, Mackeyville, PA) was used and fitted (air-backed)

inside of a custom-built plastic housing. The plastic housing and back-lid of the transducer was designed (using CAD software; Solidworks Corp., Concord, MA) and printed by three-dimensional (3D) printing (Form2; FormLabs Inc., Somerville, MA). The back-lid of the transducer contained a ball-shape structure to fit the

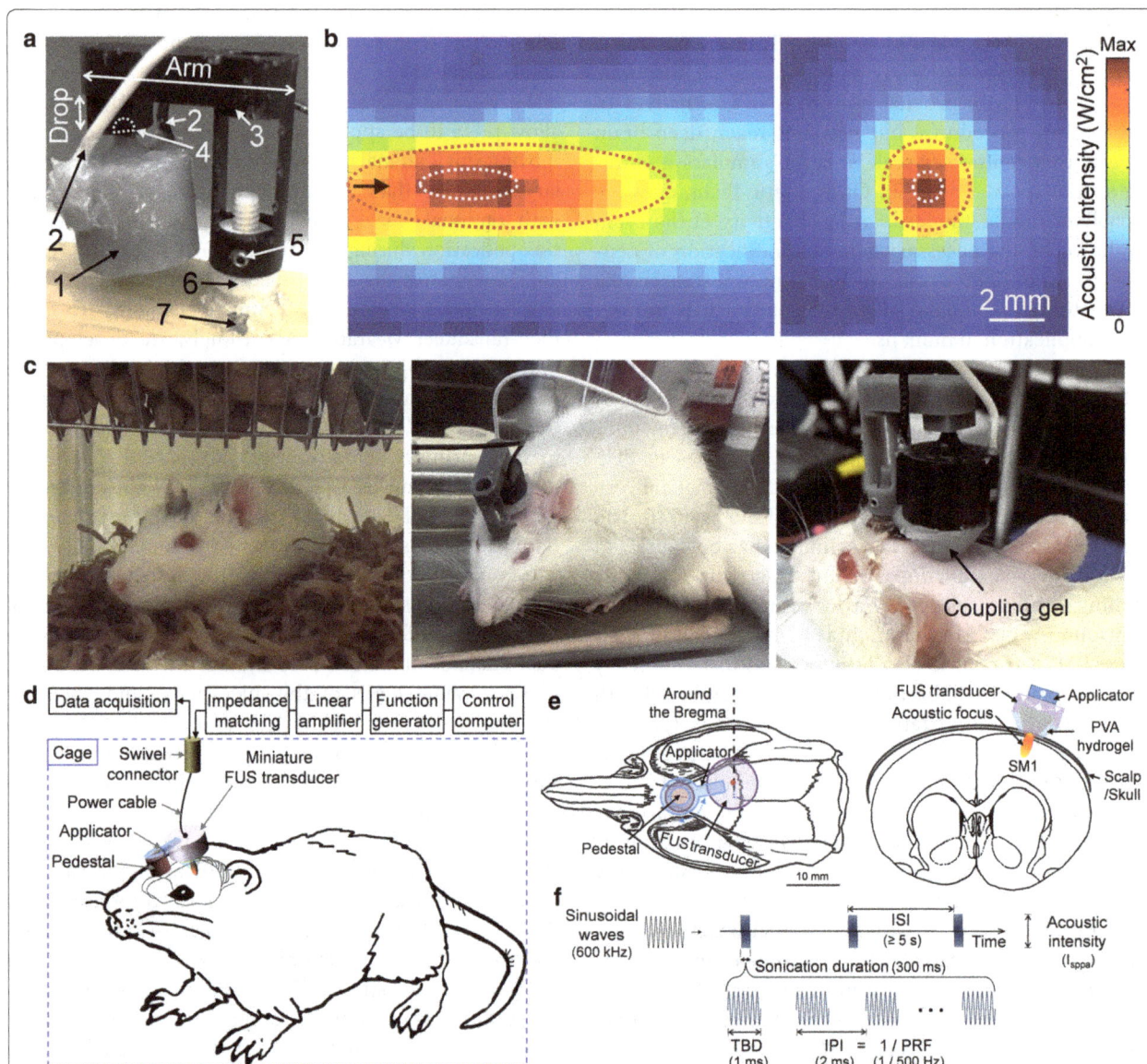

Fig. 1 The schematics for the wearable miniature transcranial FUS headgear, acoustic profile, and experimental design. **a** A demonstration of the wearable setup applied on a wood-block. 1: FUS transducer, 2: power lines, 3: detachable applicator with customizable dimensions of 'Arm' and 'Drop', 4: ball-and-socket joint, 5: set screws to securely fix the applicator, 6: skull-mounted pedestal, 7: skull-mounted screws and medical glue. The drop length of the applicator in the photo was 4.5 mm. **b** The acoustic intensity profile across (left panel) the longitudinal plane and (right panel) the transversal plane at ~ 10 mm away from exit plane of the transducer. FWHM and FW90%M of the intensity profile are depicted with a red and white dotted line, respectively. The black arrow indicates sonication direction (from the left to right). Scale bar = 2 mm. **c** A rat resting in a cage (left panel), a freely-moving rat during the awake sonication session (middle panel), and an anesthetized rat (ketamine/xylazine) with a cone-shaped coupling hydrogel (right panel). **d** Schematic drawing of the experimental settings compatible with both anesthetized and freely-moving awake rat. **e** Exemplar targeting to the rat motor cortex for the left forelimb. **f** The sonication parameters used. *TBD* tone burst duration, *IPI* inter-pulse interval, *PRF* pulse repetition frequency, sonication duration, *ISI* inter-stimulation interval

socket of an applicator (also 3D-printed), and held the transducer at a desired location/orientation (Fig. 1a). Both the transducer and applicator constituted the miniature tFUS headgear, and were attached to a pedestal (also 3D-printed), which was implanted on the skull of Sprague–Dawley rat (Charles River Laboratories, Wilmington, MA; see following section). Two set-screws were used to fasten the FUS headgear to the pedestal, ensuring a reproducible placement and orientation via lock-and-key mechanism. To accommodate the differences in individual neuroanatomy and cranial structures, applicators were customized with different 'Arm' and 'Drop' lengths (Fig. 1a).

Surgical implantation of a pedestal on the rat skull

To apply the miniature tFUS headgear in a wearable form, a pedestal was surgically implanted on the anterior region of the rat's skull. During the surgery, we measured the relative coordinates between the mounted pedestal and major skull anatomies (i.e., aural meatus, bregma, and lambda) to provide coordinates for the later FUS targeting. Two small screws were inserted (via burr holes) to the skull around the pedestal's base to provide support along with a medical-grade adhesive (Loctite 18690; Henkel, Rocky Hill, CT). The skin around the pedestal (while exposing the top portion) was sutured back (using Vicryl 5-0 polyglactin 910 suture; Ethicon Inc., Somerville, NJ). After undergoing these surgical procedures, the rats were housed for at least 2 weeks to recover from the surgery prior to the tFUS sessions. The pedestal remained in place and provided long-term mechanical stability over 8 months.

Actuation and characterization of the miniature FUS transducer

A fundamental frequency (FF) of 600 kHz was used to actuate the miniature transducer, and the acoustic intensity profile of the FUS transducer was characterized along the sonication direction as well as on the transversal plane at the focus (Fig. 1b). The detailed methods for the characterization process are described elsewhere [17]. The input signal was a sinusoidal wave generated by a function generator (33210A; Agilent, Santa Clara, CA) and amplified by a class-A linear amplifier (240 L; Electronics and Innovations Ltd., Rochester, NY) with an impedance-matching circuit. At the focus, the miniature transducer was capable of generating over 20 W/cm^2 spatial-peak pulse-average intensity (I_{sppa}). The acoustic focus was formed ~10 mm away from the exit plane of the transducer. The size of the focus, measured at full-width at half-maximum (FWHM) of acoustic intensity profile, was 11.5 mm in length and 3.0 mm in diameter. When it was measured at full-width at 90%-maximum (FW90%M), previously reported as the spatial dimension of the FUS-mediated neuromodulatory area [38, 39], the focal area was 3.5 mm in length and 1.0 mm in diameter.

Acoustic coupling using PVA gel

A cone-shaped, polyvinyl alcohol (PVA) hydrogel (7–9% weight per volume; two freeze–thaw cycles, U228-08; Avantor, Center Valley, PA) was manufactured in-house for acoustic coupling between the transducer and scalp (Fig. 1c, right) (the detailed method can be found elsewhere [46]). The hydrogel showed negligible pressure attenuation on the order of 1%. A plastic cone [28, 32] or a bag [37, 39] containing degassed water has been typically used to couple the acoustic path, but could not be used for freely-moving awake animals due to the possibility of water escaping out of the coupling path/container depending on the rat's dynamic behaviors (such as head-shaking and grooming).

Animal preparation for tFUS sessions

For the tFUS sessions using anesthesia, the Sprague–Dawley rats (all male, $n = 7$) were anesthetized with either ketamine/xylazine (80:10 mg/kg; intraperitoneal; i.p.) or isoflurane (initial induction with 3–4% followed by 0.5% for the maintenance, at oxygen flow rate of 2 L per min; inhalation). An attempt was made to decrease the maintenance isoflurane concentration under 0.1%, as used by previous investigations in mice [28, 29], but rats emerged from the anesthesia prematurely, and therefore, not used in the present study. The fur on the head was shaved prior to each sonication to prevent any potential blocking of the sonication. The rats were then placed on a custom-built plastic platform in a prone posture with their limbs and tail freely hanging. After positioning the headgear and the accompanying PVA hydrogel, a generic ultrasound gel (Aquasonic; Parker Laboratories, Fairfield, NJ) was applied at each interface. Subsequently, we used the transducer geometry to estimate the virtual focal spot of sonication in space, and aligned the acoustic focus to the motor areas of the tail, limbs, or whiskers (Fig. 1e) while referencing the functional atlas of the rat motor cortex [47, 48]. Once an adequate level of anesthetic plane was detected, such as irregular breathing, the sonication session was conducted. We allowed for slight adjustment in the orientation of the transducer (Fig. 1a) for eliciting motor responses. Also, tFUS was intentionally delivered to off-target locations (lateral or caudal to the target, few millimeters away and including unilateral auditory areas) to examine the spatial specificity in stimulation. After each sonication session, the FUS headgear was removed, and the rats were returned to the housing facility for a minimum of 48 h before the next session (Fig. 1c, left).

To conduct the tFUS experiment in an awake state, we applied the same experimental procedures with the following steps. To shave the fur and apply the tFUS headgear (with the coupling hydrogel), the animals were lightly anesthetized using isoflurane (induction with 3–4%) for ~5 min. Then, the rats were moved to an empty cage and allowed to recover until they fully regained their pre-anesthetic behaviors (we determined that ~20 min was sufficient across the animals). No additional anesthesia was given to detach the FUS headgear from the pedestal.

Experimental setup compatible with anesthetized/awake rats and data acquisition settings

We established experimental setups that accommodated both anesthetized and awake rats. The schematics of the implemented wearable tFUS headgear, with the transducer actuation systems, are shown in Fig. 1d. A swivel connector (slip ring with flange-736; Adafruit, New York, NY) was located above the middle of the cage/platform, granting unrestricted motion and access to a power source for actuating the transducer during the awake tFUS sessions. A data acquisition system (PowerLab 8/30 and LabChart 7; ADInstruments, Colorado Springs, CO) was used to acquire time-series data of sonication events (onset timing and duration), being synchronized with a video recording (29.97 frames per second; FPS, by QTH44; Q-See; Anaheim, CA) to analyze the location and onset timing of the movement elicited by the sonication. Additionally, a light-emitting diode (LED), turned on in-sync with each sonication

event, was placed within the field-of-view of the video recording as a visual indicator of the sonication timing (shown in Fig. 2a–c, upper panels).

Sonication parameters for repeated tFUS sessions with anesthetized/awake rats

We conducted repeated tFUS sessions using a pulsed sonication scheme across all conditions. Based on our previous studies [37], we used the acoustic parameters (Fig. 1f) as follows: pulse repetition frequency (PRF) of 500 Hz, tone burst duration (TBD) of 1 ms (i.e., a duty cycle of 50%), and sonication duration of 300 ms, with a 5–10 s inter-stimulation interval (ISI), with varying acoustic output (see below). The sonication was administered to the motor areas in the left or right (side randomized) hemisphere of the rat brain. At the initial phase of this study, we gave stimulatory tFUS to each rat brain, starting from an acoustic intensity of 2.1 W/cm^2 I$_{sppa}$, increasing in increments of ~1 W/cm^2, until the stimulatory response (i.e., movements from the tail, limbs or whiskers) was observed from the ketamine/xylazine as well as awake sessions. We determined that 14.9 W/cm^2 I$_{sppa}$ (for ketamine/xylazine anesthesia) and 8.8 W/cm^2 I$_{sppa}$ (for awake condition) were most suitable to elicit motor responses (regardless of their type) across all animals. These intensities were used in subsequent measurement of response rates. Acoustic intensity values at the target were estimated based on applying 17% of acoustic pressure attenuation through the rat skull [37].

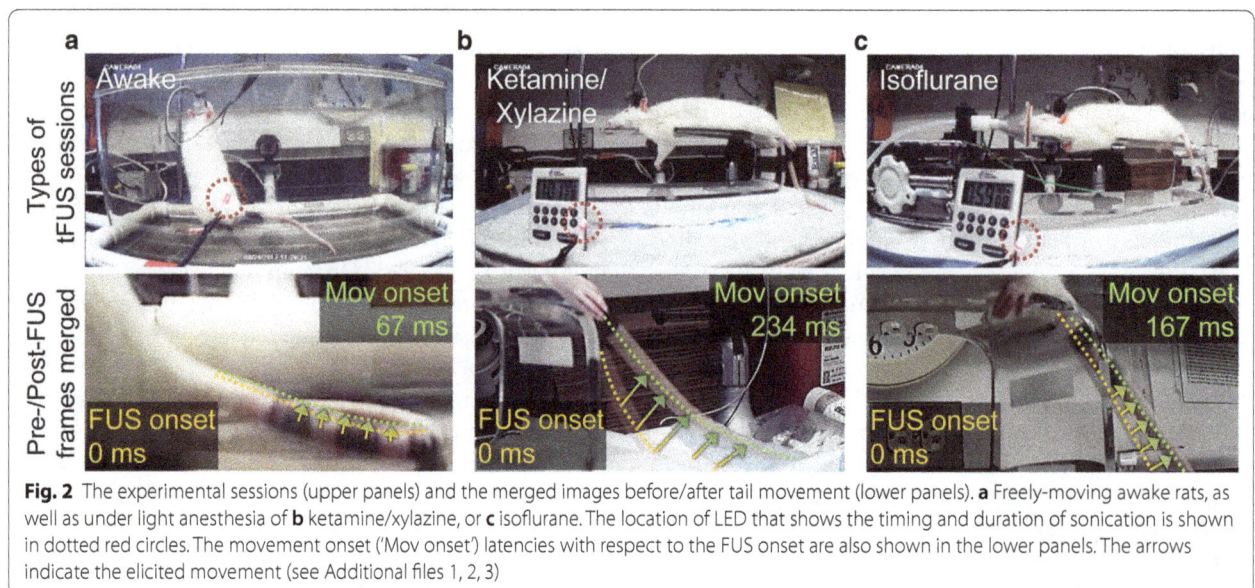

Fig. 2 The experimental sessions (upper panels) and the merged images before/after tail movement (lower panels). **a** Freely-moving awake rats, as well as under light anesthesia of **b** ketamine/xylazine, or **c** isoflurane. The location of LED that shows the timing and duration of sonication is shown in dotted red circles. The movement onset ('Mov onset') latencies with respect to the FUS onset are also shown in the lower panels. The arrows indicate the elicited movement (see Additional files 1, 2, 3)

Response rates comparison across the repeated different anesthetic/awake conditions

We examined the response rates to the sonication from the same group of animals ($n = 7$, named as 'R1' to 'R7') through three repeated tFUS sessions, under each experimental condition. The sequence of these experimental sessions was randomized and balanced. Each tFUS session consisted of a total of 10 sonication events, targeting the tail, limb, or whisker motor areas in the brain. The individual animal's mean response rates were compared using one-way analysis of variance (ANOVA) within each condition. The grand mean response rates were compared by repeated measures ANOVA and paired t-test across the conditions, with two-sample F-test for the equality of group variances.

Analysis of the FUS-mediated movement location and onset latency

The location of FUS-mediated movement and the onset latency, across all the sonication parameters, were analyzed with high-resolution videos frame-by-frame using video analysis software (Quintic Player v29; Quintic Consultancy Ltd., Sutton Coldfield, UK) by three investigators. The onset of the tFUS was identified from the frame that showed the LED light turned on. A period greater than 500 ms before and after the tFUS onset (i.e., ≥ 15 frames) was examined for each sonication event. Only frames that showed distinctive movements were used to identify the type of movement and to measure the response latency with respect to the tFUS onset. Spontaneous movements from the body (for example, breathing-related movements) or a pattern of whisker movements were excluded to isolate stimulation-specific responses for the analysis.

Examination of potential thermal effect

Potential thermal effect from the sonication was estimated using a formula of $\Delta T = 2\alpha It/(\rho_b \cdot C_p)$; where α = the absorption coefficient (0.014 cm^{-1} at ~600 kHz) [49], I = the intensity of ultrasound in the focal region, t = the ultrasound pulse duration, ρ_b = the density of brain tissue, and C_p = the specific heat of the brain tissue, where $\rho_b \cdot C_p$ is $3.796 \text{ J} \cdot \text{cm}^{-3} \cdot {}^\circ\text{C}$ [50, 51]. Using the equation, $0.016 \,^\circ\text{C}$ was the estimated thermal increase, but considering a long ISI (≥ 5 s) (Fig. 1f) and subsequent heat dissipation, in conjunction with the small size of the acoustic focus, this temperature increase was considered to be negligible. An acoustic intensity level that corresponds to the mechanical index (MI) of 1.9, maximum allowed for diagnostic ultrasound device according to the food and drug administration (FDA)-guideline [52], was 46.5 W/cm^2 I_{sppa} at 600 kHz.

Post-sonication behavior monitoring and histological assessment

The biological effects of the repeated sonication sessions were examined across the experimental conditions (awake, ketamine/xylazine, and isoflurane). During the resting and survival periods after the sonication sessions, we regularly monitored the behavior and body condition of the animal for detecting any signs that indicated undesired neurological sequelae, including pain or distress. To examine the potential tissue damage, the animals were sacrificed at short-term (sacrificed within 0.7 ± 1.2 days; $n = 3$ rats) and long-term (41.5 ± 0.6 days; $n = 4$ rats) after the end of the last sonication session using the systemic cardiac perfusion of 10% formaldehyde (i.e., the method used to euthanize the animals) under ketamine/xylazine anesthesia, and the fixed brains were harvested. The brains were sectioned along the motor cortical areas, and the presence of hemorrhage, edema, ischemia, gliosis, inflammations were examined through histological analysis. Hematoxylin & eosin (H&E) staining was used to detect cell necrosis or local recruitment of inflammatory cells. Vanadium acid fuchsin (VAF)-toluidine blue staining was used to visualize ischemic neurons. Immunohistochemistry (IHC) of glial fibrillary acidic protein (GFAP) and caspase-3 staining were performed to examine glia infiltration or signs of neurodegeneration and to detect any apoptotic activity at and around the sonicated area, respectively. Two rats belonging to the short-term assessment underwent tail vein injection of the trypan blue dye, within 1 h after the end of the last sonication session to examine the presence of BBB disruption [13].

Results

Types of elicited responses from anesthetized/awake rats

The average weight of the same group of rats ($n = 7$, 'R1–R7') was 412.7 ± 33.8 g, 395.3 ± 55.0 g, and 388.3 ± 39.6 g (mean $\pm$ SD) in the awake, ketamine/xylazine, and isoflurane conditions, respectively (no significant differences, paired t-test, two-tailed, all $p > 0.01$). Table 1 shows the types of responses elicited by sonication from the wearable tFUS headgear across the conditions. The range of acoustic intensities used for the experiment was 2.3–14.9 W/cm^2 I_{sppa} for the awake sessions, 7.5–14.9 W/cm^2 I_{sppa} for the ketamine/xylazine sessions, and 9.0–14.9 W/cm^2 I_{sppa} for the isoflurane sessions.

The responses were observed above a certain threshold of acoustic intensities, i.e., 3.4 ± 1.8 W/cm^2 I_{sppa} (mean $\pm$ SD, $n = 7$) for the awake condition, 10.2 ± 2.4 W/cm^2 I_{sppa} ($n = 7$) for the ketamine/xylazine condition, and 12.4 ± 2.8 W/cm^2 I_{sppa} ($n = 6$) for the isoflurane condition.

Table 1 FUS-mediated responses elicited during the awake (Aw), ketamine/xylazine (K/X), and isoflurane (Iso) conditions

Type of responses	Number of responsive rats		
	Aw	K/X	Iso
Tail/limbs/whiskers			
Whisker	7/7	7/7	4/7
Fore limb	5/7	7/7	6/7
Hind limb	3/7	6/7	6/7
Tail	7/7	4/7	5/7
Other responses			
Head/neck	7/7	7/7	–
Ears	7/7	1/7	–
Chewing	7/7	5/7	–

Across the experimental conditions, the number of responsive animals, out of 7 rats, was tabulated for each type of responses elicited by tFUS

The acoustic threshold levels from the awake condition were significantly lower than those observed from both anesthetic conditions (t-test, one-tailed, both $p < 0.001$) while there was no statistical difference between the ketamine/xylazine and isoflurane conditions (t-test, one-tailed, $p > 0.05$). Also, when tFUS was delivered to off-target locations (including auditory areas) or given under the effective I_{sppa}, no responses were detected.

The elicited movements were seen from either of the tail/limbs/whiskers across all experimental conditons. These movements were similar with previous rodent studies involving ketamine/xylazine anesthesia [16, 31, 37]. We also observed twitches of the head/neck/ears and chewing behaviors in the awake and ketamine/xylazine conditions (listed as 'other responses' in Table 1), individually or accompanying the movements from the tail/limbs/whiskers. Under isoflurane anesthesia, the head/neck/ears movements and chewing behaviors were not seen. In terms of their qualitative evaluation, the range of the elicited movement was generally smaller in the case of the awake condition, than those observed from the anesthetic conditions (e.g., video-frame analysis from the tail response; Fig. 2a–c; Additional files 1, 2, 3). The head/neck/ears movements and chewing behaviors in the awake condition can be found in Additional files 4, 5 and 6.

Response rates across the different conditions

The response rate was calculated from each sonication session per each rat ('R1'–'R7'), and averaged across three sessions. Each animal's mean response rates (and its standard errors) are shown in Fig. 3 across the three different conditions of (1) awake (Fig. 3a), (2) ketamine/xylazine (Fig. 3b), and (3) isoflurane sessions (Fig. 3c). In the isoflurane condition, one animal ('R2') did not show any responses to the sonication.

The mean response rate in the awake sessions ranged 56.7%–86.7% while anesthetic conditions showed much wider ranges (i.e., 36.7%–96.7% in the ketamine/xylazine sessions and 0–96.7% in the isoflurane sessions). To evaluate the inter-animal variability in mean response

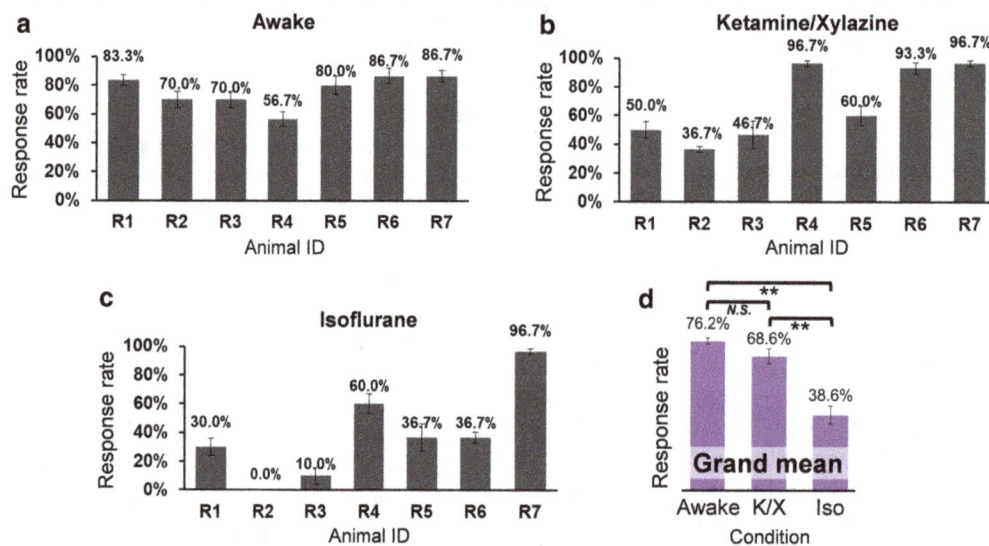

Fig. 3 Response rates of the elicited movements by sonication from the wearable FUS headgear. **a–c** Each rat's averaged response rate across three repeated sessions under each of the **a** awake, **b** ketamine/xylazine, and **c** isoflurane conditions. **d** Grand mean response rates across the same group of rats ($n = 7$ animals) under each experimental condition (paired t-test, one-tailed; $**p \leq 0.01$, N.S., non-significant; $p = 0.25$). *K/X* ketamine/xylazine, *Iso* isoflurane

rate, a one-way ANOVA was performed across the animals, and showed that the mean responses were not significantly different for the awake sessions ($p = 0.25$). On the other hand, during the anesthetic sessions, the ratio of FUS stimulation events resulted in motor response were significantly different among the animals (one-way ANOVA, $p < 0.001$ for both ketamine/xylazine and isoflurane conditions). Therefore, the data implicate that response rates were relatively even across the animals during the awake condition compared to those during the anesthetic conditions.

The overall response rate representing each condition was calculated by taking a grand mean of the response rates pooled from all rats (Fig. 3d), and revealed that both awake and ketamine/xylazine conditions showed significantly higher response rates than the isoflurane condition (repeated measures ANOVA, $p < 0.05$; augmented by paired t-test, one-tailed, $p \leq 0.01$ for both awake and ketamine/xylazine sessions compared to the isoflurane sessions). Comparisons of the grand mean response rates between the awake and ketamine/xylazine sessions did not show statistical differences (paired t-test, one-tailed, $p = 0.25$). Meanwhile, the variability of the grand mean response rate (i.e., variances or dispersions) from the awake condition was significantly decreased compared to those from both anesthetic conditions (two-sample F-test, one-tailed, both $p < 0.05$), while there was no significant difference between the ketamine/xylazine and isoflurane sessions ($p = 0.43$).

Onset latency of the elicited movements across the different conditions

The number of events describing the successful tFUS stimulation (resulting in the movement of the tail/limbs/whiskers) and the onset latency were assessed for each condition using a histogram (Fig. 4a–c). Regardless of the experimental conditions, most ($> 93\%$) of these responses were observed within a time frame of ~ 400 ms after the sonication onset. An average latency in motor responses was 139.1 ± 111.1 ms in the awake condition ($n = 510$), 212.8 ± 127.2 ms under ketamine/xylazine anesthesia ($n = 821$), and 282.9 ± 103.2 ms under isoflurane anesthesia ($n = 293$), while these latency values were significantly different to each other across the conditions (one-way ANOVA, $p < 0.001$; post hoc Tukey test, all $p < 0.001$). It is notable that the average latency of responses from the tail/limbs/whiskers in the awake condition was shorter than those under the anesthetic conditions.

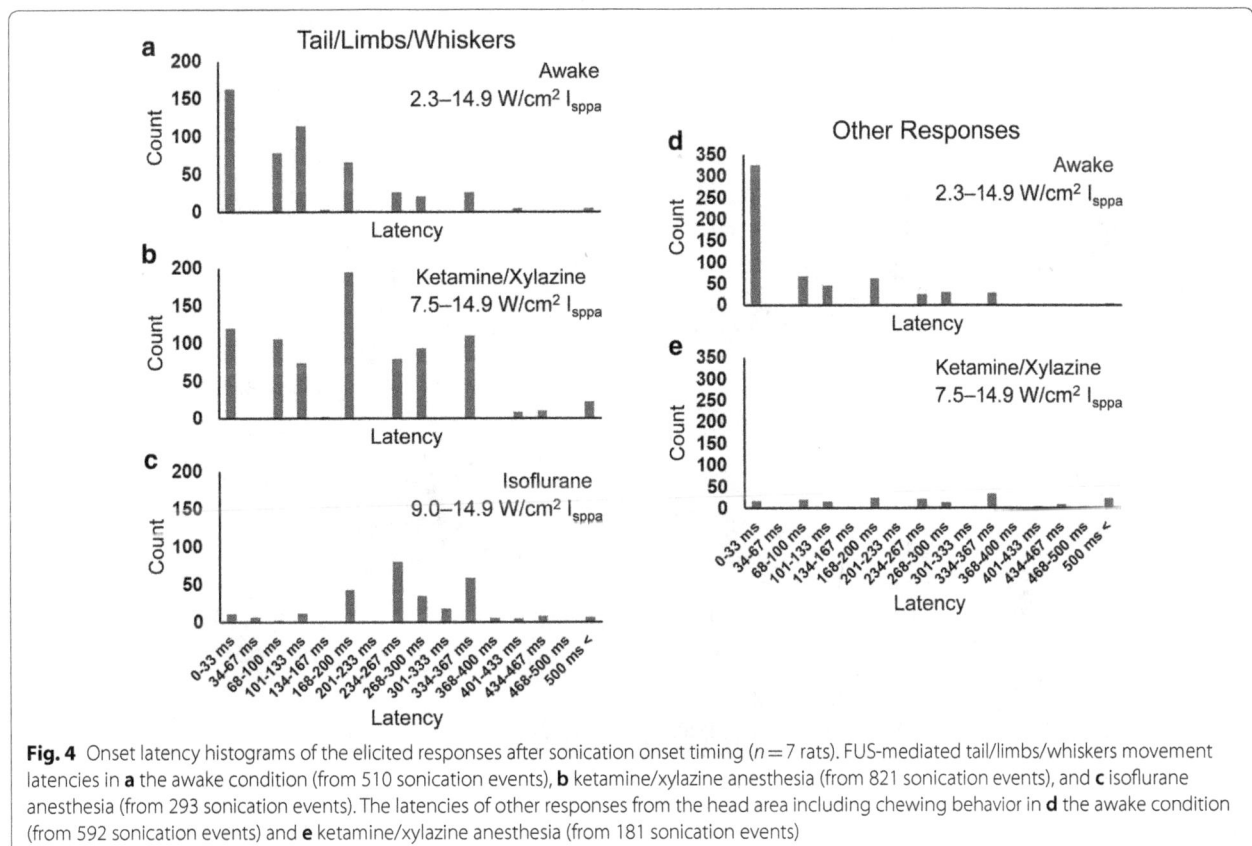

Fig. 4 Onset latency histograms of the elicited responses after sonication onset timing ($n = 7$ rats). FUS-mediated tail/limbs/whiskers movement latencies in **a** the awake condition (from 510 sonication events), **b** ketamine/xylazine anesthesia (from 821 sonication events), and **c** isoflurane anesthesia (from 293 sonication events). The latencies of other responses from the head area including chewing behavior in **d** the awake condition (from 592 sonication events) and **e** ketamine/xylazine anesthesia (from 181 sonication events)

In the awake and ketamine/xylazine conditions, we observed movements from the head/neck/ears as well as chewing behaviors (Table 1), and the same type of histogram showing its latency distributions was separately constructed (Fig. 4d and e; note that none were detected during the isoflurane sessions). The average latency of 111.9 ± 116.0 ms in the awake condition ($n = 592$) was also significantly shorter than the latency observed under ketamine/xylazine anesthesia (287.5 ± 178.0 ms; $n = 181$; t-test, one-tailed, $p < 0.001$).

To examine the presence of movement that is believed to be associated with acoustic startle responses (ASR) having short latencies (on the order of 10 ms [53–55]), we calculated the ratio of responses that occurred within 33 ms after the sonication onset (the limit of the video time frame based on 29.97 FPS), with respect to the total number of observed responses. For the tail/limbs/whiskers movements, the ratio was 32.0% in the awake condition, 14.6% under ketamine/xylazine anesthesia, and 3.8% under isoflurane anesthesia. For the head/neck/ears movements and chewing behaviors, the ratio was 55.1% in the awake condition, and 9.4% under ketamine/xylazine anesthesia. These data demonstrate that a greater portion of the responses occurred at a short latency range (< 33 ms) during the awake sessions.

Post-sonication behavioral monitoring and histological analysis

All animals showed normal behavior and health status after the sonication experiments. The histological analysis (H&E, VAF-toluidine blue, GFAP, and caspase-3 staining) performed on the sonicated brain tissues at a short-term (0.7 ± 1.2 days, $n = 3$ rats) or long-term (41.5 ± 0.6 days, $n = 4$ rats) after the last FUS session showed no apparent signs of damage (Fig. 5 shows example slides from rat 'R6'). The two rats that underwent the tail-vein trypan blue perfusion procedure did not show any signs of BBB disruption.

Discussion

A miniature FUS transducer was developed in a wearable configuration and transcranially stimulated the motor cortical areas in rats. The transducer unit was attached to an implanted pedestal for each experimental session and detached prior to returning the rats to the animal housing. The location of the acoustic focus was adjusted

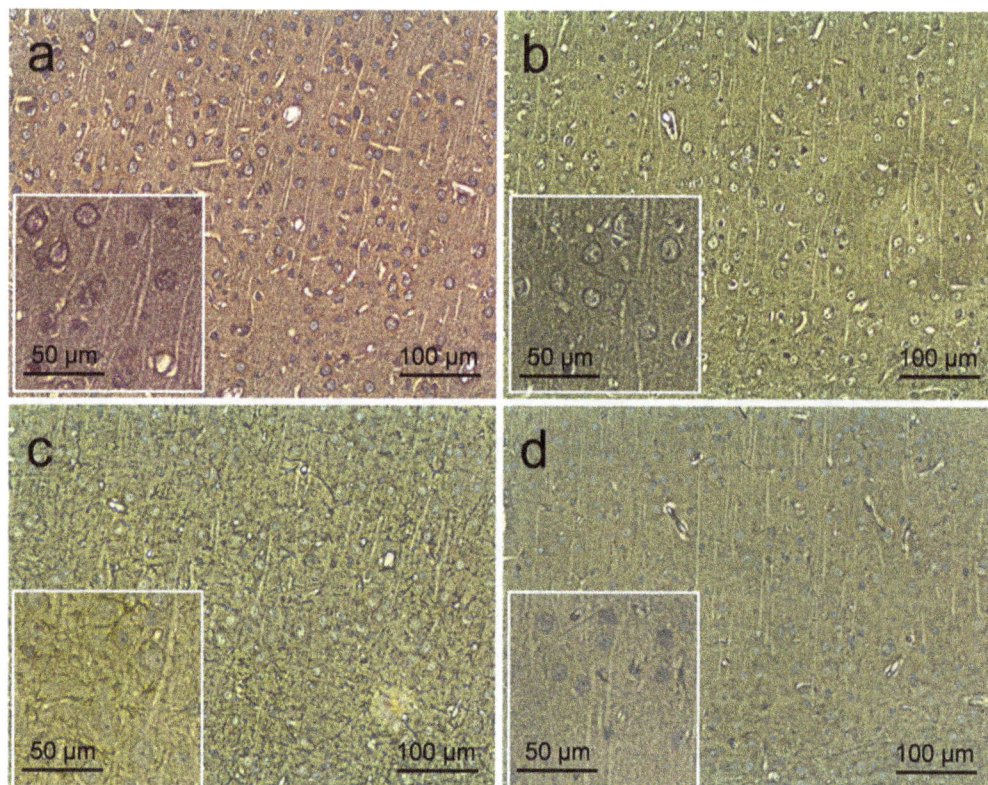

Fig. 5 Exemplar histology results from the motor cortex of one rat. The staining (for 'R6') after the repeated sonication sessions with × 100 magnification (insets with × 200 magnification) of **a** H&E, **b** VAF-toluidine blue, **c** GFAP, and **d** caspase-3. The histology revealed that all the sonicated brain tissues were normal

by the transducer applicator, having different sizes (via 3D-printing) to fit the individual cranial anatomy of the rats. The setup enabled the tFUS experiments to be conducted repeatedly in both awake and anesthetized conditions (either i.p. injection of ketamine/xylazine or isoflurane inhalation). Subsequently, it allowed for systematic condition-specific comparisons of neuromodulatory outcomes, in terms of their physical representations, and response rates/variability with onset latencies. To our knowledge, this is the first study to demonstrate the efficacy of tFUS brain stimulation in awake rats, while having comparisons with two different anesthetic conditions.

Types of elicited responses

The tFUS sonication elicited various physical motor responses across the study. Regardless of the experimental conditons, the elicited movements were seen from either of the tail/limbs/whiskers, demonstrating similiarities with previous rodent studies involving anesthesia [16, 28, 30, 31, 37]. In addition to these FUS-mediated movements, we also observed twitches from the head/neck/ears and chewing behaviors (which are new types of tFUS stimulation-related movement) in the awake and ketamine/xylazine conditions (listed as 'other responses' in Table 1). We conjecture that these new-found responses may be associated with the stimulation of corresponding motor areas due to the spatial proximity or overlap with intended motor regions for the whisker and forelimb [47, 48]. For example, imperfections in applying the sonication (e.g., mechanical slippage during application or due to the growth of cranium) can result in slight misalignments of the sonication target. Acoustic reverberation inside a small cavity of the rat skull [40, 56] with the potential to create multiple sonication foci may be another possible cause. It is also plausible that the twitches from the head/neck/ears and chewing behaviors were not seen in the previous studies due to the weight of transducer/coupling devices (water bags or plastic stand-offs were used along with much bigger/heavier transducers), which became detectable in the present study using a light-weight wearable tFUS apparatus.

Under isoflurane anesthesia, a previous mice study [29] did report neck twitching behaviors, however, head/neck/ears movements and chewing behaviors were not seen in the present study. Although the definite causes for this discrepancy is difficult to ascertain, we conjecture that the given anesthetic setting (i.e., 0.5% isoflurane) did not allow sufficient motor neuron recruitment for overt movement. Provision of adequate anesthetic planes, e.g., accomodation of much lower isoflurane concentration using sophisticated anesthetic devices supported by body temperature control [28, 29], will allow for the further exploration of physical responses to tFUS stimulation.

Acoustic intensity to elicit the responses

We found that thresholds existed, in terms of acoustic intensity, in eliciting motor responses. This is congruent with previous studies involving rodents [24, 28, 37] as well as in large animals [24] and in humans [21, 22]. The threshold acoustic intensity that started to elicit motor responses among the awake rats was much lower than those from anesthetic conditions. This finding is well-aligned with the notion that anesthesia generally suppresses neuronal excitability or dissociate the neural signal connectivity [57], which may elevate the threshold for excitation. The use of a lower acoustic intensity (in the awake condition), which will reduce overall dosimetry for the sonication, would be particularly advantageous for long and repeated FUS stimulation sessions.

Qualitative examination of the range of the elicited movements

In terms of the qualitative evaluation of the range of the elicited movement, a tail movement, for example, was smaller in the case of the awake condition than those observed from the anesthetic conditions. We speculate that the observation may be attributed to the presence of residual muscle tension during awake state or the animal's crawling postures that imposed weight to each of the limbs, which may hinder overt motor responses. Further study using measurements of strength of electromyography (EMG) or motor evoked potentials (MEP) is warranted to ascertain the electrophysiological information from FUS-mediated motor responses, especially in freely-moving awake animals.

Response rates and their variability across the different conditions

We found that there were degrees of variability in the response rates among the animals and across the experimental conditions. Existence of such variabilities in the responsiveness were congruent with previous FUS-mediated studies reporting that the types/depths of anesthesia as well as individual differences can alter response rates [24, 28, 31, 37, 40]. Further analysis of inter-animal variability on response rates, measured from the movement data for the tail/limbs/whiskers, showed that the animals during the awake sessions manifested a more consistent level of responses compared to those during the anesthetic conditions. As to the causes for this reduced variability of responses in awake condition, individual-specific responsiveness/susceptibility to the anesthetic agents [57] as well as the method of its delivery (e.g., i.p. injection of ketamine/xylazine) might have played an important role. Regarding the grand mean response rate, although there were no statistical differences between the awake and ketamine/xylazine sessions, a significant difference did exist for the awake and isoflurane settings. Taken together, the awake condition offers the advantages of higher and more consistent/reproducible response rates compared to the anesthetic conditions.

Onset latency of the elicited movements

Regarding the movement onset latency, most of the elicited responses, either from the tail/limbs/whiskers or from the head/neck/ears and chewing behaviors, were distributed within ~400 ms after the onset of the sonication event. An average latency in motor responses (from the tail/limbs/whiskers) was 139.1 ± 111.1 ms for the awake condition, 212.8 ± 127.2 ms for ketamine/xylazine, and 282.9 ± 103.2 ms for isoflurane. We note that the average onset latencies in awake rats were shorter compared to the ones from the anesthetic conditions, which may implicate that the use of anesthesia delays the onset timing of these elicited movements.

In the analysis of onset latency, intriguingly, a greater portion of responses were elicited within ~33 ms in the awake condition (over 30% for the tail/limbs/whiskers and over 50% for the head area) compared to below 15% in the anesthetic conditions. These responses having short latencies may be associated with the acoustic startle responses (ASR), known to be occurring within ~10 ms after the onset of the acoustic stimuli in rats [53–55]. Recently, Sato and colleagues reported a mice study that both ultrasound and audible sound showed similar brain activation patterns and motor response (consistent with a startle reflex) that were reduced by the chemical deafening of the animals [58], indicating that ultrasound may have an indirect link to acoustic-related (startle) effects and the elicitation of short latency responses. In this perspective, it is not surprising that awake animals, supposedly more susceptible to any external stimuli, showed a higher ratio of responses having short latencies than the anesthetic conditions. Wattiez and colleagues recently reported that cell-level acoustic neuromodulation occurs with an onset latency $\geq \sim 30$ ms [42], lending further support to the idea that responses to the sonication below this latency could be related to startle effects. In the present study, most of the stimulation-related movements were observed at much longer latency, which cannot be explained solely by the ASR. In addition, the stimulation of the auditory areas did not produce any stimulation-related movement. Taken together, our data suggests that one should be aware of the presence of ASR-like phenomena, and exert caution when interpreting the physical responses to the acoustic stimulation.

Technical limitations

In reviewing the execution of experimental settings, only the behavioral data was analyzed using video recording due to the lack of measurement of electrophysiological signals, such as EMG. As briefly discussed above, the small range of the elicited movements from awake animals made their detection difficult, which might have possibly contributed to the reduced response rates. These limitations warrant the integration of EMG measurement in future studies using freely-moving awake animals to ascertain the elicitation of the FUS-mediated motor responses. For enabling the EMG measurement from freely-moving awake animals, subdermal wires need to be implanted to the desired body/muscle parts (such as limbs or tail base) [59], whereby these wires are connected to a multi-channel electrode head pedestal that is compatible with our wearable tFUS headgear. Additional experimental modifications, such as the use of a high-speed camera, could also help to examine the response latencies with a higher time resolution.

We also note that the focal area, 3.5 mm in length and 1.0 mm in diameter measured at FW90%M of its intensity profile, can stimulate the brain regions outside the intended target (the motor cortex), reaching deeper brain structure. Since the present study did not have sufficient spatial resolutions in stimulating discrete rodent functional brain anatomy, the detailed effects of the stimulation on the response rate or the latencies could not be ascertained. We contemplate that use of large animal models (such as ovine, and corresponding larger neuroanatomy) will increase the relative spatial specificity of stimulation compared to that acquired from the rodent model, improving the assessment of region-specific effects of acoustic neuromodulation.

Safety and non-thermal mechanism

In terms of the safety profile, all the animal behaviors were normal, with no brain damage or hemorrhage, after the repeated sonication sessions during a long-term period of ~5–8 months. In our previous rat study examining sonication parameters [37], H&E histology on a rat's brain exposed to 22.4 W/cm^2 I_{sppa} (corresponding to a spatial-peak temporal-average intensity of 11.2 W/cm^2 I_{spta} with peak rarefactional pressure of 0.81 MPa, MI of 1.38) showed hemosiderin indicating potential earlier bleeding, while such signs were not observed in the present study with 14.9 W/cm^2 I_{sppa} (7.5 W/cm^2 I_{spta}, 0.67 MPa, MI of 0.86). We conjectured that the use of longer ISIs (≥ 5 s vs. previously 2 s) and lower MI, with a miniature tFUS transducer having a smaller acoustic focus, compared to those used in the previous studies, possibly prevented the occurrence of sonication related brain hemorrhage. Also, the estimated potential thermal increase of 0.016 °C (see Methods), which is believed to be negligible considering heat dissipation during the ISI (≥ 5 s) and the small size of acoustic focus, supports that the biophysical mechanism behind the tFUS stimulation of neural cells could be linked with non-thermal mechanical factors [60]. The present work utilized the sonication parameters that are compliant with safety guidelines for the diagnostic ultrasound equipment (with an exception of the maximum MI of 0.23 for ophthalmological applications). However, we note that there is neither clear consensus nor the data on the sonication parameters (such as the acoustic intensity and the MI) for safe brain tissue stimulation. Further studies are, therefore, urgently needed to establish the safety guidelines for the acoustic neuromodulation.

Conclusions

We demonstrated the application of FUS brain stimulation in a freely-moving rat model, utilizing a wearable tFUS headgear. The awake rats showed an increased response rate with reduced variability and shorter latency to FUS, in comparison with the neurostimulatory outcomes under the anesthetic conditions. Our analysis of latency distribution of responses suggests the possible involvement of ASR-like phenomena mixed with the stimulation-related physical movement. The use of small animal models, without confounding factors from anesthesia (including its unclear mechanism of action [57]), would be beneficial not only to gain further knowledge for reducing the variability (thus, may increase the reproducibility) in responsiveness to FUS but to gain more informative data regarding the potential presence of ASR. The ability to conduct FUS-mediated brain stimulation in awake small animals provides unprecedented opportunities for investigations that are not possible with anesthesia, such as sociobehavioral studies (e.g., self-administered brain stimulation [61]), or for the studies dealing with disease models that are influenced by anesthesia (e.g., epilepsy [33]).

Additional files

Additional file 1. A movie showing rat tail movement in the awake experimental condition.

Additional file 2. A movie showing rat tail movement in the ketamine/xylazine anesthetic condition.

Additional file 3. A movie showing rat tail movement in the isoflurane anesthetic condition.

Additional file 4. A movie showing rat head/neck movement in the awake experimental condition.

Additional file 5. A movie showing rat ear movement in the awake experimental condition.

Additional file 6. A movie showing rat chewing behavior in the awake experimental condition.

Abbreviations

DBS: deep brain stimulation; EpCS: epidural cortical stimulation; tDCS: transcranial direct current stimulation; TMS: transcranial magnetic stimulation; FUS: focused ultrasound; tFUS: transcranial focused ultrasound; BBB: blood–brain barrier; EEG: electroencephalographic; 3D: three-dimensional; FF: fundamental frequency; FWHM: full-width at half-maximum; FW90%M: full-width at 90%-maximum; PVA: polyvinyl alcohol; FPS: frames per second; LED: light-emitting diode; PRF: pulse repetition frequency; IPI: inter-pulse interval; TBD: tone burst duration; ISI: inter-stimulation interval; ANOVA: analysis of variance; MI: mechanical index; FDA: food and drug administration; H&E: hematoxylin & eosin; VAF: vanadium acid fuchsin; IHC: immunohistochemistry; GFAP: glial fibrillary acidic protein; N.S.: non-significant; ASR: acoustic startle responses; EMG: electromyography; MEP: motor evoked potentials; Aw: awake; K/X: ketamine/xylazine; Iso: isoflurane.

Authors' contributions

WL, PC, RWM, AC, KY, SSY participated in study design, data acquisition and analysis. WL, PC, AC, RWM performed animal surgical procedures. WL, PC, RWM, SSY prepared equipment settings. All participated in manuscript writing. All authors read and approved the final manuscript.

Acknowledgements

We thank Dr. Yongzhi Zhang for the helpful technical advice on rat surgical procedures. The initial help by Mr. Michael Y. Park is also acknowledged. We thank the Center for Comparative Medicine (CCM) of the Brigham and Women's Hospital (BWH) for the trainings on handling anesthetized and freely-moving awake animals.

Competing interests

The authors declare that they have no competing interests.

Funding

This study was supported by the Focused Ultrasound Surgery Foundation (FUS 461, to W. Lee and S.S. Yoo) and the National Institutes of Health (NIH, R01 MH111763, to S.S. Yoo).

References

1. Fregni F, Pascual-Leone A. Technology insight: noninvasive brain stimulation in neurology-perspectives on the therapeutic potential of rTMS and tDCS. Nat Clin Pract Neurol. 2007;3(7):383–93.
2. George MS, Aston-Jones G. Noninvasive techniques for probing neurocircuitry and treating illness: vagus nerve stimulation (VNS), transcranial magnetic stimulation (TMS) and transcranial direct current stimulation (tDCS). Neuropsychopharmacology. 2010;35(1).301–16.
3. Hoy KE, Fitzgerald PB. Brain stimulation in psychiatry and its effects on cognition. Nat Rev Neurol. 2010;6(5):267–75.
4. Miesenböck G. The optogenetic catechism. Science. 2009;326(5951):395–9.
5. Fry WJ, Barnard JW, Fry FJ, Brennan JF. Ultrasonically produced localized selective lesions in the central nervous system. Am J Phys Med. 1955;34(3):413–23.
6. Jolesz FA, Hynynen K, McDannold N, Tempany C. MR imaging-controlled focused ultrasound ablation: a noninvasive image-guided surgery. Magn Reson Imaging Clin N Am. 2005;13(3):545–60.
7. Lynn JG, Zwemer RL, Chick AJ, Miller AE. A new method for the generation and use of focused ultrasound in experimental biology. J Gen Physiol. 1942;26(2):179–93.

8. Hynynen K, Clement GT, McDannold N, Vykhodtseva N, King R, White PJ, Vitek S, Jolesz FA. 500-element ultrasound phased array system for non-invasive focal surgery of the brain: a preliminary rabbit study with ex vivo human skulls. Magn Reson Med. 2004;52(1):100–7.

9. Pinton G, Aubry J-F, Bossy E, Muller M, Pernot M, Tanter M. Attenuation, scattering, and absorption of ultrasound in the skull bone. Med Phys. 2012;39(1):299–307.

10. White PJ, Clement GT, Hynynen K. Longitudinal and shear mode ultrasound propagation in human skull bone. Ultrasound Med Biol. 2006;32(7):1085–96.

11. Elias WJ, Huss D, Voss T, Loomba J, Khaled M, Zadicario E, Frysinger RC, Sperling SA, Wylie S, Monteith SJ, et al. A pilot study of focused ultrasound thalamotomy for essential tremor. N Engl J Med. 2013;369(7):640–8.

12. Martin E, Jeanmonod D, Morel A, Zadicario E, Werner B. High-intensity focused ultrasound for noninvasive functional neurosurgery. Ann Neurol. 2009;66(6):858–61.

13. Cammalleri A, Croce P, Lee W, Yoon K, Yoo S-S. Therapeutic potentials of localized blood-brain barrier disruption by non-invasive transcranial focused ultrasound: A technical review. J Clin Neurophysiol. 2018; (in press).

14. Bachtold MR, Rinaldi PC, Jones JP, Reines F, Price LR. Focused ultrasound modifications of neural circuit activity in a mammalian brain. Ultrasound Med Biol. 1998;24(4):557–65.

15. Rinaldi PC, Jones JP, Reines F, Price LR. Modification by focused ultrasound pulses of electrically evoked responses from an in vitro hippocampal preparation. Brain Res. 1991;558(1):36–42.

16. Tufail Y, Matyushov A, Baldwin N, Tauchmann ML, Georges J, Yoshihiro A, Tillery SIH, Tyler WJ. Transcranial pulsed ultrasound stimulates intact brain circuits. Neuron. 2010;66(5):681–94.

17. Yoo S-S, Bystritsky A, Lee J-H, Zhang Y, Fischer K, Min B-K, McDannold NJ, Pascual-Leone A, Jolesz FA. Focused ultrasound modulates region-specific brain activity. Neuroimage. 2011;56(3):1267–75.

18. Legon W, Ai L, Bansal P, Mueller JK. Neuromodulation with single-element transcranial focused ultrasound in human thalamus. Hum Brain Mapp. 2018;39(5):1995–2006.

19. Monti MM, Schnakers C, Korb AS, Bystritsky A, Vespa PM. Non-invasive ultrasonic thalamic stimulation in disorders of consciousness after severe brain injury: a first-in-man report. Brain Stimul. 2016;9(6):940–1.

20. Lee W, Chung YA, Jung Y, Song I-U, Yoo S-S. Simultaneous acoustic stimulation of human primary and secondary somatosensory cortices using transcranial focused ultrasound. BMC Neurosci. 2016;17(1):68.

21. Lee W, Kim H, Jung Y, Song I-U, Chung YA, Yoo S-S. Image-guided transcranial focused ultrasound stimulates human primary somatosensory cortex. Sci Rep. 2015;5:8743.

22. Lee W, Kim H-C, Jung Y, Chung YA, Song I-U, Lee J-H, Yoo S-S. Transcranial focused ultrasound stimulation of human primary visual cortex. Sci Rep. 2016;6:34026.

23. Lee W, Kim S, Kim B, Lee C, Chung YA, Kim L, Yoo S-S. Non-invasive transmission of sensorimotor information in humans using an EEG/focused ultrasound brain-to-brain interface. PLoS ONE. 2017;12(6):e0178476.

24. Lee W, Lee SD, Park MY, Foley L, Purcell-Estabrook E, Kim H, Fischer K, Maeng L-S, Yoo S-S. Image-guided focused ultrasound-mediated regional brain stimulation in sheep. Ultrasound Med Biol. 2016;42(2):459–70.

25. Legon W, Sato TF, Opitz A, Mueller J, Barbour A, Williams A, Tyler WJ. Transcranial focused ultrasound modulates the activity of primary somatosensory cortex in humans. Nat Neurosci. 2014;17(2):322–9.

26. Bystritsky A, Korb AS, Douglas PK, Cohen MS, Melega WP, Mulgaonkar AP, DeSalles A, Min B-K, Yoo S-S. A review of low-intensity focused ultrasound pulsation. Brain Stimul. 2011;4(3):125–36.

27. Yoo S-S, Lee W, Jolesz FA. Chapter 23. FUS-mediated image-guided neuromodulation of the brain. In: Chen Y, Kateb B, editors. Neurophotonics and brain mapping. Boca Raton: CRC Press; 2017. p. 443–55.

28. King RL, Brown JR, Newsome WT, Pauly KB. Effective parameters for ultrasound-induced in vivo neurostimulation. Ultrasound Med Biol. 2013;39(2):312–31.

29. King RL, Brown JR, Pauly KB. Localization of ultrasound-induced in vivo neurostimulation in the mouse model. Ultrasound Med Biol. 2014;40(7):1512–22.

30. Li G-F, Zhao H-X, Zhou H, Yan F, Wang J-Y, Xu C-X, Wang C-Z, Niu L-L, Meng L, Wu S. Improved anatomical specificity of non-invasive neuro-stimulation by high frequency (5 MHz) ultrasound. Sci Rep. 2016;6:24738.

31. Mehić E, Xu JM, Caler CJ, Coulson NK, Moritz CT, Mourad PD. Increased anatomical specificity of neuromodulation via modulated focused ultrasound. PLoS ONE. 2014;9(2):e86939.

32. Ye PP, Brown JR, Pauly KB. Frequency dependence of ultrasound neuro-stimulation in the mouse brain. Ultrasound Med Biol. 2016;42(7):1512–30.

33. Min B-K, Bystritsky A, Jung K-I, Fischer K, Zhang Y, Maeng L-S, Park SI, Chung Y-A, Jolesz F, Yoo S-S. Focused ultrasound-mediated suppression of chemically-induced acute epileptic EEG activity. BMC Neurosci. 2011;12:23.

34. Min B-K, Yang PS, Bohlke M, Park S, Vago DR, Maher TJ, Yoo S-S. Focused ultrasound modulates the level of cortical neurotransmitters: potential as a new functional brain mapping technique. Int J Imaging Syst Technol. 2011;21(2):232–40.

35. Yang PS, Kim H, Lee W, Bohlke M, Park S, Maher TJ, Yoo S-S. Transcranial focused ultrasound to the thalamus is associated with reduced extracellular GABA levels in rats. Neuropsychobiology. 2012;65(3):153–60.

36. Yoo S-S, Kim H, Min B-K, Franck E, Park S. Transcranial focused ultrasound to the thalamus alters anesthesia time in rats. NeuroReport. 2011;22(15):783–7.

37. Kim H, Chiu A, Lee SD, Fischer K, Yoo S-S. Focused ultrasound-mediated non-invasive brain stimulation: examination of sonication parameters. Brain Stimul. 2014;7(5):748–56.

38. Kim H, Lee SD, Chiu A, Yoo S-S, Park S. Estimation of the spatial profile of neuromodulation and the temporal latency in motor responses induced by focused ultrasound brain stimulation. NeuroReport. 2014;25(7):475–9.

39. Kim H, Park M-A, Wang S, Chiu A, Fischer K, Yoo S-S. PET/CT imaging evidence of FUS-mediated (18)F-FDG uptake changes in rat brain. Med Phys. 2013;40(3):033501.

40. Younan Y, Deffieux T, Larrat B, Fink M, Tanter M, Aubry J-F. Influence of the pressure field distribution in transcranial ultrasonic neurostimulation. Med Phys. 2013;40(8):082902.

41. Deffieux T, Younan Y, Wattiez N, Tanter M, Pouget P, Aubry J-F. Low-intensity focused ultrasound modulates monkey visuomotor behavior. Curr Biol. 2013;23(23):2430–3.

42. Wattiez N, Constans C, Deffieux T, Daye PM, Tanter M, Aubry J-F, Pouget P. Transcranial ultrasonic stimulation modulates single-neuron discharge in macaques performing an antisaccade task. Brain Stimul. 2017;10(6):1024–31.

43. Kim H, Chiu A, Park S, Yoo S-S. Image-guided navigation of single-element focused ultrasound transducer. Int J Imaging Syst Technol. 2012;22(3):177–84.

44. Yoo S-S, Yoon K, Croce P, Cammalleri A, Margolin RW, Lee W. Focused ultrasound brain stimulation to anesthetized rats induces long-term changes in somatosensory evoked potentials. Int J Imaging Syst Technol. 2018;28(2):106–12.

45. Li G, Qiu W, Zhang Z, Jiang Q, Su M, Cai R, Li Y, Cai F, Deng Z, Xu D et al. Noninvasive ultrasonic neuromodulation in freely moving mice. IEEE Trans Biomed Eng. 2018; (in press).

46. Lee W, Lee SD, Park MY, Yang J, Yoo S-S. Evaluation of polyvinyl alcohol cryogel as an acoustic coupling medium for low-intensity transcranial focused ultrasound. Int J Imaging Syst Technol. 2014;24(4):332–8.

47. Fonoff ET, Pereira JF, Camargo LV, Dale CS, Pagano RL, Ballester G, Teixeira MJ. Functional mapping of the motor cortex of the rat using transdural electrical stimulation. Behav Brain Res. 2009;202(1):138–41.

48. Tennant KA, Adkins DL, Donlan NA, Asay AL, Thomas N, Kleim JA, Jones TA. The organization of the forelimb representation of the C57BL/6 mouse motor cortex as defined by intracortical microstimulation and cytoarchitecture. Cereb Cortex. 2011;21(4):865–76.

49. Goss SA, Frizzell LA, Dunn F. Ultrasonic absorption and attenuation in mammalian tissues. Ultrasound Med Biol. 1979;5(2):181–6.

50. Elwassif MM, Kong Q, Vazquez M, Bikson M. Bio-heat transfer model of deep brain stimulation-induced temperature changes. J Neural Eng. 2006;3(4):306–15.

51. O'Brien WD. Ultrasound—biophysics mechanisms. Prog Biophys Mol Biol. 2007;93(1–3):212–55.

52. Duck FA. Medical and non-medical protection standards for ultrasound and infrasound. Prog Biophys Mol Biol. 2007;93(1–3):176–91.

53. Gómez-Nieto R, Horta-Júnior JDAC, Castellano O, Millian-Morell L, Rubio ME, López DE. Origin and function of short-latency inputs to the

neural substrates underlying the acoustic startle reflex. Front Neurosci. 2014;8:216.

54. Pilz PK, Schnitzler HU. Habituation and sensitization of the acoustic startle response in rats: amplitude, threshold, and latency measures. Neurobiol Learn Mem. 1996;66(1):67–79.

55. Yeomans JS, Li L, Scott BW, Frankland PW. Tactile, acoustic and vestibular systems sum to elicit the startle reflex. Neurosci Biobehav Rev. 2002;26(1):1–11.

56. Yoon K, Lee W, Croce P, Cammalleri A, Yoo S-S. Multi-resolution simulation of focused ultrasound propagation through ovine skull from a single-element transducer. Phys Med Biol. 2018;63(10):105001.

57. Århem P, Klement G, Nilsson J. Mechanisms of anesthesia: towards integrating network, cellular, and molecular level modeling. Neuropsychopharmacology. 2003;28(S1):S40–7.

58. Sato T, Shapiro MG, Tsao DY. Ultrasonic neuromodulation causes widespread cortical activation via an indirect auditory mechanism. Neuron. 2018;98(5):1031–41.

59. Towne C, Montgomery KL, Iyer SM, Deisseroth K, Delp SL. Optogenetic control of targeted peripheral axons in freely moving animals. PLoS ONE. 2013;8(8):e72691.

60. Kubanek J, Shukla P, Das A, Baccus SA, Goodman MB. Ultrasound elicits behavioral responses through mechanical effects on neurons and ion channels in a simple nervous system. J Neurosci. 2018;38(12):3081–91.

61. Olds J. Pleasure centers in the brain. Sci Am. 1956;195(4):105–17.

Late administration of high-frequency electrical stimulation increases nerve regeneration without aggravating neuropathic pain in a nerve crush injury

Hong-Lin Su[1†], Chien-Yi Chiang[2†], Zong-Han Lu[2], Fu-Chou Cheng[3], Chun-Jung Chen[3], Meei-Ling Sheu[4], Jason Sheehan[5] and Hung-Chuan Pan[2,6*] [ID]

Abstract

Background: High-frequency transcutaneous neuromuscular electrical nerve stimulation (TENS) is currently used for the administration of electrical current in denervated muscle to alleviate muscle atrophy and enhance motor function; however, the time window (i.e. either immediate or delayed) for achieving benefit is still undetermined. In this study, we conducted an intervention of sciatic nerve crush injury using high-frequency TENS at different time points to assess the effect of motor and sensory functional recovery.

Results: Animals with left sciatic nerve crush injury received TENS treatment starting immediately after injury or 1 week later at a high frequency(100 Hz) or at a low frequency (2 Hz) as a control. In SFI gait analysis, either immediate or late admission of high-frequency electrical stimulation exerted significant improvement compared to either immediate or late administration of low-frequency electrical stimulation. In an assessment of allodynia, immediate high frequency electrical stimulation caused a significantly decreased pain threshold compared to late high-frequency or low-frequency stimulation at immediate or late time points. Immunohistochemistry staining and western blot analysis of S-100 and NF-200 demonstrated that both immediate and late high frequency electrical stimulation showed a similar effect; however the effect was superior to that achieved with low frequency stimulation. Immediate high frequency electrical stimulation resulted in significant expression of TNF-α and synaptophysin in the dorsal root ganglion, somatosensory cortex, and hippocampus compared to late electrical stimulation, and this trend paralleled the observed effect on somatosensory evoked potential. The CatWalk gait analysis also showed that immediate electrical stimulation led to a significantly high regularity index. In primary dorsal root ganglion cells culture, high-frequency electrical stimulation also exerted a significant increase in expression of TNF-α, synaptophysin, and NGF in accordance with the in vivo results.

Conclusion: Immediate or late transcutaneous high-frequency electrical stimulation exhibited the potential to stimulate the motor nerve regeneration. However, immediate electrical stimulation had a predilection to develop neuropathic pain. A delay in TENS initiation appears to be a reasonable approach for nerve repair and provides the appropriate time profile for its clinical application.

Keywords: Transcutaneous electrical stimulation, Nerve regeneration, Dorsal root ganglion cell, Neuropathic pain

*Correspondence: hcpan2003@yahoo.com.tw
†Hong-Lin Su and Chien-Yi Chiang contributed equally to this work.
[2] Department of Neurosurgery, Taichung Veterans General Hospital, 1650 Taiwan Boulevard Sec. 4, 40705 Taichung, Taiwan
Full list of author information is available at the end of the article

Backgrounds

Any type of nerve repair causes a period of short or long-term change in the connection between the muscle and nerve. The target muscle stayed denervated for several weeks even after immediate repair, leading to denervation-associated atrophy. A more direct method to minimize muscle atrophy is to stimulate the muscle electrically [1, 2]. In general, short-term electrical muscle stimulation after nerve repair potentially reduces muscle atrophy [3, 4]. Although several studies have reported the use of electrical stimulation after immediate nerve repair, the length and stimulation parameter was not adequately determined and these factors remain the subject of debate [5–9].

Neuromuscular electrical stimulation is performed by the application of electrical current directly to the skin surface and underlying muscle to induce a muscle contraction, as well as to retard muscle atrophy during the period of reinnervation [10]. In a prospective, nonrandomized trial, high-tone external muscle stimulation resulted in improvement of tingling, burning, pain, and numbness in diabetic and uremic neuropathy patients [11]. In another study, following external long-term muscle electrical stimulation in uremic neuropathy patients, physical capacity and ulnar motor conduction velocity were markedly improved [12]. To attenuate muscle atrophy and improve function of denervated muscle, stimuli should be applied several times a day at sufficient intensity, pulse duration, and frequency [13].

On the contrary, electrical stimulation can have a detrimental effect in nerve regeneration after crush injury. The transcutaneous electrical stimulation altered the morphology of axon with dark axoplasma, edema, and disorganized cytoarchitecture. In addition, a decrease in axon number was also observed with thinner myelination but with an increased number of Schwann cell nuclei [14]. Electrical stimulation reduced the muscle excitability, neural cell adhesion molecule expression, the integrity of neuromuscular junctions and muscle fiber cross sectional area [6, 8, 13, 15]. Furthermore, a delay of longer than 3 months for stimulation did not increase muscle re-innervation [16]. The stimulation of a partially innervated muscle can also have adverse effects for the remaining nerves because nerve connections to the muscle are formed in an asynchronizing manner, and stimulation at this time compromised functional reinnveration [3].

The timing to start electrical stimulation is very controversial. The significant improvement in twitching tension of crushed nerve was noted only when ES was applied during the middle period (day 12–21) after nerve crush, however, no difference was observed at other time points, suggesting the stimulatory effect occurred only occurred in a specific time window [17]. ES may exert an inhibitory effect on the functional neuromuscular recovery when administered daily while axons are renewed along the distal nerve stump but before they reach the muscle fibers [6].

Based on a previous review, several controversies exist, including the time profile for initiating neuromuscular stimulation, i.e., immediate, early or delay; electrical frequency; and intensity. In this study, animals with sciatic nerve injury were subjected to the electrical neuromuscular stimulation at the different time profiles and at different stimulation frequencies and intensities to assess the alteration in neurobehavior, electrophysiology, and the associated protein expression. In addition, a primary culture of dorsal root ganglion cells was used to investigate the response by the electrical current.

Methods

Nerve crush injury model

Male Sprague–Dawley rats weighing 250–300 g (bought from BioLASCO Taiwan Co.) were used and were anesthetized using isoflurane at 4% in the induction period and 1% in maintenance period. The gluteal splitting method was used to expose left sciatic nerve under the microscope, and the nerve was crushed using a vessel clamp 10 mm from the obturator [18]. The animals were randomly allocated into one of six groups as follows: Group I: sham (n=6); Group II: nerve crush injury as control (n=6); Group III (HFI): high-frequency (100 Hz) percutaneous electrical stimulation administered immediately (n=12); Group IV (HFL): high-frequency (100 Hz) percutaneous electrical stimulation administrated 7 days after nerve crush (n=12). Group V (LFI): low-frequency (5 Hz) percutaneous electrical stimulation administered immediately (n=6); Group VI (LFL): low-frequency (5 Hz) percutaneous electrical stimulation administrated 7 days after nerve crush (n=6). The electrical stimulation paradigm featured a treatment consisting of stimulation for 30 min per day for 7 consecutive days using 400 ms of biphasic pulses at 200 µs per phase and 100 or 5 Hz frequency and with 6 s of rest (ElePulsHV-F125, Omron, Japan) [19]. Food and water were provided ad libitum before and after the operation. The animal housing environment was kept under the appropriate condition with 2 animals in a single cage, in a temperature-controlled environment at 20 °C and with alternating light and dark cycles with 12-h intervals. After the experiment, all animals were euthanized using CO_2. The care and operation of all animals followed the guidelines recommended by Taichung Veterans General Hospital Institutional Animal Care and Use Committee (IACUC) (Permission No.La-1061455).

Analysis of motor function recovery

A technician blindly assessed the SFI in the various groups of animals before operation and weekly after the surgery according to our previous report [20, 21]. Several essential parameters were taken from the footprint and all measurements were taken in the experimental and control groups. An SFI of 0 indicated normal function and − 100 represented total loss of motor function.

Nociceptive behaviors

Mechanical allodynia was tested blindly by using von Frey hairs (Touch-Test Sensory Evaluator, North Coast Medical, Inc), as previously described by our group [20, 21]. Von Frey hairs were applied in a series of grams to touch the hind paw bilaterally five times for 5-s intervals when the hind paw was placed appropriately on the platform. The withdrawal threshold was considered to be the force (gram) of the hair that caused hind-paw withdrawal in at least four out of the five applications. Thermal hyperalgesia was evaluated via a hot-plate test (Technical& Scientific Equipment GmbH, TSE systems) according to the pervious procedure [21]. The withdrawal latency was recorded as the interval of the time from which the rat touched the 52 °C hotplate to the time of withdrawal of the paw. A maximal cut-off of twenty-seconds was used to prevent paw tissue injury.

Catwalk gait analysis

The CatWalk XT gait analysis has been previously described by our group [21]. Quantitative analysis of the data included the following parameters: step sequence distribution, regularity index (RI), print area, duration of swing and stance phases, and intensity. The data were presented as the ratio of the measurement for the left side divided by that for the right side.

Evoked potential of the somatosensory cortex

Evoked potential measurements have been previously published by our group [20, 21]. In brief, one active electrode was threaded into the dural surface of the somatosensory area (3 mm lateral and 2 mm posterior to the bregma). Another electrode was placed as a reference over the maxillary area at approximately 20 mm from the active electrode. A stimulation intensity of 20 mA with 20–2000 Hz filtration was applied over the sciatic nerve 1 cm proximal to the injury area. The data for conduction latency and evoked potential were presented as the ratio of the measurement for the right side to the left side, to minimize the effects of anesthesia.

Isolation and cultured dorsal root ganglion cells (DRGs) subjected to electrical stimulation

Dorsal root ganglia cells were dissected from embryonic Sprague–Dawley rat at the embryonic days 14–15 according to previous report [20, 22, 23]. The DRGs were incubated with 0.25% trypsin at 37 °C for 15 min and were dissociated, washed and re-suspended with Neurobasal medium containing 2% B27 (sigma, Inc.), 0.3% L-glutamine and 100 ng/ml nerve growth factor. Finally, these cells were cultured in the dish at a density of 1×10^4 cells per ml of medium (16-well array station, ECIS model 800). Next, the cells were maintained and cultured in an incubator at 37 °C and 5% CO_2. The cells were recognized by neuronal markers (βIII tubulin) before the experimental process and were subjected to electrical stimulation for duration of 30 min at frequencies of 5 and 100 Hz with 50 mA.

Western blot analysis

The distal end of the nerve, muscles, dorsal root ganglion cells, and brain (hippocampus/cortex) were harvested 4 weeks after the various treatment and proteins were extracted. The cell lysate of dorsal root ganglion cells after electrical stimulation were collected to determine the expression of synaptophysin, TNF-α, and NGF. Proteins (50 μg) were resolved by SDS–polyacrylamide gel electrophoresis and were transferred onto a blotting membrane [20]. After blocking with non-fat milk, the membranes were incubated with antibodies against S-100 (Neomarkers, 1:500 dilution), NF (Cellsignal, 1:1000 dilution), synaptophysin (Abcam, 1:500 dilution), TNF-α (Abcam, 1:1000 dilution), and NGF-R (1:1000, Abbiotec) overnight at 4 °C. The intensity of the protein bands was determined by a computer image analysis system (IS1000, Alpha Innotech Corporation, CA, USA).

Immunohistochemistry staining

Dorsal root ganglion cell culture after electrical stimulation and serial 8-mm-thick section of nerve, muscle, dorsal root ganglion cells, and the brain were cut using a cryostat, and mounted on superfrost/plus slides (Menzel-Glaser, Braunschweig, Germany) were subjected to immunohistochemistry using antibodies against NGF-R (1:1000, Abbiotec), S-100(1:200, Serotec), neurofilament(1:200, Millipore), anti-synaptophysin (Abcam, 1:200 dilution), and anti-TNF-α (Abcam, 1:300 dilution) to detect the inflammatory response associated with nerve regeneration in sciatic nerve, dorsal root ganglion cells, and the brain. The immunoreactive signals were observed using AF 488 donkey anti–mouse IgG and AF594 donkey anti–rabbit

(Invitrogen; 1:200 dilutions) and were then viewed using an Olympus BX40 Research Microscope.

Statistical analysis

Data are expressed as the mean $\pm$ SE (standard error). The SFI and CatWalk data were analyzed via repeated-measure ANOVA followed by Bonferroni's multiple comparison method. The statistical significance of the differences among the groups was determined via one-way analysis of variance (ANOVA) followed by Dunnett's test. A p value < 0.05 was considered significant.

Results

Immediate high-frequency electrical stimulation caused significant motor function improvement but cause a predisposition to neuropathic pain

These animals were subjected to different treatments evaluated by SFI (motor function) and mechanical withdrawal threshold (sensory function), as illustrated in Fig. 1. SFI analysis demonstrated no significant improvement after low-frequency electrical stimulation with either immediate or late treatment compared to that in the control group. High-frequency stimulation, immediate electrical stimulation exerted a significant improvement as early as at day 7 with a steeper slope compared to that in the other groups. However, late electrical stimulation delayed improvement in the beginning but reached

the effects observed with immediate high-frequency treatment at day 14. Overall, only high-frequency stimulation-either immediate or late-showed the significant improvement in motor function compared to the control or low-frequency electrical stimulation (Fig. 1a).

In the mechanical withdrawal threshold assessment, a significant decrease in mechanical withdrawal was observed after immediate high-frequency treatment compared to that observed in the other groups. There were no significant differences in mechanical withdrawal among the control, HFL, LFI, and LFL groups (Fig. 1b). These observations suggest that immediate high-frequency electrical stimulation exerted a significant enhancement of motor function from the early period that lasted to the final point of assessment; however, this stimulation carried a higher risk of neuropathic pain. The late high-frequency electrical stimulation showed delayed improvement of motor function compared to that in the HFI group but approached the final outcome of the HFI group, without the development of neuropathic pain.

Based on the above assumption and in accordance with the guidelines of NC3Rs Animal Research: Reporting In Vivo Experiments (ARRIVE), to reduce the numbers of animals used in experimental studies, the remaining part of the study focused on determining the appropriate time profile to initiate the TENS treatment of high-frequency electrical stimulation through either immediate or late administration (Additional file 1).

High-frequency electrical stimulation increased nerve myelination either immediate or late administration

For further confirmation of the nerve regeneration potential subjected to immediate or late high-frequency electrical stimulation, the sciatic nerve was harvested one month after injury. Theses nerves were subjected to immunohistochemistry analysis of S-100 and neurofilament (Fig. 2a, b). There was a significantly higher expression of myelination markers such as S-100 and neurofilament for immediate and late high-frequency electrical stimulation compared to that for the control and immediate low-frequency electrical stimulation (Fig. 2c). This result suggested that high-frequency electrical stimulation through either immediate or late administration exhibited potential for nerve regeneration.

Immediate high-frequency electrical stimulation caused higher expression of the inflammatory response in the dorsal root ganglion and brain

Synaptophysin and TNF-α expression in the dorsal root ganglion and the somatosensory cortex and hippocampus represents the severity of neuropathic pain. Immediate high-frequency electrical stimulation resulted in a significantly higher expression of synaptophysin and

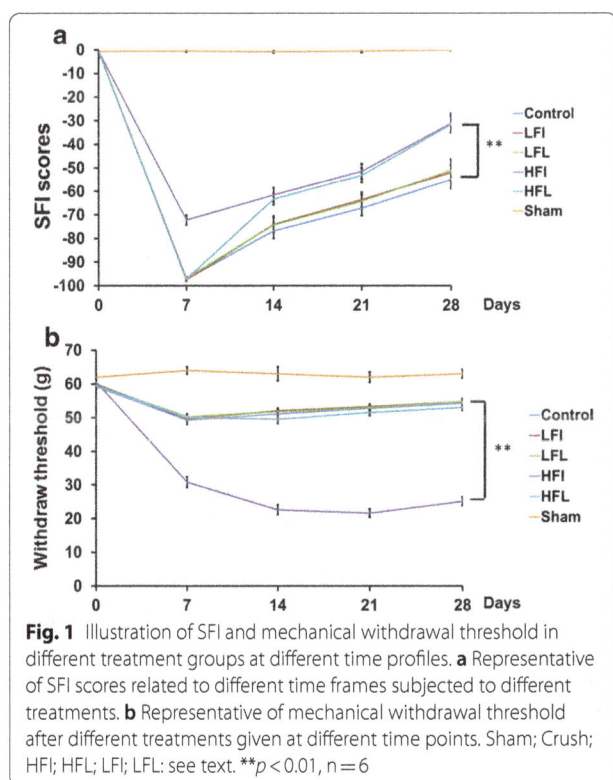

Fig. 1 Illustration of SFI and mechanical withdrawal threshold in different treatment groups at different time profiles. **a** Representative of SFI scores related to different time frames subjected to different treatments. **b** Representative of mechanical withdrawal threshold after different treatments given at different time points. Sham; Crush; HFI; HFL; LFI; LFL: see text. **$p < 0.01$, n = 6

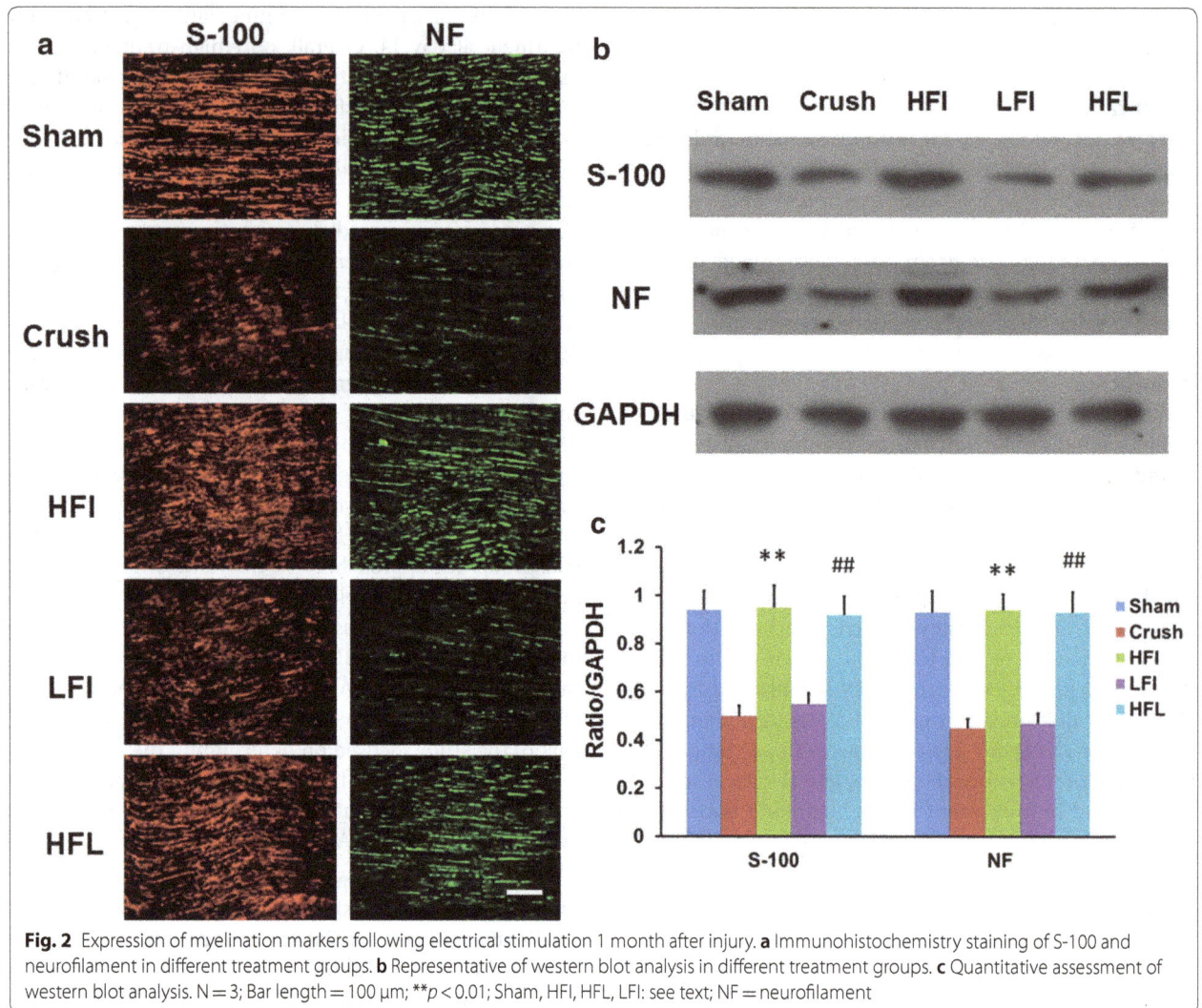

Fig. 2 Expression of myelination markers following electrical stimulation 1 month after injury. **a** Immunohistochemistry staining of S-100 and neurofilament in different treatment groups. **b** Representative of western blot analysis in different treatment groups. **c** Quantitative assessment of western blot analysis. N = 3; Bar length = 100 μm; **$p < 0.01$; Sham, HFI, HFL, LFI: see text; NF = neurofilament

TNF-α in the dorsal root ganglion compared to the control treatment or high-frequency late electrical stimulation (Fig. 3a–c). Higher expression of synaptophysin and TNF-α in the somatosensory cortex and hippocampus was also noted in the immediate group compared to that in the late high-frequency and control groups (Fig. 4a–c).

Alteration of CatWalk gait analysis and increased evoked potential in the somatosensory cortex after immediate high-frequency electrical stimulation

The Catwalk gait analysis was used to examine the motor and sensory functions. Increased intensity, decreased stance, increased swing, and decreased regularity are indicative of motor function improvement. However, increased neuropathic pain produces the opposite trend. Late high-frequency electrical stimulation produces significant improvements in intensity, stance, swing, and regularity index compared to immediate high-frequency electrical stimulation or the control groups (Fig. 5a–d). This phenomenon was because the effect of immediate high-frequency electrical stimulation in motor function was compromised by the increased sensory functional impairment.

Increased evoked potential in the central nervous system is positively correlated with a peripheral nervous system injury. The increased evoked potential amplitudes in the somatosensory cortex were significantly higher after immediate high-frequency electrical stimulation than after late high-frequency electrical stimulation or the control (Fig. 6a, b). The somatosensory evoked potential data further confirmed the alteration in the neurobehavioral and histomorphological characteristics.

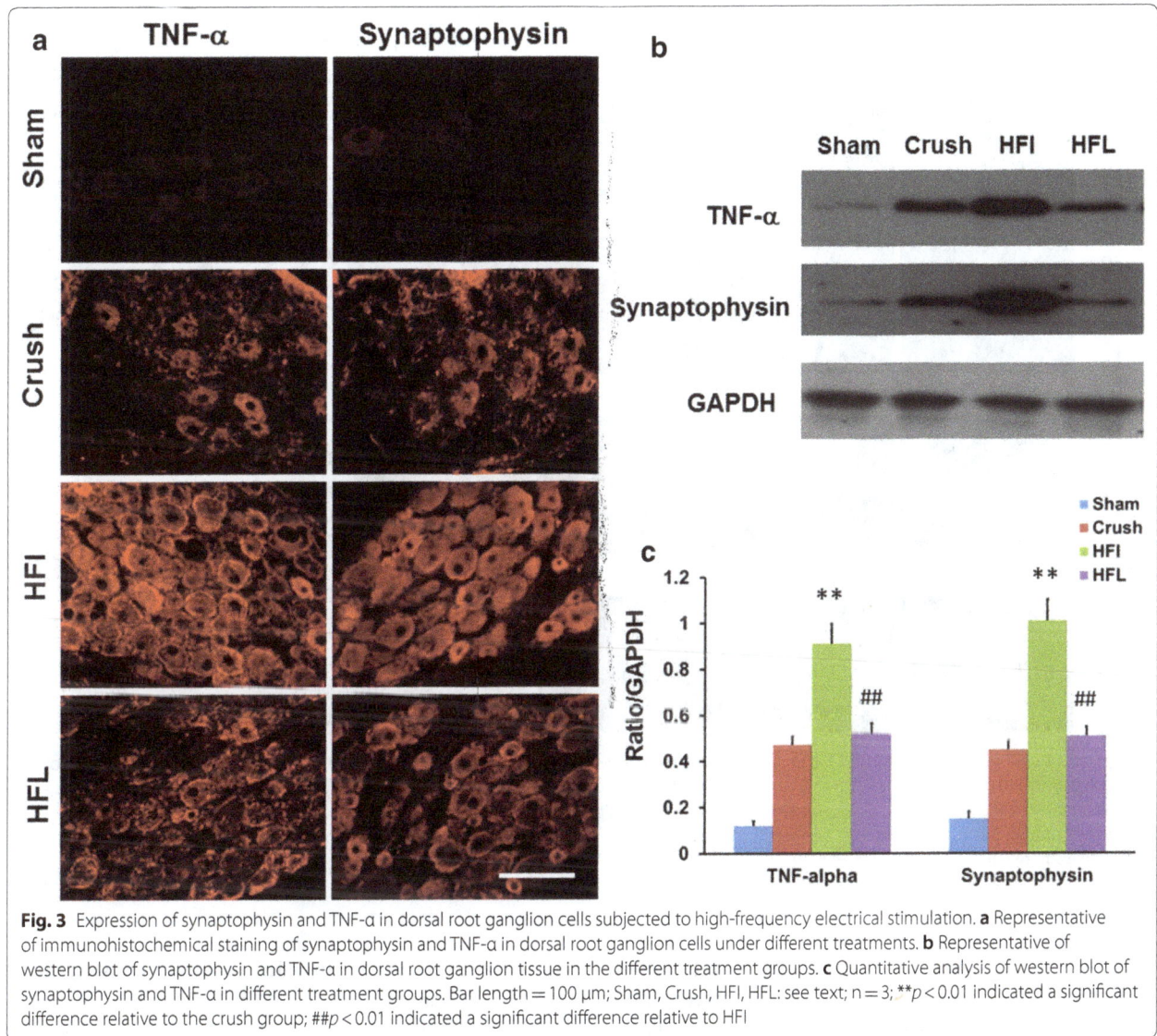

Fig. 3 Expression of synaptophysin and TNF-α in dorsal root ganglion cells subjected to high-frequency electrical stimulation. **a** Representative of immunohistochemical staining of synaptophysin and TNF-α in dorsal root ganglion cells under different treatments. **b** Representative of western blot of synaptophysin and TNF-α in dorsal root ganglion tissue in the different treatment groups. **c** Quantitative analysis of western blot of synaptophysin and TNF-α in different treatment groups. Bar length = 100 μm; Sham, Crush, HFI, HFL: see text; n = 3; **$p < 0.01$ indicated a significant difference relative to the crush group; ##$p < 0.01$ indicated a significant difference relative to HFI

Electrical stimulation induced the expression of the inflammatory response in dorsal root ganglion cell culture

To assess the inflammatory response in dorsal root ganglion cells stimulated by direct electrical stimulation, dorsal root ganglion cells were harvested and subjected to electrical stimulation. Immunohistochemistry staining demonstrated that there was increased expression of synaptophysin, TNF-α and NGF-R in the dorsal root ganglion cell culture, which was related to the difference in intensity of the electrical stimulation frequency (Fig. 7a, b). Quantitative analysis demonstrated significantly higher expression of synaptophysin, TNF-α and NGF-R after high-frequency electrical stimulation compared to that after low-frequency electrical stimulation and the

sham (Fig. 7c). Hence, high-frequency electrical stimulation harbored the potential to stimulate the dorsal root ganglion cells to express the inflammation associated proteins.

Discussion

High-frequency electrical stimulation harbored the potential to better augment nerve regeneration compared to low-frequency electrical stimulation; however, their regeneration ability was compromised by their direct electrical effect on sensory function impairment. Thus, the appropriate time profile to start the treatment after nerve injury is unclear. In this study, we found that high-frequency electrical stimulation more effectively primed dorsal root ganglion cells to express inflammatory

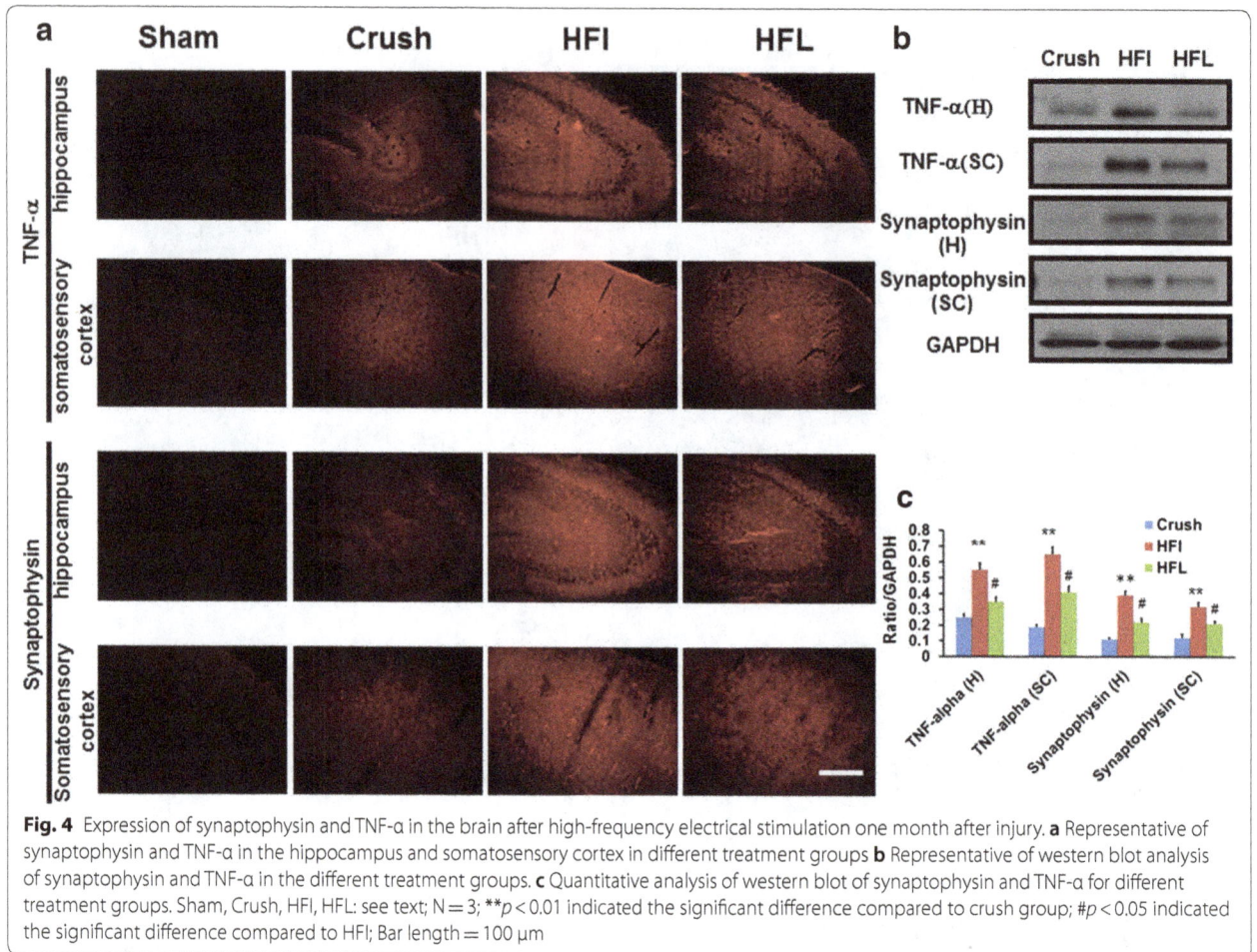

Fig. 4 Expression of synaptophysin and TNF-α in the brain after high-frequency electrical stimulation one month after injury. **a** Representative of synaptophysin and TNF-α in the hippocampus and somatosensory cortex in different treatment groups **b** Representative of western blot analysis of synaptophysin and TNF-α in the different treatment groups. **c** Quantitative analysis of western blot of synaptophysin and TNF-α for different treatment groups. Sham, Crush, HFI, HFL: see text; N = 3; **$p < 0.01$ indicated the significant difference compared to crush group; #$p < 0.05$ indicated the significant difference compared to HFI; Bar length = 100 μm

cytokines such as TNF-α, synaptophysin, and NGF. In animal studies, significantly increased nerve regeneration was noted after high-frequency electrical stimulation administrated either immediately or late; however, immediate electrical stimulation exhibited a higher potential to lead to neuropathic pain. A delay in high-frequency electrical stimulation appeared to be an appropriate time to initiate the electrical stimulation after nerve injury.

Electrical stimulation plays an important role in the treatment of neuromuscular junction disease. There are many method and types of electrical stimulation. The most common method of transcutaneous electrical stimulation used an electrical current of 90-130 Hz [24]. In another study, immediate high-frequency (100 Hz) electrical stimulation of the muscle exerted significantly a significant increase in the expression of neurotrophic factors, which contributed to neurological improvement [25]. In a diabetes animal study, high-frequency electrical stimulation (200 Hz) exerted a greater myelination effect than low-frequency stimulation (20 Hz) [26]. In contrast, a low-frequency percutaneous electrical stimulation of

2 Hz enhanced the mean value of axonal density, blood vessel number and axon outgrowth through the nerve graft [27, 28]. In our study, we found that high-frequency percutaneous electrical stimulation better improved the neurological outcome including neurobehavior and maturation of myelinization compared to low-frequency electrical stimulation. The results paralleled previous studies that demonstrated that high-frequency electrical stimulation contributing to better nerve regeneration potential than low-frequency electrical stimulation.

Percutaneous electrical stimulation was shown to alleviate pain in cases of musculoskeletal pain, arthritis pain, low back pain, neuropathic pain, and post-operative pain [22, 23, 29, 30]. Low-frequency electrical stimulation induced analgesia by inhibiting pain transmission through the recruitment of the descending inhibitory system; however, high-frequency (80–100 Hz) stimulation activated the gate control by stimulation A-beta fibers [31].There were various inconsistencies amongst previous studies with respect to the therapeutic effect according to the frequencies tested [32]. In our study,

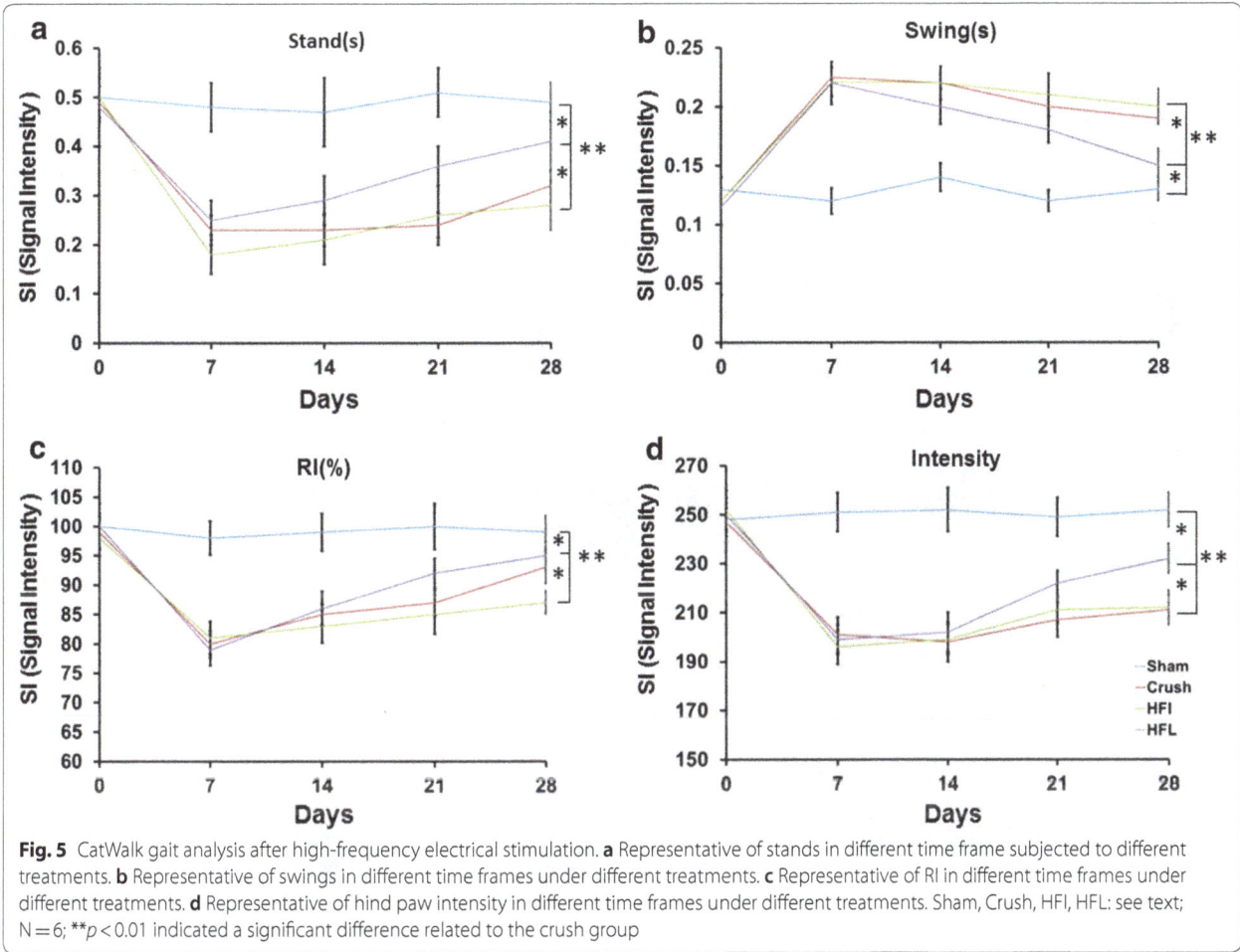

Fig. 5 CatWalk gait analysis after high-frequency electrical stimulation. **a** Representative of stands in different time frame subjected to different treatments. **b** Representative of swings in different time frames under different treatments. **c** Representative of RI in different time frames under different treatments. **d** Representative of hind paw intensity in different time frames under different treatments. Sham, Crush, HFI, HFL: see text; N=6; **p<0.01 indicated a significant difference related to the crush group

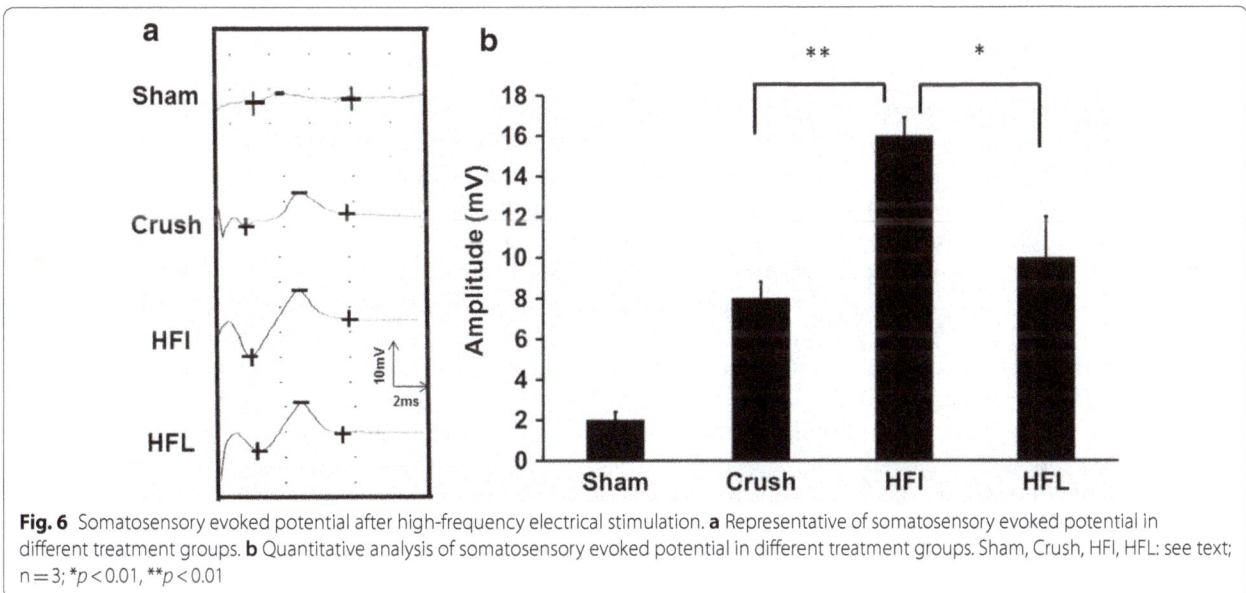

Fig. 6 Somatosensory evoked potential after high-frequency electrical stimulation. **a** Representative of somatosensory evoked potential in different treatment groups. **b** Quantitative analysis of somatosensory evoked potential in different treatment groups. Sham, Crush, HFI, HFL: see text; n=3; *p<0.01, **p<0.01

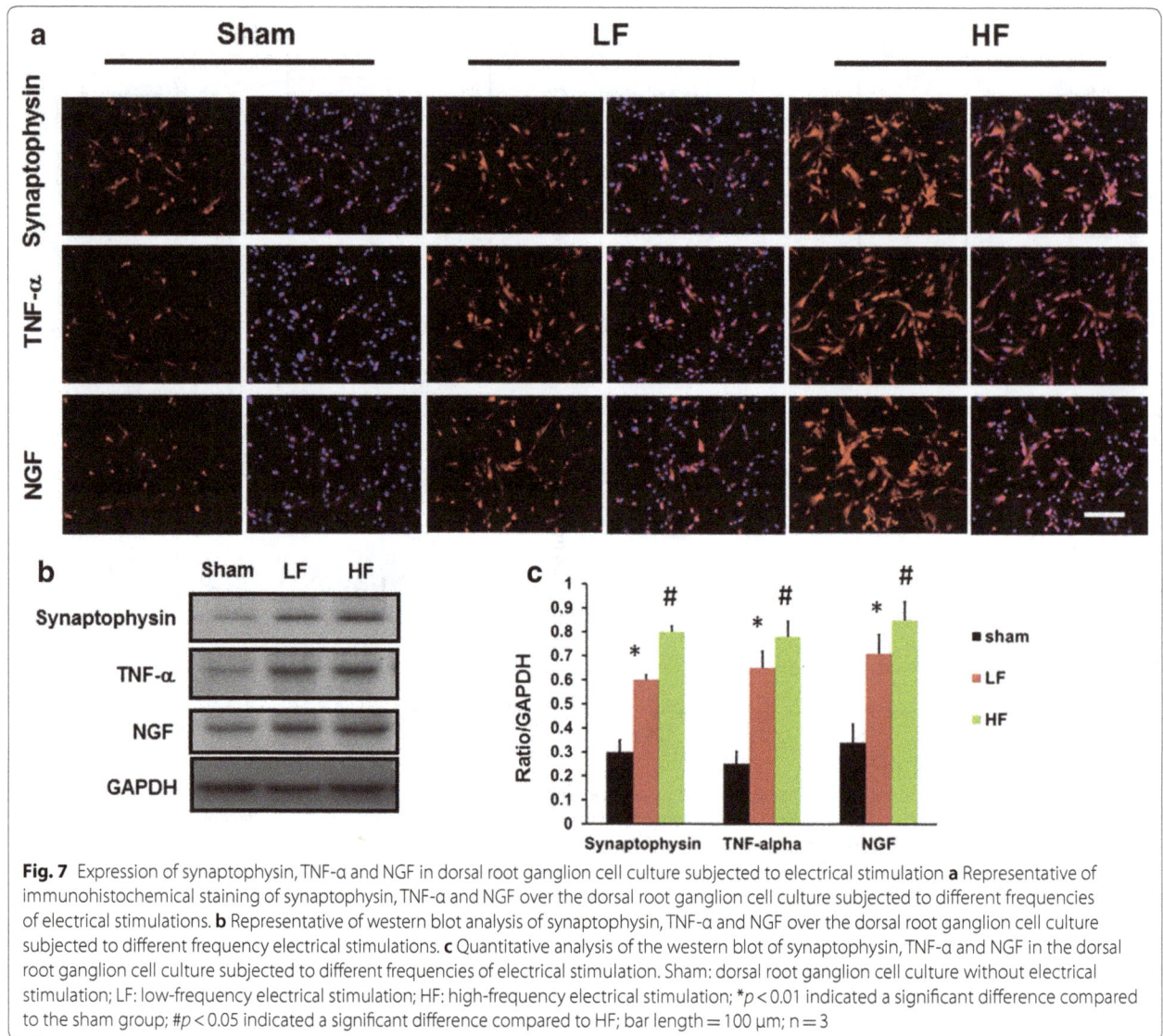

Fig. 7 Expression of synaptophysin, TNF-α and NGF in dorsal root ganglion cell culture subjected to electrical stimulation **a** Representative of immunohistochemical staining of synaptophysin, TNF-α and NGF over the dorsal root ganglion cell culture subjected to different frequencies of electrical stimulations. **b** Representative of western blot analysis of synaptophysin, TNF-α and NGF over the dorsal root ganglion cell culture subjected to different frequency electrical stimulations. **c** Quantitative analysis of the western blot of synaptophysin, TNF-α and NGF in the dorsal root ganglion cell culture subjected to different frequencies of electrical stimulation. Sham: dorsal root ganglion cell culture without electrical stimulation; LF: low-frequency electrical stimulation; HF: high-frequency electrical stimulation; $*p < 0.01$ indicated a significant difference compared to the sham group; $\#p < 0.05$ indicated a significant difference compared to HF; bar length = 100 μm; n = 3

high-frequency electrical muscle stimulation only improved the nerve regeneration without producing an analgesic effect. Furthermore, there was no pain relief following immediate electrical stimulation, however the stimulation predisposed the sensory system to inflammatory changes. Considering the nerve regeneration potential of high-frequency electrical stimulation, a delay in the initiation of stimulation appears advisable.

Dorsal root ganglion cells are located in the intervertebral foramen of the spinal cord and involve the sensory neuron; these cells respond to peripheral nerve injury. The increased expression of TNF-α, IL1β, and synaptophysin reflected the intensity of the neuropathic pain. The attenuation of these inflammatory cytokines paralleled the decreased neuropathic pain response [20,

21]. In vitro analysis demonstrated that high-frequency electrical stimulation exerted a greater potential for the dorsal root ganglion cells to express an inflammatory response compared to the low-frequency electrical stimulation. In the vivo analysis, immediate high frequency electrical stimulation resulted in a significantly higher expression of inflammatory cytokines in the dorsal root ganglion compared to late high-frequency electrical stimulation and low-frequency electrical stimulation either at the immediate or late time profiles. This result confirmed that a delay in high-frequency electrical stimulation is appropriate to facilitate nerve regeneration without increasing the risk of neuropathic pain.

Electrophysiological and biochemical alterations have been well documented to occur in the somatosensory system of the brain after peripheral nervous system injury. An increased expression of TNF-α and synaptophysin in the somatosensory cortex and hippocampus indicate a stronger response to peripheral nerve injury, and an attenuation of this response was noted during a decrease in neuropathic pain [20]. In addition, the evoked potential in the somatosensory cortex was in line with the severity of neuropathic pain with respect to both behavioral and biochemical aspects. This study showed a significantly high amplitude of the evoked potential following immediate high-frequency electrical stimulation. Both electrophysiological and molecular biology data confirmed that immediate high-frequency electrical stimulation had a potential to induce neuropathic pain.

The CatWalk gait XT system is a comprehensive and sensitive tool for the determination of gait alteration in motor and sensory function impairment at the same time profile compared to using the SFI and allodynia analyses alone [20, 33]. Motor function improvement is reflected by an increased paw intensity, increased stance, decreased swing and a decreased regularity index. However, sensory impairment is indicated by reciprocal trends [33]. Immediate high-frequency electrical stimulation showed a significant improvement in SFI but decreased the pain threshold in the mechanical allodynia test. The Catwalk gait analysis demonstrated a increased paw density, increased stance, decreased swing and reduced regularity index in motor function accompanying the sensory impairment. In the CatWalk gait analysis, we found that the increased regularity index and decreased paw intensity following immediate high-frequency electrical stimulation was due to the compromised effect of sensory and motor function alterations.

There were some limitations in this study. First, the nerve crush model cannot present the typical sensory impairment observed in well-established neuropathic models such as chronic nerve constriction injury, tibia nerve resection, or nerve root ligation model. However, we aimed to report motor function improvement without aggravation of sensory function through the investigation of different treatment time profiles and the administration of high or low electrical frequency. The nerve-crush injury model consisted of motor and sensory function impairment and was the appropriate model in this study. Second, dorsal root ganglion cell culture, subjected to either high or low-frequency electrical stimulation, did not reflect the status of late TENS biology. However, we intend to investigate the ability of high- and low-frequency electrical stimulation to prime dorsal root ganglion cells to initiate the inflammatory response to increase the nerve regeneration and improve animal behavior after high-frequency electrical stimulation but mitigate the risk of impaired sensory function.

Conclusion

Both immediate and late administration of high-frequency electrical stimulation exerted a significantly greater motor function improvement than low-frequency electrical stimulation at comparable time points. However, immediate high-frequency electrical stimulation caused a significantly lower pain threshold than late high-frequency or low-frequency stimulation delivered at the immediate or late time points. There, a delay in the initiation of TENS appears to afford a reasonable treatment approach after nerve repair and provides an appropriate time frame for clinical administration.

Abbreviations
TENS: transcutaneous neuromuscular electrical nerve stimulation; NF: neurofilament; SFI: sciatic function index; CMAP: compound muscle action potential; DRGs: dorsal root ganglion cells.

Authors' contributions
HLS: conception and design of the study, interpretation and acquisition of the immunofluorescence staining, western blot analysis, and writing the manuscript; CYC: study design, acquisition and interpretation of immunofluorescence staining and western blot analysis; ZHL: study design and interpretation of neurobehavior of motor and sensory function; FCC: design and conception of this study as well the interpretation of neurobehavioral analysis such as Catwalk gait analysis and sensory function assessment such as Von-Frey and thermal plate analysis; CJC: Interpretation of immunofluorescence staining and western blot analysis; MLS: conception and design of the study, editing the manuscript and the interpretation of western blot analysis; JS: conception and design of this study and editing the manuscript; HCP: conception and design of this study and approval of the version to be published. All authors read and approved the final manuscript.

Author details
[1] Department of Life Sciences, Agriculture Biotechnology Center, National Chung-Hsing University, Taichung, Taiwan. [2] Department of Neurosurgery, Taichung Veterans General Hospital, 1650 Taiwan Boulevard Sec. 4, 40705 Taichung, Taiwan. [3] Department of Medical Research, Taichung Veterans General Hospital, Taichung, Taiwan. [4] Institute of Biomedical Sciences, National Chung-Hsing University, Taichung, Taiwan. [5] Department of Neurosurgery, University of Virginia, Charlottesville, VA, USA. [6] Faculty of Medicine, School of Medicine, National Yang-Ming University, Taipei, Taiwan.

Acknowledgements
The authors would like to thank the research assistant of Miss Shu-Zhen Lai for the kind assistances in the manuscript preparation and the Biostatistics Task Force of Taichung Veterans General Hospital for the statistical analysis.

Competing interest
The authors declare that they have no competing interests.

Funding

The authors obtained funding through a grant from Taichung Veterans General Hospital (TCVGH-1054905C) and a joint grant from Taichung Veterans General Hospital/Providence University (TCVGH-PU1048104).

References

1. Boncompagni S, Kern H, Rossini K, Hofer C, Mayr W, Carraro U, Protasi F. Structural differentiation of skeletal muscle fibers in the absence of innervation in humans. Proc Natl Acad Sci USA. 2007;104(49):19339–44 **Epub 12007 Nov 19327**.

2. Kern H, Salmons S, Mayr W, Rossini K, Carraro U. Recovery of long-term denervated human muscles induced by electrical stimulation. Muscle Nerve. 2005;31(1):98–101.

3. Love FM, Son YJ, Thompson WJ. Activity alters muscle reinnervation and terminal sprouting by reducing the number of Schwann cell pathways that grow to link synaptic sites. J Neurobiol. 2003;54(4):566–76.

4. Willand MP, Holmes M, Bain JR, Fahnestock M, De Bruin H. Electrical muscle stimulation after immediate nerve repair reduces muscle atrophy without affecting reinnervation. Muscle Nerve. 2013;48(2):219–25. https://doi.org/10.1002/mus.23726 **(Epub 22013 May 23722)**.

5. Cole BG, Gardiner PF. Does electrical stimulation of denervated muscle, continued after reinnervation, influence recovery of contractile function? Exp Neurol. 1984;85(1):52–62.

6. Gigo-Benato D, Russo TL, Geuna S, Domingues NR, Salvini TF, Parizotto NA. Electrical stimulation impairs early functional recovery and accentuates skeletal muscle atrophy after sciatic nerve crush injury in rats. Muscle Nerve. 2010;41(5):685–93. https://doi.org/10.1002/mus.21549.

7. Marqueste T, Decherchi P, Desplanches D, Favier R, Grelot L, Jammes Y. Chronic electrostimulation after nerve repair by self-anastomosis: effects on the size, the mechanical, histochemical and biochemical muscle properties. Acta Neuropathol. 2006;111(6):589–600 **(Epub 2006 Mar 2007)**.

8. Sinis N, Horn F, Genchev B, Skouras E, Merkel D, Angelova SK, Kaidoglou K, Michael J, Pavlov S, Igelmund P. Electrical stimulation of paralyzed vibrissal muscles reduces endplate reinnervation and does not promote motor recovery after facial nerve repair in rats. Ann Anat. 2009;191(4):356–70. https://doi.org/10.1016/j.aanat.2009.1003.1004 **(Epub 2009 May 1013)**.

9. Tam SL, Archibald V, Jassar B, Tyreman N, Gordon T. Increased neuromuscular activity reduces sprouting in partially denervated muscles. J Neurosci. 2001;21(2):654–67.

10. Heidland A, Fazeli G, Klassen A, Sebekova K, Hennemann H, Bahner U, Di Iorio B. Neuromuscular electrostimulation techniques: historical aspects and current possibilities in treatment of pain and muscle waisting. Clin Nephrol. 2013;79(Suppl 1):S12–23.

11. Klassen A, Di Iorio B, Guastaferro P, Bahner U, Heidland A, De Santo N. High-tone external muscle stimulation in end-stage renal disease: effects on symptomatic diabetic and uremic peripheral neuropathy. J Ren Nutr. 2008;18(1):46–51.

12. Strempska B, Bilinska M, Weyde W, Koszewicz M, Madziarska K, Golebiowski T, Klinger M. The effect of high-tone external muscle stimulation on symptoms and electrophysiological parameters of uremic peripheral neuropathy. Clin Nephrol. 2013;79(Suppl 1):S24–7.

13. Schimrigk K, McLaughlin J, Gruninger W. The effect of electrical stimulation on the experimentally denervated rat muscle. Scand J Rehabil Med. 1977;9(2):55–60.

14. Clemente FR, Barron KW. Transcutaneous neuromuscular electrical stimulation effect on the degree of microvascular perfusion in autonomically denervated rat skeletal muscle. Arch Phys Med Rehabil. 1996;77(2):155–60.

15. Hennig R. Late reinnervation of the rat soleus muscle is differentially suppressed by chronic stimulation and by ectopic innervation. Acta Physiol Scand. 1987;130(1):153–60.

16. Willand MP, Holmes M, Bain JR, Fahnestock M, de Bruin H. Determining the effects of electrical stimulation on functional recovery of denervated rat gastrocnemius muscle using motor unit number estimation. In: Conference proceedings on IEEE Engineering in medicine and biology society 2011; 2011. p. 1977–80. https://doi.org/10.1109/iembs.2011.6090557

17. Kerns JM, Lucchinetti C. Electrical field effects on crushed nerve regeneration. Exp Neurol. 1992;117(1):71–80.

18. Pan HC, Cheng FC, Chen CJ, Lai SZ, Lee CW, Yang DY, Chang MH, Ho SP. Post-injury regeneration in rat sciatic nerve facilitated by neurotrophic factors secreted by amniotic fluid mesenchymal stem cells. J Clin Neurosci. 2007;14(11):1089–98.

19. Chen CJ, Cheng FC, Su HL, Sheu ML, Lu ZH, Chiang CY, Yang DY, Sheehan J, Pan HC. Improved neurological outcome by intramuscular injection of human amniotic fluid derived stem cells in a muscle denervation model. PLoS ONE. 2015;10(5):e0124624. https://doi.org/10.1371/journal.pone.0124624 **(eCollection 0122015)**.

20. Chiang CY, Liu SA, Sheu ML, Chen FC, Chen CJ, Su HL, Pan HC. Feasibility of human amniotic fluid derived stem cells in alleviation of neuropathic pain in chronic constrictive injury nerve model. PLoS ONE. 2016;11(7):e0159482. https://doi.org/10.1371/journal.pone.0159482 **(eCollection 0152016)**.

21. Chiang CY, Sheu ML, Cheng FC, Chen CJ, Su HL, Sheehan J, Pan HC. Comprehensive analysis of neurobehavior associated with histomorphological alterations in a chronic constrictive nerve injury model through use of the CatWalk XT system. J Neurosurg. 2014;120(1):250–62. https://doi.org/10.3171/2013.9.JNS13353 **(Epub 12013 Nov 13351)**.

22. Cho HY, Suh HR, Han HC. A single trial of transcutaneous electrical nerve stimulation reduces chronic neuropathic pain following median nerve injury in rats. Tohoku J Exp Med. 2014;232(3):207–14.

23. Correa JB, Costa LO, de Oliveira NT, Sluka KA, Liebano RE. Effects of the carrier frequency of interferential current on pain modulation in patients with chronic nonspecific low back pain: a protocol of a randomised controlled trial. BMC Musculoskelet Disord. 2013;14:195. https://doi.org/10.1186/1471-2474-1114-1195.

24. Suszynski K, Marcol W, Gorka D. Physiotherapeutic techniques used in the management of patients with peripheral nerve injuries. Neural Regen Res. 2015;10(11):1770–2. https://doi.org/10.4103/1673-5374.170299.

25. Willand MP. Electrical stimulation enhances reinnervation after nerve injury. Eur J Transl Myol. 2015;25(4):243–8. https://doi.org/10.4081/ejtm.2015.5243 **(eCollection 2015 Aug 4024)**.

26. Kao CH, Chen JJ, Hsu YM, Bau DT, Yao CH, Chen YS. High-frequency electrical stimulation can be a complementary therapy to promote nerve regeneration in diabetic rats. PLoS ONE. 2013;8(11):e79078. https://doi.org/10.71371/journal.pone.0079078 **(eCollection 0072013)**.

27. Chen YS, Hu CL, Hsieh CL, Lin JG, Tsai CC, Chen TH, Yao CH. Effects of percutaneous electrical stimulation on peripheral nerve regeneration using silicone rubber chambers. J Biomed Mater Res. 2001;57(4):541–9.

28. Gordon T, Sulaiman O, Boyd JG. Experimental strategies to promote functional recovery after peripheral nerve injuries. J Peripher Nerv Syst. 2003;8(4):236–50.

29. Robinson AJ. Transcutaneous electrical nerve stimulation for the control of pain in musculoskeletal disorders. J Orthop Sports Phys Ther. 1996;24(4):208–26.

30. Vance CG, Rakel BA, Blodgett NP, DeSantana JM, Amendola A, Zimmerman MB, Walsh DM, Sluka KA. Effects of transcutaneous electrical nerve stimulation on pain, pain sensitivity, and function in people with knee osteoarthritis: a randomized controlled trial. Phys Ther. 2012;92(7):898–910. https://doi.org/10.2522/ptj.20110183 **(Epub 20112012 Mar 20110130)**.

31. Carbonario F, Matsutani LA, Yuan SL, Marques AP. Effectiveness of high-frequency transcutaneous electrical nerve stimulation at tender points as adjuvant therapy for patients with fibromyalgia. Eur J Phys Rehabil Med. 2013;49(2):197–204 **(Epub 2013 Mar 2013)**.

32. Nnoaham KE, Kumbang J. Transcutaneous electrical nerve stimulation (TENS) for chronic pain. Cochrane Database Syst Rev. 2008;3:CD003222. https://doi.org/10.1002/14651858.CD003222.pub2.

33. Chen YJ, Cheng FC, Sheu ML, Su HL, Chen CJ, Sheehan J, Pan HC. Detection of subtle neurological alterations by the Catwalk XT gait analysis system. J Neuroeng Rehabil. 2014;11:62. https://doi.org/10.1186/1743-0003-1111-1162.

17

Identification of the neurotransmitter profile of AmFoxP expressing neurons in the honeybee brain using double-label in situ hybridization

Adriana Schatton[1]* ⓘD, Julia Agoro[1,2], Janis Mardink[1], Gérard Leboulle[2] and Constance Scharff[1]

Abstract

Background: FoxP transcription factors play crucial roles for the development and function of vertebrate brains. In humans the neurally expressed FOXPs, FOXP1, FOXP2, and FOXP4 are implicated in cognition, including language. Neural FoxP expression is specific to particular brain regions but FoxP1, FoxP2 and FoxP4 are not limited to a particular neuron or neurotransmitter type. Motor- or sensory activity can regulate FoxP2 expression, e.g. in the striatal nucleus Area X of songbirds and in the auditory thalamus of mice. The DNA-binding domain of FoxP proteins is highly conserved within metazoa, raising the possibility that cellular functions were preserved across deep evolutionary time. We have previously shown in bee brains that FoxP is expressed in eleven specific neuron populations, seven tightly packed clusters and four loosely arranged groups.

Results: The present study examined the co-expression of honeybee FoxP (AmFoxP) with markers for glutamatergic, GABAergic, cholinergic and monoaminergic transmission. We found that AmFoxP could co-occur with any one of those markers. Interestingly, AmFoxP clusters and AmFoxP groups differed with respect to homogeneity of marker co-expression; within a cluster, all neurons co-expressed the same neurotransmitter marker, within a group co-expression varied. We also assessed qualitatively whether age or housing conditions providing different sensory and motor experiences affected the AmFoxP neuron populations, but found no differences.

Conclusions: Based on the neurotransmitter homogeneity we conclude that AmFoxP neurons within the clusters might have a common projection and function whereas the AmFoxP groups are more diverse and could be further sub-divided. The obtained information about the neurotransmitters co-expressed in the AmFoxP neuron populations facilitated the search of similar neurons described in the literature. These comparisons revealed e.g. a possible function of AmFoxP neurons in the central complex. Our findings provide opportunities to focus future functional studies on invertebrate FoxP expressing neurons. In a broader context, our data will contribute to the ongoing efforts to discern in which cases relationships between molecular and phenotypic signatures are linked evolutionary.

Keywords: FoxP, FoxP1, Honeybee, Acetylcholine, Glutamate, GABA, Monoamine, Songbird, Deep homology, In situ hybridization

*Correspondence: a.schatton@fu-berlin.de
[1] Department of Animal Behavior, Freie Universität Berlin, Takustraße 6, 14195 Berlin, Germany
Full list of author information is available at the end of the article

Background

Transcription factors of the FOXP family are intensively investigated because of their role in human disease [1]. Human patients with mutations in FOXP1, FOXP2 or FOXP4 show several cognitive deficits such as autistic features, mental retardation and language impairments [2–6]. A point mutation in FOXP2, initially discovered in one large family, impairs speech perception and production while non-language-related behaviors are less affected [7, 8]. More than 30 genetic alterations of FOXP2 in other individuals also affect language in similar ways, and are additionally associated with autistic spectrum disorders [5, 9–11]. In the following text we adopted the nomenclature proposed by Kaestner et al. [12], e.g. human gene *FOXP* and protein FOXP, mouse (*Foxp2*/Foxp2) and all other species (*FoxP2*/FoxP2).

FoxP gene expression in the CNS is overall similar in all vertebrates analyzed and includes regions involved in sensory-motor and multimodal integration [13–23].

Invertebrate genomes harbor only one *FoxP* gene locus that contains a highly conserved DNA-binding domain [24, 25]. In sponges FoxP is upregulated in vitro during the formation of cell aggregates [26]. In *Drosophila*, FoxP (dFoxP) has been implicated in decision-making, locomotion and motor learning [27–30]. In honeybees, FoxP (AmFoxP) is expressed in the cortical areas of all major neuropils, either in dense neuron clusters or more widely dispersed neuron groups [25, 31, 32]. The *FoxP* gene is most similar to vertebrate *FoxP1*, based on particular alternative splice forms in bilaterians [25, 33].

We previously described eleven AmFoxP expressing neuron populations in particular locations of the honeybee brain [25]. We chose to study the role of FoxP in the honeybee *Apis mellifera* because it is a well-established animal model to study insect cognition [34, 35] such as memory formation [36], navigation [37], symbolic communication [38–41] or conceptual learning [42–44].

For one of the described AmFoxP clusters, the posterior cluster medioventral to the lobula (mvLO-p), we proposed, based on location and connectivity, a functional role in visual processing [25, 31], consistent with FoxP expressing neurons in the mammalian visual thalamus [45, 46]. Here we further characterize the AmFoxP neuron populations in the honeybee brain in terms of their neurotransmitters to better compare them with neurons of known function in the insect CNS. Moreover, we also studied whether environmental stimuli affected *AmFoxP* expression in honeybees, because FoxP2 can be regulated by activity in some vertebrate neurons, e.g. by light, mtor behavior and/or sound [13, 47–49].

In honeybees, neurotransmitter systems were described by various means, including the detection of the neurotransmitters themselves [50–55], of the

enzymes implicated in their metabolism [56–58], of molecules that transport the neurotransmitters into cellular compartments [59] and of specific receptors [60–67].

We concentrated on the most relevant neurotransmitters by means of their markers: the honeybee (Am) vesicular transporters for acetylcholine (AmVAchT), glutamate (AmVGluT) and monoamines (AmVMAT) as well as glutamate decarboxylase (AmGad). These markers were chosen because they are exclusively associated with presynaptic release (transporters) or synthesis (Gad) of the respective neurotransmitter. To our knowledge, VAchT, VGluT and Gad have not been reported to be expressed endogenously in glia cells. *Drosophila* VMAT is also expressed in glia cells, however restricted to serotonin and histamine containing neurons in a relatively thin layer between the retina and the optic lobe [68] where we did not detect AmFoxP. Acetylcholine (Ach) is the main excitatory neurotransmitter in insects, in contrast to vertebrates that predominantly use glutamate for excitatory transmission [69, 70]. Excitatory currents induced by Ach are characterized [71, 72]. Glutamatergic signaling in honeybees is important for particular memory mechanisms [63, 73, 74]. Inhibitory currents induced by Glutamate (Glu) through glutamate chloride channels (GluCl) have also been described [72, 75]. The detection of receptors homologous to their vertebrate counterparts (AMPA/kainate, NMDA) suggests that Glu also acts as an excitatory neurotransmitter in the CNS [61]. Another major inhibitory neurotransmitter in the bilaterian brain is GABA [72, 76, 77]. GluCl and GABA receptors are both involved in honeybee long term memory [78, 79]. AmVMAT transports the biogenic amines octopamin, dopamine, histamine and serotonin [68, 80] and thus serves as a marker for modulatory neurons. In insects, modulatory neurons are crucial for different learning processes [81–83], involved in the division of labour [84, 85] and mediate the biological state of the organism like aggression, sleep or hunger [86–88]. For the quantitative PCR analysis of neurotrasmitters expressed in the Kenyon cells of the mushroom bodies, we used, beside AmVachT, AmVGluT and AmVMAT, also AmVIAAT (the honeybee vesicular transporter for inhibitory amino acids). AmVIAAT is a presynaptic marker for glycinergic and GABAergic neurons.

Although insect and vertebrate brains demonstrate fundamental differences in terms of development, anatomy, structure, design and complexity, they also have many principle features in common [89]. Some of those might be convergent whereas others, like the regulatory networks and molecular architecture of specific neurons could date back to their last common bilaterian ancestor and are therefore 'deeply homologous' [90]. In the framework of deep homology between insect and vertebrate brains [90, 91], we are interested in potentially conserved features of FoxP expressing neurons with implications for similarities and differences in behavior.

Methods

Animals

All honeybees of the species *A. mellifera* were collected between July and September from apiaries located at the department of Neurobiology, FU Berlin (Königin-Luise-Str. 1-3, 14195 Berlin). Access was generously provided by Professors Randolf Menzel and Dorothea Eisenhardt.

Sampling method

To address whether differences in experience or life history affected *AmFoxP* expression we created four conditions that varied with respect to sensory experience and opportunity for motor activity. From each condition we sampled bees of different ages. In condition 1 bees were kept in an observation hive with two frames (W × D × H: 53.5 × 18 × 65 cm), in the presence of the queen and siblings (~ 4000 individuals), a honeycomb and the possibility to fly and forage outside of the hive ('unmanipulated' group). In order to sample bees of the unmanipulated group at specific ages, they were marked with acrylic color on their thorax within 16 h after emergence. In the other three conditions one or more variables were altered (Table 1): In condition 2 ('honeycomb' group) ~ 100 individuals were kept in a caged honeycomb frame (22 cm × 37 cm × 5 cm). In condition 3 ('mini-cage' group) ~ 30 bees were kept separately within the hive, enclosed in a small cage (10 cm × 3 cm × 10 cm) without an own honeycomb. In condition 4 ('incubator' group) ~ 30 bees were kept in an empty cage (13 cm × 20 cm × 8 cm) within an incubator at 29 °C in constant darkness and supplied with 30% sucrose.

Preparation of in situ hybridization probes

Table 2 provides an overview of the primers used to prepare in situ hybridization (*ISH*) probes. In the following text, nucleotide sequences (*ISH*-probes, primers) are written in *italics* and '*Am*' as a prefix refers to '*Apis mellifera*'. The *AmFoxP* probe-containing pGemT-easy plasmid was kindly provided by Prof. Taketoshi Kiya (Kanazawa University, Japan). The same probe was used

Table 1 Treatment and sample size of the four experimental groups

Condition/group	Sisters	Queen	Honeycomb	Foraging/light	Number and ages of individuals sampled
'Unmanipulated'	+	+	+	+	3 (age: 1 × 1 days, 1 × 15 days, 1 × 50 days)
'Honeycomb'	+	+	+	–	4 (age: 1 × 4 days, 1 × 11 days, 1 × 15 days, 1 × 19 days)
'Mini-cage'	+	+	–	–	3 (age: 2 × 23 days, 1 × 26 days)
'Incubator'	+	–	–	–	5 (age: 2 × 15 days, 1 × 27 days, 1 × 31 days, 1 × 40 days)

The manipulated features are indicated by symbols. The column on the right lists the sample size. The detailed distribution of age (d = days after emergence) within the group is given in brackets

Table 2 RNA probe names used for in situ hybridization

Probe name	Primers 5'–3'	Ref. seq of cds	Length (nt)
AmFoxP	GAGAAACCGCTGGACGTTTC CGTTGCGCCGGAAGTAGCAG	NM_001104949	847
AmVGlut	GGCCCCCATTGCGTCACA AATGCCAGCCACAACCAGAAACAGTA	XM_016914051.1	631
AmGad	AATGGTGAACGTCTGCTTCTGGTAT ACTTACGTGCTATGAGTATCCTTTG	XM_391979	806
AmVAchT	CTCGGGCGCGTTGATAGACAGGAT CGCCGAACACGTGGGGGAAGAA	XM_006562557.2	605
AmVMAT	AAGGCGTTGGTTCGTCGTGCTC CTTCTTTCGTTGGCGGTGCTCGTAA	XM_392061.6	855
D2-like/AmDop3	CAGCGCATTCGTTAATCTGA GCCCAGACCAACAGTATCGT	NM_001014983.1	534

Primer sequences, reference sequence IDs and probe length are given. The AmFoxP-probe sequence containing plasmid was kindly given by Prof. Taketoshi Kiya, Kanazawa University (Japan). The AmGad primer pair was adopted from Kiya et al. [58]

previously [25] and does not discriminate between the two the Forkhead domain—affecting isoforms [25]. The *AmGad*-probe was produced according to Kiya and Kubo [58]. Honeybee sequences were identified with BLASTN 2.7.0+ using the 'blastn' algorithm [92] (RRID: 196SCR_001010) and phylogenetic analysis (clustal omega, EMBL-EBI, RRID:SCR_001591) by comparing to *Drosophila* and mammalian orthologous genes available in sequence databases. Primers (mwg Eurofins Genomics, Ebersberg, Germany) were identified with 'primer3' software [93] (RRID:SCR_002285) and used to PCR-amplify sequences between 500 and 1000 nt to serve as *ISH* templates. Template cDNA was prepared as follows: freshly dissected honeybee brains were homogenized with a pellet pestle (Sigma-Aldrich, Germany) in 400 µl TriZol®. After adding 80 µl of chloroform the solution was vortexed and centrifuged (15 min at 12,000 g at 4 °C), the RNA-containing upper layer was collected and purified on columns ('RNeasy MinElute Cleanup' by Qiagen, Hilden, Germany) according to the manufacturer's protocol. Residual DNA was restricted with TurboDNase® (Thermo Fisher, Braunschweig, Germany). RNA concentration was measured with a NanoDrop 1000 Spectrophotometer. 200 ng of total RNA were transcribed into cDNA by using oligo-dT-primers and SuperScript® III Reverse Transcriptase (Thermo Fisher, Braunschweig, Germany).

PCR-amplified fragments were purified with a purification kit (Macherey–Nagel, Düren, Germany) and ligated into pGemT-easy plasmids (Promega, Wisconsin, USA) which were transformed in *E. coli* bacteria (Top 10). DNA-templates for RNA-probe synthesis were PCR-amplified with pGemt-easy M13 primers, detected by gel electrophoresis and purified again. SP6 and T7 polymerases (Roche, Mannheim, Germany) were used for in vitro transcription with Dig- and FITC-labeled UTP containing RNA Labeling Mix (Roche, Mannheim, Germany) and 200 ng of the cDNA template. Probes were purified with mini Quick Spin Columns (Roche, Mannheim, Germany), diluted 1:1 in formamid and stored at − 80 °C.

Tissue preparation

Honeybee brains were quickly dissected in DEPC-treated water, immediately embedded in TissueTek® (Sakura, Staufen, Germany), frozen on dry ice and kept at − 80 °C until use.

Staining protocol—fluorescent double label

The double-label *ISH* (*dISH*) protocol was kindly provided by Prof. T. Kiya (Kanazawa University), published in Kiya and Kubo [58] and was slightly modified. Briefly, 12 µm frontal cryosections were fixed 15 min in 4% PFA in DEPC-treated water at room temperature (RT),

washed in 0.1 M phosphate buffer pH 7.4 (PB: 18 mM NaH₂PO₄, 82 mM Na₂HPO₄), permeabilized and covered with the respective Dig- and FITC-labeled RNA probes. Per slide 0.3 µl *AmFoxP* and 1 µl neurotransmission marker probes were diluted in 150 µl hybridization buffer [58]. Slides were covered with coverslips (24 × 60 mm, Carl Roth, Karlsruhe, Germany) and hybridized overnight at 60 °C in a mineral oil bath. The next day, slides were washed sequentially in 5×, 2× and 0.2× saline-sodium citrate buffer pH 7.0 (20× SSC: 3 M NaCl, 0.3 M trisodium citrate), blocked in blocking reagent (Roche, Mannheim, Germany) and incubated 2 h at RT with anti-Dig-POD antibody (1:500, Roche, Mannheim, Germany). RNAse A treatment was not applied. After several washes, slides were incubated 15 min at RT in Cy5-labeled tyramids ('TSA-system' by Perkin Elmer, Rodgau, Germany) according to the manufacturer's protocol. Peroxidase was reduced by 3% hydrogen peroxide, the slides blocked again and incubated overnight at 4 °C with anti-FITC-POD (1:500, Roche, Mannheim, Germany). The next day, slides were washed and incubated in Cy3-labeled tyramids ('TSA-system' by Perkin Elmer, Rodgau, Germany), counterstained with DAPI for 10 min at RT (1:20,000) and embedded in 'Immu-Mount™' (Thermo Fisher, Braunschweig, Germany).

Adjacent cryosections were incubated each with the *AmFoxP*-specific Dig-labeled probe and a second FITC-labeled probe specific for one of the four neurotransmitter markers, which were the honeybee (*Am*) *vesicular transporters* of either (1) *acetylcholine* (*AmVAchT*), (2) *glutamate* (*AmVGluT*) and (3) *monoamines* (*AmVMAT*) or (4) *glutamate decarboxylase* (*AmGad*) (Tables 2, 4).

We also performed one *dISH* with the FITC-labeled *AmVAchT* and a Dig-labeled *AmVGluT* probe on a newly emerged bee. Sample sizes for bees analyzed for neurotransmitter markers are listed in Table 1. For the analysis of the monoaminergic receptor *AmDop3* in the KC, one unmanipulated adult forager of undetermined age was analyzed using *dISH*.

Probes were chosen for *dISH* if two conditions were met: for each probe, the corresponding control ('sense') probe produced no specific staining and the 'antisense' probe labeled neurons known to express the particular neurotransmitter, e.g.: the octopaminergic VUMmx neurons located ventrally to the gnathal ganglia (GNG) for *AmVMAT* [53], the glutamatergic cortex of the optic lobes for *AmVGluT* [52], the inhibitory local interneurons and inhibitory projection neurons lateral and dorsal to the antennal lobes (AL) [50, 57, 94] as well as the neurons of the protocerebral-calycal tract (p.c.t.) [95, 96] for *AmGad* and the uniglomerular projection neurons (uPNs) of the antennal lobes [57, 97, 98] for *AmVAchT*.

Chromogen single label

Tissue was dissected as described for *dISH* above but incubated with biotinylated (instead of fluorescently labeled) tyramids and DAB was used as the chromogen according to the manufacturer's protocol (DAKO/agilent, Santa Clara, USA). All sense and antisense probes were first used in a single-label protocol to check for specificity.

Immuno-labeling of AmFoxP protein

AmFoxP protein was detected using the custom-made AmFoxP^{42kDa} antiserum (RRID: AB_2722599). Antiserum specificity was shown previously [25, 32], immuno-labeling protocol, microscopy and data analysis was performed as described previously [25, 32]. Figure 7b was prepared from an immuno-labeled brain that was previously injected (in vivo) with Lucifer yellow (Life Technologies L453, CH lithium salt, MW 457.24; 5%) as described in [25].

RT-qPCR and statistics

Animals were captured from an observation hive composed of marked bee as described above ('unmanipulated' group, see "Sampling method" section). They were immobilized on ice and decapitated. The head capsule was fixed on wax, the brain was exposed and covered with 0.1 M PBS (137 mM NaCl, 2.7 mM KCl, 8.1 mM Na$_2$HPO$_4$ (2H$_2$O), 1.47 mM KH$_2$PO$_4$), the calyces were visually identified, removed with forceps and homogenized with a Teflon pestle and a glass homogenizer filled with 200 µl Trizol (Braunschweig, Germany). One sample consisted of 8–10 animals. The precision of the dissection was evaluated by staining brains with SYTOX Green diluted 1:2000 to reveal cell bodies (Fig. 14k, l). Total RNA was extracted and cDNA was synthetized from 1 µg of total RNA (see "Preparation of in situ hybridization probes" section). For the RT-qPCR experiments, 5 µl of diluted cDNA, 1 µl of the forward and reverse primers (10 µM, TIB Molbiol, Berlin, Germany), 10 µl Kapa Sybr Fast qPCR mastermix (PeqLab, Erlangen, Germany), 0.4 µl low Rox (50 nM) adjusted to 25 µl with

water and analyzed on a Stratagene MX3000P (Agilent Technologies, Santa Clara, USA). Primers are listed in Table 3, *AmViaat* is the vesicular transporter for inhibitory amino-acids that is specific in vertebrates for GABA and glycine. This candidate was selected instead of *AmGad* because its expression levels can be better compared to the other vesicular transporters. *AmRpL32* and *AmGapDH* were chosen as reference genes. Primer efficiency was calculated on serial dilutions (10, 10^2, 10^3 and 10^4) of the cDNA, primer interactions or the formation of unspecific products evaluated by melting curve analysis at the end of the amplification. On each plate, 'no template controls' (NTC) were analyzed by replacing cDNA with water for each parameter. Each sample was analyzed in triplicate. In Fig. 14l, the PCR profile was 2 min 95 °C, 40 amplification cycles 30 s at 95 °C, 30 s at 59 °C, 30 s at 72 °C and the melting curve analysis: 1 min 95 °C, 30 s at 55 °C, increasing to 95 °C and 30 s at 95 °C. The Cts were calculated by amplification based threshold. Fold change was calculated with the corrected amplification rate: e^{-Ct} (e = 10$^{-1/slope}$) and the data were normalized to the geometric mean of the housekeeper genes, which did not vary over age groups (Kruskal–Walli statistic H(2) = 0.6, $p = 0.74$). Plots and statistics were performed with GraphPad Prism version 5.00 for Windows (GraphPad Software, La Jolla California USA) (RRID: SCR_015807). Data was tested for normal distribution using D'Agostino & Pearson omnibus normality test. Two means were compared for statistical differences using two-tailed Student's t test.

Results

AmFoxP expressing neuron populations (clusters and groups)

We determined which of the four investigated neurotransmitter markers, *AmVAchT*, *AmVGLuT*, *AmVMAT* and *AmGad*, were co-expressed in the 11 AmFoxP neuron populations. We identified these population previously based on mRNA in situ hybridization and immunoreactivity to a custom-made antiserum ('anti-AmFoxP^{42kDa}') [25, 32]. The anatomical nomenclature

Table 3 RT-qPCR primer list and amplification efficiency

mRNA	Forward 5′ 3′	Reverse 5′ 3′	Efficiency (%)
AmVAchT	AGGGCGTCGGTTCCGCTTTC	CAGCATCACTCCGTCCGCCA	89.7
AmVGluT	AACGCCCCGTGAGGGTAGCA	GACGCAATGGGGGCCGTTCA	96.3
AmVMAT	ATTGTCGGCCCCCTCACCCA	GAGCACGACGAACCAACGCC	99.7
AmVIAAT	CGCCGTATTGCGAGGCGGTT	CGCGTTGTCCAGTCGTCGTGT	99.8
AmRpL32	TGTGCTGAAATTGCTCATGGGGG	AGAACGTAACCTTGCACTGGCATAA	100.3
AmGapDH	CGGTTTTGGCCGTATTGGCCGT	AATGGCAACAACCTGAGCACCGAA	99.4

follows Ito et al. [99], Table 5. For ease of reading, we will use the terms AmFoxP neuron, AmFoxP cluster and AmFoxP group. We previously showed these cells to produce both *AmFoxP* mRNA and AmFoxP protein [25, 32]. Here we use immunohistochemistry and in situ hybridization (ISH) interchangeably. Neurons that were neither immunoreactive to the AmFoxP[42kDa] antiserum nor labeled by the *AmFoxP* ISH probe are referred to as AmFoxP-negative.

We previously described seven AmFoxP 'clusters', which consist of densely packed neurons and four 'groups', in which the AmFoxP neurons are more broadly distributed ([25], Fig. 1, Table 3). In the present study, we found that each of the seven AmFoxP clusters homogeneously co-expressed only one of the used neurotransmitter markers. In contrast, all AmFoxP groups co-expressed two or even three of the transmitter markers, but not *AmVMAT*. This difference between clusters and groups was observed in all treatment groups and ages.

Neurotransmitter expression

All four neurotransmitter markers used in the present study were detected in cortical areas around all major neuropils (Figs. 2, 3, 4, 5, 6, 7, 8, 9, 10, 11, 12, 13).

The mRNA of *AmVAchT* and *AmVGluT* as well as *AmGad* were very abundant in cortical areas surrounding the antennal (AL) (Fig. 3) and optic lobes (OL) (Fig. 4), as well as the gnathal ganglia (GNG) (Fig. 7). The markers of the two excitatory neurotransmitters *AmVAchT* and *AmVGluT* had similar expression patterns. However double labeling showed that both *AmVAchT* and *AmV-GluT* mRNAs were not co-expressed in the same neurons (Fig. 2).

AmVMAT expression was scarce and found in cell clusters (Figs. 3d, 5d) as well as in single cells (Figs. 4d, 7d, l, 8d, h, 10e, i, k, 11).

Cholinergic AmFoxP neurons
AmVAchT was detected in large cell clusters dorsal and dorso-lateral to the AL (Fig. 3c)—most likely

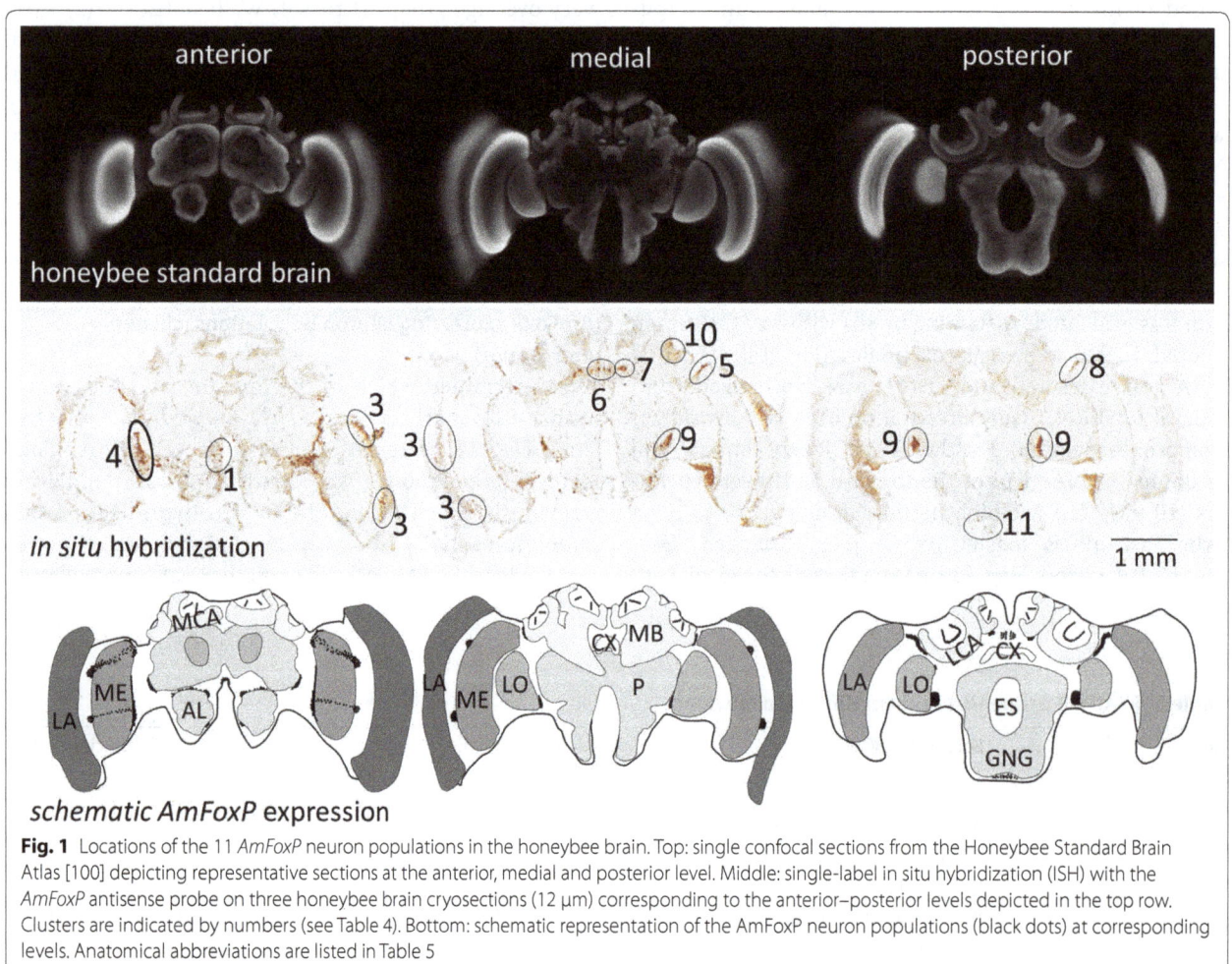

Fig. 1 Locations of the 11 *AmFoxP* neuron populations in the honeybee brain. Top: single confocal sections from the Honeybee Standard Brain Atlas [100] depicting representative sections at the anterior, medial and posterior level. Middle: single-label in situ hybridization (ISH) with the *AmFoxP* antisense probe on three honeybee brain cryosections (12 μm) corresponding to the anterior–posterior levels depicted in the top row. Clusters are indicated by numbers (see Table 4). Bottom: schematic representation of the AmFoxP neuron populations (black dots) at corresponding levels. Anatomical abbreviations are listed in Table 5

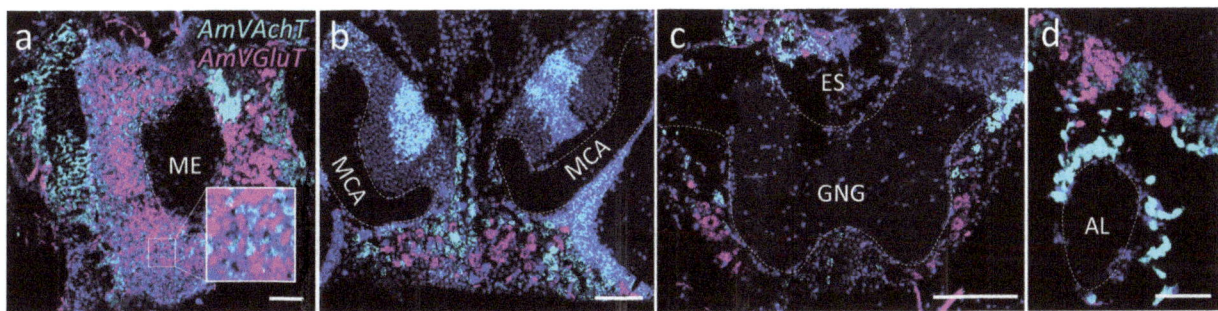

Fig. 2 AmVAchT (cyan) and *AmVGluT* (magenta) do not co-localize within the same neurons. Double ISH (dISH) stainings on 12 μm cryosections from the brain of a newly emerged worker honeybee depict somatic areas surrounding different neuropils: **a** the area around the medulla (ME), **b** the area ventral to the medial calices (MCA) in the posterior brain, **c** the area ventral and lateral to the gnathal ganglia (GNG) and **d** the area around the antennal lobes (AL). Rectangular inset in **a** shows higher magnifications of small boxed region. Scale bars: 100 μm

uniglomerular projection neurons (uPNs) [57], in cortical areas around the OL and in the KC (Fig. 14a–e). The cholinergic marker was co-expressed in five of the seven AmFoxP clusters (Table 4), i.e. the lLH (Fig. 5), the plLCA (Fig. 6), the vMCA (Fig. 8), the large mvLO (Fig. 10) and the mKC (Fig. 12b–e). The mvLO cluster has a higher cell density than the surrounding tissue, clearly visible in nuclear DAPI staining (Fig. 10i, k). However, by AmFoxP labeling, this cluster could be further subdivided in two subdivisions, an anterior (mvLO-a) and a posterior (mvLO-p) part; each subdivision projects to a different brain area, as described previously [25]. Both subdivisions expressed *AmVAchT*. The mvLO-a and mvLO-p are separated by a layer of AmFoxP-negative neurons that expressed *AmGad* (Fig. 10f). *AmVAchT* was also clearly expressed in the region of the mKC and coincided with *AmFoxP* expression. However, due to the subcellular punctate staining in the KC (Fig. 12bIII–V), the two colors representing *AmFoxP* and *AmVAchT* did not coincide to the same extent as in other neurons. We therefore considered KC to co-express two probes as long as any punctate label was located within the area of a DAPI-positive nucleus, which was the case for *AmVAchT* in essentially all *AmFoxP*-expressing KC (but different in the *AmDop3/AmFoxP dISH*, Fig. 12g). In the AmFoxP groups, with less densely clustered cells and co-expression of more than one neurotransmitter, *AmVAchT* was expressed in neurons around the AL (pAL, Fig. 3c, j), around the medulla (pMe, Fig. 4c, g, j) and ventral to the GNG (vGNG, Fig. 7c, g) but not dorsal to the central complex (dCX, Fig. 8). The pME could be further subdivided in at least three local groups. Two of them wrap around the anterior medulla; one ventrally and one dorsally (Fig. 4a–g). The ventral AmFoxP neurons co-expressed only *AmVAchT* (Fig. 4c, g), whereas the dorsal one co-expressed *AmVAchT*, *AmVGluT* and

AmGad (Fig. 4c, e–g) and the group lateral to the ME co-expressed *AmGad* and *AmVGluT* (Fig. 4e, f, I, k, l).

GABA-ergic AmFoxP neurons

Our stainings confirmed the *AmGad* expression pattern shown by Kiya and Kubo [58]. We also found GABAergic neurons particularly in the cortical regions of the AL, the OL, the CX, but not in the KC of the MB, which is also corroborated by our RT-qPCR data (Fig. 14m). *AmGad* was detected in large clusters lateral to the AL (Fig. 3g, h, o), most likely inhibitory PNs (iPNs) [94, 101] or inhibitory local interneurons [50, 57]. The A3-v neuron cluster of the PCT [58, 95, 96] was also labeled (not shown). Only one AmFoxP cluster expressed *AmGad* exclusively, the alLCA (Fig. 6). *AmGad* expressing AmFoxP neurons were also observed in all four AmFoxP groups; around the AL (pAL, Fig. 3e, g, h, l, o), around the ME (pME, Fig. 4e, I, k), ventral to the GNG (vGNG, Fig. 7e, h, j) and dorsal to the CX (dCX, Fig. 8e, k, i). Within the pME, GABAergic AmFoxP neurons accumulated medioventral to the ME (Fig. 4e, i, k).

Glutamatergic AmFoxP neurons

AmVGluT was strongly expressed in large somata lateral to the GNG (Fig. 2c), most likely motor neurons as described previously [52], as well as in cortical areas around the medulla (Fig. 2a, Fig. 4f, l) and in clusters dorsal to the AL (Fig. 3f, n, m). Within the pAL glutamatergic AmFoxP neurons were detected anterio-mediodorsal (Fig. 3n) and posterioventral to the AL (Fig. 3i). In seven samples (Fig. 14f–j) there was also very weak *AmVGluT* signal in the small and middle KC (sKC and mKC) of the MB. In the other eight *AmVGluT* samples the KC signal did not differ from background. The adES cluster was the only AmFoxP cluster that exclusively co-expressed *AmVGlut* (Fig. 3f, m). Only few *AmVGluT* neurons were detected in the vGNG (Fig. 7f) and dorsal to the central

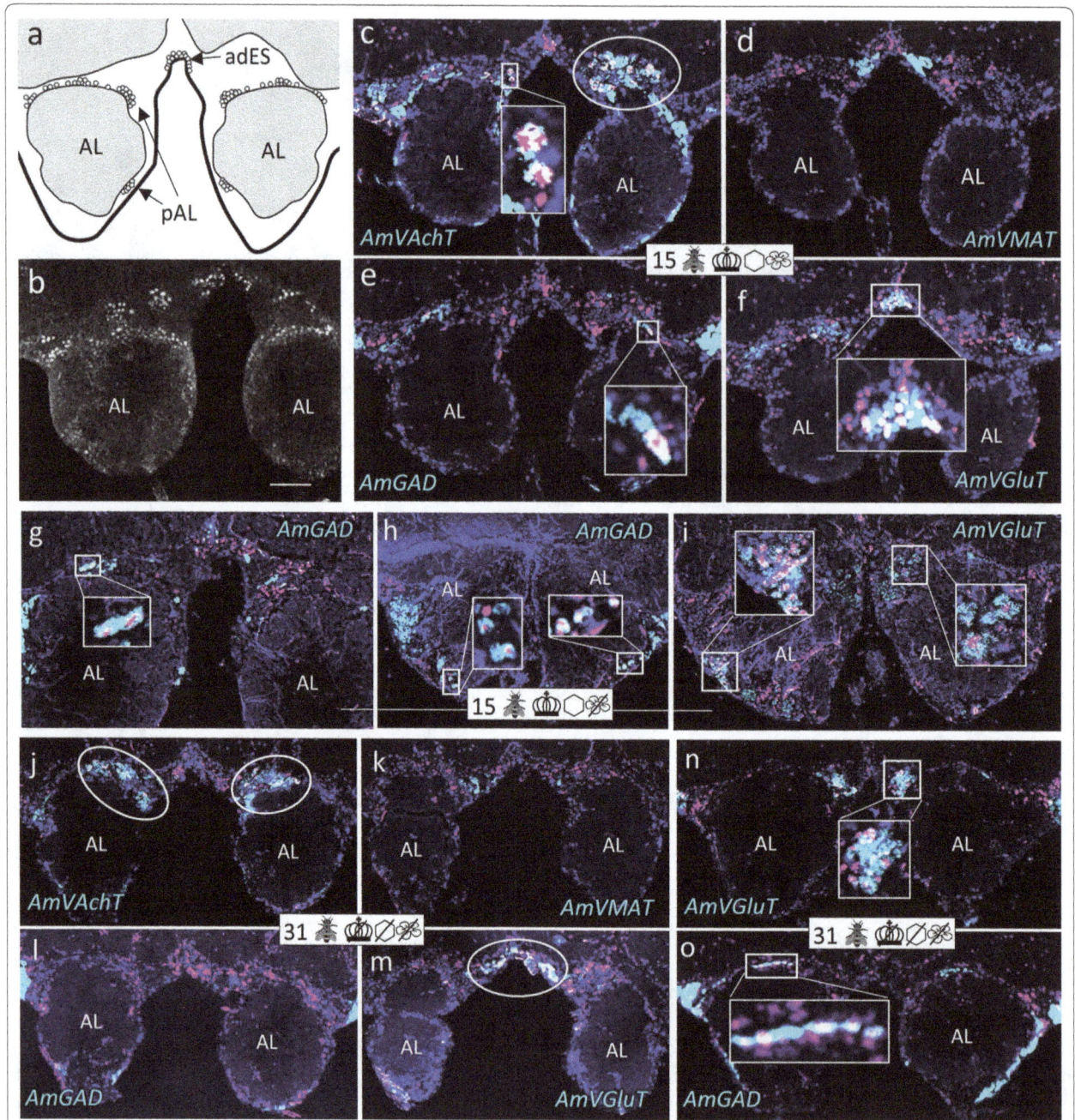

Fig. 3 Group 'around (peri) antennal lobe' (pAL) and cluster 'anteriodorsal to the esophageal hole' (adES). **a** Schematic drawing of the honeybee AL. AmFoxP neurons are depicted as empty circles, arrows point to the two neuron populations. **b** Confocal image (2 μm confocal section) of a pupal brain stained with the AmFoxP[42kDa] antiserum (white label). **c–o** dISH stainings show *AmFoxP* transcript (magenta), neurotransmitter marker transcript (cyan) and DAPI-stained nuclei (blue). Large rectangular insets show higher magnifications of small boxed regions, with white label reflecting co-expressing neurons. Some double-labeled neurons are also visible in circled areas in **c**, **j**, **m**. **c–f** Adjacent cryosections of a 15 days old individual from the 'unmanipulated' condition. **g–i** Adjacent cryosections of a 15 days old individual from the 'honeycomb' condition, anterior (**g**) and posterior (**h**, **i**). **j–o** Adjacent cryosections of a 31 days old individual from the 'incubator' condition, anterior (**j–m**) and posterior (**n**, **o**). Pictograms refer to the conditions outlined in Table 1. Anatomical abbreviations see Table 5. Scale bar **b**: 100 μm, as orientation for all other panels

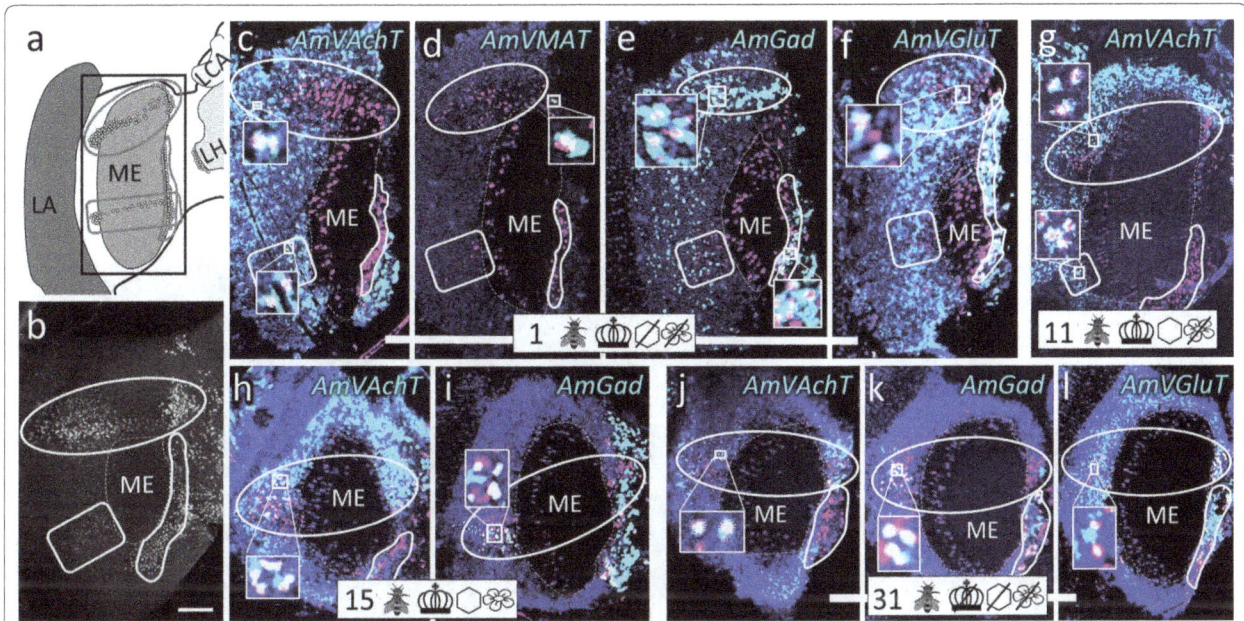

Fig. 4 Group 'around (peri) medulla' (pME). **a** Honeybee brain schematic drawing focuses on the ME. AmFoxP neurons are depicted as empty circles which surround the ME in three subsets: a dorsal (gray circle) and a ventral (gray rectangle with rounded corners) subset wrap around the anterior ME, a third subset (outlined in gray) is bordering the ME medially in a thin strip. The black rectangle indicates the localization of panels (**c–l**). **b** Confocal image (60 μm confocal stack) of a pupal brain stained with the AmFoxP^{42kDa} antiserum (white label). The outlined areas refer to the AmFoxP subsets as in **a**, the ME is indicated with a dashed line. **c–l** dISH stainings showing *AmFoxP* transcript (magenta), neurotransmitter transcript (cyan) and DAPI-stained nuclei (blue). Rectangular insets show co-localization of the two probes, resulting in white label. **c–f** Adjacent cryosections of a newly emerged individual. **g** Cryosections of an 11 days old individual from the 'honeycomb' group. **h, i** Adjacent cryosections of a 15 days old individual from the 'unmanipulated' group. **j–l** Adjacent cryosections of a 31 days old individual of the 'incubator' group. For explanations of pictograms see Table 1, for anatomical abbreviations see Table 5. Scale bar **b**: 100 μm, as orientation for all other panels

complex (dCX, Fig. 8h). *AmVGluT*-expressing AmFoxP neurons in the dCX were located medial to *AmGad*-expressing ones. The *AmVGlut* neurons in the pAL, pME and vGNG were intermingled with AmFoxP neurons expressing *AmGad* and *AmVAchT*.

Monoaminergic AmFoxP neurons

The monoaminergic marker VMAT labels neurons that express histamine (HA), octopamine (OA), dopamine (DA) or serotonin (5-HT). Large clusters were located in the region of the antennal commissure (Fig. 3e, i) and ventral to the lateral calyx (LCA) (Figs. 5d, 11b), likely corresponding to the dopaminergic C1 and C3 clusters previously described [51, 102, 103]. Further large *AmV-MAT* positive cells were localized in the somatic region ventral to the GNG, probably corresponding to the octopaminergic VUMmx neurons described previously [53, 83, 103]. Only a few isolated AmFoxP neurons co-localized with *AmVMAT*. They did not belong to any of the above described neuron populations (Fig. 1; Table 3). Because there were only individual neurons co-labeled by *AmFoxP* and *AmVMAT* we decided to name them 'MF neurons'; monoaminergic AmFoxP neurons. They were detected in four regions: dorsolateral to the AL ('MF1'),

anteriomedial to the medulla ('MF2'), dorsomedial to the lobula ('MF3') and lateral to the upper division of the central body (CBU), part of the CX ('MF4') (Figs. 4d, 11).

AmFoxP neuron populations and co-expressed neurotransmitters were consistently detected in all sampled brains

We qualitatively compared brains from individuals aged 1–50 days after emergence from the differently treated groups (Table 1). All 11 AmFoxP neuron populations were consistently detected, independent of age or treatment. The type of neurotransmitter being co-expressed was also stable and did not change (Figs. 3, 4, 5, 6, 7, 8, 9, 10).

Monoaminergic receptors in the KC

To further refine the identity of the AmFoxP-expressing mKC [32] we checked for co-expression of the D2-like dopamine receptor AmDop3 that was shown to be restricted to the lKC [150]. While the AmDop3 sense-probe (control) did not show any unspecific staining (Fig. 12f), our *dISH* stainings with the AmDop3 antisense probe revealed no coincidence with AmFoxP label within

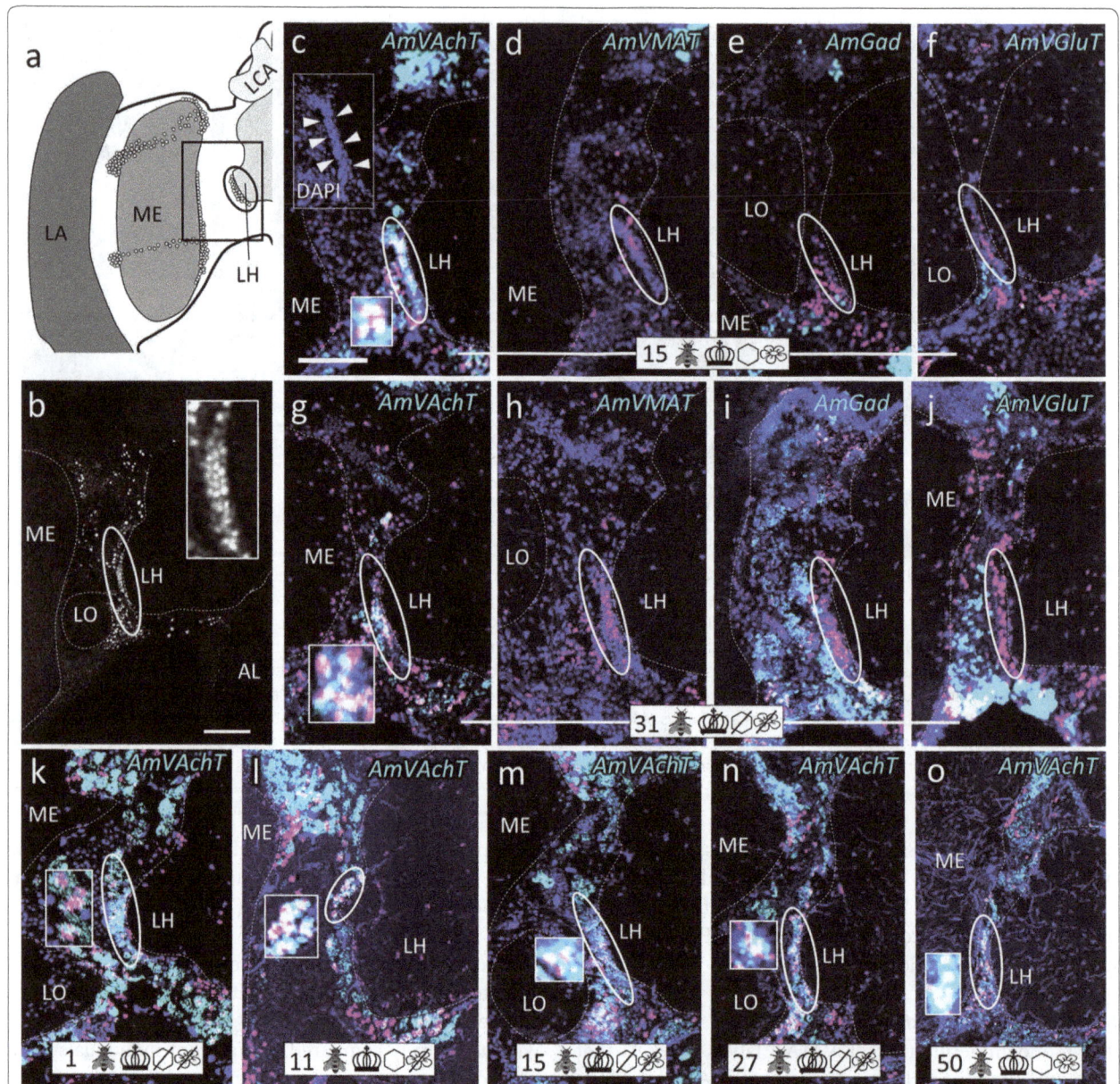

Fig. 5 Cluster 'lateral to the lateral horn' (lLH). **a** Honeybee brain schematic drawing focuses on the LH and ME. AmFoxP neurons are indicated with small empty circles. Rectangle indicates the localization of panels (**c–o**). **b** Confocal image (2 µm confocal section) of a forager brain stained with the AmFoxP[42kDa] antiserum (white label). **c–o** dISH stainings showing *AmFoxP* transcript (magenta), neurotransmitter transcript (cyan) and DAPI-stained nuclei (blue) on 12 µm brain cryosections. Small rectangular insets in **c**, **g**, **k–o** show co-localization of the two probes. Larger rectangular insets in **b**, **c** show densely-packed small nuclei of the lLH, stained with AmFoxP[42kDa] antiserum (**b**) and DAPI (**c**). **c–f** Adjacent cryosections of a 15 days old individual from the 'unmanipulated' group. **g–j** Adjacent cryosections of a 31 days old individual from the 'incubator' group. **k** Newly emerged individual. **l** 11 days old individual from the 'honeycomb' group. **m** 15 days old individual from the 'incubator' group. **n** 27 days old individual of the 'incubator' group. **o** Cryosection of a 50 days old individual from the 'unmanipulated' group. For explanations of pictograms see Table 1, for anatomical abbreviations see Table 5. Scale bar **b**, **c**: 100 µm, as orientation for all other panels

the same neurons, but juxtaposed populations of neurons expressing AmFoxP or AmDop3 (Fig. 12g).

Figure 13 schematically summarizes the neurotransmitter profiles of AmFoxP neuron populations in the honeybee brain described above.

AmVAchT and *AmVGluT* expression pattern in the KC varied in bee samples of different age

Our stainings consistently revealed AmVAchT-expression in the class I KC across all samples. This was confirmed by RT-qPCR data that revealed ten

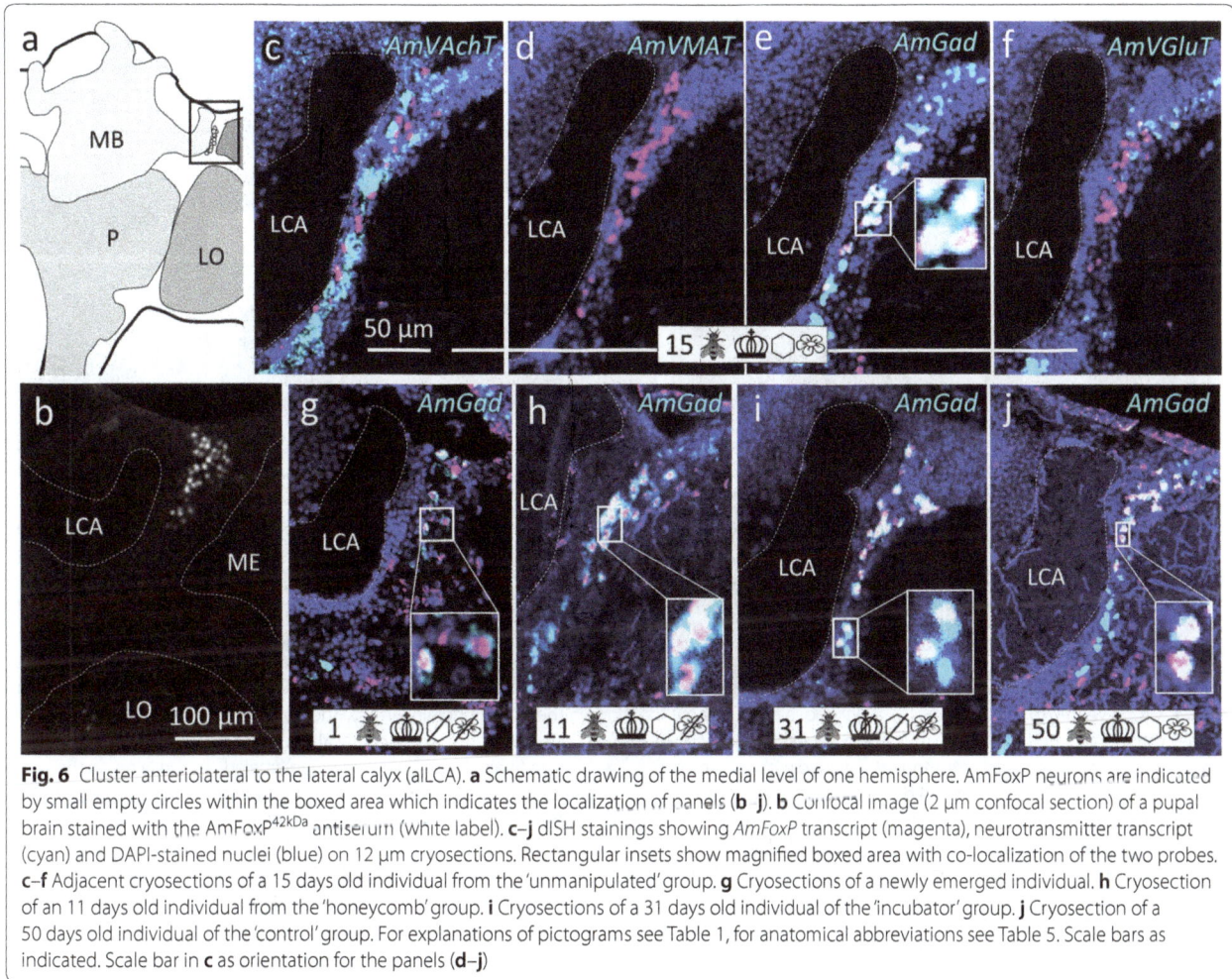

Fig. 6 Cluster anteriolateral to the lateral calyx (alLCA). **a** Schematic drawing of the medial level of one hemisphere. AmFoxP neurons are indicated by small empty circles within the boxed area which indicates the localization of panels (**b j**). **b** Confocal image (2 μm confocal section) of a pupal brain stained with the AmFoxP[42kDa] antiserum (white label). **c–j** dISH stainings showing *AmFoxP* transcript (magenta), neurotransmitter transcript (cyan) and DAPI-stained nuclei (blue) on 12 μm cryosections. Rectangular insets show magnified boxed area with co-localization of the two probes. **c–f** Adjacent cryosections of a 15 days old individual from the 'unmanipulated' group. **g** Cryosections of a newly emerged individual. **h** Cryosection of an 11 days old individual from the 'honeycomb' group. **i** Cryosections of a 31 days old individual of the 'incubator' group. **j** Cryosection of a 50 days old individual of the 'control' group. For explanations of pictograms see Table 1, for anatomical abbreviations see Table 5. Scale bars as indicated. Scale bar in **c** as orientation for the panels (**d–j**)

times more AmVAchT than AmVGluT mRNA levels in extracts prepared from calyces (Fig. 14m). AmVMAT and AmVIAAT levels were very low compared to AmVAchT (AmVMAT: 100 times less, AmVIAAT: 70 times less).

Interestingly, in younger bees (age 1–4) AmVAchT expression was restricted to the small and middle KC (sKC and mKC) (Figs. 2, 14a, b) whereas the large KC (lKC) only started expressing AmVAchT between the ages 11–15 (Fig. 14c, d). In very old bees (aged 40 and 50 days) the intensity of AmVAchT-expression in the sKC decreased but did no longer differ between the different types of class I KCs (Fig. 14e). Although very low in general and only visible with increased brightness and contrast (FIJI), AmVGluT expression levels in the small and medial KC were comparatively higher between 1 and 19 days after emergence than in older bees (Fig. 14f–j). Low AmVGluT levels in the KC were also detected with RT-qPCR and 7–11 times higher than AmVIAAT and AmVMAT levels (Fig. 14m).

Discussion

The transcription factors FOXP1, FOXP2 and FOXP4 are relevant for human cognition including language [104]. They are strongly conserved in vertebrates where they play a role in sensory processing, motor behaviors and learning [105–110]. The genomes of other animals harbor only a single *FoxP* gene locus encoding a gene with a highly conserved DNA-binding domain [25, 33, 111, 112]. The fact that the neural expression pattern in vertebrates and the Forkhead box sequence in bilateria are so highly conserved raises the question whether FoxP might bestow neurons with particular properties and functions that might have been conserved since the last common ancestor of the bilateria. This type of 'deep homology' has been noted for a number of other transcription factors [90, 91, 113–116]. Alternatively, honeybee FoxP (AmFoxP) might have very different functions than vertebrate FoxPs, depending on the evolution of the *FoxP* gene's regulatory sequences and differences in binding of

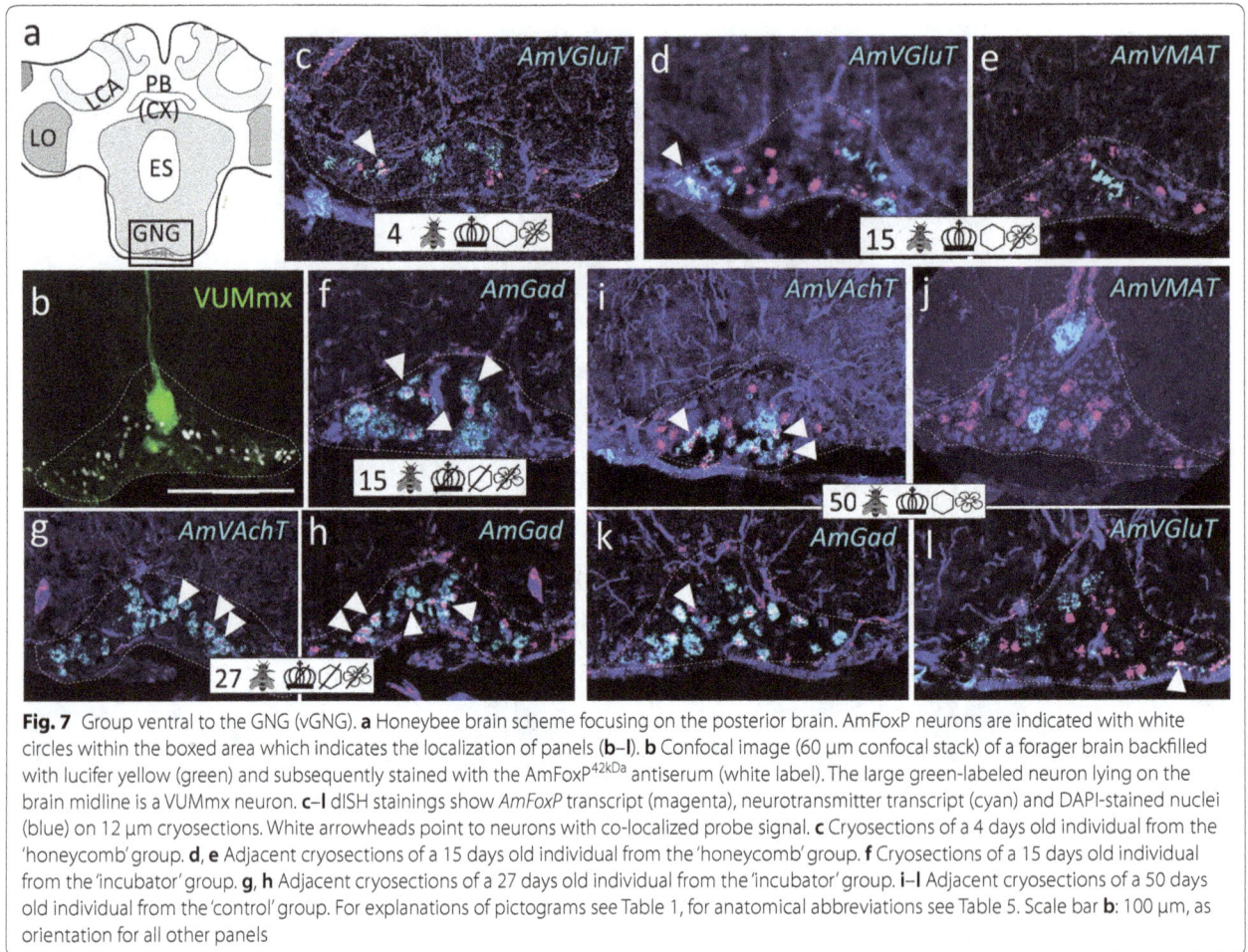

Fig. 7 Group ventral to the GNG (vGNG). **a** Honeybee brain scheme focusing on the posterior brain. AmFoxP neurons are indicated with white circles within the boxed area which indicates the localization of panels (**b–l**). **b** Confocal image (60 μm confocal stack) of a forager brain backfilled with lucifer yellow (green) and subsequently stained with the AmFoxP[42kDa] antiserum (white label). The large green-labeled neuron lying on the brain midline is a VUMmx neuron. **c–l** dISH stainings show *AmFoxP* transcript (magenta), neurotransmitter transcript (cyan) and DAPI-stained nuclei (blue) on 12 μm cryosections. White arrowheads point to neurons with co-localized probe signal. **c** Cryosections of a 4 days old individual from the 'honeycomb' group. **d, e** Adjacent cryosections of a 15 days old individual from the 'honeycomb' group. **f** Cryosections of a 15 days old individual from the 'incubator' group. **g, h** Adjacent cryosections of a 27 days old individual from the 'incubator' group. **i–l** Adjacent cryosections of a 50 days old individual from the 'control' group. For explanations of pictograms see Table 1, for anatomical abbreviations see Table 5. Scale bar **b**: 100 μm, as orientation for all other panels

the FoxP proteins to their target genes and other proteins [117].

As a first step towards the evaluation of these hypotheses, we used bee brains to map the distribution of isoform-specific AmFoxP expressing neurons and for some of them their projection pattern [25]. AmFoxP is expressed in particular sets of neurons in most cortical regions of the honeybee brain, many of them densely clustered, whereas others are found in a more distributed fashion [25].

In the present report we classified AmFoxP neurons by their neurotransmitters without discriminating between the two previously described AmFoxP isoforms. We examined individuals of different age and treatments to qualitatively assess whether the number of populations was rather robust or susceptible to different sensory and motor experience. FoxP2 can be regulated developmentally as well as by motor activity and sensory stimuli [13, 14, 47–49]. Overall, we found that AmFoxP neurons in the honeybee co-expressed a variety of neurotransmitters, similar to what has been reported in vertebrates.

Below we will discuss the transmitter profile of different neurons in honeybee and other insect brains based on the markers we used, and propose how these neurons might relate to already described neurons and their function.

Neurotransmitters

Neurotransmitters are essential for the identity and function of neurons. In honeybees their expression levels have been correlated to certain behaviors, e.g. novelty-seeking [118] or learning and memory [119]. Some of the proteins involved in neurotransmitter release are conserved and date back to the last common ancestor of eukaryotes [120, 121]. We focused on the most abundant neurotransmitters in the insect brain, i.e. glutamate, GABA, acetylcholine and monoamines. Using double-label in situ hybridization we revealed differential expression of their markers in AmFoxP neuron populations. The seven previously defined AmFoxP neuron clusters (adES, lLH, alLCA, vMCA, mKC, plLCA, mvLO) co-expressed only one of the four neurotransmitter markers whereas the four groups (pAL,

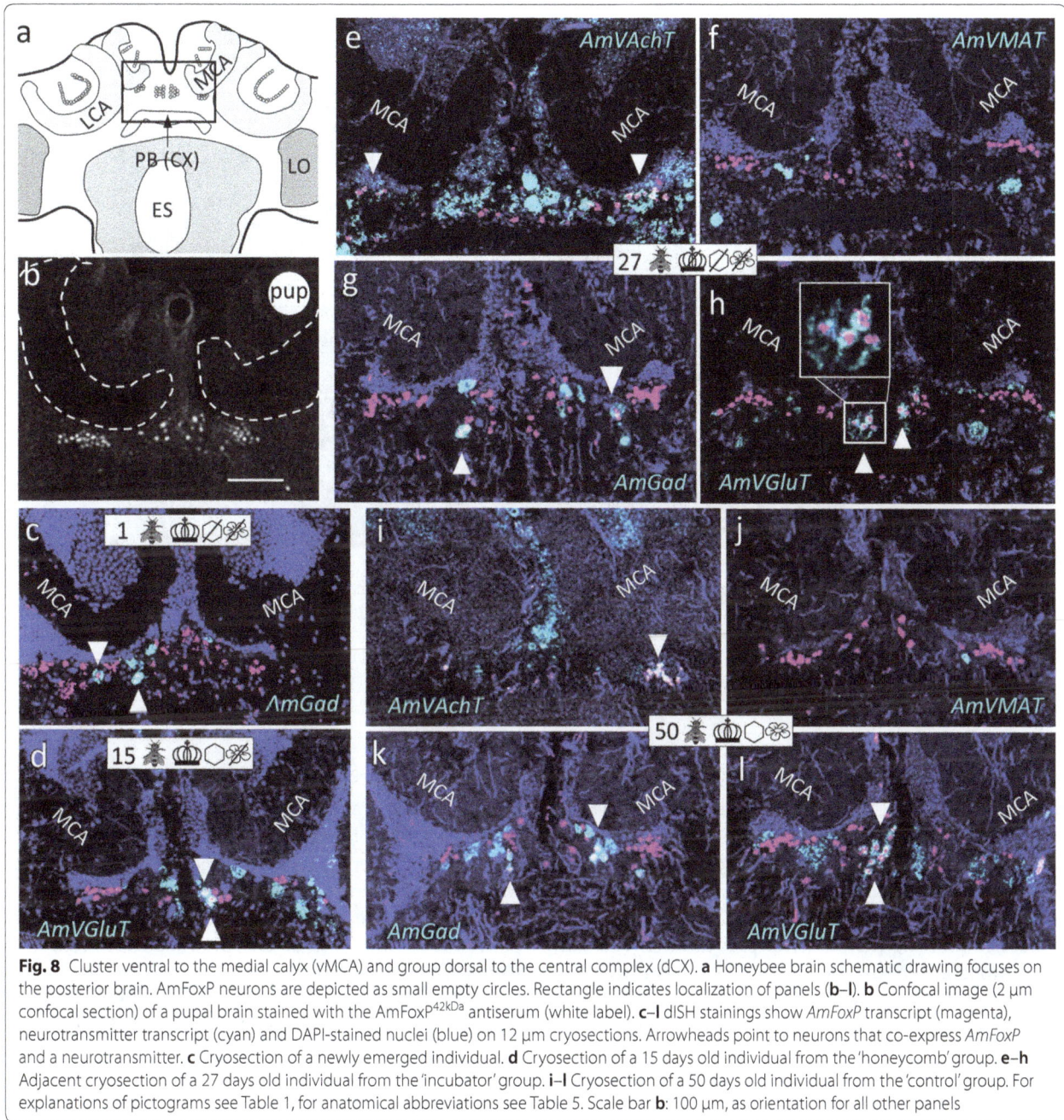

Fig. 8 Cluster ventral to the medial calyx (vMCA) and group dorsal to the central complex (dCX). **a** Honeybee brain schematic drawing focuses on the posterior brain. AmFoxP neurons are depicted as small empty circles. Rectangle indicates localization of panels (**b–l**). **b** Confocal image (2 μm confocal section) of a pupal brain stained with the AmFoxP^{42kDa} antiserum (white label). **c–l** dISH stainings show *AmFoxP* transcript (magenta), neurotransmitter transcript (cyan) and DAPI-stained nuclei (blue) on 12 μm cryosections. Arrowheads point to neurons that co-express *AmFoxP* and a neurotransmitter. **c** Cryosection of a newly emerged individual. **d** Cryosection of a 15 days old individual from the 'honeycomb' group. **e–h** Adjacent cryosection of a 27 days old individual from the 'incubator' group. **i–l** Cryosection of a 50 days old individual from the 'control' group. For explanations of pictograms see Table 1, for anatomical abbreviations see Table 5. Scale bar **b**: 100 μm, as orientation for all other panels

pME, dCX, vGNG) showed a rather heterogeneous neurotransmitter profile. This finding corroborates the differentiation between the two AmFoxP neuron population classes, i.e. 'groups' and 'clusters'. Within the 'groups' there might be smaller subunits that project to the same areas and co-express only one neurotransmitter. The pAL could certainly be further subdivided into smaller clusters lateral, medial, ventral and dorsal to the AL, being glutamatergic, GABAergic or cholinergic.

Acetylcholine

Three of the four AmFoxP groups (pAL, pME, vGNG) and five of the seven clusters (lLH, mvLO, plLCA, vMCA, mKC) expressed *AmVAchT*. The largest cluster, the mvLO, consists of two divisions, an anterior (mvLO-a) and a posterior (mvLO-p) part that project to different areas of the brain [25]. The neurites of the mvLO-p somata converge onto a tract that connects the lobula with the posteriolateral protocerebrum

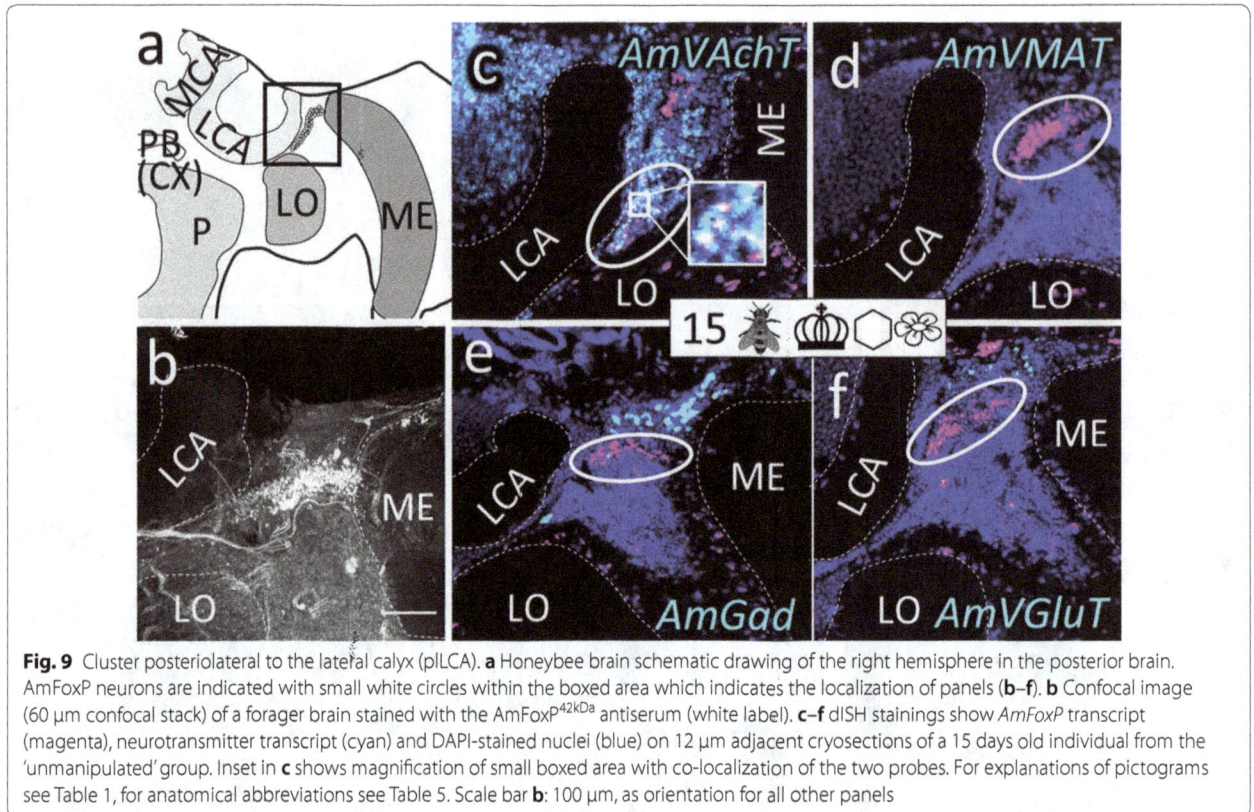

Fig. 9 Cluster posteriolateral to the lateral calyx (plLCA). **a** Honeybee brain schematic drawing of the right hemisphere in the posterior brain. AmFoxP neurons are indicated with small white circles within the boxed area which indicates the localization of panels (**b–f**). **b** Confocal image (60 μm confocal stack) of a forager brain stained with the AmFoxP[42kDa] antiserum (white label). **c–f** dISH stainings show *AmFoxP* transcript (magenta), neurotransmitter transcript (cyan) and DAPI-stained nuclei (blue) on 12 μm adjacent cryosections of a 15 days old individual from the 'unmanipulated' group. Inset in **c** shows magnification of small boxed area with co-localization of the two probes. For explanations of pictograms see Table 1, for anatomical abbreviations see Table 5. Scale bar **b**: 100 μm, as orientation for all other panels

(PLP). Such a posterior cholinergic tract was previously seen with AChE histochemistry [56]. Whether the GABAergic, AmFoxP-negative neurons between the two subdivisions of the cluster converge onto the same tracts as the mvLO-a or mvLO-p requires further studies. Schäfer and Bicker [50] showed a GABA-ir tract connecting the posterior part of the lobula and the protocerebrum that could be intermingled with the AchE-tract. If this were the case the PLP would receive inhibitory and excitatory input from the lobula. The circuitry involved might be thus important to extract oscillating, like temporal features of sensory signals [122–124].

The cholinergic vMCA is reminiscent of a cluster with AchE activity ventral to the medial calyx and dorsal to the anterior optic tract (AOT) described by Kreissl and Bicker [56]. This cluster connects to the fan-shaped body/CBU, a major subdivision of the central complex which is important for polarized vision, motor control and spatial memory [125, 126]. In future studies, neuronal tracing will help to further identify the other two cholinergic AmFoxP clusters; i.e. the lLH and the plLCA.

Interestingly, *AmVachT* was highly expressed in the KC, as shown by both RT-qPCR and *dISH*. Staining was punctate and coincided less with cell bodies, in contrast

to the *AmVachT* staining observed in the rest of the brain. Because we do not assume local translation and the puncta were numerous we do not think that these signals are located synapses contacting the KC somata which were described only for dopaminergic synapses [127]. Due to the concentrated and punctuate staining pattern it is difficult to determine whether *AmFoxP* and *AmVachT* co-localized in all mKC. Based on our analysis (see "Cholinergic AmFoxP neurons" section) we conclude that they predominantly do. Until recently there was no strong evidence about the identity of KC neurotransmitters, one of the main limitations being the difficulty to isolate postsynaptic neurons to KC to characterize physiologically their neurotransmitter profiles. Previous studies in the honeybee described the expression of *Acetylcholinesterase (AchE)* in KC [56, 128]. Shapira et al. [128] showed expression in all class I KC in nurses, but restricted signal in the lKC in foragers. *AmVachT* expression in our study was restricted to the sKC and mKC in young bees and expanded to all class I KC in older bees. These differences could be explained by the different biosynthetic origins of the AchE enzyme and the vesicular transporter VAchT. AchE is associated to the neurotransmitter cycle by degrading acetylcholine in the synaptic cleft. In vertebrate neuromuscular junctions it can be

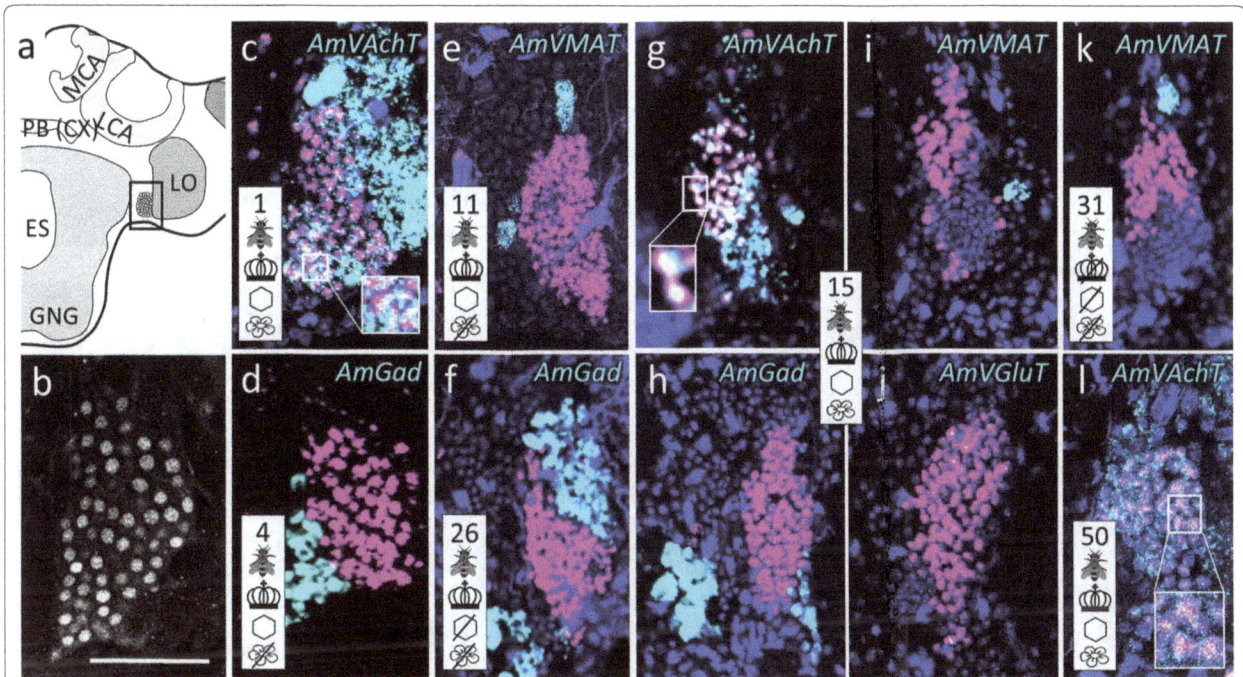

Fig. 10 Cluster medioventral to the lobula-posterior part (mvLO-p). **a** Honeybee brain schematic drawing focuses on a posterior brain hemisphere. AmFoxP neurons are indicated by small empty circles within the boxed area which indicates localization of panels (**b–j**). **b** Confocal image (2 μm confocal section) of a forager brain stained with the AmFoxP[42kDa] antiserum (white label) shows the mvLO-p. **c–l** dISH stainings showing AmFoxP transcript (magenta), neurotransmitter transcript (cyan) and DAPI-stained nuclei (blue) on 12 μm cryosections. **c** Cryosection of a newly emerged individual. **d** Cryosection of a 4 days old individual from the 'honeycomb' group, **e** Cryosection of a 11 days old individual of the 'honeycomb' group. **f** Cryosection of a 26 days old individual of the 'mini-cage' group. **g–j** Adjacent cryosections of a 15 days old individual from the 'unmanipulated' group. **k** Cryosection of a 31 days old individual of the 'incubator' group. **l** Cryosection of a 50 days old individual of the 'unmanipulated' group. Inset in **c, g, l** show magnification of boxed area with co-localization of the two probes. For explanations of pictograms see Table 1, for anatomical abbreviations see Table 5. Scale bar **b**: 50 μm, as orientation for all other panels

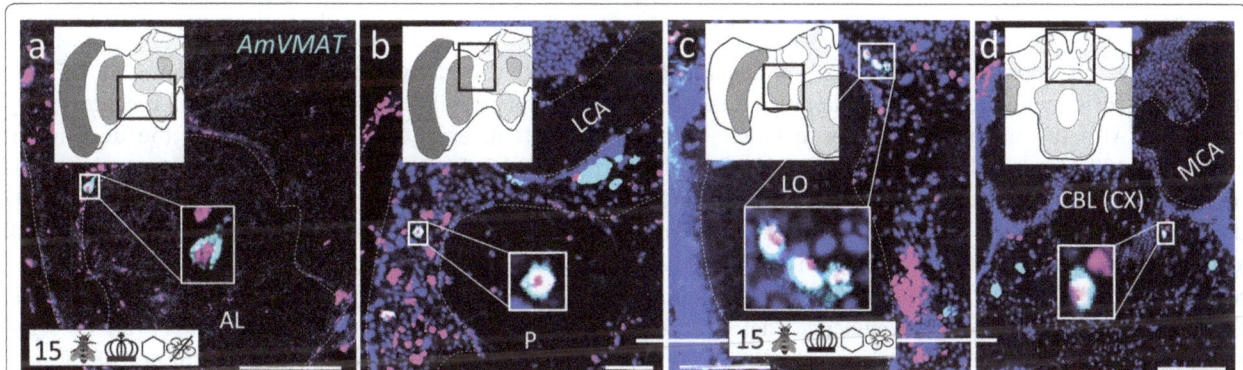

Fig. 11 Individudal 'MF' neurons (monoaminergic AmFoxP neurons) that co-express AmFoxP and *AmVMAT*. **a–d** dISH stainings showing AmFoxP transcript (magenta), *AmVMAT* (cyan) and nuclei (blue) in honeybee brain cryosections, anterior (**a**) to posterior (**d**). Insets outlined by white boxes show co-localization of the two probes. Locations in the brain where photomicrographs were taken are outlined (black line) in the schematic drawing in the insets at the top of each panel. **a** 'MF1' neurons dorsolateral to the antennal lobe (AL) of a 15 days old individual from the 'encaged honeycomb' group. **b** 'MF2' neuron medial to the medulla (ME). **c** 'MF3' neurons dorso-medial to the lobula (LO). **d** 'MF4' neurons close to the fan-shaped body (FB) of the central complex (CX). **b–d** Cryosections of a 15 days old individual from the 'control' group. For explanations of pictograms see Table 1, for anatomical abbreviations see Table 5. Scale bars: 100 μm

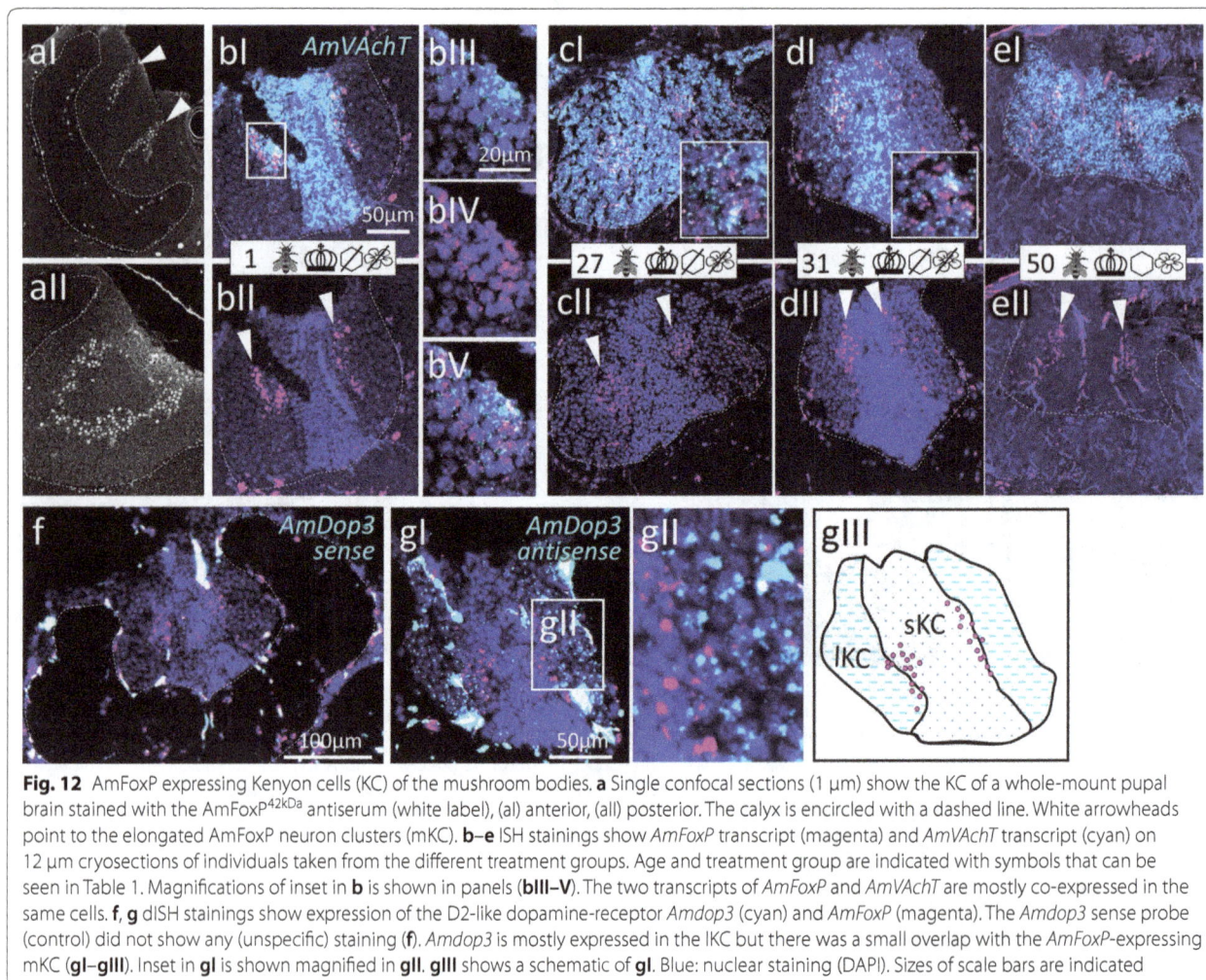

Fig. 12 AmFoxP expressing Kenyon cells (KC) of the mushroom bodies. **a** Single confocal sections (1 μm) show the KC of a whole-mount pupal brain stained with the AmFoxP[42kDa] antiserum (white label), (aI) anterior, (aII) posterior. The calyx is encircled with a dashed line. White arrowheads point to the elongated AmFoxP neuron clusters (mKC). **b–e** ISH stainings show *AmFoxP* transcript (magenta) and *AmVAchT* transcript (cyan) on 12 μm cryosections of individuals taken from the different treatment groups. Age and treatment group are indicated with symbols that can be seen in Table 1. Magnifications of inset in **b** is shown in panels (**bIII–V**). The two transcripts of *AmFoxP* and *AmVAchT* are mostly co-expressed in the same cells. **f, g** dISH stainings show expression of the D2-like dopamine-receptor *Amdop3* (cyan) and *AmFoxP* (magenta). The *Amdop3* sense probe (control) did not show any (unspecific) staining (**f**). *Amdop3* is mostly expressed in the lKC but there was a small overlap with the *AmFoxP*-expressing mKC (**gI–gIII**). Inset in **gI** is shown magnified in **gII**. **gIII** shows a schematic of **gI**. Blue: nuclear staining (DAPI). Sizes of scale bars are indicated

released pre- and post-synaptically [129] which makes it a marker for cholinergic as well as cholireceptive neurons [130]. Also, it is implicated in other metabolic pathways [131, 132]. Thus AchE produced by the KC might be predominantly transported to the microglomeruli in the calyx neuropil to hydrolyze Ach transmitted by projection neurons. Barnstedt et al. [133] demonstrated that some KC are cholinergic in *Drosophila* and our finding constitute the first unequivocal evidence that KC are cholinergic in the honeybee.

Glutamate

All four AmFoxP groups and one cluster, the adES, expressed *AmVGluT*. In VGlut-reporter *Drosophila* lines, several large glutamatergic neurons with a similar distribution as the neurons of the honeybee dCX cluster were shown to project into the central complex (CX) [134]. Thus, the AmFoxP neurons of the dCX might be a subset of glutamatergic neurons also projecting into the CX. This proposition is supported by the study on *Drosophila*

dFoxP gene activity in the CX by Lawton et al. [27]. As the CX neuropils strongly express GluCl receptors [64], the glutamatergic AmFoxP neurons of the dCX might transmit inhibitory input. Based on location, the glutamatergic AmFoxP neurons in the vGNG cluster might be descending (motor) neurons, possibly innervating neck muscles [135, 136].

In some sections, especially in newly emerged bees, sparse and very weak signals of *AmVGluT* were detected in the sKC. This was corroborated by the RT-qPCR data showing that the KC expressed small amounts of *AmVGluT*, ten times less than *AmVAchT*, but 7–11 times more than *AmVIAAT* and *AmVMAT*. The very low levels of the latter two markers might be due to contamination of the samples with cells other than KC. Very weak glu-ir signals [52] and high mRNA amounts of *AmEAAT* [59] in the sKC of the MB have been described before [52, 59]. In crickets, glu-like-ir signal was reported only in the (inner) KII and (outer) K III but not in the (inner) KI KC [54]. In *Drosophila*, glu-like-ir was detected in

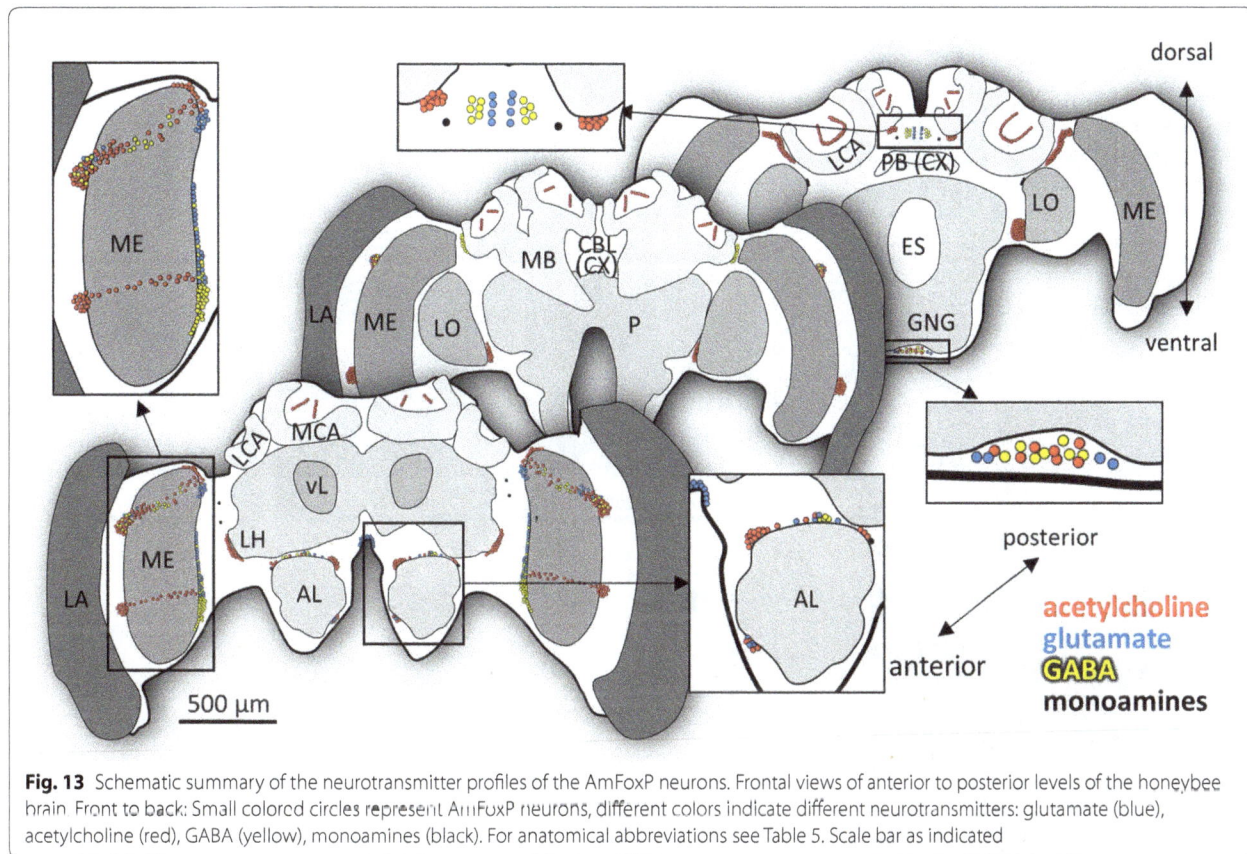

Fig. 13 Schematic summary of the neurotransmitter profiles of the AmFoxP neurons. Frontal views of anterior to posterior levels of the honeybee brain. Front to back: Small colored circles represent AmFoxP neurons, different colors indicate different neurotransmitters: glutamate (blue), acetylcholine (red), GABA (yellow), monoamines (black). For anatomical abbreviations see Table 5. Scale bar as indicated

the $\alpha\beta_c$—KC subset, which is developmentally generated last and expresses dFoxP [28, 32], but not dVGluT [55]. These authors discuss that neurotransmitter expression in the KC could vary over lifetime and that glutamate might be expressed only transiently. This is in line with our data, as we see weak signals in younger bees at the age of 1–19 days, but less distinctive or not at all in older bees, aged 23–50 days. This age-dependent difference could mirror the behavioral switch from nurses to foragers which is accompanied by gene expression differences [137].

GABA

The four AmFoxP groups and the alLCA cluster express *AmGad*. AmFoxP neurons dorsal to the CX (dCX) that co-express *AmGad* might correspond to neurons described by GABA-like-ir [50] and project to the CX. If the glutamatergic AmFoxP neurons connected to postsynaptic neurons with GluCl receptors in the CX, as mentioned above, then the dCX cluster would transmit only inhibitory input to the CX. Strausfeld and Hirth [91] have compared the CX to the vertebrate basal ganglia, based on similar developmental

gene expression profiles, similar function in the selection and maintenance of adaptive behavior and because both constitute a 'midline brain structure' [91]. Interestingly the striatum of the basal ganglia express FoxP1, 2 and 4 [14, 21, 23, 138–140]; and plays a role in adaptive sensorimotor behavior [141–144]. Similarly, the CX is important for sensorimotor integration and motor control [91, 145–147] and it will be interesting for future studies to examine a possible corresponding role of the inhibitory AmFoxP neurons that might project to the CX.

The single *AmGad*-expressing AmFoxP neurons in the pAL neuron group are located anterio-dorsal and posterio-ventral to the AL but not in the larger *AmGad*-labeled clusters lateral to the AL which are most likely inhibitory projection neurons [94, 101]. The GABAergic AmFoxP neurons within the pAL might be local interneurons [57, 148]. We also showed that the AmFoxP neurons in the mvLO are not GABAergic and thus confirmed that they do not correspond to the (more anteriorly located) A3v cluster as suggested by Kiya et al. [31].

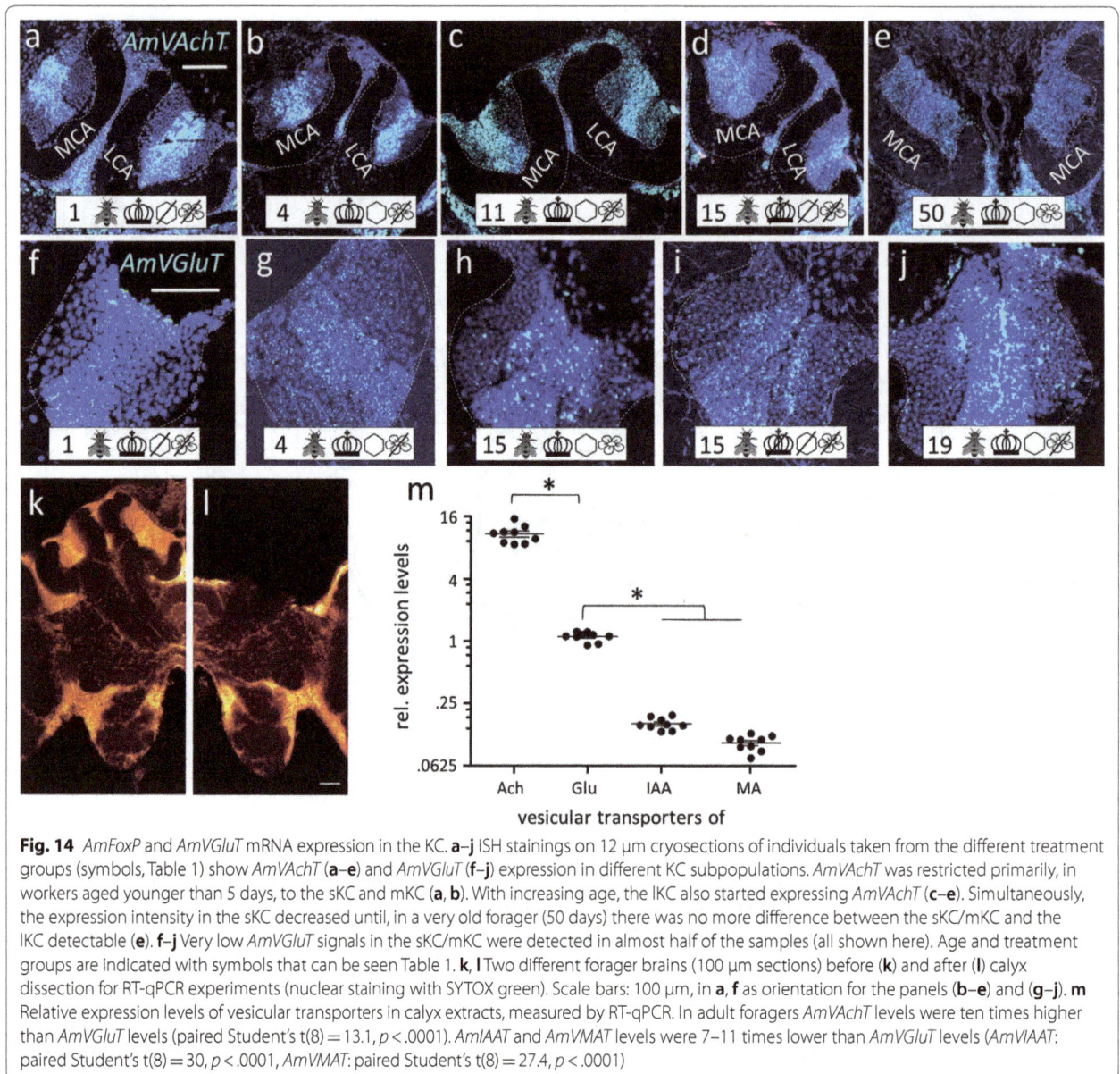

Fig. 14 *AmFoxP* and *AmVGluT* mRNA expression in the KC. **a–j** ISH stainings on 12 µm cryosections of individuals taken from the different treatment groups (symbols, Table 1) show *AmVAchT* (**a–e**) and *AmVGluT* (**f–j**) expression in different KC subpopulations. *AmVAchT* was restricted primarily, in workers aged younger than 5 days, to the sKC and mKC (**a, b**). With increasing age, the lKC also started expressing *AmVAchT* (**c–e**). Simultaneously, the expression intensity in the sKC decreased until, in a very old forager (50 days) there was no more difference between the sKC/mKC and the lKC detectable (**e**). **f–j** Very low *AmVGluT* signals in the sKC/mKC were detected in almost half of the samples (all shown here). Age and treatment groups are indicated with symbols that can be seen Table 1. **k, l** Two different forager brains (100 µm sections) before (**k**) and after (**l**) calyx dissection for RT-qPCR experiments (nuclear staining with SYTOX green). Scale bars: 100 µm, in **a, f** as orientation for the panels (**b–e**) and (**g–j**). **m** Relative expression levels of vesicular transporters in calyx extracts, measured by RT-qPCR. In adult foragers *AmVAchT* levels were ten times higher than *AmVGluT* levels (paired Student's t(8) = 13.1, $p < .0001$). *AmIAAT* and *AmVMAT* levels were 7–11 times lower than *AmVGluT* levels (*AmVIAAT*: paired Student's t(8) = 30, $p < .0001$, *AmVMAT*: paired Student's t(8) = 27.4, $p < .0001$)

Monoamines

We found overlap between *AmVMAT* and *AmFoxP* expression only in less than ten isolated *AmVMAT*-expressing AmFoxP neurons throughout the brain whereas none of the eleven described AmFoxP neuron populations expressed *AmVMAT*. The isolated *AmVMAT*-expressing neurons around the mvLO might be part of the S_L cluster that projects dorsally [51, 102]. The MF1 might correspond to the 2–3 dopaminergic soma between the AOTU and the AL described by Tedjakumala et al. [102]. Because of their localization rather dorso-lateral to the lobula, the MF3 neurons could not be part of the dopaminergic C4 cluster [102].

Mercer et al. [103] also located a catecholamine-labeled neuron cluster dorso-medial to the lobula, as did Nässel et al. [149] for serotonin. The MF4 might belong to the 'S_P-cluster' that projects into the central body and the noduli [51].

We also used *AmDop3* to detect the dopaminergic D2-like receptor, previously reported to be expressed in the lKC [150]. There were only individual—DAPI identified—KC nuclei being labeled by both, the *AmFoxP* and the *AmDop3* probes which supports the suggestion by Suenami et al. [151] that AmFoxP expressing KC could belong to the lKC. However, mostly, *AmDop3* and *AmFoxP* did not overlap. This is consistent with

Table 4 List of the 11 AmFoxP expressing neuron populations (clusters or groups) and their co-expressed neurotransmitter(s) (Glut: glutamate, Ach: acetylcholine) ordered from anterior to posterior

#	Type of AmFoxP neuron population	Localization	Name	Neurotransmitter	Figures
1	Group	Around (peri) antennal lobe	pAL	GABA, Glut, Ach	Figure 3
2	Cluster	Anteriodorsal to esophageal hole	adES	Glu	Figure 3
3	Group	Around (peri) medulla	pME	GABA, Glut, Ach	Figure 4
4	Cluster	Lateral to the lateral horn	lLH	Ach	Figure 5
5	Cluster	Anteriolateral to the lateral calyx	alLCA	GABA	Figure 6
6	Group	Dorsal to the central complex	dCX	Glu, GABA	Figure 8
7	Cluster	Ventral to the medial calyx	vMCA	Ach	Figure 8
8	cluster	Posteriolateral to the lateral calyx	plLCA	Ach	Figure 10
9.1	Cluster	Medioventral to the lobula, anterior	mvLO-a	Ach	Figure 10
9.2	Cluster	Medioventral to the lobula, posterior	mvLO-p	Ach	Figure 10
10	Cluster	Middle Kenyon cells	mKC	Ach	Figure 12
11	Group	Ventral to the gnathal ganglia	vGNG	GABA, Glut, Ach	Figure 7

the idea that there is a separation between different KC subgroups, but it is not always sharp.

We did detect monoamines also in the previously described dopaminergic clusters C1, C3 and the S-clusters, which we found to be strongly labeled by *AmVMAT*, whereas C2 and C4 were not labeled. This could be due to differential sensitivity of the markers used. The previous studies detected immunoreactivity for Tyrosine Hydroxylase (TH) the enzyme that catalyzes l-tyrosine to L-DOPA, the precursor for dopamine [51] and immunoreactivity for GABA [102]. Furthermore, our staining labeled the large and strongly expressing octopaminergic VUMmx neurons ventral to the GNG [53]. We unambiguously identified the VUMmx neurons by their projection pattern using neuronal backfilling [53, 83]. We also observed some very weakly-labeled *AmVMAT* neurons close to the AL that might express serotonin as described in Dacks et al. [152].

In vertebrates, FoxP2 is expressed in the ventral tegmental area and substantia nigra [20, 23] which are the main sources of striatal and limbic forebrain dopamine. However, explicit cellular co-localization of dopamine and FoxP2 has not been reported for these regions.

Neurotransmitter profile of vertebrate FoxP neurons

Some developmentally relevant transcription factors are only expressed in neurons of a particular neurotransmitter type [153, 154]. This is not the case in our study of honeybees and also not in vertebrates. For instance, FoxP2 and GABA co-occur in the Purkinje cells, striatal medium spiny neurons [14, 20], 'arkypallidal' neurons of the external Globus pallidus [155], neurons ventromedial to the 'Barrington' nucleus ('Bar', pons, brain stem)

[156] and in the parabrachial nucleus ('PB', pons, brain stem) [157]. FoxP2 and glutamate co-occur in pyramidal neurons in the cortex [20], the dLGN (thalamus) [46], neurons dorsolateral to the Bar nucleus [156], in the subparabrachial nucleus [158] and in the PB (pons, brain stem) [157]. Cholinergic spinal motor neurons express FoxP1, FoxP2 and FoxP4 during neuronal differentiation [159–162]. FoxP2-expressing neurons in the substantia nigra [20] are likely to be dopaminergic. Which of these neuron populations might have similarities (beyond FoxP and a specific neurotransmitter profile) to neurons in honeybee, requires more comparative information on molecular profiles of particular AmFoxP expressing neurons, their anatomical connections and their function.

Aging/environmental stimulus manipulation

Age and environmental factors determine many aspects of life in honeybees. For this reason, we investigated whether age or environmental conditions play a role in the co-expression of neurotransmitters and AmFoxP in the analyzed neuron populations. After emerging from their cells, honeybee workers stay in the hive for about 3 weeks and perform tasks sequentially, i.e. cell cleaning, nursing, wax production and guarding. Subsequently, they start to forage for water, nectar or pollen and communicate their findings with the highly sophisticated 'waggle dance' behavior to their sisters in the hive [38–41, 163]. They die about 6 weeks after emersion. Honeybee brain anatomy [164] and the expression levels of certain proteins like CREB [165], bruchpilot [166] vitellogenin [167], synapsin [168] or neuropeptides [169] vary with age and experience. Seasonal changes in gene expression were also observed

[170–172]. FoxP2 levels also change in a specific brain area of songbirds with age [14] and as a result of singing [47–49]. For this reason, we hypothesized that some AmFoxP clusters and groups might be dynamic in terms of *AmFoxP* and neurotransmitter expression. However, we could identify the clusters and groups based on FoxP expression reliably in all brain samples analyzed, regardless of age and environmental condition. While this finding is not quantitative it suggests that under the housing and seasonal conditions we used *AmFoxP* and the associated neurotransmitters did not vary noticeably. We conclude that the neuron populations, we identified, are not functionally restricted to certain life-cycle phases, but instead needed for behavior that might be constantly relevant. Using RT-qPCR Kiya et al. [31] detected an age-dependent increase of *AmFoxP* expression in whole-brain samples from eclosion to age 34 days but no significant differences between nurse and worker bees. We also found an increase of *AmFoxP* transcript from pupae to workers aged 33 days [25]. We conclude that the results of Kiya et al. [31] and ours reflect a different sensitivity than our in situ hybridization protocol affords. A combination of laser-capture and RT-qPCR could more precisely quantify the actual *AmFoxP* amounts within the eleven clusters and groups at different life history stages.

Conclusion

In summary we showed that each of the seven AmFoxP neuron *clusters* co-expressed only one particular neurotransmitter whereas the four *groups* co-expressed more than one neurotransmitter and might therefore be further sub-divided. Five clusters expressed *AmVAchT* and are therefore excitatory whereas one cluster (alLCA) co-expressed *AmGad* and is therefore inhibitory. The glutamatergic adES cluster could be inhibitory or excitatory, depending on the receptor type in the postsynapse. None of the eleven AmFoxP neuron populations co-expressed *AmVMAT*, they are therefore not modulatory. However, a small number of isolated neurons in different parts of the central brain showed co-expression of *AmFoxP* and *AmVMAT*.

All eleven AmFoxP neuron populations kept their neurotransmitter profiles across ages and under different conditions of sensory and motor deprivation. This indicates that the FoxP expressing neurons in honeybees do not undergo neurotransmitter switching [173]. Our present data provide a framework to pursue further comparative studies on the function of particular populations of invertebrate and vertebrate FoxP neurons in the context of 'deep homology', which can lead to insights to questions of evolutionary conservation and novelty.

Abbreviations
See Table 5.

Table 5 List of anatomical and molecular abbreviations

Anatomical abbreviations

AL	Antennal lobe
CX	Central complex
CBU/CBL	Central body, upper and lower division
ES	Esophageal hole
GNG	Gnathal ganglia
KC (sKC, IKC, mKC)	Small, large and middle Kenyon cells
LA	Lamina
LCA	Lateral calyx
LH	Lateral horn
LO	Lobula
MCA	Medial calyx
ME	Medulla
OL	Optic lobe
P	Protocerebrum
PB	Protocerebral bridge
PLP	Posteriolateral protocerebrum
Am	*Apis mellifera*

Molecular abbreviations

AmVAchT	The honeybee vesicular transporter for acetylcholine
AmDop3	The honeybee D2-like dopamine receptor
AmVGluT	The honeybee vesicular transporter for glutamate
AmGad	The honeybee glutamate decarboxylase
AmVIAAT	The honeybee vesicular transporter of inhibitory amino acids
AmVMAT	The honeybee vesicular transporter for monoamines
dISH	Double-lable in situ hybridization
GABA	Gamma-aminobutyric acid
glu	Glutamate
-ir	Immunoreactive immunoreactive

Authors' contributions

CS, AS and GL designed the study. AS, JA and JM generated *dISH* data. AS performed confocal imaging. GL designed and performed the RT-qPCR experiments. AS and CS analyzed the data and wrote the manuscript. GL contributed to the analysis and writing. All authors read and approved the final manuscript.

Author details

[1] Department of Animal Behavior, Freie Universität Berlin, Takustraße 6, 14195 Berlin, Germany. [2] Department of Neurobiology, Freie Universität Berlin, Königin-Luise-Straße 28-30, 14195 Berlin, Germany.

Acknowledgements

We thank Peter Knoll for his help with handling the bees, especially for the manipulation experiments. We thank Anja Slowinski for help with generating RT-qPCR data. For providing figure artwork we thank Marco Schubert and for confocal microscope equipment we would like to acknowledge the assistance of the Core Facility BioSupraMol supported by the DFG.

Authors' information

The present study is part of AS Doctoral project under the supervision of CS, in collaboration with GL. JM did his BA thesis with AS and CS, JA contributed as a student assistant to the laboratory work of GL and AS.

Competing interests

The authors declare that they have no competing interests.

Funding

AS was funded by a Ph.D. scholarship of the International Research School in Molecular Neurobiology (MolNeuro), part of the Helmholtz foundation. GL and JA were funded by a Research Grant of the DFG: "Molecular correlates of memory phases and development of molecular tools to modify brain physiology in the honeybee" (219171051).

References

1. Golson ML, Kaestner KH. Fox transcription factors: from development to disease. Development. 2016;143(24):4558–70.
2. Konopka G, Roberts TF. Insights into the neural and genetic basis of vocal communication. Cell. 2016;164(6):1269–76.
3. Bowers JM, Konopka G. The role of the FOXP family of transcription factors in ASD. Dis Mark. 2012;33(5):251–60.
4. Le Fevre AK, Taylor S, Malek NH, Horn D, Carr CW, Abdul-Rahman OA, et al. FOXP1 mutations cause intellectual disability and a recognizable phenotype. Am J Med Genet Part A. 2013;161(12):3166–75.
5. Reuter MS, Riess A, Moog U, Briggs TA, Chandler KE, Rauch A, et al. FOXP2 variants in 14 individuals with developmental speech and language disorders broaden the mutational and clinical spectrum. J Med Genet. 2017;54(1):64–72.
6. Charng WL, Karaca E, Coban Akdemir Z, Gambin T, Atik MM, Gu S, et al. Exome sequencing in mostly consanguineous Arab families with neurologic disease provides a high potential molecular diagnosis rate. BMC Med Genom. 2016;9(1):42.
7. Lai CSL, Fisher SE, Hurst JA, Vargha-Khadem F, Monaco AP. A forkhead-domain gene is mutated in a severe speech and language disorder. Nature. 2001;413(6855):519–23.
8. Schulze K, Vargha-Khadem F, Mishkin M. Phonological working memory and FOXP2. Neuropsychologia. 2018;108:147–52.
9. Gong X, Jia M, Ruan Y, Shuang M, Liu J, Wu S, et al. Association between the FOXP2 gene and autistic disorder in Chinese population. Am J Med Genet Part B Neuropsychiatr Genet. 2004;127B(1):113–6.
10. Chien YL, Wu YY, Chen HI, Tsai WC, Chiu YN, Liu SK, et al. The central nervous system patterning gene variants associated with clinical symptom severity of autism spectrum disorders. J Formos Med Assoc. 2017;116(10):755–64.
11. Morgan A, Fisher S, Scheffer I, Hildebrand M. FOXP2-related speech and language disorders. In: Adam MPAH, Pagon RA, et al., editors. June 23 2016 ed. GeneReviews®; 2016.
12. Kaestner KH, Knöchel W, Martínez DE. Unified nomenclature for the winged helix/forkhead transcription factors. Genes Dev. 2000;14(2):142–6.
13. Horng S, Kreiman G, Ellsworth C, Page D, Blank M, Millen K, et al. Differential gene expression in the developing lateral geniculate nucleus and medial geniculate nucleus reveals novel roles for Zic4 and Foxp2 in visual and auditory pathway development. J Neurosci. 2009;29(43):13672–83.
14. Haesler S, Wada K, Nshdejan A, Morrisey EE, Lints T, Jarvis ED, et al. FoxP2 expression in avian vocal learners and non-learners. J Neurosci. 2004;24(13):3164.
15. Wohlgemuth S, Adam I, Scharff C. FoxP2 in songbirds. Curr Opin Neurobiol. 2014;28:86–93.
16. Hannenhalli S, Kaestner KH. The evolution of Fox genes and their role in development and disease. Nat Rev Genet. 2009;10(4):233–40.
17. Takahashi H, Takahashi K, Liu F-C. FOXP genes, neural development, speech and language disorders. In: Maiese K, editor. Forkhead transcription factors: vital elements in biology and medicine. New York: Springer; 2010. p. 117–29.
18. Lai CSL, Gerrelli D, Monaco AP, Fisher SE, Copp AJ. FOXP2 expression during brain development coincides with adult sites of pathology in a severe speech and language disorder. Brain. 2003;126(11):2455–62.
19. Shu W, Yang H, Zhang L, Lu MM, Morrisey EE. Characterization of a new subfamily of winged-helix/forkhead (fox) genes that are expressed in the lung and act as transcriptional repressors. J Biol Chem. 2001;276(29):27488–97.
20. Campbell P, Reep RL, Stoll ML, Ophir AG, Phelps SM. Conservation and diversity of Foxp2 expression in muroid rodents: functional implications. J Comp Neurol. 2009;512(1):84–100.
21. Mendoza E, Tokarev K, Düring DN, Retamosa EC, Weiss M, Arpenik N, et al. Differential coexpression of FoxP1, FoxP2, and FoxP4 in the Zebra Finch (*Taeniopygia guttata*) song system. J Comp Neurol. 2015;523(9):1318–40.
22. Chen Q, Heston JB, Burkett ZD, White SA. Expression analysis of the speech-related genes FoxP1 and FoxP2 and their relation to singing behavior in two songbird species. J Exp Biol. 2013;216(19):3682–92.
23. Ferland RJ, Cherry TJ, Preware PO, Morrisey EE, Walsh CA. Characterization of Foxp2 and Foxp1 mRNA and protein in the developing and mature brain. J Comp Neurol. 2003;460(2):266–79.
24. Shimeld SM, Degnan B, Luke GN. Evolutionary genomics of the Fox genes: origin of gene families and the ancestry of gene clusters. Genomics. 2010;95(5):256–60.
25. Schatton A, Mendoza E, Grube K, Scharff C. FoxP in bees: a comparative study on the developmental and adult expression pattern in three bee species considering isoforms and circuitry. J Comp Neurol. 2018;526(9):1589–610.
26. Adell T, Muller WE. Isolation and characterization of five Fox (Forkhead) genes from the sponge *Suberites domuncula*. Gene. 2004;334:35–46.
27. Lawton KJ, Wassmer TL, Deitcher DL. Conserved role of *Drosophila melanogaster* FoxP in motor coordination and courtship song. Behav Brain Res. 2014;268:213–21.

28. DasGupta S, Ferreira CH, Miesenböck G. FoxP influences the speed and accuracy of a perceptual decision in Drosophila. Science. 2014;344(6186):901–4.

29. Mendoza E, Colomb J, Rybak J, Pflüger H-J, Zars T, Scharff C, et al. Drosophila FoxP mutants are deficient in operant self-learning. PLoS ONE. 2014;9(6):e100648.

30. Groschner LN, Chan WHL, Bogacz R, DasGupta S, Miesenbock G. Dendritic integration of sensory evidence in perceptual decision-making. Cell. 2018;173(4):894.e13–905.e13.

31. Kiya T, Itoh Y, Kubo T. Expression analysis of the FoxP homologue in the brain of the honeybee Apis mellifera. Insect Mol Biol. 2008;17(1):53–60.

32. Schatton A, Scharff C. FoxP expression identifies a Kenyon cell subtype in the honeybee mushroom bodies linking them to fruit fly αβc neurons. Eur J Neurosci. 2017;46(9):2534–41.

33. Santos ME, Athanasiadis A, Leitão AB, DuPasquier L, Sucena É. Alternative splicing and gene duplication in the evolution of the FoxP gene subfamily. Mol Biol Evol. 2011;28(1):237–47.

34. Srinivasan MV. Honey bees as a model for vision, perception, and cognition. Annu Rev Entomol. 2010;55(1):267–84.

35. Menzel R. The honeybee as a model for understanding the basis of cognition. Nat Rev Neurosci. 2012;13(11):758–68.

36. Eisenhardt D. Molecular mechanisms underlying formation of long-term reward memories and extinction memories in the honeybee (Apis mellifera). Learn Memory. 2014;21(10):534–42.

37. Menzel R, Greggers U, Smith A, Berger S, Brandt R, Brunke S, et al. Honey bees navigate according to a map-like spatial memory. Proc Natl Acad Sci USA. 2005;102(8):3040–5.

38. von Frisch K. Decoding the language of the bee. Science. 1974;185:663–8.

39. von Frisch K. Die Tänze der Bienen. Österr Zool Zeit. 1946;1:1–48.

40. Schürch R, Couvillon MJ, Beekman M. Ballroom biology: recent insights into honey bee waggle dance communications. Front Ecol Evol. 2016;3:147.

41. von Frisch K. Über die "Sprache" der Bienen, eine tier-psychologische Untersuchung. Zool Jahrb. 1923;40:1–186.

42. Avargues-Weber A, Giurfa M. Conceptual learning by miniature brains. Proc Biol Sci. 2013;280(1772):20131907.

43. Perry CJ, Barron AB. Honey bees selectively avoid difficult choices. Proc Natl Acad Sci. 2013;110(47):19155–9.

44. Howard SR, Avarguès-Weber A, Garcia JE, Greentree AD, Dyer AG. Numerical ordering of zero in honey bees. Science. 2018;360(6393):1124–6.

45. Duffy KR, Holman KD, Mitchell DE. Shrinkage of X cells in the lateral geniculate nucleus after monocular deprivation revealed by FoxP2 labeling. Vis Neurosci. 2014;31(3):253–61.

46. Iwai L, Ohashi Y, van der List D, Usrey WM, Miyashita Y, Kawasaki H. FoxP2 is a Parvocellular-specific transcription factor in the visual thalamus of monkeys and ferrets. Cereb Cortex (New York, NY). 2013;23(9):2204–12.

47. Miller JE, Spiteri E, Condro MC, Dosumu-Johnson RT, Geschwind DH, White SA. Birdsong decreases protein levels of FoxP2, a molecule required for human speech. J Neurophysiol. 2008;100(4):2015–25.

48. Teramitsu I, White SA. FoxP2 regulation during undirected singing in adult songbirds. J Neurosci. 2006;26(28):7390–4.

49. Adam I, Mendoza E, Kobalz U, Wohlgemuth S, Scharff C. FoxP2 directly regulates the reelin receptor VLDLR developmentally and by singing. Mol Cell Neurosci. 2016;74:96–105.

50. Schäfer S, Bicker G. Distribution of GABA-like immunoreactivity in the brain of the honeybee. J Comp Neurol. 1986;246(3):287–300.

51. Schäfer S, Rehder V. Dopamine-like immunoreactivity in the brain and suboesophageal ganglion of the honeybee. J Comp Neurol. 1989;280(1):43–58.

52. Bicker G, Schafer S, Ottersen O, Storm-Mathisen J. Glutamate-like immunoreactivity in identified neuronal populations of insect nervous systems. J Neurosci. 1988;8(6):2108–22.

53. Kreissl S, Eichmüller S, Bicker G, Rapus J, Eckert M. Octopamine-like immunoreactivity in the brain and subesophageal ganglion of the honeybee. J Comp Neurol. 1994;348(4):583–95.

54. Schürmann F-W, Ottersen OP, Honegger H-W. Glutamate-like immunoreactivity marks compartments of the mushroom bodies in the brain of the cricket. J Comp Neurol. 2000;418(2):227–39.

55. Sinakevitch I, Farris SM, Strausfeld NJ. Taurine-, aspartate- and glutamate-like immunoreactivity identifies chemically distinct subdivisions of Kenyon cells in the cockroach mushroom body. J Comp Neurol. 2001;439(3):352–67.

56. Kreissl S, Bicker G. Histochemistry of acetylcholinesterase and immunocytochemistry of an acetylcholine receptor-like antigen in the brain of the honeybee. J Comp Neurol. 1989;286(1):71–84.

57. Fusca D, Husch A, Baumann A, Kloppenburg P. Choline acetyltransferase-like immunoreactivity in a physiologically distinct subtype of olfactory nonspiking local interneurons in the cockroach (Periplaneta americana). J Comp Neurol. 2013;521(15):3556–69.

58. Kiya T, Kubo T. Analysis of GABAergic and non-GABAergic neuron activity in the optic lobes of the forager and re-orienting worker honeybee (Apis mellifera L.). PLoS ONE. 2010;5(1):e8833.

59. Kucharski R, Ball EE, Hayward DC, Maleszka R. Molecular cloning and expression analysis of a cDNA encoding a glutamate transporter in the honeybee brain. Gene. 2000;242(1–2):399–405.

60. Thany SH, Lenaers G, Crozatier M, Armengaud C, Gauthier M. Identification and localization of the nicotinic acetylcholine receptor alpha3 mRNA in the brain of the honeybee Apis mellifera. Insect Mol Biol. 2003;12(3):255–62.

61. Zannat MT, Locatelli F, Rybak J, Menzel R, Leboulle G. Identification and localisation of the NR1 sub-unit homologue of the NMDA glutamate receptor in the honeybee brain. Neurosci Lett. 2006;398(3):274–9.

62. Sinakevitch I, Mustard JA, Smith BH. Distribution of the octopamine receptor AmOA1 in the honey bee brain. PLoS ONE. 2011;6(1):e14536.

63. El Hassani AK, Schuster S, Dyck Y, Demares F, Leboulle G, Armengaud C. Identification, localization and function of glutamate-gated chloride channel receptors in the honeybee brain. Eur J Neurosci. 2012;36(4):2409–20.

64. Démares F, Raymond V, Armengaud C. Expression and localization of glutamate-gated chloride channel variants in honeybee brain (Apis mellifera). Insect Biochem Mol Biol. 2013;43(1):115–24.

65. Humphries MA, Mustard JA, Hunter SJ, Mercer A, Ward V, Ebert PR. Invertebrate D2 type dopamine receptor exhibits age-based plasticity of expression in the mushroom bodies of the honeybee brain. J Neurobiol. 2003;55(3):315–30.

66. Ultsch A, Schuster CM, Laube B, Schloss P, Schmitt B, Betz H. Glutamate receptors of Drosophila melanogaster: cloning of a kainate-selective subunit expressed in the central nervous system. Proc Natl Acad Sci. 1992;89(21):10484–8.

67. Ultsch A, Schuster CM, Laube B, Betz H, Schmitt B. Glutamate receptors of Drosophila melanogaster. FEBS Lett. 1993;324(2):171–7.

68. Romero-Calderón R, Uhlenbrock G, Borycz J, Simon AF, Grygoruk A, Yee SK, et al. A glial variant of the vesicular monoamine transporter is required to store histamine in the drosophila visual system. PLoS Genet. 2008;4(11):e1000245.

69. Homberg U. Neurotransmitters and neuropeptides in the brain of the locust. Microsc Res Tech. 2002;56(3):189–209.

70. Breer H. Neurochemistry of cholinergic synapses in insects. In: von Keyserlingk HC, Jäger A, von Szczepanski C, editors. Approaches to new leads for insecticides. Berlin: Springer; 1985. p. 89–99.

71. Goldberg F, Grünewald B, Rosenboom H, Menzel R. Nicotinic acetylcholine currents of cultured Kenyon cells from the mushroom bodies of the honey bee Apis mellifera. J Physiol. 1999;514(Pt 3):759–68.

72. Barbara GS, Zube C, Rybak J, Gauthier M, Grünewald B. Acetylcholine, GABA and glutamate induce ionic currents in cultured antennal lobe neurons of the honeybee, Apis mellifera. J Comp Physiol A. 2005;191(9):823–36.

73. Müßig L, Richlitzki A, Rößler R, Eisenhardt D, Menzel R, Leboulle G. Acute disruption of the NMDA receptor subunit NR1 in the honeybee brain selectively impairs memory formation. J Neurosci. 2010;30(23):7817–25.

74. Démares F, Drouard F, Massou I, Crattelet C, Lœuillet A, Bettiol C, et al. Differential involvement of glutamate-gated chloride channel splice variants in the olfactory memory processes of the honeybee Apis mellifera. Pharmacol Biochem Behav. 2014;124:137–44.

75. Liu WW, Wilson RI. Glutamate is an inhibitory neurotransmitter in the Drosophila olfactory system. Proc Natl Acad Sci USA. 2013;110(25):10294–9.

76. Enell L, Hamasaka Y, Kolodziejczyk A, Nässel DR. γ-Aminobutyric acid (GABA) signaling components in Drosophila: immunocytochemical localization of GABAB receptors in relation to the GABAA receptor subunit RDL and a vesicular GABA transporter. J Comp Neurol. 2007;505(1):18–31.

77. Sattelle DB, Lummis SCR, Wong JFH, Rauh JJ. Pharmacology of insect GABA receptors. Neurochem Res. 1991;16(3):363–74.

78. El Hassani AK, Giurfa M, Gauthier M, Armengaud C. Inhibitory neurotransmission and olfactory memory in honeybees. Neurobiol Learn Memory. 2008;90(4):589–95.

79. Raccuglia D, Mueller U. Focal uncaging of GABA reveals a temporally defined role for GABAergic inhibition during appetitive associative olfactory conditioning in honeybees. Learn Memory. 2013;20(8):410–6.

80. Greer CL, Grygoruk A, Patton DE, Ley B, Romero-Calderon R, Chang H-Y, et al. A splice variant of the Drosophila vesicular monoamine transporter contains a conserved trafficking domain and functions in the storage of dopamine, serotonin, and octopamine. J Neurobiol. 2005;64(3):239–58.

81. Waddell S. Reinforcement signalling in Drosophila; dopamine does it all after all. Curr Opin Neurobiol. 2013;23(3):324–9.

82. Kaneko T, Macara AM, Li R, Hu Y, Iwasaki K, Dunnings Z, et al. Serotonergic Modulation enables pathway-specific plasticity in a developing sensory circuit in Drosophila. Neuron. 2017;95(3):623.e4–38.e4.

83. Hammer M. An identified neuron mediates the unconditioned stimulus in associative olfactory learning in honeybees. Nature. 1993;366:59.

84. Kamhi JF, Traniello JFA. Biogenic amines and collective organization in a superorganism: neuromodulation of social behavior in ants. Brain Behav Evol. 2013;82(4):220–36.

85. Schulz DJ, Barron AB, Robinson GE. A Role for octopamine in honey bee division of labor. Brain Behav Evol. 2002;60(6):350–9.

86. Damrau C, Toshima N, Tanimura T, Brembs B, Colomb J. Octopamine and tyramine contribute separately to the counter-regulatory response to sugar deficit in Drosophila. Front Syst Neurosci. 2017;11:100.

87. Stevenson PA, Dyakonova V, Rillich J, Schildberger K. Octopamine and experience-dependent modulation of aggression in crickets. J Neurosci. 2005;25(6):1431–41.

88. Nall AH, Sehgal A. Small-molecule screen in adult Drosophila identifies VMAT as a regulator of sleep. J Neurosci. 2013;33(19):8534–40.

89. Katz P, Grillner S, Wilson R, Borst A, Greenspan R, Buzsáki G, et al. Vertebrate versus invertebrate neural circuits. Curr Biol. 2013;23(12):R504–6.

90. Shubin N, Tabin C, Carroll S. Deep homology and the origins of evolutionary novelty. Nature. 2009;457:818.

91. Strausfeld NJ, Hirth F. Deep homology of arthropod central complex and vertebrate basal ganglia. Science. 2013;340(6129):157–61.

92. Altschul SF, Madden TL, Schäffer AA, Zhang J, Zhang Z, Miller W, et al. Gapped BLAST and PSI-BLAST: a new generation of protein database search programs. Nucleic Acids Res. 1997;25(17):3389–402.

93. Koressaar T, Remm M. Enhancements and modifications of primer design program Primer3. Bioinformatics. 2007;23(10):1289–91.

94. Strutz A, Soelter J, Baschwitz A, Farhan A, Grabe V, Rybak J, et al. Decoding odor quality and intensity in the Drosophila brain. ELife. 2014;3:e04147.

95. Bicker G, Schäfer S, Kingan TG. Mushroom body feedback interneurones in the honeybee show GABA-like immunoreactivity. Brain Res. 1985;360(1–2):394–7.

96. Rybak J, Menzel R. Anatomy of the mushroom bodies in the honey bee brain: the neuronal connections of the alpha-lobe. J Comp Neurol. 1993;334(3):444–65.

97. Bicker G. Histochemistry of classical neurotransmitters in antennal lobes and mushroom bodies of the honeybee. Microsc Res Tech. 1999;45(3):174–83.

98. Warren B, Kloppenburg P. Rapid and Slow chemical synaptic interactions of cholinergic projection neurons and GABAergic local interneurons in the insect antennal lobe. J Neurosci. 2014;34(39):13039–46.

99. Ito K, Shinomiya K, Ito M, Armstrong JD, Boyan G, Hartenstein V, et al. A systematic nomenclature for the insect brain. Neuron. 2014;81(4):755–65.

100. Brandt R, Rohlfing T, Rybak J, Krofczik S, Maye A, Westerhoff M, et al. Three-dimensional average-shape atlas of the honeybee brain and its applications. J Comp Neurol. 2005;492(1):1–19.

101. Lai S-L, Awasaki T, Ito K, Lee T. Clonal analysis of Drosophila antennal lobe neurons: diverse neuronal architectures in the lateral neuroblast lineage. Development. 2008;135(17):2883–93.

102. Tedjakumala SR, Rouquette J, Boizeau ML, Mesce KA, Hotier L, Massou I, et al. A tyrosine-hydroxylase characterization of dopaminergic neurons in the honey bee brain. Front Syst Neurosci. 2017;11(47):47.

103. Mercer AR, Mobbs PG, Davenport AP, Evans PD. Biogenic amines in the brain of the honeybee Apis mellifera. Cell Tissue Res. 1983;234(3):655–77.

104. Graham SA, Fisher SE. Understanding language from a genomic perspective. Annu Rev Genet. 2015;49(1):131–60.

105. Haesler S, Rochefort C, Georgi B, Licznerski P, Osten P, Scharff C. Incomplete and inaccurate vocal imitation after knockdown of FoxP2 in Songbird basal ganglia nucleus area X. PLoS Biol. 2007;5(12):e321.

106. Schreiweis C, Bornschein U, Burguière E, Kerimoglu C, Schreiter S, Dannemann M, et al. Humanized Foxp2 accelerates learning by enhancing transitions from declarative to procedural performance. Proc Natl Acad Sci. 2014;111(39):14253–8.

107. Gaub S, Fisher SE, Ehret G. Ultrasonic vocalizations of adult male Foxp2-mutant mice: behavioral contexts of arousal and emotion. Genes Brain Behav. 2016;15(2):243–59.

108. Chabout J, Sarkar A, Patel SR, Radden T, Dunson DB, Fisher SE, et al. A Foxp2 mutation implicated in human speech deficits alters sequencing of ultrasonic vocalizations in adult male mice. Front Behav Neurosci. 2016;10:197.

109. Heston JB, White SA. Behavior-linked FoxP2 regulation enables zebra finch vocal learning. J Neurosci. 2015;35(7):2885–94.

110. Kurt S, Fisher SE, Ehret G. Foxp2 mutations impair auditory-motor association learning. PLoS ONE. 2012;7(3):e33130.

111. Lee HH, Frasch M. Survey of forkhead domain encoding genes in the Drosophila genome: classification and embryonic expression patterns. Dev Dyn. 2004;229(2):357–66.

112. Song X, Tang Y, Wang Y. Genesis of the vertebrate FoxP subfamily member genes occurred during two ancestral whole genome duplication events. Gene. 2016;588(2):156–62.

113. Wang VY, Hassan BA, Bellen HJ, Zoghbi HY. Drosophila atonal fully rescues the phenotype of math1 null mice: new functions evolve in new cellular contexts. Curr Biol. 2002;12(18):1611–6.

114. Quiring R, Walldorf U, Kloter U, Gehring W. Homology of the eyeless gene of Drosophila to the small eye gene in mice and Aniridia in humans. Science. 1994;265(5173):785–9.

115. Williams MJ, Goergen P, Rajendran J, Zheleznyakova G, Hägglund MG, Perland E, et al. Obesity-linked homologues TfAP-2 and Twz establish meal frequency in Drosophila melanogaster. PLoS Genet. 2014;10(9):e1004499.

116. Kalousova A, Mavropoulos A, Adams BA, Nekrep N, Li Z, Krauss S, et al. Dachshund homologues play a conserved role in islet cell development. Dev Biol. 2010;348(2):143–52.

117. Villar D, Flicek P, Odom DT. Evolution of transcription factor binding in metazoans—mechanisms and functional implications. Nat Rev Genet. 2014;15:221.

118. Liang ZS, Nguyen T, Mattila HR, Rodriguez-Zas SL, Seeley TD, Robinson GE. Molecular determinants of scouting behavior in honey bees. Science. 2012;335(6073):1225–8.

119. Dupuis J, Louis T, Gauthier M, Raymond V. Insights from honeybee (Apis mellifera) and fly (Drosophila melanogaster) nicotinic acetylcholine receptors: from genes to behavioral functions. Neurosci Biobehav Rev. 2012;36(6):1553–64.

120. Liebeskind BJ, Hillis DM, Zakon HH, Hofmann HA. Complex homology and the evolution of nervous systems. Trends Ecol Evol. 2016;31(2):127–35.

121. Kloepper TH, Kienle CN, Fasshauer D. An elaborate classification of SNARE proteins sheds light on the conservation of the eukaryotic endomembrane system. Mol Biol Cell. 2007;18(9):3463–71.

122. Ai H, Kai K, Kumaraswamy A, Ikeno H, Wachtler T. Interneurons in the honeybee primary auditory center responding to waggle dance-like vibration pulses. J Neurosci. 2017;37(44):10624–35.

123. Pollack GS. Analysis of temporal patterns of communication signals. Curr Opin Neurobiol. 2001;11(6):734–8.

124. Alluri RK, Rose GJ, Hanson JL, Leary CJ, Vasquez-Opazo GA, Graham JA, et al. Phasic, suprathreshold excitation and sustained inhibition underlie

neuronal selectivity for short-duration sounds. Proc Natl Acad Sci USA. 2016;113(13):E1927–35.

125. Pfeiffer K, Homberg U. Organization and functional roles of the central complex in the insect brain. Annu Rev Entomol. 2014;59(1):165–84.

126. Stone T, Webb B, Adden A, Weddig NB, Honkanen A, Templin R, et al. An anatomically constrained model for path integration in the bee brain. Curr Biol. 2017;27(20):3069.e11–85.e11.

127. Blenau W, Schmidt M, Faensen D, Schürmann F-W. Neurons with dopamine-like immunoreactivity target mushroom body Kenyon cell somata in the brain of some hymenopteran insects. Int J Insect Morphol Embryol. 1999;28(3):203–10.

128. Shapira M, Thompson CK, Soreq H, Robinson GE. Changes in neuronal acetylcholinesterase gene expression and division of labor in honey bee colonies. J Mol Neurosci. 2001;17(1):1–12.

129. De La Porte S, Vallette FM, Grassi J, Vigny M, Koenig J. Presynaptic or postsynaptic origin of acetylcholinesterase at neuromuscular junctions? An immunological study in heterologous nerve-muscle cultures. Dev Biol. 1986;116(1):69–77.

130. Zoli M. Distribution of cholinergic neurons in the mammalian brain with special reference to their relationship with neuronal nicotinic acetylcholine receptors. In: Clementi F, Fornasari D, Gotti C, editors. Neuronal nicotinic receptors. Berlin: Springer; 2000. p. 13–30.

131. Kim YH, Kim JH, Kim K, Lee SH. Expression of acetylcholinesterase 1 is associated with brood rearing status in the honey bee Apis mellifera. Sci Rep. 2017;7:39864.

132. Zimmermann M. Neuronal AChE splice variants and their non-hydrolytic functions: redefining a target of AChE inhibitors? Br J Pharmacol. 2013;170(5):953–67.

133. Barnstedt O, Owald D, Felsenberg J, Brain R, Moszynski J-P, Talbot Clifford B, et al. Memory-relevant mushroom body output synapses are cholinergic. Neuron. 2016;89(6):1237–47.

134. Kahsai L, Carlsson MA, Winther ÅME, Nässel DR. Distribution of metabotropic receptors of serotonin, dopamine, GABA, glutamate, and short neuropeptide F in the central complex of Drosophila. Neuroscience. 2012;208:11–26.

135. Hsu CT, Bhandawat V. Organization of descending neurons in Drosophila melanogaster. Sci Rep. 2016;6:20259.

136. Hasegawa E, Truman JW, Nose A. Identification of excitatory premotor interneurons which regulate local muscle contraction during Drosophila larval locomotion. Sci Rep. 2016;6:30806.

137. Whitfield CW, Cziko A-M, Robinson GE. Gene expression profiles in the brain predict behavior in individual honey bees. Science. 2003;302(5643):296–9.

138. Kaoru T, Fu-Chin L, Katsuiku H, Hiroshi T. Expression of Foxp4 in the developing and adult rat forebrain. J Neurosci Res. 2008;86(14):3106–16.

139. Teramitsu I, Kudo LC, London SE, Geschwind DH, White SA. Parallel oxP1 and FoxP2 expression in songbird and human brain predicts functional interaction. J Neurosci. 2004;24(13):3152–63.

140. Kaoru T, Fu-Chin L, Katsuiku H, Hiroshi T. Expression of Foxp2, a gene involved in speech and language, in the developing and adult striatum. J Neurosci Res. 2003;73(1):61–72.

141. Graybiel AM, Aosaki T, Flaherty AW, Kimura M. The basal ganglia and adaptive motor control. Science. 1994;265(5180):1826.

142. DeLong MR, Georgopoulos AP. Motor functions of the basal ganglia. London: Wiley; 2011.

143. Tewari A, Jog R, Jog MS. The striatum and subthalamic nucleus as independent and collaborative structures in motor control. Front Syst Neurosci. 2016;10:17.

144. Tecuapetla F, Jin X, Lima SQ, Costa RM. Complementary contributions of striatal projection pathways to action initiation and execution. Cell. 2016;166(3):703–15.

145. Varga AG, Kathman ND, Martin JP, Guo P, Ritzmann RE. Spatial navigation and the central complex: sensory acquisition, orientation, and motor control. Front Behav Neurosci. 2017;11:4.

146. Martin JP, Guo P, Mu L, Harley CM, Ritzmann RE. Central-complex control of movement in the freely walking cockroach. Curr Biol. 2015;25(21):2795–803.

147. Strauss R. The central complex and the genetic dissection of locomotor behaviour. Curr Opin Neurobiol. 2002;12(6):633–8.

148. Christensen TA, Waldrop BR, Harrow ID, Hildebrand JG. Local interneurons and information processing in the olfactory glomeruli of the moth Manduca sexta. J Comp Physiol A. 1993;173(4):385–99.

149. Nässel DR. Histamine in the brain of insects: a review. Microsc Res Tech. 1999;44(2–3):121–36.

150. McQuillan HJ, Nakagawa S, Mercer AR. Mushroom bodies of the honeybee brain show cell population-specific plasticity in expression of amine-receptor genes. Learn Memory. 2012;19(4):151–8.

151. Suenami S, Oya S, Kohno H, Kubo T. Kenyon cell subtypes/populations in the honeybee mushroom bodies: possible function based on their gene expression profiles, differentiation, possible evolution, and application of genome editing. Front Psychol. 2018;9:1717.

152. Dacks AM, Reisenman CE, Paulk AC, Nighorn AJ. Histamine-immunoreactive local neurons in the antennal lobes of the hymenoptera. J Comp Neurol. 2010;518(15):2917–33.

153. Juárez-Morales JL, Schulte CJ, Pezoa SA, Vallejo GK, Hilinski WC, England SJ, et al. Evx1 and Evx2 specify excitatory neurotransmitter fates and suppress inhibitory fates through a Pax2-independent mechanism. Neural Dev. 2016;11(1):5.

154. Borromeo MD, Meredith DM, Castro DS, Chang JC, Tung K-C, Guillemot F, et al. A transcription factor network specifying inhibitory versus excitatory neurons in the dorsal spinal cord. Development. 2014;141(14):2803–12.

155. Abdi A, Mallet N, Mohamed FY, Sharott A, Dodson PD, Nakamura KC, et al. Prototypic and arkypallidal neurons in the dopamine-intact external globus pallidus. J Neurosci. 2015;35(17):6667–88.

156. Verstegen AMJ, Vanderhorst V, Gray PA, Zeidel ML, Geerling JC. Barrington's nucleus: neuroanatomic landscape of the mouse "pontine micturition center". J Comp Neurol. 2017;525(10):2287–309.

157. Geerling JC, Kim M, Mahoney CE, Abbott SBG, Agostinelli LJ, Garfield AS, et al. Genetic identity of thermosensory relay neurons in the lateral parabrachial nucleus. Am J Physiol Regul Integr Comp Physiol. 2016;310(1):R41–54.

158. Geerling JC, Yokota S, Rukhadze I, Roe D, Chamberlin NL. Kölliker-Fuse GABAergic and glutamatergic neurons project to distinct targets. J Comp Neurol. 2017;525(8):1844–60.

159. Rousso David L, Pearson Caroline A, Gaber ZB, Miquelajauregui A, Li S, Portera-Cailliau C, et al. Foxp-mediated suppression of N-cadherin regulates neuroepithelial character and progenitor maintenance in the CNS. Neuron. 2012;74(2):314–30.

160. Rousso DL, Gaber ZB, Wellik D, Morrisey EE, Novitch BG. Coordinated actions of the Forkhead protein Foxp1 and hox proteins in the columnar organization of spinal motor neurons. Neuron. 2008;59(2):226–40.

161. Dasen JS, De Camilli A, Wang B, Tucker PW, Jessell TM. Hox repertoires for motor neuron diversity and connectivity gated by a single accessory factor, FoxP1. Cell. 2008;134(2):304–16.

162. Morikawa Y, Komori T, Hisaoka T, Senba E. Detailed expression pattern of Foxp1 and Its possible roles in neurons of the spinal cord during embryogenesis. Dev Neurosci. 2009;31(6):511–22.

163. Seeley TD. Honeybee democracy. Princeton: Princeton University Press; 2010.

164. Groh C, Lu Z, Meinertzhagen IA, Rössler W. Age-related plasticity in the synaptic ultrastructure of neurons in the mushroom body calyx of the adult honeybee Apis mellifera. J Comp Neurol. 2012;520(15):3509–27.

165. Gehring KB, Heufelder K, Kersting I, Eisenhardt D. Abundance of phosphorylated Apis mellifera CREB in the honeybee's mushroom body inner compact cells varies with age. J Comp Neurol. 2016;524(6):1165–80.

166. Gehring KB, Heufelder K, Depner H, Kersting I, Sigrist SJ, Eisenhardt D. Age-associated increase of the active zone protein Bruchpilot within the honeybee mushroom body. PLoS ONE. 2017;12(4):e0175894.

167. Amdam GV, Omholt SW. The regulatory anatomy of honeybee lifespan. J Theor Biol. 2002;216(2):209–28.

168. Fahrbach SE, Van Nest BN. Synapsin-based approaches to brain plasticity in adult social insects. Curr Opin Insect Sci. 2016;18(Supplement C):27–34.

169. Han B, Fang Y, Feng M, Hu H, Qi Y, Huo X, et al. Quantitative Neuropeptidome analysis reveals neuropeptides are correlated with social behavior regulation of the honeybee workers. J Proteome Res. 2015;14(10):4382–93.

170. Steinmann N, Corona M, Neumann P, Dainat B. Overwintering is associated with reduced expression of immune genes and higher susceptibility to virus infection in honey bees. PLoS ONE. 2015;10(6):e0129956.

171. Bonnafé E, Alayrangues J, Hotier L, Massou I, Renom A, Souesme G, et al. Monoterpenoid-based preparations in beehives affect learning, memory, and gene expression in the bee brain. Environ Toxicol Chem. 2017;36(2):337–45.

172. Cardoso-Júnior CAM, Eyer M, Dainat B, Hartfelder K, Dietemann V. Social context influences the expression of DNA methyltransferase genes in the honeybee. Sci Rep. 2018;8(1):11076.

173. Spitzer NC. Neurotransmitter switching in the developing and adult brain. Annu Rev Neurosci. 2017;40(1):1–19.

18

Downregulation of calcium-dependent NMDA receptor desensitization by sodium-calcium exchangers: a role of membrane cholesterol

Dmitry A. Sibarov, Ekaterina E. Poguzhelskaya and Sergei M. Antonov[*] (iD)

Abstract

Background: The plasma membrane Na^+/Ca^{2+}-exchanger (NCX) has recently been shown to regulate Ca^{2+}-dependent *N*-methyl-D-aspartate receptor (NMDAR) desensitization, suggesting a tight interaction of NCXs and NMDARs in lipid nanoclasters or "rafts". To evaluate possible role of this interaction we studied effects of Li^+ on NMDA-elicited whole-cell currents and Ca^{2+} responses of rat cortical neurons in vitro before and after cholesterol extraction by methyl-β-cyclodextrin (MβCD).

Results: Substitution Li^+ for Na^+ in the external solution caused a concentration-dependent decrease of steady-state NMDAR currents from 440 ± 71 pA to 111 ± 29 pA in 140 mM Na^+ and 140 mM Li^+, respectively. The Li^+ inhibition of NMDAR currents disappeared in the absence of Ca^{2+} in the external solution (Ca^{2+}-free), suggesting that Li^+ enhanced Ca^{2+}-dependent NMDAR desensitization. Whereas the cholesterol extraction with MβCD induced a decrease of NMDAR currents to 136 ± 32 pA in 140 mM Na^+ and 46 ± 15 pA in 140 mM Li^+, the IC_{50} values for the Li^+ inhibition were similar (about 44 mM Li^+) before and after this procedure. In the Ca^{2+}-free Na^+ solution the steady-state NMDAR currents after the cholesterol extraction were $47 \pm 6\%$ of control values. Apparently this amplitude decrease was not Ca^{2+}-dependent. In the Na^+ solution containing 1 mM Ca^{2+} the Ca^{2+}-dependent NMDAR desensitization was greater when cholesterol was extracted. Obviously, this procedure promoted its development. In agreement, Li^+ and KB-R7943, an inhibitor of NCX, both considerably reduced NMDA-activated Ca^{2+} responses. The cholesterol extraction itself caused a decrease of NMDA-activated Ca^{2+} responses and, in addition, abolished the effects of Li^+ and KB-R7943. The cholesterol loading into the plasma membrane caused a recovery of the KB-R7943 effects.

Conclusions: Taken together our data suggest that NCXs downregulate the Ca^{2+}-dependent NMDAR desensitization. Most likely, this is determined by a tight functional interaction of NCX and NMDAR molecules because of their co-localization in membrane lipid rafts. The destruction of these rafts is accompanied by an enhancement of NMDAR desensitization and a loss of NCX-selective agent effects on NMDARs.

Keywords: NMDA receptors, Sodium-calcium exchanger, Lipid rafts, Desensitization, Glutamate

*Correspondence: antonov452002@yahoo.com
Sechenov Institute of Evolutionary Physiology and Biochemistry, Russian
Academy of Sciences, pr. Torez 44 Saint-Petersburg, Russia

Background

N-methyl-D-aspartate activated glutamate receptors (NMDARs) are ligand gated ion channels which naturally transfer currents determined by Na^+, K^+ and Ca^{2+} permeation. High permeability of NMDARs to Ca^{2+} makes them involved in synaptic plasticity [1, 2], while their hyperactivation during ischemia or stroke causes neuronal Ca^{2+} overload and apoptosis [3]. Ca^{2+}-dependent desensitization of NMDARs represents a feedback regulation of the NMDAR open probability by the Ca^{2+} entry into neurons [4–8]. The Ca^{2+} entry via NMDAR pores produces a local increase of Ca^{2+} concentration (up to micromolar range) in a close proximity of receptor intracellular domains. Calmodulin binds free Ca^{2+} and then interacts with C-terminal domains of NMDAR GluN1 subunits causing the decrease of the channel open probability in the Ca^{2+} concentration-dependent manner because of Ca^{2+}-dependent NMDAR desensitization [9, for review see 10].

Recently it has been demonstrated that the inhibition of the plasma membrane Na^+/Ca^{2+} exchanger (NCX) either by KB-R7943 (2-[2-[4-(4-nitrobenzyloxy) phenyl] ethyl] isothiourea methanesulfonate) or by the substitution of Li^+ for Na^+ in the external physiological solution considerably enhances the Ca^{2+}-dependent desensitization of NMDARs [11]. As Li^+ is a substrate inhibitor of Na^+-dependent neurotransmitter transporters [12, 13] and exchangers [for review see 14] the substitution of Li^+ for Na^+ in the external solution decreases the efficacy of Ca^{2+} extrusion via NCX. The direct effects of Li^+ on NMDAR kinetics and conductance is negligible, because NMDARs have similar Li^+ and Na^+ channel permeabilities [15]. These observations suggest that NCX is involved in regulation of Ca^{2+}-dependent desensitization of NMDARs that could be achieved in the case of close location and interaction of NCX and NMDAR molecules in the plasma membrane.

The Li^+ therapy is widely used to stabilize mood disorders, including bipolar disorders and depression as well as suicidal behaviors [13]. There are some experimental indications that KB-R7943 reduces 4-aminopyridine-induced epileptiform activity in adult rats [16]. It is still not clear whether NCXs could represent a target of pharmacological action to compensate NMDAR-related neuronal pathologies and whether an acceleration of Ca^{2+}-dependent NMDAR desensitization by Li^+ is at least partially contributed to the Li^+ therapeutic effects. To provide more clues for understanding of these aspects of the NMDAR pharmacology here we study the concentration dependence of Li^+ effects on NMDAR currents and the role of functional interaction between NCXs and NMDARs that presumably requires their close spatial localization in lipid rafts.

Results

Lithium inhibition of NMDA-elicited currents

Cortical neurons in cultures express a variety of NCXs including NCX1-3 and NCKX isoforms [14]. Extracellular Li^+ represents a tool to cause the substrate inhibition of Na^+-dependent Ca^{2+} extrusion by all sodium-calcium exchanger subtypes. The stepwise proportional substitution of Li^+ for Na^+ in the bathing solution was used to obtain the dose-inhibition curve of NMDA-evoked currents for Li^+. With this particular aim the NMDA-activated currents were measured at 0, 21, 42, 70, 112 and 140 mM Li^+ in the bathing solution in the same experiment, where 140 mM Li^+ corresponded to 100% substitution of Li^+ for Na^+. An application of Li^+-containing solutions without agonists always preceded the application of the corresponding solution with NMDA. An increase of Li^+ concentrations in the external solution caused a decrease of NMDA-activated currents at the steady state (Fig. 1a). The control NMDA-evoked currents, measured at the steady state in the bathing solutions (140 mM Na^+) had the amplitude of 440.4 ± 71.9 pA ($n = 10$), that was significantly ($p < 0.001$, Student's two-tailed t test) larger compared to the corresponding value of 111.4 ± 29.1 pA ($n = 10$) measured at 140 mM Li^+ in the external solution. Dose-inhibition curves obtained from experiments were well fitted by Hill equation with IC_{50} of 46 ± 21 mM (Fig. 1b). Previously, we demonstrated that the inhibition of NMDA-activated currents by Li^+ is Ca^{2+}-dependent, because it could not be observed in the nominal absence of Ca^{2+} in the external solution [11]. Since Li^+ does not directly affect the NMDAR conductance and activation kinetics, as a substrate inhibitor of NCXs it could sufficiently decrease the efficacy of Ca^{2+} extrusion from neurons due to breaking ion transport by NCXs. The decrease of NMDAR current by Li^+ suggests that NCX contributes to the regulation of free Ca^{2+} concentration close to the inner membrane surface and the Ca^{2+}-dependent desensitization of NMDARs. This requires some functional interaction between NCXs and NMDARs that could occur if these molecules are located closely and interact within lipid nanoclasters or rafts.

The extraction of cholesterol from the plasma membrane by MβCD [17] is a widely used conventional procedure to destroy lipid nanoclusters. The treatment of neurons with 1.5 mM MβCD for 5 min was undertaken to extract cholesterol from membrane lipid rafts to achieve spatial uncoupling of NMDARs and NCXs. This procedure did not significantly alter the current–voltage relationships (I/V), suggesting the lack of its effect on the input resistance of neurons ($n = 5$, Fig. 1a). After the cholesterol extraction the mean amplitude of NMDA-evoked currents at the steady state in the Na^+-containing bathing

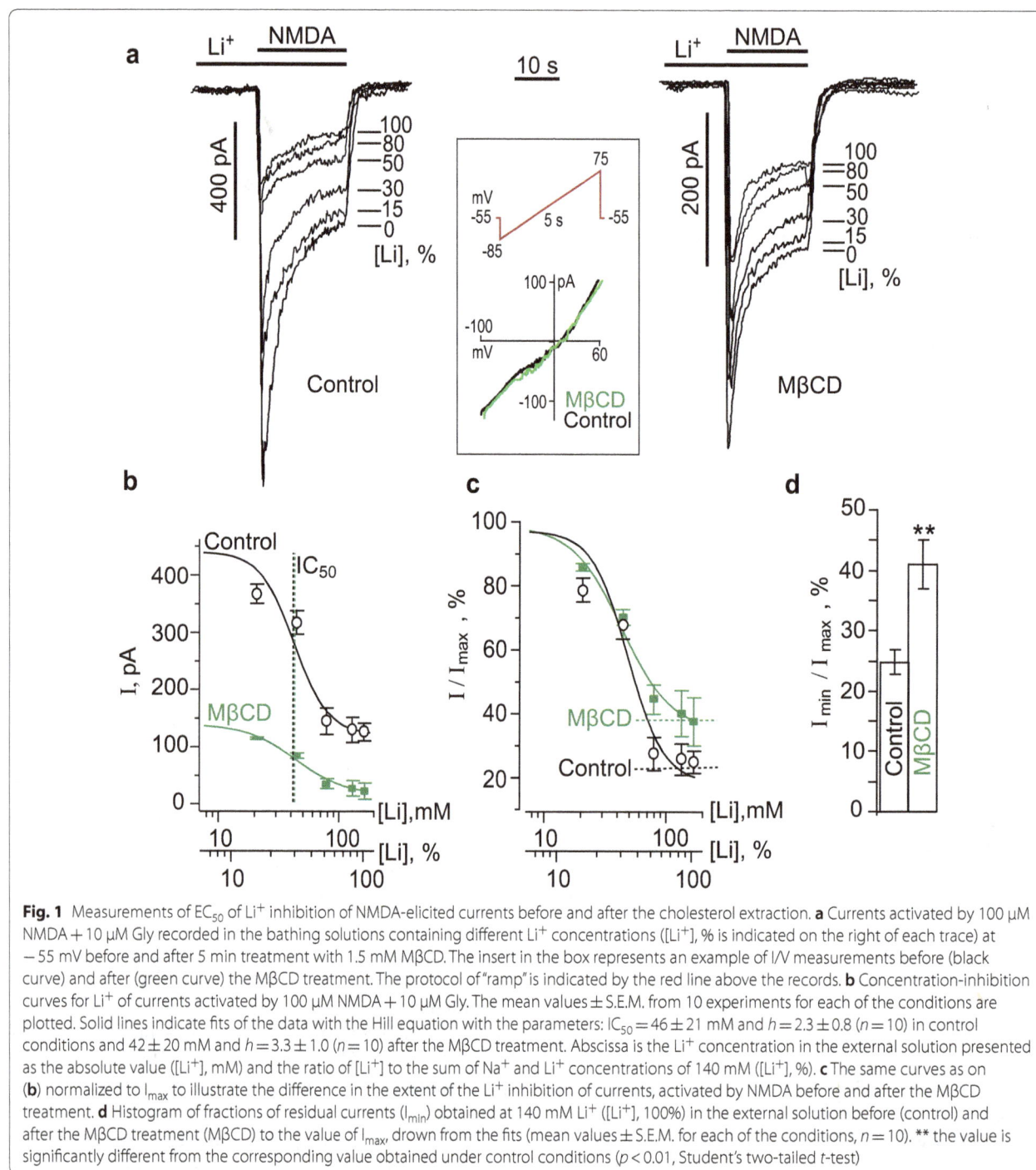

Fig. 1 Measurements of EC_{50} of Li^+ inhibition of NMDA-elicited currents before and after the cholesterol extraction. **a** Currents activated by 100 μM NMDA + 10 μM Gly recorded in the bathing solutions containing different Li^+ concentrations ([Li^+], % is indicated on the right of each trace) at − 55 mV before and after 5 min treatment with 1.5 mM MβCD. The insert in the box represents an example of I/V measurements before (black curve) and after (green curve) the MβCD treatment. The protocol of "ramp" is indicated by the red line above the records. **b** Concentration-inhibition curves for Li^+ of currents activated by 100 μM NMDA + 10 μM Gly. The mean values ± S.E.M. from 10 experiments for each of the conditions are plotted. Solid lines indicate fits of the data with the Hill equation with the parameters: $IC_{50} = 46 \pm 21$ mM and $h = 2.3 \pm 0.8$ ($n = 10$) in control conditions and 42 ± 20 mM and $h = 3.3 \pm 1.0$ ($n = 10$) after the MβCD treatment. Abscissa is the Li^+ concentration in the external solution presented as the absolute value ([Li^+], mM) and the ratio of [Li^+] to the sum of Na^+ and Li^+ concentrations of 140 mM ([Li^+], %). **c** The same curves as on (**b**) normalized to I_{max} to illustrate the difference in the extent of the Li^+ inhibition of currents, activated by NMDA before and after the MβCD treatment. **d** Histogram of fractions of residual currents (I_{min}) obtained at 140 mM Li^+ ([Li^+], 100%) in the external solution before (control) and after the MβCD treatment (MβCD) to the value of I_{max}, drown from the fits (mean values ± S.E.M. for each of the conditions, $n = 10$). ** the value is significantly different from the corresponding value obtained under control conditions ($p < 0.01$, Student's two-tailed t-test)

solution was 136.8 ± 32.8 pA ($n = 10$), revealing its decrease in comparison to MβCD untreated neurons as control conditions ($p < 0.007$, Student's two-tailed t test, Fig. 1a, b). The stepwise substitution of Li^+ for Na^+ in the external solution after the MβCD treatment further decreased the NMDA-evoked currents to the mean steady-state amplitude of 46.8 ± 15.3 pA ($n = 10$, $p < 0.008$, Student's

two-tailed t-test). The IC_{50} value for the Li^+ inhibition of NMDA-activated currents after the MβCD treatment was 42 ± 20 mM (Fig. 1b, c) which did not differ significantly from the value obtained under the control conditions (on MβCD untreated neurons). It should be noted, however, that the degree of the NMDAR current inhibition in the Li^+-containing bathing solution was less pronounced after the MβCD treatment than before this procedure and were 59±4% ($n=10$) and 77±3% ($n=10$) inhibition ($p<0.03$, Student's two-tailed t-test), respectively (Fig. 1d). Presumably, spatial uncoupling of NCXs and NMDARs limits the effect of the NCX inhibition on NMDAR currents. This could be the case, if NCXs maintain low intracellular free Ca^{2+} concentration in the close proximity of NMDARs, which prevents the development of Ca^{2+}-dependent inactivation of NMDARs.

Calcium-dependent and -independent effects of cholesterol extraction on NMDARs

The interpretation of the above data that the cholesterol extraction may accelerate the Ca^{2+}-dependent desensitization destroying membrane lipid rafts and NCX-NMDAR interplay becomes less evident in a view of the recent observation that cholesterol is important for the NMDAR functioning and its extraction provokes the ligand-dependent desensitization of NMDARs [17]. In order to distinguish between Ca^{2+}-dependent and -independent mechanisms the effects of cholesterol extraction by MβCD on NMDA-activated currents were evaluated in the presence of 1 mM Ca^{2+} and in the nominal absence of Ca^{2+} in the bathing solution (Fig. 2a).

In the absence of Ca^{2+} in the external solution the ratio of amplitudes of NMDA-activated steady-state currents, recorded after and before 5 min MβCD treatment was 47±6% ($n=6$). The decrease of the steady-state amplitudes of NMDAR currents after the treatment is caused by the direct effect of the cholesterol extraction on NMDARs, because under these particular conditions the Ca^{2+}-dependent desensitization was not observed (Fig. 2a). In the presence of 1 mM Ca^{2+} in the bathing solution, however, the Ca^{2+}-dependent desensitization of NMDARs, measured as the ratio of the steady-state amplitudes of currents in the presence and absence of Ca^{2+} before and after the MβCD treatment was significantly greater when cholesterol was extracted (Fig. 2a, b), suggesting that this procedure enhanced the Ca^{2+}-dependent NMDAR desensitization. In addition, we performed similar experiments on neurons patched with 1 mM BAPTA in the pipette solution. Under these particular conditions the Ca^{2+}-dependent desensitization of NMDARs was not observed both in the presence and absence of Ca^{2+} in the external bathing solution (Fig. 2c). The direct effect of MβCD treatment on NMDARs was pronounced and the ratio values obtained in the presence and absence of external Ca^{2+} were similar (Fig. 2c, d). In 1 mM intrapipette BAPTA the steady-state NMDAR currents decreased after the extraction to about 10% of their amplitudes (Fig. 2d), whereas in experiments when the intracellular media was

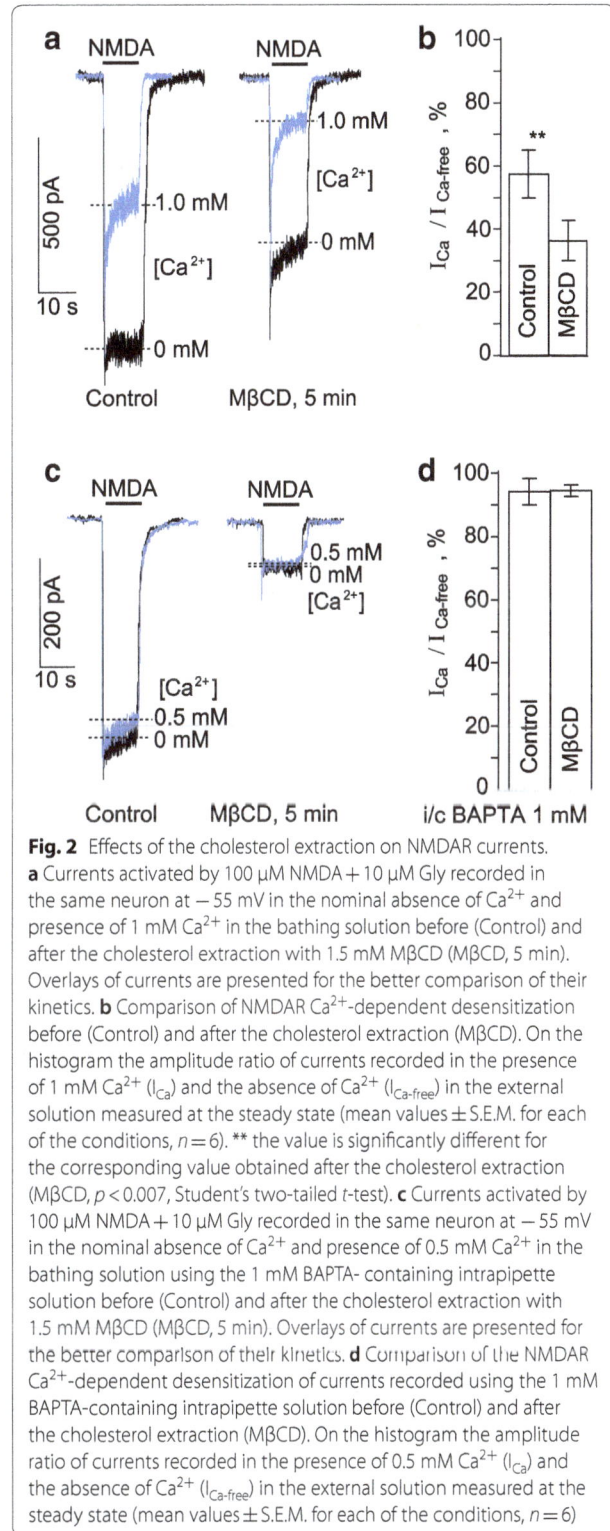

Fig. 2 Effects of the cholesterol extraction on NMDAR currents. **a** Currents activated by 100 µM NMDA + 10 µM Gly recorded in the same neuron at − 55 mV in the nominal absence of Ca^{2+} and presence of 1 mM Ca^{2+} in the bathing solution before (Control) and after the cholesterol extraction with 1.5 mM MβCD (MβCD, 5 min). Overlays of currents are presented for the better comparison of their kinetics. **b** Comparison of NMDAR Ca^{2+}-dependent desensitization before (Control) and after the cholesterol extraction (MβCD). On the histogram the amplitude ratio of currents recorded in the presence of 1 mM Ca^{2+} (I_{Ca}) and the absence of Ca^{2+} ($I_{Ca\text{-}free}$) in the external solution measured at the steady state (mean values ± S.E.M. for each of the conditions, $n=6$). ** the value is significantly different for the corresponding value obtained after the cholesterol extraction (MβCD, $p<0.007$, Student's two-tailed t-test). **c** Currents activated by 100 µM NMDA + 10 µM Gly recorded in the same neuron at − 55 mV in the nominal absence of Ca^{2+} and presence of 0.5 mM Ca^{2+} in the bathing solution before (Control) and after the cholesterol extraction with 1.5 mM MβCD (MβCD, 5 min). Overlays of currents are presented for the better comparison of their kinetics. **d** Comparison of the NMDAR Ca^{2+}-dependent desensitization of currents recorded using the 1 mM BAPTA-containing intrapipette solution before (Control) and after the cholesterol extraction (MβCD). On the histogram the amplitude ratio of currents recorded in the presence of 0.5 mM Ca^{2+} (I_{Ca}) and the absence of Ca^{2+} ($I_{Ca\text{-}free}$) in the external solution measured at the steady state (mean values ± S.E.M. for each of the conditions, $n=6$)

natural in terms of Ca^{2+} buffering the NMDAR currents decreased in a much lesser extent (about 47%, Fig. 2a).

Based on these experiments we may assume that in lipid rafts NCX weakens Ca^{2+}-dependent desensitization of NMDARs by quick extrusion of local intracellular Ca^{2+} entering neurons via open NMDAR pores. It is likely, that the destruction of lipid rafts increases the distance between NCXs and NMDARs allowing intracellular Ca^{2+} accumulation close to the NMDAR intracellular domains which enhances their Ca^{2+}-dependent desensitization. Pronounced Ca^{2+}-dependent desensitization of NMDARs, however, should provide a feed back regulation to limit the cytoplasmic Ca^{2+} accumulation during the NMDA action on neurons.

NCX inhibition and NMDA-elicited cytoplasmic Ca^{2+} accumulation

To provide additional experimental support in favor of mechanisms suggested, the effects of NCX inhibition with 140 mM Li^+ or KB-R7943 before and after the cholesterol extraction by MβCD (1.5 mM for 5 min) on intracellular Ca^{2+} responses to 2 min NMDA applications were studied. For quantitative comparison of effects we evaluated an integral of Ca^{2+}-induced fluorescence, which has to be proportional to the Ca^{2+} entry through open NMDAR channels and, therefore, to the amplitudes of NMDA-activated currents. As in electrophysiological experiments, the Li^+-containing bathing solution was applied alone and than with NMDA to equilibrate neurons and check pure Li^+ effects for possible further data correction (Fig. 3a). When NMDA was applied in the Li^+-containing bathing solution Ca^{2+} responses of neurons decreased to $54 \pm 2\%$ (overall 98 neurons, $n = 3$) of Ca^{2+} responses recorded in the Na^+-containing bathing solution ($p < 0.001$, Student's t test). This observation is consistent with the Li^+ effect on NMDA-activated currents. After the MβCD treatment the Ca^{2+} responses to NMDA in the Na^+-containing solution were $35 \pm 9\%$ (overall 98 neurons, $n = 3$) and in the Li^+-containing solution were $36 \pm 9\%$ (overall 98 neurons, $n = 3$) of the Ca^{2+} responses, obtained before the treatment in the Na^+-containing solution (Fig. 3a and b). Because these values were significantly smaller, than those obtained before the treatment in the Na^+ solution ($p < 0.0001$, one-way paired ANOVA) and did not differ between each other (Bonferroni post hoc test) we conclude that the MβCD treatment abolished the effects of Li^+ on NMDARs.

Thus, spatial uncoupling of NMDARs and NCXs resulted in the decrease of Ca^{2+} entry via NMDARs. Inhibition of NCX with Li^+ after the cholesterol extraction was not able to decrease NMDAR mediated Ca^{2+} accumulation.

We further performed the Ca^{2+} imaging experiments in which KB-R7943 (10 μM) as a specific NCX

inhibitor, was utilized instead of the Li^+ solution. In the Na^+-containing external solution combined applications of NMDA with KB-R7943 induced Ca^{2+} responses that corresponded to $59 \pm 5\%$ (overall 91 neurons, $n = 3$) of NMDA-elicited Ca^{2+} responses and differed from them significantly ($p < 0.001$, one-way paired ANOVA) (Fig. 3c). This observation is consistent with the KB-R7943 effect on NMDA-activated currents [11]. The MβCD treatment decreased the NMDA-elicited Ca^{2+} responses both in the absence and presence of KB-R7943 to $32 \pm 8\%$ and $24 \pm 7\%$ (overall 91 neurons, $n = 3$), respectively (Fig. 3d). These values are not significantly different (Bonferroni post hoc test) suggesting that the cholesterol extraction abolished the KB-R7943 effects on NMDA-activated currents. To validate that the effects of MβCD treatment are actually caused by the cholesterol loss from the plasma membrane, cholesterol-MβCD, as a cholesterol donor, was applied for 30 min after the effects of MβCD were achieved (Fig. 3c). Loading of cholesterol into the plasma membrane both increased the amplitudes of Ca^{2+}-responses to NMDA and recovered the inhibitory effect of KBR (Fig. 3c, d).

Therefore, the effects of Li^+ and KB-R7943 on NMDA-elicited Ca^{2+} responses of neurons coincide well suggesting that they both are realizing through the influence of NCX on the Ca^{2+}-dependent desensitization of NMDARs.

Discussion

In spite of a large number of novel pharmacological agents has recently appeared, Li^+ has still broad usage as a tool of neuroscience researches, since it can affect key functional processes of the central nervous system (CNS) including different enzymes [for review see 13] and Na^+-dependent neurotransmitter transporters [12] and exchangers [for review see 14]. Diverse and complex action of Li^+ on the human CNS is highlighted by the Li^+ therapy which is widely utilized to stabilize many mental disorders. Usually therapeutic Li^+ concentrations in the blood vary within the range of 0.6–1.2 mM and the concentrations over 1.5 mM are thought to become toxic [for review see 13]. In addition it has been demonstrated recently that the substitution of Li^+ for Na^+ in the external solution in the presence of Ca^{2+} causes considerable decrease of currents activated by NMDA [11]. This somehow contradicts to the lack of the NMDAR Li^+ inhibition in the absence of Ca^{2+} in the external solution [11] and to the observation that Li^+ does not influence the NMDAR conductance and activation kinetics [15]. The IC_{50} value for the Li^+ inhibition of NMDA-activated currents measured here is about 44 mM. It is, therefore, unlikely that the Li^+ inhibition of NMDAR currents in some extent

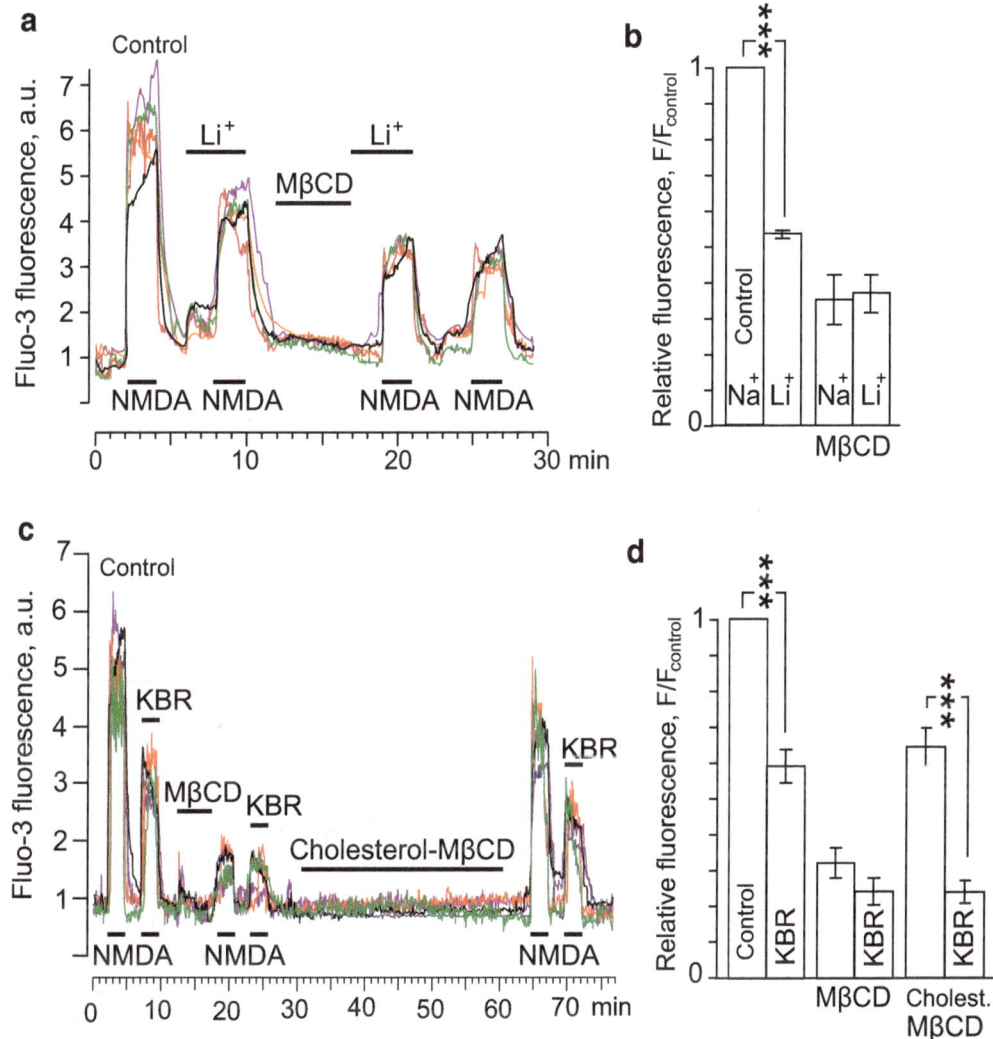

Fig. 3 Effects of the cholesterol extraction and loading on Ca^{2+} responses induced by NMDA. **a** Neuronal Ca^{2+} responses evoked by 100 μM NMDA + 10 μM Gly in the 140 mM Na^+-containing (Control) and 140 mM Li^+-containing external solutions before and after the cholesterol extraction. Applications of 100 μM NMDA + 10 μM Gly, 140 mM Li^+ and 1.5 mM MβCD are indicated by bars. Examples of Ca^{2+} responses of 4 neurons are shown. **b** The histogram represents the ratio of squares of Ca^{2+} responses to the square of Ca^{2+} response obtained under control (140 mM Na^+-containing external solution). Mean values ± S.E.M. for each of the conditions (overall 98 neurons, $n = 3$) are plotted. *** the value is significantly different from other data ($p < 0.0001$, one-way paired ANOVA, Bonferroni post hoc test). **c** Neuronal Ca^{2+} responses recorded in 140 mM Na^+-containing external solution evoked by 100 μM NMDA + 10 μM Gly (Control) and 100 μM NMDA + 10 μM Gly + 10 μM KB-R7943 (KBR) before cholesterol extraction, after cholesterol depletion with MβCD and then after cholesterol restoration with cholesterol-MβCD. Applications of 100 μM NMDA + 10 μM Gly, 10 μM KB-R7943, 1.5 mM MβCD and 1.5 mM cholesterol-MβCD are indicated by bars. Examples of Ca^{2+} responses of 6 neurons are shown. **d** The histogram represents the ratio of squares of Ca^{2+} responses to the square of Ca^{2+} response obtained under control (NMDA). Mean values ± S.E.M. for each of the conditions (overall 91 neurons, $n = 3$) are plotted. *** the value is significantly different from other data ($p < 0.0001$, one-way paired ANOVA, Bonferroni post hoc test)

contributes in the therapeutic effect during the Li^+ therapy, whereas the mechanism of the Ca^{2+}-dependent Li^+ inhibition of NMDARs requires further consideration.

The critical dependence of Li^+ inhibition of NMDAR currents on extracellular Ca^{2+} forced us to the conclusion that Li^+ inhibits NMDARs indirectly breaking the Ca^{2+} extrusion from neurons by NCXs, which are involved in regulation of pre-membrane Ca^{2+} concentration in the close proximity to the NMDAR intracellular domains during Ca^{2+} entry through the channels of activated NMDARs. By the other words Li^+ promotes Ca^{2+}-dependent desensitization of NMDARs inhibiting the NCX transport of Ca^{2+} from neurons [11]. If this is the case then NMDARs and NCXs should co-localize

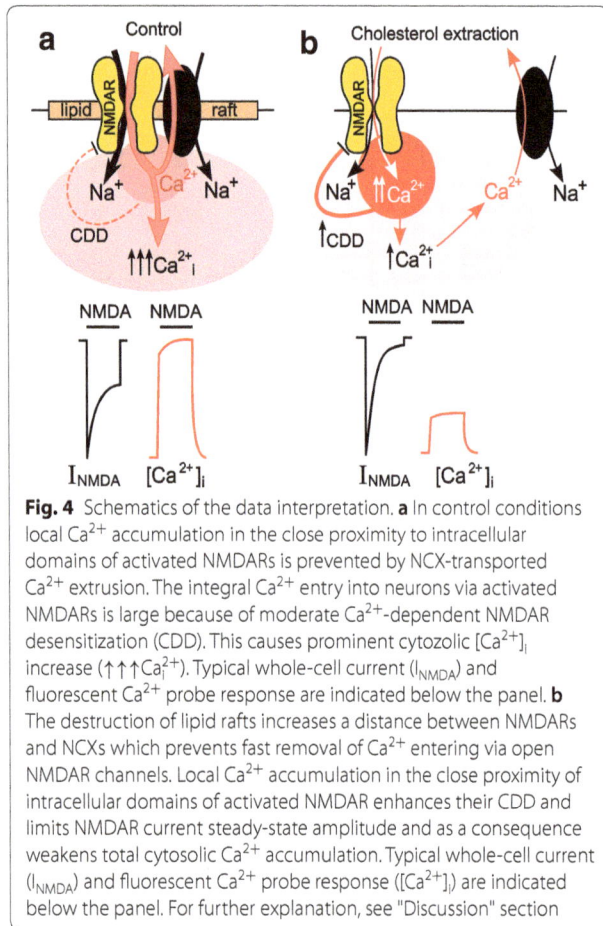

Fig. 4 Schematics of the data interpretation. **a** In control conditions local Ca^{2+} accumulation in the close proximity to intracellular domains of activated NMDARs is prevented by NCX-transported Ca^{2+} extrusion. The integral Ca^{2+} entry into neurons via activated NMDARs is large because of moderate Ca^{2+}-dependent NMDAR desensitization (CDD). This causes prominent cytozolic [Ca^{2+}]$_i$ increase ($\uparrow\uparrow\uparrow$Ca$_i^{2+}$). Typical whole-cell current (I$_{NMDA}$) and fluorescent Ca^{2+} probe response are indicated below the panel. **b** The destruction of lipid rafts increases a distance between NMDARs and NCXs which prevents fast removal of Ca^{2+} entering via open NMDAR channels. Local Ca^{2+} accumulation in the close proximity of intracellular domains of activated NMDAR enhances their CDD and limits NMDAR current steady-state amplitude and as a consequence weakens total cytosolic Ca^{2+} accumulation. Typical whole-cell current (I$_{NMDA}$) and fluorescent Ca^{2+} probe response ([Ca^{2+}]$_i$) are indicated below the panel. For further explanation, see "Discussion" section

and interact that could be achieved in membrane cholesterol rich nanoclusters or lipid rafts (Fig. 4a). Actually the co-localization of NMDARs and NCXs in lipid rafts at the distance less than 80 nm was recently demonstrated using FRET (Förster Resonance Energy Transfer) experiments [18, 19]. In our experiments the cholesterol extraction, that is known to destruct lipid rafts, resulted in a substantial decrease of NMDAR currents, which is consistent to the earlier observation [17], but did not cause significantly changes of the IC$_{50}$ value for the Li$^+$ inhibition of NMDAR currents. This may suggest that the cholesterol extraction does not influence the transport by NCXs [20] and similar Li$^+$ concentrations are required to inhibit NCXs before and after the MβCD treatment.

The requirement of cholesterol for functioning of NMDARs was recently demonstrated [17], because its extraction induced fast ligand-dependent NMDAR desensitization. In agreement when we used 1 mM BAPTA containing intrapipette solution (calculated free Ca^{2+} concentration is 13 nM) a tenfold decrease of NMDAR currents and a lack of Ca^{2+}-dependent NMDAR desensitization were

observed. NMDA-activated currents recorded in the absence of Ca^{2+} in the external solution using the BAPTA-free intrapipette solution did not reveal the NMDAR Ca^{2+}-dependent desensitization as well. The cholesterol extraction under these conditions, however, induced a twofold decrease of the NMDAR currents. The lesser extent of the ligand-dependent desensitization obtained without BAPTA may suggest that some normal level of free Ca^{2+} in the cytoplasm is required for NMDAR functioning. In addition the extraction caused an enforcement of Ca^{2+}-dependent NMDAR desensitization suggesting that the disaggregation of molecules within destructed lipid rafts is accompanied by the disruption of NCX regulated Ca^{2+} pre-membrane balance.

Measurements of intracellular Ca^{2+} dynamics revealed that the NCX inhibition with Li$^+$ or KB-R7943 significantly decreased the NMDA-elicited Ca^{2+} responses, which is consistent to their effects on currents, activated by NMDA. In agreement to previous observations [21] the cholesterol extraction caused the decrease of the cytoplasm Ca^{2+} accumulation, and furthermore abolished the effects of both Li$^+$ and KB-R7943 on the neuronal Ca^{2+} cytoplasmic responses. The cholesterol loading into the plasma membrane was followed by the recovery of Ca^{2+}-response amplitudes and, most importantly, restored the NCX effects on the Ca^{2+}-dependent NMDAR desensitization. These further support our conclusion that the destruction of lipid rafts abolishes the influence of NCXs on NMDARs (Fig. 4b), which is consistent to modeling of interaction between CaM and C-terminal of NMDAR GluN1 subunits that requires molecule co-localization within the distance of tens of nanometers [22].

Thus, our observations considerably widen the range of pharmacological agents which may indirectly influence NMDAR functioning through the metabolism of cholesterol or the inhibition of NCX, that presumably could potentiate the Ca^{2+}-desensitization of NMDARs.

Conclusions

Thus, the NCX inhibition prevents the maintainance of low Ca^{2+} level in the proximity of the intracellular domains of NMDARs by the Ca^{2+} extrusion to the outside, which elevates pre-membrane local Ca^{2+} concentration, but limits total Ca^{2+} entry into neurons. Spatial uncoupling of NCXs and NMDARs by cholesterol extraction enhances the NMDAR Ca^{2+}-dependent desensitization abolishing its regulation by NCXs and is accompanied by a loss of NCX-selective agent effects on NMDARs. As a consequence the inhibition of NCXs with Li$^+$ or KB-R7943 after the cholesterol extraction does not significantly influence the cytoplasmic Ca^{2+} accumulation in response to NMDAR activation.

Methods

Primary culture of cortical neurons

The culture preparation from rat embryos was previously described [23, 24]. All procedures using animals were in accordance with recommendations of the Federation for Laboratory Animal Science Associations and approved by the Bioethics Committee of Sechenov Institute of Evolutionary Physiology and Biochemistry of the Russian Academy of Sciences (IEPhB RAS). Wistar rats were maintained on a 12 h day/night cycle at constant room temperature with ad libitum access to water and standard rat fodder in the animal facility of the IEPhB RAS. Experiments were designed to minimize the number of animals used in research.

Overall 12 Wistar rats 16 days pregnant were used for experiments. The pregnant rat was placed into the plastic box connected by a tube with CO_2 tank and then sacrificed by 30–40 s CO_2 inhalation. Immediately after cardiac arrest fetuses were removed and their cerebral cortices were isolated, enzymatically dissociated and used to prepare primary neuronal cultures. Cells were used for experiments after 10–15 days in culture [24, 25]. Cells were grown in Neurobasal™ culture media supplemented with B-27 (Gibco-Invitrogen, UK) on glass coverslips coated with poly-D-lysine.

Patch clamp recordings

Whole-cell currents were recorded on rat cortical neurons in primary culture (10–15 days in vitro) by patch clamp technique using a MultiClamp 700B amplifier with Digidata 1440A acquisition system. Details of recording and fast perfusion system were described previously [26]. Unless otherwise specified, the following extracellular medium was used for recording (external bathing solution, in mM): 140 NaCl; 2.8 KCl; 1.0 $CaCl_2$; 10 HEPES, at pH 7.2–7.4. The patch-pipette solution contained (in mM): 120 CsF, 10 CsCl, 10 EGTA, and 10 HEPES. In some experiments BAPTA ((1,2-bis(o-aminophenoxy) ethane-N,N,N',N'-tetraacetic acid) was added to path-pipette solution to prevent calcium-dependent desensitization of NMDARs. This solution contained (in mM): 120 CsF, 10 CsCl, 10 EGTA, 10 HEPES, 0.1 $CaCl_2$, 1 BAPTA to achieve calculated free $[Ca^{2+}]$ of 13 nM. The pH was adjusted to 7.4 with CsOH. Measured osmolarities of the external bathing solution and the patch-pipette solution were 310 and 300 mOsm, respectively. Patch pipettes (2–4 MΩ) were pulled from 1.5-mm (outer diameter) borosilicate standard wall capillaries with inner filament (Sutter Instrument, Novato, CA, USA). In whole-cell configuration the series resistances did

not exceed 10 MΩ. Holding membrane voltage (V_m) was corrected for the liquid junction potential between the Na^+-containing external bathing solution and the Cs^+-containing pipette solution of − 15 mV.

Loading of Fluo-3 AM and Ca^{2+} imaging

Cells were loaded with Fluo-3 AM (4 mM, Life Technologies, Foster City, CA, USA) using conventional protocols as described previously [27]. Coverslips with Fluo-3-loaded neurons were placed in the perfusion chamber, which was mounted on the stage of a Leica TCS SP5 MP inverted microscope (Leica Microsystems, Germany). Fluorescence was activated with 488 nm laser light and emission was measured within the wavelength range from 500 to 560 nm. Images were captured every 1.5 s during 30 min experiments.

Drugs

Functional activity of NMDARs requires binding of both glutamate and a co-agonist, glycine. Unless otherwise stated, to activate NMDARs we applied 100 μM NMDA with 10 μM L-glycine (Gly). KB-R7943 (2-[4-[(4-nitrophenyl)methoxy]phenyl]ethyl ester, methanesulfonate, 10 μM) application or proportional substitution of Li^+ for Na^+ in the external bathing solution were used to inhibit NCX. Methyl-β-cyclodextrin (MβCD, 1.5 mM) application for 5 min was used to destruct lipid rafts by extracting cholesterol from the plasma membrane. The complex of cholesterol with methyl-β-cyclodextrin (cholesterol-MβCD, 1.5 mM) as a donor of cholesterol was applied for 30 min to restore the cholesterol content of the plasma membrane. All compounds were from Sigma-Aldrich, St. Louis, MO, USA or Tocris Bioscience, UK.

Data analysis

Quantitative data are expressed as mean ± SEM. ANOVA and Bonferroni multiple comparison methods as well as Student's two-tailed t-test were used for statistical analysis. Number of experiments is indicated by n throughout. In the patch-clamp experiments n represents a number of recorded neurons. In the Ca^{2+}-imaging experiments n represents a number of used culture coverslips. From every coverslip a single mean value obtained from many cells was utilized for statistics. The data were considered as significantly different based on a confidence level of 0.05. Current measurements were plotted using ClampFit 10.2 (Molecular Devices). The IC_{50} (half maximal inhibitory concentration) and Hill coefficient (h) for inhibition of NMDA-evoked currents with Li^+ were estimated by fitting of concentration–response curves with the Hill equation, $I = I_{min} + (I_{max} - I_{min})/(1 + [Li^+]^h/IC_{50}^h)$, where the I_{max} and I_{min} are the current of maximal and minimal amplitudes elicited by NMDA at different $[Li^+]$.

Abbreviations

KB-R7943: (2-[4-[(4-nitrophenyl)methoxy]phenyl]ethyl ester, methanesulfonate; MβCD: Methyl-β-cyclodextrin; NCX: Na$^+$/Ca^{2+}-exchanger; NMDAR: N-methyl-D-aspartate receptor.

Authors' contributions

EEP and DAS performed experiments. DAS supervised data acquisition and statistical analysis. DAS and SMA are responsible for the data interpretation and wrote the paper. SMA is responsible for critically revising the manuscript for intellectual content. All authors read and approved the final manuscript.

Acknowledgements

Imaging experiments were performed at Center for Collective Use of Sechenov Institute of Evolutionary Physiology and Biochemistry of the Russian Academy of Sciences.

Competing interests

The authors declare that they have no competing interests.

Funding

This work was supported by Russian Science Foundation Grant #16-15-10192.

References

1. Bliss TVP, Collingridge GL. A synaptic model of memory: long-term potentiation in the hippocampus. Nature. 1993;361:31–9. https://doi.org/10.1038/361031a0.

2. Bear MF. Mechanism for a sliding synaptic modification threshold. Neuron. 1995;15:1–4. https://doi.org/10.1016/0896-6273(95)90056-X.

3. Choi DW. Calcium: still center-stage in hypoxic-ischemic neuronal death. Trends Neurosci. 1995;18:58–60. https://doi.org/10.1016/0166-2236(95)80018-W.

4. Mayer ML, Westbrook GL. The action of N-methyl-D-aspartic acid on mouse spinal neurones in culture. J Physiol. 1985;361:65–90. https://doi.org/10.1113/jphysiol.1985.sp015633.

5. Zorumski CF, Yang J, Fischbach GD. Calcium dependent, slow desensitization distinguishes different types of glutamate receptors. Cell Mol Neurobiol. 1989;9:95–104. https://doi.org/10.1007/BF00711446.

6. Legendre P, Rosenmund C, Westbrook GL. Inactivation of NMDA channels on hippocampal neurons by intracellular calcium. J Neurosci. 1993;13:674–84. https://doi.org/10.1523/JNEUROSCI.13-02-00674.1993.

7. Vyklický LJ. Calcium-mediated modulation of N-methyl-D-aspartate (NMDA) responses in cultured rat hippocampal neurones. J Physiol. 1993;470:575–600. https://doi.org/10.1113/jphysiol.1993.sp019876.

8. Medina I, Filippova N, Charton G, Rougeole S, Ben-Ari Y, Khrestchatisky M, Bregestovski P. Calcium-dependent inactivation of heteromeric NMDA receptor-channels expressed in human embryonic kidney cells. J Physiol. 1995;482:567–73. https://doi.org/10.1113/jphysiol.1995.sp020540.

9. Ehlers MD, Zhang S, Bernhadt JP, Huganir RL. Inactivation of NMDA receptors by direct interaction of calmodulin with the NR1 subunit. Cell. 1996;84(5):745–55. https://doi.org/10.1016/S0092-8674(00)81052-1.

10. Sibarov DA, Antonov SM. Calcium dependent desensitization of NMDA receptors. Biochemistry (Moscow). 2018;83(10):1173–83.

11. Sibarov DA, Abushik PA, Poguzhelskaya EE, Bolshakov KV, Antonov SM. Inhibition of plasma membrane Na/Ca-exchanger by KB-R7943 or lithium reveals its role in Ca-dependent NMDAR inactivation. J Pharmacol Exp Ther. 2015;355(3):484–95. https://doi.org/10.1124/jpet.115.227173.

12. Antonov SM, Magazanik LG. Intense non-quantal release of glutamate in an insect neuromuscular junction. Neurosci Lett. 1988;93:204–8. https://doi.org/10.1016/0304-3940(88)90082-1.

13. Can A, Schulze TG, Gould TD. Molecular actions and clinical pharmacogenetics of lithium therapy. Pharmacol Biochem Behav. 2014;123:3–16. https://doi.org/10.1016/j.pbb.2014.02.004.

14. Török TL. Electrogenic Na$^+$/Ca^{2+}-exchange of nerve and muscle cells. Prog Neurobiol. 2007;82:287–347. https://doi.org/10.1016/j.pneurobio.2007.06.003.

15. Karkanias NB, Papke RL. Subtype-specific effects of lithium on glutamate receptor function. J Neurophysiol. 1999;81:1506–12. https://doi.org/10.1152/jn.1999.81.4.1506.

16. Hernandez-Ojeda M, Ureña-Guerrero ME, Gutierrez-Barajas PE, Cardenas-Castillo JA, Camins A, Beas-Zarate C. KB-R7943 reduces 4-aminopyridine-induced epileptiform activity in adult rats after neuronal damage induced by neonatal monosodium glutamate treatment. J Biomed Sci. 2017;24(1):27. https://doi.org/10.1186/s12929-017-0335-y.

17. Korinek M, Vyklicky V, Borovska J, Lichnerova K, Kaniakova M, Krausova B, et al. Cholesterol modulates open probability and desensitization of NMDA receptors. J Physiol. 2015;593(10):2279–93. https://doi.org/10.1113/jphysiol.2014.288209.

18. Marques-da-Silva D, Gutierrez-Merino C. L-type voltage-operated calcium channels, N-methyl-D-aspartate receptors and neuronal nitric-oxide synthase form a calcium/redox nano-transducer within lipid rafts. Biochem Biophys Res Commun. 2012;420:257–62. https://doi.org/10.1016/j.bbrc.2012.02.145.

19. Marques-da-Silva D, Gutierrez-Merino C. Caveolin-rich lipid rafts of the plasma membrane of mature cerebellar granule neurons are microcompartments for calcium/reactive oxygen and nitrogen species cross-talk signaling. Cell Calcium. 2014;56(2):108–23. https://doi.org/10.1016/j.ceca.2014.06.002.

20. Bossuyt J, Taylor BE, James-Kracke M, Hale CC. Evidence for cardiac sodium-calcium exchanger association with caveolin-3. FEBS Lett. 2002;511(1–3):113–7. https://doi.org/10.1016/S0014-5793(01)03323-3.

21. Frank C, Giammarioli AM, Pepponi R, Fiorentini C, Rufini S. Cholesterol perturbing agents inhibit NMDA-dependent calcium influx in rat hippocampal primary culture. FEBS Lett. 2004;566(1–3):25–9. https://doi.org/10.1016/j.febslet.2004.03.113.

22. Iacobucci GJ, Popescu GK. Resident calmodulin primes NMDA receptors for Ca-dependent inactivation. Biophys J. 2017;113(10):2236–48. https://doi.org/10.1016/j.bpj.2017.06.035.

23. Antonov SM, Gmiro VE, Johnson JW. Binding sites for permeant ions in the channel of NMDA receptors and their effects on channel block. Nat Neurosci. 1998;1:451–61. https://doi.org/10.1038/2167.

24. Mironova EV, Evstratova AA, Antonov SM. A fluorescence vital assay for the recognition and quantification of excitotoxic cell death by necrosis and apoptosis using confocal microscopy on neurons in culture. J Neurosci Methods. 2007;163:1–8. https://doi.org/10.1016/j.jneumeth.2007.02.010.

25. Han EB, Stevens CF. Development regulates a switch between post- and presynaptic strengthening in response to activity deprivation. Proc Natl Acad Sci USA. 2009;106:10817–22. https://doi.org/10.1073/pnas.0903603106.

26. Sibarov DA, Abushik PA, Giniatullin R, Antonov SM. GluN2A Subunit-containing NMDA receptors are the preferential neuronal targets of homocysteine. Front Cell Neurosci. 2016;10:246. https://doi.org/10.3389/fncel.2016.00246.

27. Abushik PA, Sibarov DA, Eaton MJ, Skatchkov SN, Antonov SM. Kainate-induced calcium overload of cortical neurons in vitro: dependence on expression of AMPAR GluA2-subunit and down-regulation by subnanomolar ouabain. Cell Calcium. 2013;54:95–104. https://doi.org/10.1016/j.ceca.2013.05.002

19

The significance of anti-neuronal antibodies for acute psychiatric disorders

Morten B. Schou[1,2*†], Sverre Georg Sæther[1,3†], Ole Kristian Drange[1,2], Karoline Krane-Gartiser[1,2], Solveig K. Reitan[1,4], Arne E. Vaaler[1,2] and Daniel Kondziella[1,5]

Abstract

Background: The clinical significance of anti-neuronal antibodies in patients with psychiatric disorders, but without encephalitis, remains unknown. In patients admitted to acute psychiatric inpatient care we aimed to identify clinical features distinguishing anti-neuronal antibody positive patients from matched controls.

Results: Patients who were serum-positive to N-methyl D-aspartate receptor (NMDAR) (n = 21), contactin-associated protein 2 (CASPR2) (n = 14) and/or glutamic acid decarboxylase 65 (GAD65) (n = 9) antibodies (cases) were age and sex matched (1:2) with serum-negative patients from the same cohort (controls). The prevalence and severity of psychiatric symptoms frequently encountered in NMDAR, CASPR2 and GAD65 antibody associated disorders were compared in cases and controls. NMDAR, CASPR2 and GAD65 antibody positive patients did not differ in their clinical presentation from matched serum negative controls.

Conclusion: In this cohort, patients with and without NMDAR, CASPR2 and GAD65 antibodies admitted to acute psychiatric inpatient care had similar psychiatric phenotypes. This does not exclude their clinical relevance in subgroups of patients, and studies further investigating the clinical significance of anti-neuronal antibodies in patients with psychiatric symptomatology are needed.

Keywords: Mental disorders, Psychoneuroimmunology, Anti-neuronal antibodies, NMDA receptor antibodies

Background

Anti-neuronal antibodies are associated with autoimmune encephalitis, which often presents with psychiatric symptoms [1]. We recently found serum anti-neuronal antibodies [Immunoglobulin (Ig) G, IgA and/or IgM] in 12% of 925 patients consecutively admitted to acute psychiatric inpatient care [N-methyl D-aspartate receptor (NMDAR) antibodies in 7.6%, contactin-associated protein 2 (CASPR2) antibodies in 2.5%, and glutamic acid decarboxylase 65 (GAD65) antibodies in 1.9%] [2]. The

IgG isotype of NMDAR, CASPR2 and GAD65 antibodies has been associated with autoimmune encephalitis with prominent psychiatric features [1]. The IgA and IgM isotypes of NMDAR antibodies have been associated with psychotic symptoms in dementia [3, 4], and there is some evidence that they have pathogenic potential [5]. In a recent meta-analysis, Grain et al. found that GAD65 antibodies are more prevalent in patients with psychotic disorders compared to controls [6]. The role of any of these antibodies in psychiatric patients without evidence of autoimmune encephalitis is, however, not clear. This is an important issue to address because these patients might benefit from immunotherapy [7].

The prevalence of anti-neuronal antibodies in patients with psychiatric disorders has been investigated in several studies [2, 8–10]. However, it might be that the traditional psychiatric diagnostic classifications [e.g.

*Correspondence: morten.b.schou@ntnu.no
†Morten B. Schou and Sverre Georg Sæther contributed equally to this work
[2] Division of Mental Health Care, St Olavs Hospital HF, avd Østmarka, Trondheim University Hospital, Postboks 3250, Torgarden, 7006 Trondheim, Norway
Full list of author information is available at the end of the article

International Classification of Diseases-10 (ICD-10)] are inadequate for the plethora of autoimmune psychiatric symptoms [11, 12]. Consequently, we chose a different approach. In this large single-center study, we searched for differences in the clinical phenotypes of patients admitted to acute psychiatric inpatient care who tested either positive or negative for three well-known anti-neuronal antibodies (NMDAR, CASPR2 and GAD65). We hypothesized that psychiatric patients testing positive to a specific antibody (e.g. anti-NMDAR) would have an increased frequency and/or severity of psychiatric symptoms typically seen in neurological syndromes associated with that antibody (e.g. anti-NMDAR encephalitis).

Methods

Setting

This case-controlled study was performed in an acute psychiatric inpatient clinic in a university center (St. Olavs Hospital, Trondheim University Hospital, Trondheim, Norway). The hospital receives all patients (≥ 18 years) admitted to acute psychiatric inpatient care in the catchment area. The most common reasons for referral include major depression, bipolar disorder, schizophrenia spectrum disorders, personality disorders, anxiety disorders or substance induced psychiatric disorders. The only inclusion criterion was admission to acute psychiatric inpatient care. Exclusion criteria were inability to give informed consent, discharge before consent could be obtained, or lack of proficiency in Norwegian or English.

Patients

A total of 654 consecutive patients were admitted during 7 months in 2011–2012. Three hundred and forty patients (52%) consented to participate in the study, of which 41 tested positive for NMDAR, CASPR2 and/or GAD65 antibodies (IgA, IgG or IgM). None tested positive for antibodies directed to Leucine-rich glioma-inactivated protein 1 (LGI1), α-amino-3-hydroxy-5-methyl-4-isoxazolepropionic acid receptor (AMPAR) or γ-aminobutyric acid B receptor (GABA$_B$R) [2]. Eighty-two anti-neuronal antibody negative controls were chosen from the same cohort (i.e. 2 controls for each case) (Fig. 1). Controls were selected randomly among patients with the same sex and age (± 5 years) as each case. If no such patient was present in the cohort, the age interval was increased (± 10 years, ± 15 years).

Variables

Variables of symptomatology were selected following a systematic literature search for psychiatric symptomatology in disorders associated with NMDAR, CASPR2 and GAD65 antibodies. Comparisons were made only for symptoms associated with each specific anti-neuronal antibody. See Additional file 1 for search strategy

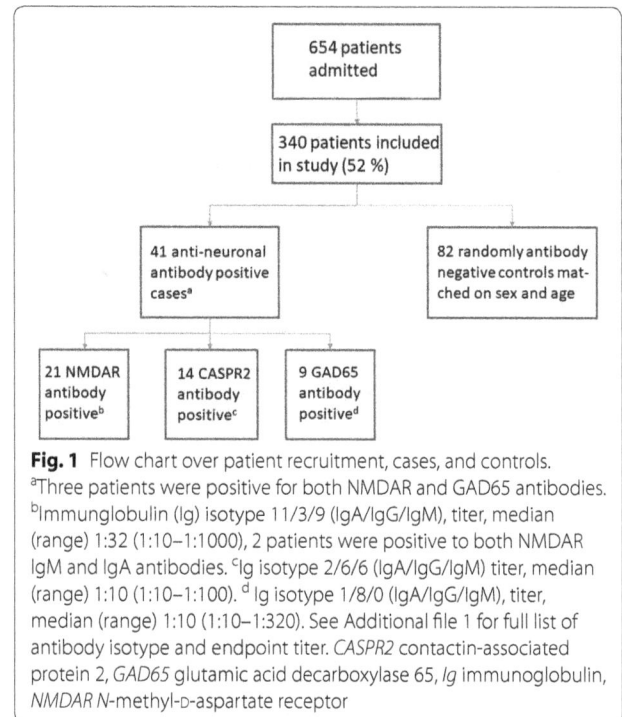

Fig. 1 Flow chart over patient recruitment, cases, and controls. [a]Three patients were positive for both NMDAR and GAD65 antibodies. [b]Immunglobulin (Ig) isotype 11/3/9 (IgA/IgG/IgM), titer, median (range) 1:32 (1:10–1:1000), 2 patients were positive to both NMDAR IgM and IgA antibodies. [c]Ig isotype 2/6/6 (IgA/IgG/IgM) titer, median (range) 1:10 (1:10–1:100). [d] Ig isotype 1/8/0 (IgA/IgG/IgM), titer, median (range) 1:10 (1:10–1:320). See Additional file 1 for full list of antibody isotype and endpoint titer. *CASPR2* contactin-associated protein 2, *GAD65* glutamic acid decarboxylase 65, *Ig* immunoglobulin, *NMDAR* N-methyl-ᴅ-aspartate receptor

and citations on the papers reviewed. Symptom variables were included only if they either were available from the data collected during the inclusion period (2011–2012) or could be reliably assessed during retrospective chart review. Symptom variables included were; hallucinations, delusions, lowered mood, elevated mood, irritability, disinhibition, agitation, disorientation, symptom fluctuation, and sleep problems. The symptom variables anxiety, catatonia and apathy were also extracted in the literature review but were deemed too unreliable to be assessed by retrospective chart review. A subset of symptom variables was associated with exclusively one or two of the antibodies assessed in this study (Table 1).

On the first day following admission, the attending physicians evaluated the degree of agitation with the Positive and Negative Syndrome Scale-Excited Component (PANSS-EC) [13], impulse control as a measure of disinhibition with the use of PANSS item G14 and the degree of fluctuation of psychiatric symptoms with Symptomatic Organic Mental Disorder Assessment Scale (SOMAS) item A [14]. In addition, the nursing staff evaluated the degree of irritability and disorientation with the Brøset Violence checklist (BVC) [15]. Sleep variables were recorded by an actigraph worn around the wrist for 24 h soon after admission (Actiwatch Spectrum, Philips Respironics Inc., Murrysville PA, USA) [16], mean time until the actigraphy recording started was 2.2 (SD 2.2) days after admission. A blinded assessor

Table 1 Patients with and without anti-neuronal antibodies were compared on the following clinical characteristics

Clinical characteristic	NMDAR	CASPR2	GAD65	Variable	Obtained	Definitions
Hallucinations	X	X	n/a	Dichotome (Yes/No)	Retrospective	Vis., aud., tact. and/or olf.
Delusions	X	X	n/a	Dichotome (Yes/No)	Retrospective	Described in chart
Lowered mood	X	X	X	Dichotome (Yes/No)	Retrospective	Described in chart
Elevated mood	X	n/a	n/a	Dichotome (Yes/No)	Retrospective	Described in chart
Irritability	X	n/a	X	Dichotome (Yes/No)	Prospective	Brøset Violence Checklist
Disorientation	X	X	X	Dichotome (Yes/No)	Prospective	Brøset Violence Checklist
Disinhibition	X	n/a	n/a	Continuous (1–7)	Prospective	PANSS Item G14
Agitation	X	X	X	Continuous (5–35)	Prospective	PANSS-EC
Symptom fluctuation	X	n/a	n/a	Continuous (1–10)	Prospective	SOMAS Item A
Total sleep time (actigraphy)	X	X	n/a	Continuous (min)	Prospective	According to actigraphy software algorithms
Wake after sleep onset (actigraphy)	X	X	n/a	Continuous (min)	Prospective	According to actigraphy software algorithms

aud auditive, *CASPR2* contactin-associated protein 2, *GAD65* glutamic acid decarboxylase 65, *n/a* not applicable (because the systematic literature search did not reveal associations between the symptom variable and the specific antibody), *NMDAR* N-methyl-D-aspartate receptor, *olf* olfactory, *PANSS* positive and negative syndrome scale, *PANSS-EC* positive and negative syndrome scale- excited component, *SOMAS* Symptomatic Organic Mental Disorder Assessment Scale, *tact* tactile, *Vis* visual

scored the actigraphy recordings. For each patient a rest interval at nighttime was set by visual inspection. The actigraphy software (Actiware, version 5.70.1) then automatically calculated the variables "total sleep time" and "wake after sleep onset" during the rest interval using the Immobile Minutes algorithm of 10 min, and a wake threshold after sleep onset of 40 activity counts (medium sensitivity), which has been used in validation studies [17, 18]. All other clinical characteristics were extracted from patient charts by blinded examiners who reviewed charts from the 24 h following admission. Psychiatric diagnoses were set according to the International Classification of Diseases (ICD)-10 criteria for research [19] in a consensus meeting including the physician or psychologist in charge of the treatment of the patient and at least two psychiatrists and/or senior clinical psychologist. The main diagnosis was registered in this study. Patients were asked for life-time history of seizures and evaluated with regards to whether or not alcohol or illegal substances had been consumed during the days/weeks prior to admission. This evaluation consisted of patient interviews, alcohol breathing tests and urine analyses of alcohol, benzodiazcpines (oxazepam, desmethyldiazepam, nitrazepam, flunitrazepam, clonazepam, and alprazolam), zopiclone, stimulants (amphetamine, metamphetamine, 3,4-methylendioksymetamphetamine, 3,4-methyl-dioxy-amphetamine, ephedrine, and benzoylecgonine), opioids (morphine, codeine, etylmorphine, methadone, buprenorphine, pholcodine, and oxycodone) carisoprodol, meprobamate, cannabis, and phencyclidine (Liquid chromatography with mass spectroscopy).

Serological analysis

Sera were tested for the presence of anti-neuronal antibodies directed against NMDAR, LGI1, CASPR2, AMPAR, GABA_BR and GAD65 (IgA, IgG and IgM) using transfected HEK293 cells expressing the respective recombinant target antigens (Euroimmun, Lübeck, Germany) [20, 21]. Samples were classified as positive or negative based on fluorescence intensity of the transfected cells in direct comparison with non-transfected cells and control samples. Endpoint titers were defined as the last dilution showing a measurable degree of fluorescence, with 1:10 being the cut-off for positivity [20, 21].

Ethics

On the day after admission a psychiatrist or senior clinical psychologist evaluated each patient's ability to consent. Patients without ability to consent were excluded. Included patients gave written, informed consent. The study was conducted in accordance with the Declaration of Helsinki and approved by The Regional Committee for Medical Research Ethics, Central Norway (2011/137). The data for the present study were collected as part of a previous clinical trial, "Agitation in the Acute Psychiatric Department", which was prospectively registered on https://clinicaltrials.gov/ on August 11th 2011 (NCT01415323).

Statistics

We compared patients with a positive serology for NMDAR, CASPR2 or GAD65 antibodies with their respective age- and sex-matched controls for the presence and degree of psychiatric symptoms as outlined in Tables 1 and 3. Categorical variables were analyzed using the Chi square test or Fisher's exact test. Continuous variables were compared using the T test or Mann–Whitney U-test. Alpha level was set at 0.05. Adjustment for multiple comparisons was not performed due to the exploratory study design. Statistical analyses were done in SPSS 21 (SPSS, Chicago, US-IL).

Results

Demographic and clinical data

The inclusion rate was 52% (340 out of 654 admitted patients). There were no significant differences in age ($p = 0.64$, Mann–Whitney U test) or sex ($p = 0.67$, chi-square test) between included and non-included patients. However, there was a difference in diagnostic distribution between the groups ($p < 0.001$, Chi square test). This was attributable to overrepresentation of patients suffering from depressive and bipolar disorders, and underrepresentation of patients suffering from psychotic disorders and patients not fulfilling ICD-10 criteria for a specific psychiatric disorder (Z-diagnosis) among the included patients (data not shown).

Demographic and clinical data of cases and controls are presented in Table 2. Compared to controls, NMDAR antibody positive patients had a higher prevalence of alcohol and substance use prior to admission (76 vs. 50%, $p = 0.047$) and received antidepressant drugs more often at discharge (43 vs. 17%, $p = 0.024$). GAD65 antibody

Table 2 Demographic and clinical data of patients with NMDAR, CASPR2 or GAD65 antibodies and of their controls

	NMDAR		CASPR2		GAD65	
	Cases (n = 21)	Controls (n = 42)	Cases (n = 14)	Controls (n = 28)	Cases (n = 9)	Controls (n = 18)
Age, mean (SD)	48.6 (16.3)	46.7 (14.2)	45.0 (16.1)	43.4 (14.7)	47.1 (14.0)	45.8 (11.8)
Sex, men (%)	62	62	71	71	56	56
Education, n (%)						
≤ 9 years	9 (43)	20 (48)	6 (43)	9 (32)	4 (44)	7 (39)
10–12 years	7 (33)	14 (33)	2 (14)	13 (46)	4 (44)	9 (50)
> 12 years	5 (24)	8 (19)	6 (43)	6 (21)	1 (11)	2 (11)
Psychiatric diagnosis, n (%)						
Substance use disorder (F10–19)	4 (19)	7 (17)	3 (21)	6 (21)	2 (22)	3 (17)
Psychotic disorder (F20–29)	1 (6)	6 (14)	2 (14)	6 (21)	1 (11)	1 (6)
Affective disorder (F30–39)	8 (38)	20 (48)	5 (36)	12 (43)	3 (33)	9 (50)
Other psychiatric disorders[a]	8 (38)	9 (21)	4 (29)	4 (14)	3 (33)	5 (28)
Psychopharmacological med. at admission, n (%)						
Antipsychotic med.	6 (29)	13 (31)	5 (36)	10 (36)	3 (33)	5 (28)
Antipsychotic dose, mean (SD)[b]	482 (422)	458 (302)	241 (185)	324 (170)	1071 (124)	469 (276)*
Antidepressive med.	8 (38)	9 (21)	4 (29)	8 (29)	3 (33)	6 (33)
Mood stabilizing med.	3 (14)	10 (24)	2 (14)	4 (14)	2 (22)	3 (17)
No psychopharmacological med.	10 (48)	18 (43)	5 (36)	12 (43)	4 (44)	8 (44)
Psychopharmacological med. at discharge, n (%)						
Antipsychotic med.	9 (43)	26 (62)	6 (43)	18 (64)	5 (56)	11 (61)
Antipsychotic dose, mean (SD)[b]	418 (449)	408 (331)	222 (203)	342 (226)	784 (403)	331 (254)*
Antidepressive med.	9 (43)	7 (17)*	4 (29)	7 (25)	2 (22)	6 (33)
Mood stabilizing med.	6 (29)	15 (36)	5 (36)	6 (21)	2 (22)	5 (28)
No psychopharmacological med.	5 (24)	10 (24)	3 (21)	5 (18)	2 (22)	5 (28)
Number of days admitted, mean (SD)	9.5 (11.4)	9.9 (9.1)	9.5 (6.1)	10.1 (11.6)	9.6 (9.3)	9.1 (8.3)
Alcohol or substance use days/weeks prior to admission, n (%)	16 (76)	21 (50)*	10 (71)	18 (64)	7 (78)	10 (56)
History of seizures[c]	1 (6)	9 (25)	4 (40)	3 (13)	2 (22)	3 (18)

CASPR2 contactin-associated protein 2, *eq* equivalents, *GAD65* glutamic acid decarboxylase 65, *med* medication, *NMDAR* N-methyl-ᴅ-aspartate receptor, *SD* standard deviation

*p < 0.05

[a] 3 patients with organic mental disorder (F00–09), 13 patients with anxiety disorders (F40–49), 7 patients with personality disorders (F60–69), 1 patient with mental retardation (F70–79), 1 patient with ADHD (F90–98) and 5 patients without specific psychiatric disorder (Z00–99); [b]chlorpromazine equivalents; [c]self-reported at admission (missing data; NMDAR, 3 cases and 6 controls; CASPR2, 4 cases and 5 controls; GAD, 1 control)

positive patients received higher doses of antipsychotic medication compared to controls both at admission and discharge [Chlorpromazine equivalents mean (SD) 1071 (124) vs. 469 (276), p = 0.013, and 784 (403) versus 331 (254), p-value = 0.015, respectively]. None of the anti-GAD65 positive cases or controls had diabetes mellitus type I.

Clinical characteristics

None of the clinical parameters differed between patients with NMDAR, CASPR2 and GAD65 antibodies and their respective controls (Table 3). None of the NMDAR IgG positive patients had symptoms or signs of NMDAR encephalitis.

Discussion

In this large cohort of patients admitted to acute psychiatric inpatient care, patients who were serum positive or negative to anti-neuronal antibodies had a similar psychiatric phenotype. Specifically, patients with NMDAR, CASPR2 and GAD65 antibodies did *not* exhibit psychiatric symptoms suggestive of autoimmune encephalitis more frequently than controls.

Previous studies in patients with psychiatric disorders have explored the prevalence of anti-neuronal antibodies in different diagnostic groups. It is still controversial whether or not the prevalence of anti-neuronal antibodies is increased in patients with first episode or chronic psychosis [2, 8–10, 22, 23]. A limited number of studies have addressed clinical characteristics in anti-neuronal antibody-positive and -negative psychiatric patients irrespective of diagnostic categories. Hammer et al. [24]

did not find any differences in PANSS or Global Assessment of Function (GAF) when comparing patients with schizophrenia who were positive or negative for NMDAR antibodies. Similarly, in a cohort of patients with first-episode psychosis PANSS scores, cognitive testing and catatonia symptoms were not clinically significant different in anti-neuronal antibody positive (NMDAR, CASPR2, LGI1 or GABA$_A$ receptor antibodies) and negative patients [9]. The authors of a study including patients with both first episode and chronic schizophrenia found more severe psychotic symptoms (PANSS scores) in NMDAR antibody positive compared to negative patients [10]. The studies in this field are heterogeneous and the results depend to a certain degree on the antibody detection method used. Fixed and live cell-based assays are the most commonly used methods for anti-neuronal antibody detection. Using a novel single molecule-based imaging approach, Jezequel et al. [10] recently showed that NMDAR antibodies from schizophrenia patients alter the surface dynamics of the NMDAR in contrast to NMDAR antibodies from healthy controls. Jezequel et al. [25] found that fixed cell-based assays (such as the one used in this study) have a lower sensitivity for detection of IgG antibodies in psychotic patients compared to live cell-based assays. Hence, it is possible that the use of other antibody detection methods in the present study would have yielded slightly different results. Another possible explanation for the lack of phenotypic differences is the low antibody titers found in our patients; alternatively, the lack of significant findings in our study could reflect a lack of clinical significance of these antibodies for acute psychiatric patients in general.

Table 3 Psychiatric symptoms in antibody positive cases (+) and controls (−)

Clinical characteristic	NMDAR		p^a	CASPR2		p^a	GAD65		
	+ n = 21	− n = 42		+ n = 14	− n = 28		+ n = 9	− n = 18	p^a
Hallucinations, n (%)	3 (14.3)	1 (2.4)	0.10	0 (0)	3 (10.7)	0.54			
Delusions, n (%)	2 (9.5)	7 (16.7)	0.71	2 (14.3)	3 (10.7)	1.00			
Lowered mood^b, n (%)	10 (55.6)	16 (39.0)	0.24^i	8 (61.5)	15 (60.0)	0.93^i	5 (55.6)	11 (64.7)	0.69
Elevated mood^c, n (%)	2 (11.1)	7 (17.1)	0.71						
Irritability^d, n (%)	3 (15.0)	6 (14.3)	1.00	3 (23.1)	5 (18.5)	1.00	1 (12.5)	5 (27.8)	0.63
Disorientation^e, n (%)	1 (5.0)	7 (16.7)	0.26	4 (30.8)	4 (15.4)	0.40	0 (0)	2 (11.1)	1.00
Disinhibition (median (range))	1 (1–6)	1 (1–6)	0.57^j						
Agitation (median (range))^f	8 (5–31)	8 (5–32)	0.62^j	7 (5–27)	10 (5–21)	0.34^j	10 (5–17)	8 (5–23)	0.98^j
Symptom fluctuation (median (range))^g	2 (1–7)	3 (1–8)	0.89^j						
Total sleep time (min) (mean (SD))^h	458 (115)	476 (112)	0.66^k	438 (109)	442 (114)	0.93^k			
Time awake after sleep onset (min) (mean (SD))^h	39 (23)	37 (35)	0.90^k	47 (18)	40 (24)	0.51^k			

CASPR2 contactin-associated protein 2, *GAD65* glutamic acid decarboxylase 65, *NMDAR* N-methyl-ᴅ-aspartate receptor, *SD* standard deviation

^{a} Fisher's exact test if not stated otherwise. Data missing on ^{b}NMDAR (3 cases, 1 control), CASPR2 (1 case, 3 controls), GAD65 (1 control); ^{c}NMDAR (3 cases, 1 control); ^{d}NMDAR (1 case), CASPR2 (1 case, 1 control), GAD65 (1 case); ^{e}NMDAR (1 case), CASPR2 (1 case, 2 controls), GAD65 (1 case); ^{f}CASPR2 (1 case, 1 control); ^{g}NMDAR (3 cases, 7 controls); ^{h}NMDAR (10 cases, 16 controls), CASPR2 (6 cases, 14 controls); ^{i}Chi square; ^{j}Mann Whitney U test; ^{k}T-test

Hence, whether or not phenotypical differences are present in psychiatric patients with higher antibody titers is an important question for further research. To further investigate this, future studies should include cerebrospinal fluid (CSF) analyses, electroencephalography (EEG) and brain imaging.

NMDAR antibody positive patients were treated more often with antidepressants than controls. These findings could be coincidental. However, it is also possible that excessive use of antidepressants indicates a higher burden of depressive and/or anxious symptoms in NMDAR positive patients, although we were unable to detect such differences in our retrospective chart assessment. The increased frequency of alcohol and substance use prior to admission in NMDAR antibody positive patients may suggest self-medication for depressive and/or anxious symptoms. However, an influence of alcohol and substance use on NMDAR antibody titers cannot be ruled out. The NMDAR is implicated in addiction in several ways. For instance, associations have been found between addiction and genes coding for NMDAR subunits [26]; alcohol has acute and chronic effects on NMDAR functioning [27]; and NMDAR modulators are used to treat alcohol dependency [28]. Interestingly, alcohol and illicit substances can cause blood brain barrier dysfunction [29, 30], which might facilitate the occurrence of NMDAR antibodies by exposing NMDAR to lymphoid cells. However, the exact reasons for the observed association between NMDAR antibodies and alcohol and substance remains unknown. GAD65 antibody positive patients used higher doses of antipsychotic drugs compared to antibody negative patients, which could imply a more severe symptomatology in these patients. Alternatively, antipsychotic medication might also lead to enhanced production of GAD65 antibodies. A similar association is known for chlorpromazine and antinuclear antibodies [31, 32].

The present study has limitations. The inclusion rate of 52% is similar to other studies in this setting [33, 34]. However, there is a risk of selection bias (i.e. patients with a higher severity of symptoms may decline participation or lack ability to consent more often than patients with less severe phenotypes). Patients with affective disorders were overrepresented and psychotic disorders underrepresented in our study. We included patients with all isotypes of NMDAR, CASPR2 and GAD65 antibodies (IgG, IgA and IgM). Whereas most known relevant antineuronal antibodies are of the IgG isotype, the results of pathogenicity studies of NMDAR IgA and IgM antibodies show their pathogenic potential in vitro [5, 24, 35, 36] and in a study of patients with stroke [37], although authors from another study concluded that NMDAR IgA and IgM antibodies do not alter NMDAR levels [38]. It is possible that our study would have yielded a different result if we had focused exclusively on IgG positive patients. Also, small group sizes and the categorical nature of several of the variables may have resulted in a lower sensitivity for detecting clinical differences. Although age- and sex-matched control subjects were randomly selected, some differences in diagnostic distribution and psychopharmacological treatment between the case and control group were present (Table 3).

Conclusion

Based on our findings, patients admitted to acute psychiatric care with and without NMDAR, CASPR2 and GAD65 antibodies have a similar clinical phenotype. However, of note, absence of phenotypic differences between patients with and without anti-neuronal antibodies is not evidence that these antibodies lack clinical significance. Even if anti-neuronal antibodies played a role in only a minor subset of psychiatric patients, this would have important clinical implications as these patients might benefit from immunomodulatory treatment. This area must be further investigated by large prospective longitudinal multicenter studies that include cerebrospinal fluid analyses, brain imaging and electrophysiological investigations.

Abbreviations
BVC: Brøset violence checklist; CASPR2: contactin-associated protein 2; GAD65: glutamic acid decarboxylase 65; ICD: international classification of diseases; Ig: immunoglobulin; NMDAR: N-methyl D-aspartate receptor; PANSS-EC: Positive and Negative Syndrome Scale-Excited Component; SOMAS: Symptomatic Organic Mental Disorder Assessment Scale.

Authors' contributions
MS, SGS and DK designed the study. MS and OKD collected the retrospective data. MS, SGS, OKD, SKR and AV collected the prospective data. KKG analyzed the actigraphy data. MS and SGS analyzed all other data. MS, SGS and DK drafted the manuscript. All authors read and approved the final manuscript.

Author details
[1] Department of Mental Health, Norwegian University of Science and Technology (NTNU), Trondheim, Norway. [2] Division of Mental Health Care, St Olavs Hospital HF, avd Østmarka, Trondheim University Hospital, Postboks 3250, Torgarden, 7006 Trondheim, Norway. [3] Division of Mental Health Care, St Olavs Hospital HF, Nidaros DPS, Trondheim University Hospital, Postboks 3250, Torgarden, 7006 Trondheim, Norway. [4] Division of Mental Health Care, Tiller DPS, St Olavs Hospital HF, Trondheim University Hospital, Postboks 3250, Torgarden, 7006 Trondheim, Norway. [5] Neurology Department, Rigshospitalet, Copenhagen University Hospital, Blegdamsvei 9, 2100 København Ø, Denmark.

Acknowledgements
None.

Competing interests
The authors declare that they have no competing interests.

Funding
No direct funding were given for this project.

References
1. Herken J, Pruss H. Red flags: clinical signs for identifying autoimmune encephalitis in psychiatric patients. Front Psychiatry/Front Res Found. 2017;8:25.
2. Schou M, Saether SG, Borowski K, Teegen B, Kondziella D, Stoecker W, et al. Prevalence of serum anti-neuronal autoantibodies in patients admitted to acute psychiatric care. Psychol Med. 2016;46:3303–13.
3. Busse S, Busse M, Brix B, Probst C, Genz A, Bogerts B, et al. Seroprevalence of N-methyl-D-aspartate glutamate receptor (NMDA-R) autoantibodies in aging subjects without neuropsychiatric disorders and in dementia patients. Eur Arch Psychiatry Clin Neurosci. 2014;264(6):545–50.
4. Busse S, Brix B, Kunschmann R, Bogerts B, Stoecker W, Busse M. N-methyl-D-aspartate glutamate receptor (NMDA-R) antibodies in mild cognitive impairment and dementias. Neurosci Res. 2014;85:58–64.
5. Castillo-Gomez E, Oliveira B, Tapken D, Bertrand S, Klein-Schmidt C, Pan H, et al. All naturally occurring autoantibodies against the NMDA receptor subunit NR1 have pathogenic potential irrespective of epitope and immunoglobulin class. Mol Psychiatry. 2017;22:1776–84.
6. Grain R, Lally J, Stubbs B, Malik S, LeMince A, Nicholson TR, et al. Autoantibodies against voltage-gated potassium channel and glutamic acid decarboxylase in psychosis: a systematic review, meta-analysis, and case series. Psychiatry Clin Neurosci. 2017;71(10):678–89.
7. Zandi MS, Deakin JB, Morris K, Buckley C, Jacobson L, Scoriels L, et al. Immunotherapy for patients with acute psychosis and serum N-methyl-D-Aspartate receptor (NMDAR) antibodies: a description of a treated case series. Schizophr Res. 2014;160(1–3):193–5.
8. Dahm L, Ott C, Steiner J, Stepniak B, Teegen B, Saschenbrecker S, et al. Seroprevalence of autoantibodies against brain antigens in health and disease. Ann Neurol. 2014;76(1):82–94.
9. Lennox BR, Palmer-Cooper EC, Pollak T, Hainsworth J, Marks J, Jacobson L, et al. Prevalence and clinical characteristics of serum neuronal cell surface antibodies in first-episode psychosis: a case–control study. Lancet Psychiatry. 2017;4(1):42–8.
10. Jezequel J, Johansson EM, Dupuis JP, Rogemond V, Grea H, Kellermayer B, et al. Dynamic disorganization of synaptic NMDA receptors triggered by autoantibodies from psychotic patients. Nat Commun. 2017;8(1):1791.
11. Pollak TA, Beck K, Irani SR, Howes OD, David AS, McGuire PK. Autoantibodies to central nervous system neuronal surface antigens: psychiatric symptoms and psychopharmacological implications. Psychopharmacology. 2016;233(9):1605–21.
12. Pearlman DM, Najjar S. Meta-analysis of the association between N-methyl-D-aspartate receptor antibodies and schizophrenia, schizoaffective disorder, bipolar disorder, and major depressive disorder. Schizophr Res. 2014;157(1–3):249–58.
13. Montoya A, Valladares A, Lizan L, San L, Escobar R, Paz S. Validation of the Excited Component of the Positive and Negative Syndrome Scale (PANSS-EC) in a naturalistic sample of 278 patients with acute psychosis and agitation in a psychiatric emergency room. Health Qual Life Outcomes. 2011;9:18.
14. Vaaler AE, Morken G, Iversen VC, Kondziella D, Linaker OM. Acute Unstable Depressive Syndrome (AUDS) is associated more frequently with epilepsy than major depression. BMC Neurol. 2010;10:67.
15. Woods P, Almvik R. The Broset violence checklist (BVC). Acta Psychiatr Scand Suppl. 2002;412:103–5.
16. Ancoli-Israel S, Cole R, Alessi C, Chambers M, Moorcroft W, Pollak CP. The role of actigraphy in the study of sleep and circadian rhythms. Sleep. 2003;26(3):342–92.
17. Paquet J, Kawinska A, Carrier J. Wake detection capacity of actigraphy during sleep. Sleep. 2007;30(10):1362–9.
18. Kaplan KA, Talbot LS, Gruber J, Harvey AG. Evaluating sleep in bipolar disorder: comparison between actigraphy, polysomnography, and sleep diary. Bipolar Disord. 2012;14(8):870–9.
19. WHO. The ICD-10 classification of mental and behavioural disorders: diagnostic criteria for research. Geneva, Switzerland: World Health Organization; 1993.
20. Probst C, Saschenbrecker S, Stoecker W, Komorowski L. Anti-neuronal autoantibodies: current diagnostic challenges. Mul Scler Relat Disord. 2014;3(3):303–20.
21. Wandinger KP, Saschenbrecker S, Stoecker W, Dalmau J. Anti-NMDA-receptor encephalitis: a severe, multistage, treatable disorder presenting with psychosis. J Neuroimmunol. 2011;231(1–2):86–91.
22. Masdeu JC, Gonzalez-Pinto A, Matute C, Ruiz De Azua S, Palomino A, De Leon J, et al. Serum IgG antibodies against the NR1 subunit of the NMDA receptor not detected in schizophrenia. Am J Psychiatry. 2012;169(10):1120–1.
23. Pathmanandavel K, Starling J, Merheb V, Ramanathan S, Sinmaz N, Dale RC, et al. Antibodies to surface dopamine-2 receptor and N-methyl-D-aspartate receptor in the first episode of acute psychosis in children. Biol Psychiat. 2015;77(6):537–47.
24. Hammer C, Stepniak B, Schneider A, Papiol S, Tantra M, Begemann M, et al. Neuropsychiatric disease relevance of circulating anti-NMDA receptor autoantibodies depends on blood-brain barrier integrity. Mol Psychiatry. 2014;19(10):1143–9.
25. Jezequel J, Rogemond V, Pollak T, Lepleux M, Jacobson L, Grea H, et al. Cell- and single molecule-based methods to detect anti-N-methyl-D-aspartate receptor autoantibodies in patients with first-episode psychosis from the OPTiMiSE Project. Biol Psychiat. 2017;82(10):766–72.
26. Chen J, Ma Y, Fan R, Yang Z, Li MD. Implication of genes for the N-methyl-D-aspartate (NMDA) receptor in substance addictions. Mol Neurobiol. 2018;55(9):7567–78.
27. Ron D, Wang J. The NMDA receptor and alcohol addiction. In: Van Dongen AM, editor. Biology of the NMDA receptor. Boca Raton: CRC Press; 2009.
28. Tomek SE, Lacrosse AL, Nemirovsky NE, Olive MF. NMDA receptor modulators in the treatment of drug addiction. Pharmaceuticals (Basel). 2013;6(2):251–68.
29. Kousik SM, Napier TC, Carvey PM. The effects of psychostimulant drugs on blood brain barrier function and neuroinflammation. Front Pharmacol. 2012;3:121.
30. Rubio-Araiz A, Porcu F, Perez-Hernandez M, Garcia-Gutierrez MS, Aracil-Fernandez MA, Gutierrez-Lopez MD, et al. Disruption of blood-brain barrier integrity in postmortem alcoholic brain: preclinical evidence of TLR4 involvement from a binge-like drinking model. Addict Biol. 2017;22:1103–16.
31. Canoso RT, Sise HS. Chlorpromazine-induced lupus anticoagulant and associated immunologic abnormalities. Am J Hematol. 1982;13(2):121–9.
32. Canoso RT, de Oliveira RM. Characterization and antigenic specificity of chlorpromazine-induced antinuclear antibodies. J Lab Clin Med. 1986;108(3):213–6.
33. Mordal J, Medhus S, Holm B, Morland J, Bramness JG. Influence of drugs of abuse and alcohol upon patients admitted to acute psychiatric wards: physician's assessment compared to blood drug concentrations. J Clin Psychopharmacol. 2013;33(3):415–9.
34. Kohigashi M, Kitabayashi Y, Okamura A, Nakamura M, Hoshiyama A, Kunizawa M, et al. Relationship between patients' quality of life and coercion in psychiatric acute wards. Psychiatry Res. 2013;208(1):88–90.
35. Pruss H, Holtje M, Maier N, Gomez A, Buchert R, Harms L, et al. IgA NMDA receptor antibodies are markers of synaptic immunity in slow cognitive impairment. Neurology. 2012;78(22):1743–53.
36. Pruss H, Finke C, Holtje M, Hofmann J, Klingbeil C, Probst C, et al. N-methyl-D-aspartate receptor antibodies in herpes simplex encephalitis. Ann Neurol. 2012;72(6):902–11.
37. Zerche M, Weissenborn K, Ott C, Dere E, Asif AR, Worthmann H, et al. Preexisting serum autoantibodies against the NMDAR Subunit NR1 modulate evolution of lesion size in acute ischemic stroke. Stroke. 2015;46(5):1180–6.
38. Hara M, Martinez-Hernandez E, Arino H, Armangue T, Spatola M, Petit-Pedrol M, et al. Clinical and pathogenic significance of IgG, IgA, and IgM antibodies against the NMDA receptor. Neurology. 2018;90(16):e1386–94.

20

Biaryl scaffold-focused virtual screening for anti-aggregatory and neuroprotective effects in Alzheimer's disease

Sidra Khalid[1], Muhammad Ammar Zahid[1,3], Hussain Ali[1], Yeong S. Kim[2] and Salman Khan[1]* (iD)

Abstract

Background: Alzheimer's disease (AD) is a primary cause of dementia in ageing population affecting more than 35 million people around the globe. It is a chronic neurodegenerative disease caused by defected folding and aggregation of amyloid beta (Aβ) protein. Aβ is formed by the cleavage of membrane embedded amyloid precursor protein (APP) by using enzyme 'transmembrane aspartyl protease, β-secretase'. Inhibition of β-secretase is a viable strategy to prevent neurotoxicity in AD. Another strategy in the treatment of AD is inhibition of acetylcholinesterase. This inhibition reduces the degradation of acetylcholine and temporarily restores the cholinergic function of neurons and improves cognitive function. Monoamine oxidase and higher glutamate levels are also found to be linked with Aβ peptide related oxidative stress. Oxidative stress leads to reduced activity of glutamate synthase resulting in significantly higher level of glutamate in brain. The aim of this study is to perform in silico screening of a virtual library of biaryl scaffold containing compounds potentially used for the treatment of AD. Screening was done against the primary targets of AD therapeutics, acetylcholinesterase, β-secretase (BACE1), Monoamine oxidases (MAO) and N-Methyl-D-aspartate (NMDA) receptor. Compounds were screened for their inhibitory potential by employing molecular docking approach using AutoDock vina. Binding energy scores were embodied in the heatmap to display varies strengths of interactions of the ligands targeting AD.

Results: Several ligands showed notable interaction with at least two targets, but the strong interaction with all the targets is shown by very few ligands. The pharmacokinetics of the interacting ligands was also predicted. The interacting ligands have good drug-likeness and brain availability essential for drugs with intracranial targets.

Conclusion: These results suggest that biaryl scaffold may be pliable to drug development for neuroprotection in AD and that the synthesis of further analogues to optimize these properties should be considered.

Keywords: Computational analysis, Alzheimer, Biaryl scaffold, Neuroprotection

Background

Alzheimer disease (AD) is the primary cause of dementia worldwide. Currently, more than 35 million people are suffering from this disease around the globe. By the year 2050, the diseases burden is excepted to raise four times i.e. almost 1 out of 85 persons will be suffering from AD [1]. The major pathological hallmarks of AD include widespread neuronal and synaptic loss, excessive presence of astrocytes, and aggregation of multiple proteinaceous deposits for instance β-amyloid plaques and neurofibrillary tangles (NFT) [2]. The number of hypotheses are proposed along the years to describe the root cause of AD such as the production of β-amyloid, cholinergic hypothesis, excitotoxicity and oxidative stress hypothesis [3] as summarized in Fig. 1. Senile plaques are the main and distinguished neurological feature of the AD directly related to its onset and progression [4]. The production of amyloid beta (Aβ) takes place by the proteolytic cleavage of beta-secretase protein on amyloid

---
*Correspondence: skhan@qau.edu.pk
[1] Department of Pharmacy, Faculty of Biological Sciences, Quaid-i-Azam University, Islamabad 45320, Pakistan
Full list of author information is available at the end of the article

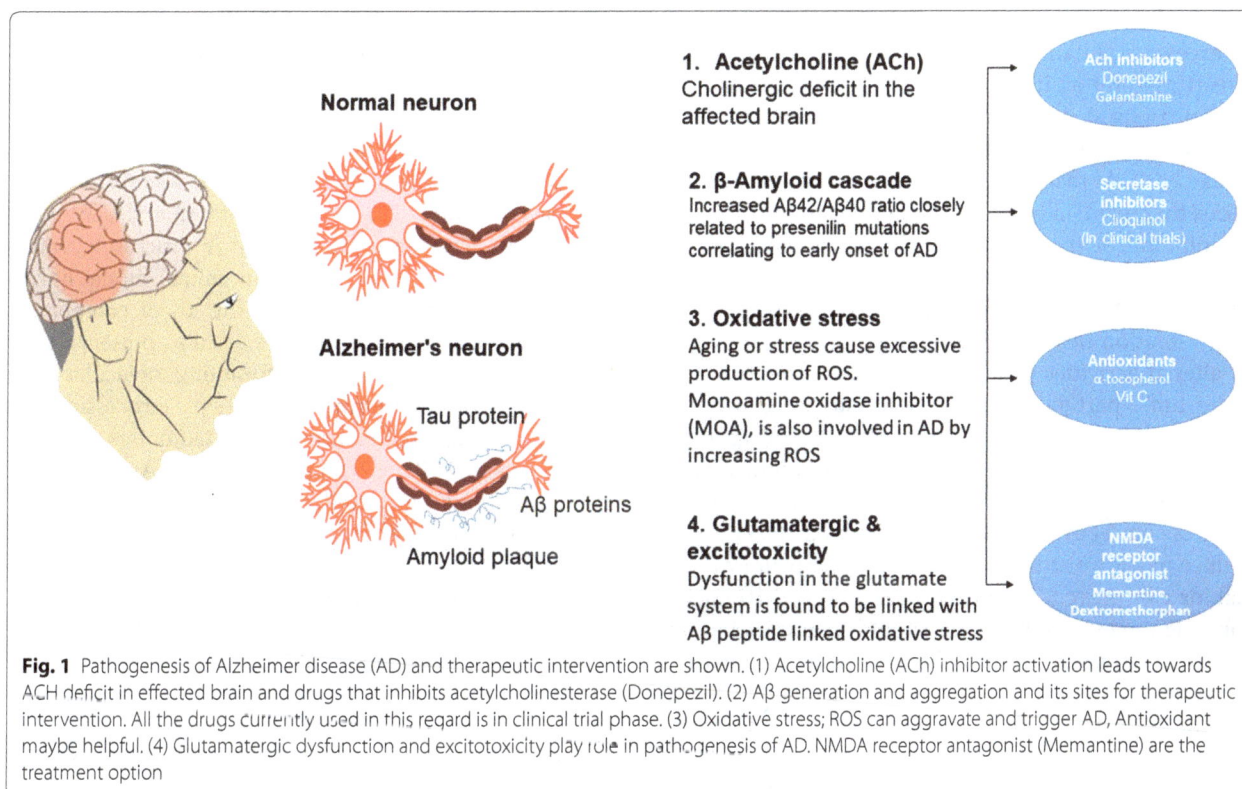

Fig. 1 Pathogenesis of Alzheimer disease (AD) and therapeutic intervention are shown. (1) Acetylcholine (ACh) inhibitor activation leads towards ACH deficit in effected brain and drugs that inhibits acetylcholinesterase (Donepezil). (2) Aβ generation and aggregation and its sites for therapeutic intervention. All the drugs currently used in this regard is in clinical trial phase. (3) Oxidative stress; ROS can aggravate and trigger AD, Antioxidant maybe helpful. (4) Glutamatergic dysfunction and excitotoxicity play role in pathogenesis of AD. NMDA receptor antagonist (Memantine) are the treatment option

precursor protein (APP) whereas in AD, a pathogenic mutations affects the protease cleavage sites in APP and aid its cleavage [5]. The Aβ are mainly divided into two isoforms, based upon the length of amino acids, Aβ of 40 amino acid residues (Aβ40) and Aβ of 42 amino acid residues (Aβ42) are the two isoforms. Although Aβ42 differ in only 2 amino acids, it is much more neurotoxic and aggregates faster as compared to Aβ40. In the cerebrospinal fluid (CSF) presence of Aβ42 is a well-known biomarker of AD, and is used both in AD research and increasingly in clinical practice [6]. The increased level of Aβ42 as compare to Aβ40 has been generally considered to play a critical role. The increased Aβ42/Aβ40 ratio is closely related to presenilin mutations correlating to early onset of AD [7]. Although Aβ40 is several-fold more abundant in the brain Aβ42 is the major and sometimes exclusive component in amyloid plaques, due to its more aggregation prone nature [7].

AD is also characterized by the cholinergic deficit in the affected brain. The acetylcholine-releasing neurons especially there cell bodies which lied in basal forebrain degrades selectively in AD affecting cognitive functions and memory as these neurons are vital in the normal functioning of cerebral cortex and related structures. In AD there is a modification and alteration in polymorphism of acetylcholinesterase (AChE) in brain [8]. An increased amount of AChE levels around the Aβ plaques and NFT is commonly reported feature of AD. The current therapy of AD is mainly based on the use of AChE (AChE-I) inhibitors. The effect of these AChE-I is modest and transient due to up-regulation of AChE activity following chronic AChE-I therapy [9].

Another mechanism by which AD can develop is by excessive presence of the reactive oxygen species (ROS) in the mitochondria. This rise in ROS is due to aging or stress and if the antioxidant system of the body fails to cope with this condition AD may develop. The role of oxidative stress in AD is evident from the fact that brain of these patients shows a substantial oxidative damage [10]. Monoamine oxidase (MOA), is also involved in AD by increasing ROS in brain. MAO and its isoenzymes i.e. MAO-A and MAO-B are liable for the catalysis of biogenic amines, like serotonin, dopamine and norepinephrine so its inhibition results in an augmented level of neurotransmitters in the CNS [11].

Similarly, the key excitatory neurotransmitter glutamate which is involved in synaptic plasticity and learning, is also linked to AD. Dysfunction in the glutamate system is found to be linked with Aβ peptide linked oxidative stress. Oxidative stress leads to reduced activity of glutamate synthase resulting in significantly higher level of glutamate in brain [12]. The over-activation of

N-methyl-D-aspartate receptor (NMDA) receptor due to excessive glutamate leads to the continuous calcium ions (Ca^2+) influx into the nerve cells, generating a slow excitotoxicity at post synaptic level ultimately leading to a gradual neurodegenerative effect in AD patients [13]. Thus, NMDA receptor antagonists could be advantageous therapeutically in the management of AD.

Inhibition of these targets individually with currently approved or developing drugs has been proved relatively unsuccessful at reversing the progression of AD. A likely solution lies in a multi-pharmacological approach to altered activities of numerous of these targets at the same time, particularly those associated with the progression of the disease. Such multiple target drugs developed for AD have targeted two or more of known targets (cholinesterases, BACE1, MAO, NMDA) or have disease progression retarding properties, such as metal chelation, reduce oxidative stress or have anti-inflammatory potential, or can prevent Aβ or tau aggregation [14]. Ligands for drug targets combinations should be assessed against disease progression to define best possible combinations.

Molecular docking; a computational technique, is used for the estimation of the binding affinity between two molecules like the protein–protein and ligands-protein [15]. Virtual screening or computer-aided drug design (CADD) combined with wet lab techniques contributes towards the development of new drug molecules [16]. CADD is particularly useful especially in three major areas: (1) selection of most suitable compounds from large libraries of possibly actives compounds (2) Addition of an appropriate functional groups in the lead compounds for making it more suitable for new drug development (3) By adding pharmacophore features, designing the new molecules from a target structure. In light of current study the interactions of selected compounds with the various targets of AD was determined, using docking and in silico absorption, distribution metabolism and excretion (ADME) pharmacokinetics studies [15].

Methods
Preparation of protein targets
The target proteins i.e. AChE (4EY7) [17], BACE-1 (2HM1) [18], MAO-A (2Z5X) [19] and NMDA (1PBQ) [20] were selected. These X-ray crystallographic structures were downloaded from protein data bank (PDB). Preparation of all the protein structure was done in Chimera by using 'Dockprep' workflow [21]. The preparation includes addition of hydrogen to the protein, assignment of bond orders, and unnecessary associated molecules deletion. Addition of side chains was done, partial charges were assigned, disulphide bonds were made and missing atoms were added. Optimized Potentials for

Liquid Simulations (OPLS_2005) force field was used for energy minimization. The active sites of the proteins were determined by the co-crystallized ligands.

Ligand dataset preparation
The zinc database (zinc15.docking.com) was searched for the biaryl scaffold. The hits were filtered and only those compounds were selected for further processing which was ever tested in vivo (neither in animal model nor in man) and available for free sale. The ids of compounds along with their binding affinities are also present in the attached file (Additional file 1). Resulting molecules were downloaded in mol2 format. Ligand's pre-processing was done, using Ligprep, the formation of tautomers and ionization states (pH 7.0 ± 2.0) using Epik [22]. An addition of hydrogen atoms was also done, neutralization of charged groups and geometry of the ligands were also optimized.

Virtual screening: binding mode analysis
Computational analysis was performed by firstly downloading mol2 structures of the ligands from ZINC database and then converted to PDBQT formats after assigning Gastegier charges and merging non-polar hydrogens by using AutoDock Tools 1.5.4. PyRX software was used for virtual screening. Both Autodock and Auto-Dock Vina are included in the PyRX [24]. The binding site for docking analysis was determined by the position of the co-crystallized ligand. The grid box was centered on the experimentally docked ligands with the dimension given in Table 1. Docking was performed using Auto-Dock Vina (version 1.1.2) by considering all the bonds in the ligands as rotatable and the proteins as the rigid structures. Rest of the parameters were kept as default and docking scores were calculated by the default scoring

Table 1 Grid box centre and dimension for docking of the ligands against target protein

Protein	Grid box centre	Grid box dimensions
4EY7	X: − 2.91	X:59.75
	Y: − 40.11	Y:61.25
	Z: 30.86	Z:72.51
2HM1	X: 16.08	X:57.15
	Y: − 0.07	Y:68.97
	Z: 10.02	Z:48.99
1PBQ	X: 2.535	X:55.36
	Y: 39.35	Y:49.88
	Z: − 17.65	Z:48.12
2Z5X	X: 34.6965	X:88.4415
	Y: 28.131	Y:75.9847
	Z: − 20.0943	Z:62.8238

Where: acetylcholinesterase (4EY7), beta-secretase cleavage enzyme (2HM1), monoamine oxidase (2Z5X) and *N*-methyl-D-aspartate receptor receptor (1PBQ) function [23]. The best binding modes of the ligands were exported as mol2 files and the interaction of the best binding modes with the protein target were investigated by using discovery studio visualizer. Ligands with best binding scores were redocked using the glide/SP docking algorithm in Maestro https://pubs.acs.org/doi/10.1021/jm0306430. The binding poses generated by glide were matched with the best binding poses from AutoDock Vina using an RMSD cutoff of Å. All RMSD values were calculated using the python script "rmsd.py". Data warrior was used for data handling and visualization [25]. To find out compounds with multi-target binding efficiency, the heatmap was generated using chemmines numerical clustering tool based on binding scores [26].

Pharmacokinetic parameters

The calculation of the physiochemical properties of the drugs is done by SwissADME. Physiochemical properties like, octanol/water partition coefficient (XPlogPo/w), compound's molecular weight (MW), the number of hydrogen bond acceptors (accptHB), hydrogen bond donors (donorHB), and percentage human oral absorption, blood brain penetration was predicted. Violations of Lipinski's rule of five by any drug was also analyzed. Based on these molecular descriptors, the intestinal absorption and blood–brain barrier penetration were represented by using a BOILED-egg model [27].

Result

The key focus of the current study is to identify new compounds containing biaryl scaffold for the treatment of AD. Around, 107 compounds were screened using in silico molecular docking technique by AutoDock Vina. Out of the screened compounds, ZINC000003872600, ZINC000002010548, ZINC000000390492 and ZINC000043014847 interacted significantly with chosen protein targets of AD in the chosen active sites. The docking score was obtained in the range of − 10.8 to − 6.4 for AChE (4EY7), − 8.7 to − 6.1 in BACE 1 (2HM1), − 10.5 to − 6.3 in MAO-A (2Z5X), and − 8.7 to − 6.2 with NMDA (1PBQ). Among these compounds, against each target the best hit was selected on the basis of docking score and binding energy. The best binding ligands were redocked using glide and the docking scores of the comparable binding poses were determined. Comparison between target protein with potent known drugs/inhibitors in the crystal structures for binding modes and the molecular interactions was done. The binding energies of both hydrophilic as well as hydrophobic interacting residues and their bond length of the best predicted mode with each protein target residue are shown in Table 2. The heatmaps based on binding scores are presented in Fig. 2.

Validation of docking

The co-crystallized ligands were extracted from the PDB files of target proteins. Theses extracted ligands were re-docked into the proteins by using same parameters and workflow to validate the reliability and reproducibility of the docking results. The RMSD values of the docked ligand and the co-crystallized ligand was calculated by using all atoms in discovery studio visualizer v17.2. The docked ligand and the co-crystallized structures almost superimpose (Fig. 3) each other and RMSD values ranges from 0.0184 to 0.0992 Å. These results indicate that the docking experiment has produced correct docking poses thus validating the results.

Molecular interaction of ZINC000000593414 with acetylcholinesterase (4EY7)

Against AChE, the lowest binding energy was observed with ZINC000000593414 with binding energy of−10.8 which is comparable with known inhibitor donepezil whosebinding energy was − 11.9. ZINC000000593414 forms hydrogen bonding with Tyr124, Ser125 and Trp286 (PAS residue); pi–pi stacking with Ser293 and Trp341 (PAS residue). Pi-sigma interactions were observed with Trp86 (quaternary ammonium binding locus) and Phe338 (Fig. 4). When redocked with glide, the binding score of the best binding pose was found to be − 8.547.

Molecular interaction of ZINC000002010548 with β-secretase cleavage enzyme (2HM1)

The BACE-1 ligand interaction largely depends on the conformation of the active site residues, which consisted of the catalytic dyad (Asp32 and Asp 228), composition of the 10 s loop consist of residues from 9 to 14, flap consisting of 67–77 amino acid and all other residues within 8 Å from aspartates. With BACE-1, ZINC000002010548 exhibited lowest binding energy of−8.7. Hydrogen bonding was formed with Thr329, Thr72, Thr231, Arg235 and Ser327. Salt bridge with Asp32 (catalytic residue) was observed at Phe108 (Fig. 5). When redocked using glide, the docking score was − 5.443.

Molecular interaction of ZINC000000390492 with monoamine oxidase (2Z5X)

The results of MAO-A docking showed the least docking score at − 10.5 with ZINC000000390492. Docking results showed hydrogen bonding with Tyr69, Pi–Pi stack with Phe352 and Tyr407 and Pi-alkyl interactions with Ile335 (Fig. 6). When redocked by using glide, the docking score was found to be − 10.498.

Table 2 The structures generated through ChemDraw and binding scores of the best predicted compounds along with their Zinc-ID against each protein target

Zinc_ID	Structure	Binding score			
		4EY7	2HM1	2Z5X	1PBQ
Control		−11.9	−9.1	−7.5	−8.7
ZINC000043014847		−10.3	−8.4	−8.3	−8.6
ZINC000002010548		−10.3	−8.7	−10.1	−8.3
ZINC000000593414		−10.8	−7.3	−8.2	−8
ZINC000000390492		−10.1	−7.9	−10.5	−7.9

Where: acetylcholinesterase (4EY7), beta-secretase cleavage enzyme (2HM1), monoamine oxidase (2Z5X) and *N*-methyl-D-aspartate receptor receptor (1PBQ) (Structures are drawn fromChemDraw)

Molecular interaction of ZINC000043014847 with *N*-methyl-D-aspartate receptor receptor (1PBQ)

ZINC000043014847 showed the best docking score of—8.6 whereas DCKA showed a docking score of −8.7. Hydrogen bonding was observed between the ligand and Gly93, Thr94, Asn107, Arg131 whereas pi–pi stacking was observed with Phe92 of 1PBQ (Fig. 7). When redocked by using glide, the docking score was found to be −6.233.

Prediction of pharmacokinetic properties

In regards to prediction of pharmacokinetic properties, none of the compounds in current study demonstrate violation of the Lipinski's rule of five. The percentage of oral absorption of drug in human was calculated on the scale of 0–100% to predict the oral absorption of the drug. Absorption of more than 80% was considered as good absorption whereas any compound having less than 25% absorption is poor. According to this principle; all the drugs when given via oral route have medium to high absorption. Brain availability by crossing the blood brain barrier was also found to be from medium to high

as represented by boiled egg model (Fig. 8). This model gives a nice and simple graphical representation of intestinal absorption and brain penetration of the ligands as a function of lipophilic nature (WLOGP) and polarity of the molecules (TPSA).

Discussion

Molecular docking is an important technique. It is actually not a standalone technique but works best if treated as a supplementary technique along with other in silico methods as well as in vitro and in vivo experiments [28]. While there is a dire need for new pharmaceutical research in this field, in silico drug analysis is an effective and promising tool for discovering therapeutic utility of both new and already existing drugs [29]. There are number of examples of repurposed drugs which were discovered by the in silico approach and are now being used in many diseases [23] including AD [30].

The main focus of the present study is to signify importance of docking analysis and identify compounds containing biaryl scaffold for the management of AD. About, 107 compounds were screened using docking. Among screened compounds significantly interacting

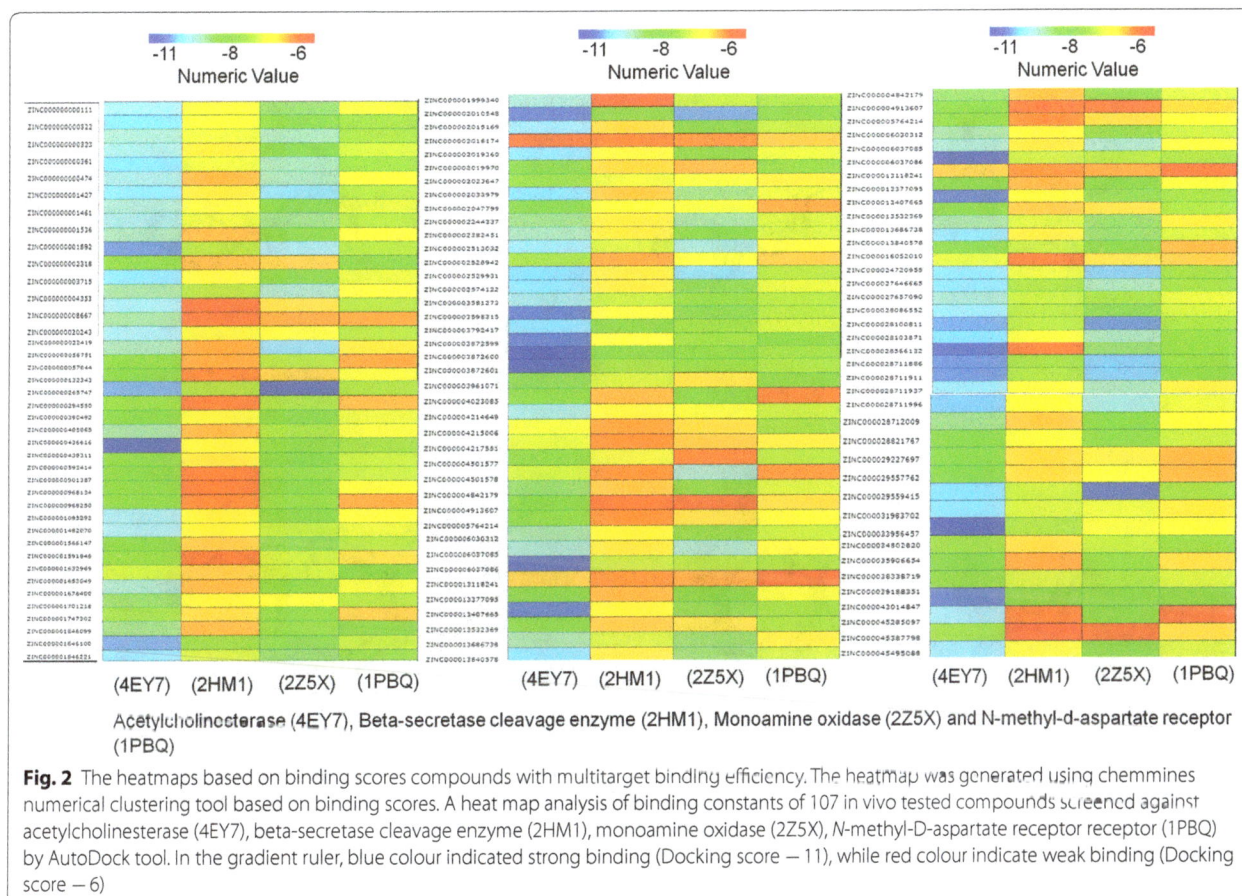

Fig. 2 The heatmaps based on binding scores compounds with multitarget binding efficiency. The heatmap was generated using chemmines numerical clustering tool based on binding scores. A heat map analysis of binding constants of 107 in vivo tested compounds screened against acetylcholinesterase (4EY7), beta-secretase cleavage enzyme (2HM1), monoamine oxidase (2Z5X), N-methyl-D-aspartate receptor receptor (1PBQ) by AutoDock tool. In the gradient ruler, blue colour indicated strong binding (Docking score — 11), while red colour indicate weak binding (Docking score — 6)

compounds with selected protein targets of AD were identified.

Some previous studies showed the possible potential of marketed antipsychotic drugs against various targets associated with AD by using docking approach [23]. Previously conventional structure-based docking method for the identification of drug molecules for BACE were largely futile [31]. By using in silico computer-aided drug design approaches, the activity of biaryl compounds against AD targets BACE1 and BACE2 was also determined and interestingly it was found that the fused-ring compounds are in general more active than the biaryl-based ligands [32].

In present study 4 targets of AD were chosen. The results of docking were firstly validated. As a general rule, the success of the docking scoring function is validated if the conformation of the bound ligand in the crystal structure resembles the conformation of the docked ligand [33].

One of the selected targets was AChe. An enzyme Ache catalyzes the metabolism of acetylcholine and some other choline esters neurotransmitters. Number of well-known drugs interact with acetylcholinesterase [34]. The human AChE's active site is 20 Å deep. The active site comprises of catalytic site of AChE (Glu334,Ser 203 and His447), acyl-binding pocket (Phe297and Phe295), oxyanion hole (Ala204, Gly120 and Gly121), quaternary ammonium binding locus (Trp86) and finally, PAS (Tyr341, Trp286, Tyr124, Tyr72 and Asp74), which groups at the active site gorge's entry [35].

Similarly, monoamine oxidase (MAO) an enzyme majorly involves in the oxidation of numerous vital monoamine hormones and neurotransmitters such as adrenaline, noradrenaline, dopamine, and serotonin [36]. There is a hydrophobic cavity in MAO-A which has a volume of ~400 Å. The structure of MAO-A consist of one larger cavity or a bipartite cavity depending upon the conformation of Phe208, but in this case it fails to work as gating residue. The MAO-A has conserved active site residues which comprise of a pair of Tyr of the "aromatic sandwich" and a Lys-hydrogen bonded to the N(5) position of the Flavin i.e. Lys305 in enzyme [37]. There are additional non-conserved active site residues primarily Ile180 and Asn181in MAO-A. The Phe208–Ile335 in MAO-A is the main factor in controlling the differential inhibitor and substrate specificities of these enzymes

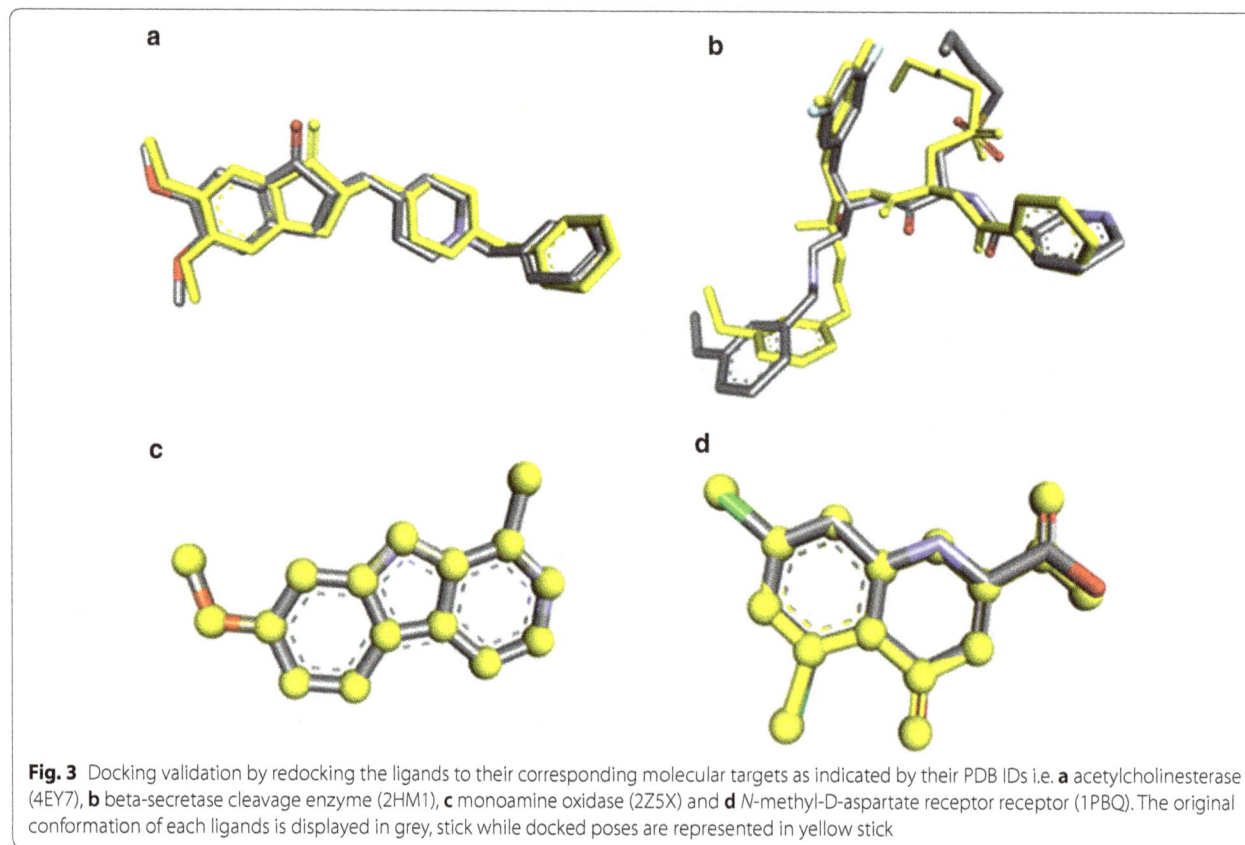

Fig. 3 Docking validation by redocking the ligands to their corresponding molecular targets as indicated by their PDB IDs i.e. **a** acetylcholinesterase (4EY7), **b** beta-secretase cleavage enzyme (2HM1), **c** monoamine oxidase (2Z5X) and **d** *N*-methyl-D-aspartate receptor receptor (1PBQ). The original conformation of each ligands is displayed in grey, stick while docked poses are represented in yellow stick

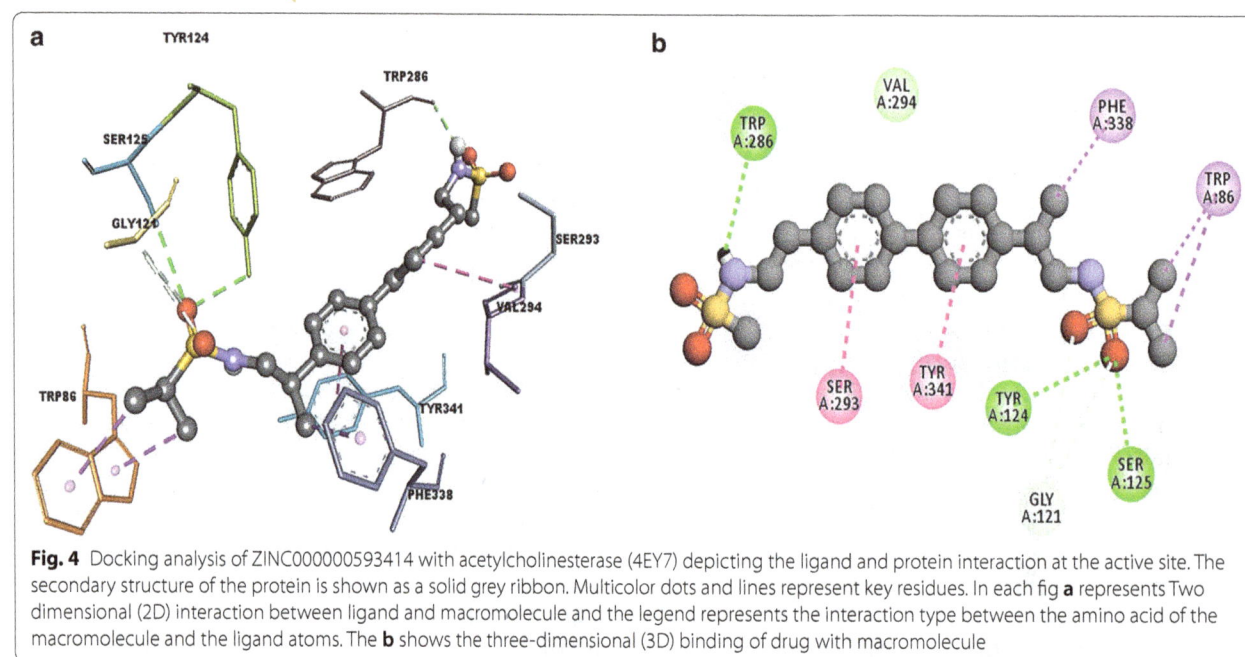

Fig. 4 Docking analysis of ZINC000000593414 with acetylcholinesterase (4EY7) depicting the ligand and protein interaction at the active site. The secondary structure of the protein is shown as a solid grey ribbon. Multicolor dots and lines represent key residues. In each fig **a** represents Two dimensional (2D) interaction between ligand and macromolecule and the legend represents the interaction type between the amino acid of the macromolecule and the ligand atoms. The **b** shows the three-dimensional (3D) binding of drug with macromolecule

[38]. In MAO-A, the least docking score was − 10.5 with ZINC000000390492 and in the case of known inhibitor, Hermine, the docking score was − 7.5.

The inhibition of BACE1 through the development of selective and potent inhibitors has been in a limelight in the quest for treatment of AD. BACE an enzyme playing vital role in the proteolytic cleavage of APP is an

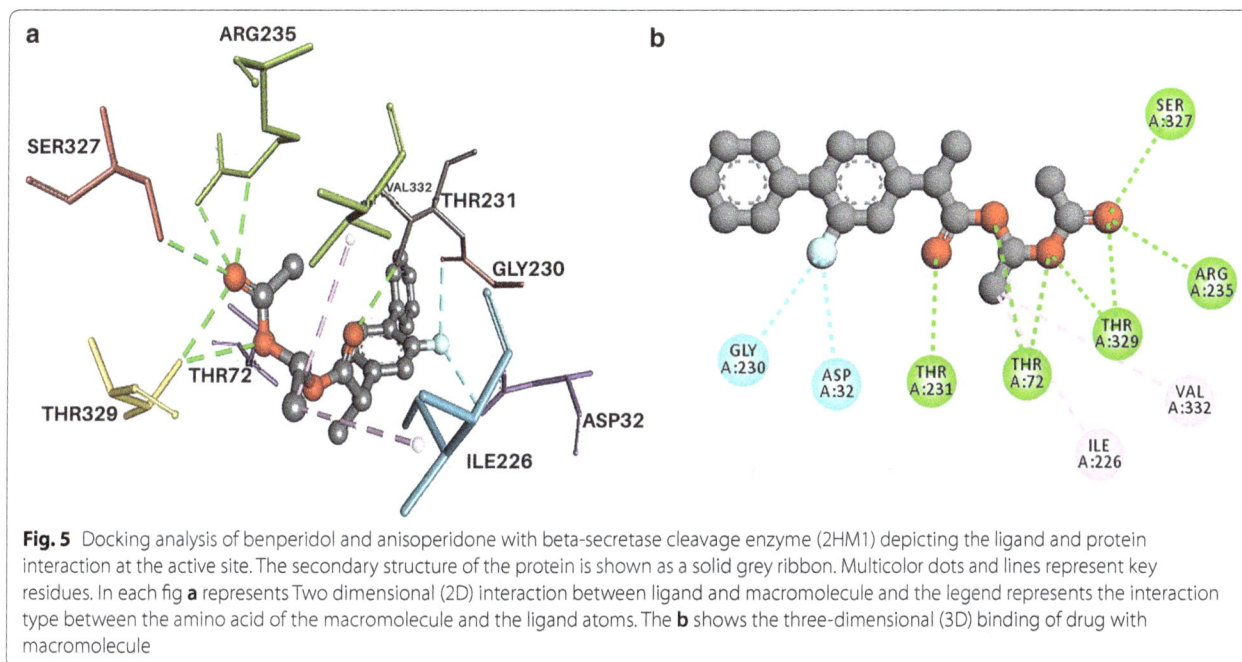

Fig. 5 Docking analysis of benperidol and anisoperidone with beta-secretase cleavage enzyme (2HM1) depicting the ligand and protein interaction at the active site. The secondary structure of the protein is shown as a solid grey ribbon. Multicolor dots and lines represent key residues. In each fig **a** represents Two dimensional (2D) interaction between ligand and macromolecule and the legend represents the interaction type between the amino acid of the macromolecule and the ligand atoms. The **b** shows the three-dimensional (3D) binding of drug with macromolecule

important target of AD management [39]. The BACE-1

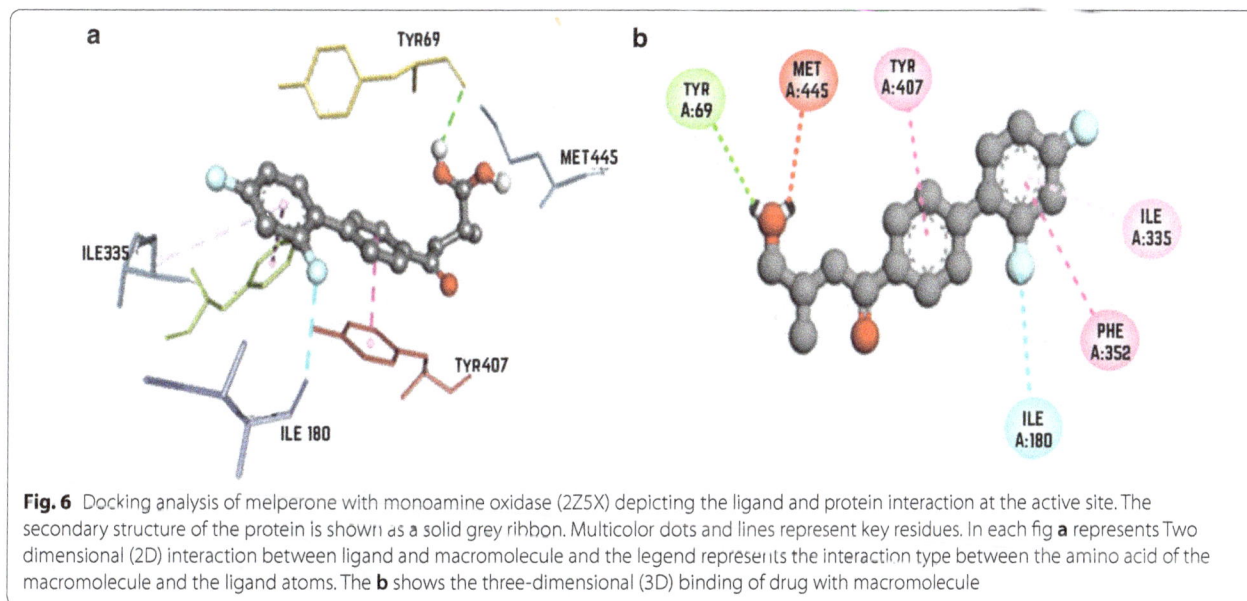

Fig. 6 Docking analysis of melperone with monoamine oxidase (2Z5X) depicting the ligand and protein interaction at the active site. The secondary structure of the protein is shown as a solid grey ribbon. Multicolor dots and lines represent key residues. In each fig **a** represents Two dimensional (2D) interaction between ligand and macromolecule and the legend represents the interaction type between the amino acid of the macromolecule and the ligand atoms. The **b** shows the three-dimensional (3D) binding of drug with macromolecule

ligand ZINC000002010548 exhibited highest docking score of—8.7 and known inhibitor LY2886721 had docking score of − 9.1 in the previous study [40]

Another target, for protein 1PBQ an ion channel protein and glutamate receptor found in nerve cells, has vital interacting residues with 5,7-Dichlorokynurenic acid (DCKA); a selective NMDA antagonist. DCKA:

The co-crystallized ligand interacts with Pro124, Ser180, Arg131 and Thr126. 1PBQ's hydrophobic pocket has following amino acid residues: Phe92, Phe16, Phe250 and Trp223 [41].

Pharmacokinetic properties of drugs is a significant parameter in drug selection and to determine its utility as a clinically beneficial agent. Docking models have been simulated as a useful alternative to wet lab research

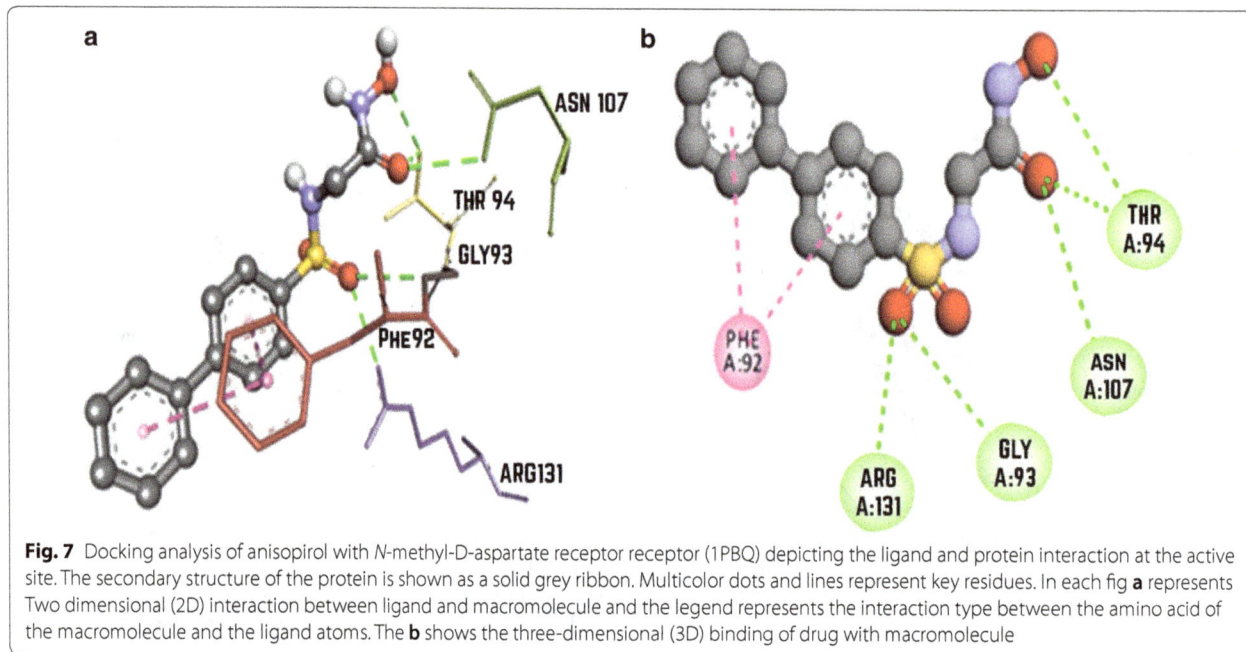

Fig. 7 Docking analysis of anisopirol with *N*-methyl-D-aspartate receptor receptor (1PBQ) depicting the ligand and protein interaction at the active site. The secondary structure of the protein is shown as a solid grey ribbon. Multicolor dots and lines represent key residues. In each fig **a** represents Two dimensional (2D) interaction between ligand and macromolecule and the legend represents the interaction type between the amino acid of the macromolecule and the ligand atoms. The **b** shows the three-dimensional (3D) binding of drug with macromolecule

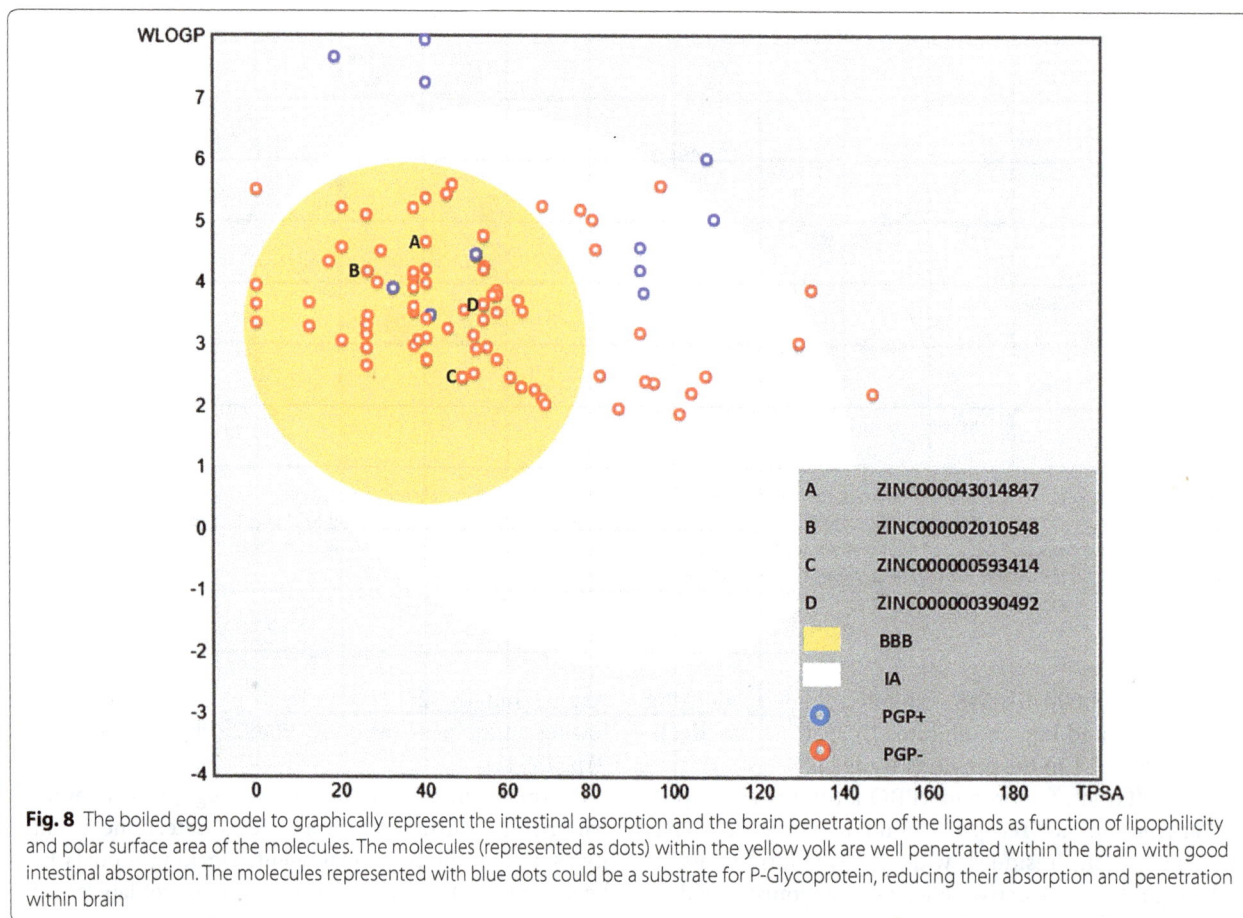

Fig. 8 The boiled egg model to graphically represent the intestinal absorption and the brain penetration of the ligands as function of lipophilicity and polar surface area of the molecules. The molecules (represented as dots) within the yellow yolk are well penetrated within the brain with good intestinal absorption. The molecules represented with blue dots could be a substrate for P-Glycoprotein, reducing their absorption and penetration within brain

procedures especially at initial stages were chemical structures are numerous but resources are scarce [42]. Hence, in present study the physio-chemical factors were determine to assess the ADME properties of the drugs. Lipinski's rule of five required that the drug must have molecular weight of 500 Da or less, donorHB ≤ 5, accptHB ≤ 10 and octanol–water partition coefficient log P < 5. If drug follow these rules then it's considered as an orally active drug. The molecules which fails to follow more than one of above stated rules may face difficulty with bioavailability. In current study none of the compounds is violating Lipinski rule of 5. Therefore, in silico computational analysis has been able to identify some encouraging compounds which may prove to be useful in the management of AD. Further research is needed in this regard.

Conclusion

AD is a complex disease involving many different pathways and drug targets, for instance, AChE, BACE-1, MAO-A and NMDA. In addition to these targets, anti-inflammatory and antioxidant drugs are also proved to be beneficial. Several molecules belonging to different chemical classes have already been developed against these individual targets to relieve the symptoms of this ailment but a multi-target approach is required. In this context the present study explored the potential of biaryl scaffold to inhibit these multiple targets. Of all the compounds screened, biaryl sulphonamides were found to be the top candidate for the cholinergic (AChE), beta-secretase cleavage enzyme (BACE-1), monoaminergic (MAO-A) and glutamatergic system (NMDA). Further analogues can also be computationally designed and tested against these druggable targets. Hence, virtual screening can successfully identify auspicious compounds which might be worthwhile therapeutically in AD.

Abbreviations
ADME: absorption, distribution, metabolism, and excretion; AcceltHB: number of hydrogen bond acceptors; 4EY7: acetylcholinesterase; AChE: acetylcholinesterase; Ala: alanine; AD: Alzheimer's disease; Aβ: amyloid beta; APP: amyloid precursor protein; Arg: arginine; Asn: asparagine; Asp: aspartic acid; Aβ40: Aβ of 40 amino acid residues; BACE1: beta-secretase-1; 2HM1: beta-secretase cleavage enzyme; CSF: cerebrospinal fluid; CADD: computer-aided drug design; Cys: cysteine; DCKA: 5,7-Dichlorokynurenic acid; DonorHB: number of hydrogen bond donors; Glu: glutamic acid; Gln: glutamine; Gly: glycine; His: histidine; Ile: isoleucine; Leu: leucin; Lys: lysine; Met: methionine; 2Z5X: monoamine oxidase; 1PBQ: N-methyl-D-aspartate receptor; MAO: monoamine oxidases; MW: molecular weight; NFT: neurofibrillary tangles; NMDA: N-methyl-D-aspartate receptor; Phe: phenylalanine; Pro: proline; PDB: Protein Data Bank; QPlogPo/w: predicted octanol/water partition coefficient; ROS: reactive oxygen species; Ser: serine; Thr: threonine; Trp: tryptophan; Tyr: tyrosine; Val: valine.

Authors' contributions
S. K and M.A Z performed the analyses of the results. S.K* and YSK conceived and designed the project. H Ali made substantial contribution in analysis and writing of manuscript. We further confirm that the order of authors listed in the manuscript has been approved by all of us. All authors wrote the manuscript. All authors reviewed the manuscript. All authors read and approved the final manuscript.

Author details
[1] Department of Pharmacy, Faculty of Biological Sciences, Quaid-i-Azam University, Islamabad 45320, Pakistan. [2] Natural Products Research Institute, College of Pharmacy, Seoul National University, Seoul, South Korea. [3] Department of Biotechnology, Faculty of Biological Sciences, Quaid-i-Azam University, Islamabad, Pakistan.

Acknowledgements
This work was supported by the Higher Education Commission (HEC), Pakistan under the SRGP funding (No. 357 SRGP/HEC/2014). The authors are grateful to the National Research Foundation of Korea (NRF), Seoul National University, grant funded by the Korean Government (MSIP) (No. 2009-0083533).

Competing interests
The authors declare that they have no competing interests.

Funding
The project was funded by Quaid-i-Azam University Islamabad under Faculty Research Grant scheme.

References
1. Brookmeyer R, Johnson E, Ziegler-Graham K, Arrighi HM. Forecasting the global burden of Alzheimer's disease. Alzheimers Dement. 2007;3:186–91.
2. Murphy MP, LeVine H. Alzheimer's disease and the amyloid-β peptide. J Alzheimers Dis. 2010;19:311–23.
3. Kumar S, Chowdhury S, Kumar S. In silico repurposing of antipsychotic drugs for Alzheimer's disease. BMC Neurosci. 2017. https://doi.org/10.1186/s12868-017-0394-8.
4. Basile L. Virtual screening in the search of new and potent anti-alzheimer agents. In: Roy K, editor. Computational modeling of drugs against Alzheimer's disease. New York, NY: Springer New York; 2018. p. 107–37. http://link.springer.com/10.1007/978-1-4939-7404-7_4. Accessed 25 Aug 2018.
5. Kalaria RN, Galloway PG, Perry G. Widespread serum amyloid P immunoreactivity in cortical amyloid deposits and the neurofibrillary pathology of Alzheimer's disease and other degenerative disorders. Neuropathol Appl Neurobiol. 1991;17:189–201.
6. Janelidze S, Zetterberg H, Mattsson N, Palmqvist S, Vanderstichele H, Lindberg O, et al. CSF Ab42/Ab40 and Ab42/Ab38 ratios: better diagnostic markers of Alzheimer disease. Ann Clin Transl Neurol. 2016;3:154–65.
7. Gu L, Guo Z. Alzheimer's Aβ42 and Aβ40 peptides form interlaced amyloid fibrils. J Neurochem. 2013;126:305–11.
8. Coyle JT, Price DL, DeLong MR. Alzheimer's disease: a disorder of cortical cholinergic innervation. Am Assoc Adv Sci. 1983;219:1184–90.
9. García-Ayllón M-S. Revisiting the role of acetylcholinesterase in Alzheimer's disease: cross-talk with P-tau and β-amyloid. Front Mol Neurosci. 2011. https://doi.org/10.3389/fnmol.2011.00022.
10. Huang WJ, Zhang X, Chen WW. Role of oxidative stress in Alzheimer's disease. Biomed Res Int. 2016;4:519–22.
11. Son SY, Tsukihara T, Ma J, Kondou Y, Yoshimura M, Yamashita E. Structure

of human monoamine oxidase A at 2.2-Å resolution: the control of opening the entry for substrates/inhibitors. Proc Natl Acad. 2008;105:5739–44.

12. Butterfield DA, Pocernich CB. The glutamatergic system and Alzheimer's disease: therapeutic implications. CNS Drugs. 2003;17:641–52.

13. Parsons CG, Danysz W, Dekundy A, Pulte I. Memantine and cholinesterase inhibitors: complementary mechanisms in the treatment of Alzheimer's disease. Neurotox Res. 2013;24:358–69.

14. Zhang Y, Li P, Feng J, Wu M. Dysfunction of NMDA receptors in Alzheimer's disease. Neurol Sci. 2016;37:1039–47.

15. Goodsell DS, Morris GM, Olson AJ. Automated docking of flexible ligands: applications of AutoDock. J Mol Recognit. 1996;9:1–5.

16. Baig MH, Ahmad K, Roy S, Ashraf JM, Adil M, Siddiqui MH, et al. Computer aided drug design: success and limitations. Curr Pharm Des. 2016;22:572–81.

17. Cheung J, Rudolph MJ, Burshteyn F, Cassidy MS, Gary EN, Love J, et al. Structures of human acetylcholinesterase in complex with pharmacologically important ligands. J Med Chem. 2012;55:10282–6.

18. Mirsafian H, Mat Ripen A, Merican AF, Bin Mohamad S. Amino acid sequence and structural comparison of BACE1 and BACE2 using evolutionary trace method. Sci World J. 2014;2014:482463.

19. De Colibus L, Li M, Binda C, Lustig A, Edmondson DE, Mattevi A. Three-dimensional structure of human monoamine oxidase A (MAO A): relation to the structures of rat MAO A and human MAO B. Proc Natl Acad Sci U S A. 2005;102:12684–9.

20. Hedegaard M, Hansen KB, Andersen KT, Bräuner-Osborne H, Traynelis SF. Molecular pharmacology of human NMDA receptors. Neurochem Int. 2012;61:601–9.

21. Pettersen EF, Goddard TD, Huang CC, Couch GS, Greenblatt DM, Meng EC, et al. UCSF Chimera–a visualization system for exploratory research and analysis. J Comput Chem. 2004;25:1605–12.

22. Shelley JC, Cholleti A, Frye LL, Greenwood JR, Timlin MR, Uchimaya M. Epik: a software program for pK(a) prediction and protonation state generation for drug-like molecules. J Comput Aided Mol Des. 2007;21:681–91.

23. Kumar A, Bora U. In silico inhibition studies of NF-κB p50 subunit by curcumin and its natural derivatives. Med Chem Res. 2012;21:3281–7.

24. Dallakyan S, Olson AJ. Small-molecule library screening by docking with PyRx. Methods Mol Biol Clifton NJ. 2015;1263:243–50.

25. Sander T, Freyss J, von Korff M, Rufener C. DataWarrior: an open-source program for chemistry aware data visualization and analysis. J Chem Inf Model. 2015;55:460–73.

26. Backman TWH, Cao Y, Girke T. ChemMine tools: an online service for analyzing and clustering small molecules. Nucleic Acids Res. 2011;39:W486–91.

27. Daina A, Michielin O, Zoete V. SwissADME: a free web tool to evaluate pharmacokinetics, drug-likeness and medicinal chemistry friendliness of small molecules. Sci Rep. 2017. https://doi.org/10.1038/srep42717.

28. Goodsell David S, Morris Garrett M, Olson Arthur J. Automated docking of flexible ligands: applications of AutoDock. J Mol Recognit. 1996;9:1–5.

29. Merk D, Grisoni F, Friedrich L, Gelzinyte E, Schneider G. Scaffold hopping from synthetic RXR modulators by virtual screening and *de novo* design. MedChemComm. 2018;9:1289–92.

30. Roy S, Kumar A, Baig MH, Masařík M, Provazník I. Virtual screening, ADMET profiling, molecular docking and dynamics approaches to search for potent selective natural molecules based inhibitors against metallothionein-III to study Alzheimer's disease. Methods San Diego Calif. 2015;83:105–10.

31. Manoharan P, Ghoshal N. Fragment-based virtual screening approach and molecular dynamics simulation studies for identification of BACE1 inhibitor leads. J Biomol Struct Dyn. 2018;36:1878–92.

32. Chirapu SR, Pachaiyappan B, Nural HF, Cheng X, Yuan H, Lankin DC, et al. Molecular modeling, synthesis, and activity studies of novel biaryl and fused-ring BACE1 inhibitors. Bioorg Med Chem Lett. 2009;19:264–74.

33. Hevener KE, Zhao W, Ball DM, Babaoglu K, Qi J, White SW, et al. Validation of molecular docking programs for virtual screening against dihydropteroate synthase. J Chem Inf Model. 2009;49:444–60.

34. Baig MH, Rizvi SMD, Shakil S, Kamal MA, Khan S. A neuroinformatics study describing molecular interaction of Cisplatin with acetylcholinesterase: a plausible cause for anticancer drug induced neurotoxicity. CNS Neurol Disord Drug Targets. 2014;13:265–70.

35. Johnson G, Moore SW. The peripheral anionic site of acetylcholinesterase: structure, functions and potential role in rational drug design. Curr Pharm Des. 2006;12:217–25.

36. Nagatsu T. Progress in monoamine oxidase (MAO) research in relation to genetic engineering. Neurotoxicology. 2004;25:11–20.

37. Geha RM, Chen K, Wouters J, Ooms F, Shih JC. Analysis of conserved active site residues in monoamine oxidase A and B and their three-dimensional molecular modeling. J Biol Chem. 2002;277:17209–16.

38. Edmondson DE, Binda C, Wang J, Upadhyay AK, Mattevi A. Molecular and mechanistic properties of the membrane-bound mitochondrial monoamine oxidases. Biochemistry (Mosc). 2009;48:4220–30.

39. John V. Human β-secretase (BACE) and BACE Inhibitors: progress Report. Curr Top Med Chem. 2006;6:569–78.

40. May PC, Willis BA, Lowe SL, Dean RA, Monk SA, Cocke PJ, et al. The potent BACE1 Inhibitor LY2886721 elicits robust central A pharmacodynamic responses in mice, dogs, and humans. J Neurosci. 2015;35:1199–210.

41. Furukawa H, Gouaux E. Mechanisms of activation, inhibition and specificity: crystal structures of the NMDA receptor NR1 ligand-binding core. EMBO J. 2003;22:2873–85.

42. Daina A, Michielin O, Zoete V. SwissADME: a free web tool to evaluate pharmacokinetics, drug-likeness and medicinal chemistry friendliness of small molecules. Sci Rep. 2017;7:42717.

Permissions

All chapters in this book were first published in NEUROSCIENCE, by BioMed Central; hereby published with permission under the Creative Commons Attribution License or equivalent. Every chapter published in this book has been scrutinized by our experts. Their significance has been extensively debated. The topics covered herein carry significant findings which will fuel the growth of the discipline. They may even be implemented as practical applications or may be referred to as a beginning point for another development.

The contributors of this book come from diverse backgrounds, making this book a truly international effort. This book will bring forth new frontiers with its revolutionizing research information and detailed analysis of the nascent developments around the world.

We would like to thank all the contributing authors for lending their expertise to make the book truly unique. They have played a crucial role in the development of this book. Without their invaluable contributions this book wouldn't have been possible. They have made vital efforts to compile up to date information on the varied aspects of this subject to make this book a valuable addition to the collection of many professionals and students.

This book was conceptualized with the vision of imparting up-to-date information and advanced data in this field. To ensure the same, a matchless editorial board was set up. Every individual on the board went through rigorous rounds of assessment to prove their worth. After which they invested a large part of their time researching and compiling the most relevant data for our readers.

The editorial board has been involved in producing this book since its inception. They have spent rigorous hours researching and exploring the diverse topics which have resulted in the successful publishing of this book. They have passed on their knowledge of decades through this book. To expedite this challenging task, the publisher supported the team at every step. A small team of assistant editors was also appointed to further simplify the editing procedure and attain best results for the readers.

Apart from the editorial board, the designing team has also invested a significant amount of their time in understanding the subject and creating the most relevant covers. They scrutinized every image to scout for the most suitable representation of the subject and create an appropriate cover for the book.

The publishing team has been an ardent support to the editorial, designing and production team. Their endless efforts to recruit the best for this project, has resulted in the accomplishment of this book. They are a veteran in the field of academics and their pool of knowledge is as vast as their experience in printing. Their expertise and guidance has proved useful at every step. Their uncompromising quality standards have made this book an exceptional effort. Their encouragement from time to time has been an inspiration for everyone.

The publisher and the editorial board hope that this book will prove to be a valuable piece of knowledge for researchers, students, practitioners and scholars across the globe.

List of Contributors

Monica J. Chau, Todd C. Deveau, Xiaohuan Gu and Yo Sup Kim
Department of Anesthesiology, Emory University School of Medicine, Atlanta, GA 30322, USA

Yun Xu
Department of Neurology, Nanjing University School of Medicine, Nanjing, China

Shan Ping Yu
Department of Anesthesiology, Emory University School of Medicine, Atlanta, GA 30322, USA
Center for Visual and Neurocognitive Rehabilitation, Veteran's Affair Medical Center, Atlanta, GA, USA

Ling Wei
Department of Anesthesiology, Emory University School of Medicine, Atlanta, GA 30322, USA
Department of Neurology, Emory University School of Medicine, Atlanta, GA 30322, USA
Woodruff Memorial Research Building, Suite 617, Emory University School of Medicine, 101 Woodruff Circle, Atlanta, GA 30322, USA

Vera Clemens, Francesca Regen, Nathalie Le Bret, Isabella Heuser and Julian Hellmann-Regen
Section Clinical Neurobiology, Department of Psychiatry and Psychotherapy, Campus Benjamin Franklin, Charité – University Medicine Berlin, Hindenburgdamm 30, 12203 Berlin, Germany

Katrin Giglhuber, Stefanie Maurer and Sandro M. Krieg
Department of Neurosurgery, Klinikum rechts der Isar, Technische Universität München, Ismaninger Str. 22, 81675 Munich, Germany
TUM-Neuroimaging Center, Klinikum rechts der Isar, Technische Universität München, Munich, Germany

Bernhard Meyer
Department of Neurosurgery, Klinikum rechts der Isar, Technische Universität München, Ismaninger Str. 22, 81675 Munich, Germany

Claus Zimmer
Section of Neuroradiology, Department of Radiology, Klinikum rechts der Isar, Technische Universität München, Ismaninger Str. 22, 81675 Munich, Germany

Saeedeh Asadi, Masoud Fereidoni, Elham Kordijaz and Ali Moghimi
Department of Biology, Rayan Center for Neuroscience and Behavior, Faculty of Science, Ferdowsi University of Mashhad, Mashhad, Iran

Ali Roohbakhsh
Pharmaceutical Research Center, Pharmaceutical Technology Institute, Mashhad University of Medical Sciences, Mashhad, Iran

Ali Shamsizadeh
Physiology-Pharmacology Research Center, Rafsanjan University of Medical Sciences, Rafsanjan, Iran

Leo Ai, Priya Bansal and Jerel K. Mueller
Division of Physical Therapy and Division of Rehabilitation Science, Department of Rehabilitation Medicine, Medical School, University of Minnesota, 426 Church St. SE Rm 361, Minneapolis, MN 55455, USA

Wynn Legon
Division of Physical Therapy and Division of Rehabilitation Science, Department of Rehabilitation Medicine, Medical School, University of Minnesota, 426 Church St. SE Rm 361, Minneapolis, MN 55455, USA
Department of Neurological Surgery, School of Medicine, University of Virginia, 409 Lane Rd. Rm 1031, Charlottesville, VA 22901, USA

Tammy R. Chaudoin and Stephen J. Bonasera
Division of Geriatrics, Department of Internal Medicine, University of Nebraska Medical Center, 3028 Durham Research Center II, Omaha, NE 68198-5039, USA

Ping Xie, Sa Zhou, Xingran Wang, Yibo Wang and Yi Yuan
Institute of Electric Engineering, Yanshan University, Qinhuangdao 066004, Hebei, China

Yasufumi Sakakibara and Michiko Sekiya
Department of Alzheimer's Disease Research, Center for Development of Advanced Medicine for Dementia, National Center for Geriatrics and Gerontology, Obu, Aichi 474-8511, Japan

Takashi Saito and Takaomi C. Saido
Laboratory for Proteolytic Neuroscience, RIKEN Center for Brain Science, Wako, Saitama 351-0198, Japan

Koichi M. Iijima
Department of Alzheimer's Disease Research, Center for Development of Advanced Medicine for Dementia, National Center for Geriatrics and Gerontology, Obu, Aichi 474-8511, Japan
Department of Experimental Gerontology, Graduate School of Pharmaceutical Sciences, Nagoya City University, Nagoya 467-8603, Japan

Tifei Yuan
Shanghai Key Laboratory of Psychotic Disorders, Shanghai Mental Health Center, Shanghai Jiao Tong University School of Medicine, Shanghai, China
Co-innovation Center of Neuroregeneration, Nantong University, Nantong, Jiangsu, China

Ali Yadollahpour
Department of Medical Physics, School of Medicine, Ahvaz Jundishapur University of Medical Sciences, Golestan Blvd, Ahvaz 61357-33118, Iran

Julio Salgado-Ramírez and Rocío Ortega-Palacios
Biomedical Engineering Department, Polytechnic University of Pachuca, Zempoala, Mexico

Daniel Robles-Camarillo
Graduate and Research Department, Polytechnic University of Pachuca, Zempoala, Mexico

Ernesto Alberto Rendón-Ochoa, Teresa Hernández-Flores, Victor Hugo Avilés-Rosas, Verónica Alejandra Cáceres-Chávez, Mariana Duhne, Antonio Laville, Dagoberto Tapia, Elvira Galarraga and José Bargas
División de Neurociencias, Instituto de Fisiología Celular, Universidad Nacional Autónoma de México, Circuito Exterior s/n Ciudad Universitaria, Col. Coyoacán, 04510 Ciudad de México, México

Xinshi Huang, Wei Qin, Ting Zhang, Xiaofang Zhu, Xiaochun Zhu and Xiaobing Wang
Rheumatology Department, The First Affiliated Hospital of Wenzhou Medical University, Wenzhou, China

Wenjing Ye
Rheumatology Department, The First Affiliated Hospital of Wenzhou Medical University, Wenzhou, China
Rheumatology Department, Ruian People's Hospital, Wenzhou, China

Siyan Chen
Neurology Department, The First Affiliated Hospital of Wenzhou Medical University, Wenzhou, China

Chongxiang Lin
Stomatological Department, The First Affiliated Hospital of Wenzhou Medical University, Wenzhou, China

Anne Petersen and Madeleine Zetterberg
Department of Clinical Neuroscience, Institute of Neuroscience and Physiology, Sahlgrenska Academy at the University of Gothenburg, Gothenburg, Sweden

Michelle Porritt and John Wiseman
IMED Biotech Unit, Discovery Biology, Discovery Sciences, AstraZeneca, Gothenburg, Sweden

Julia Adelöf and Malin Hernebring
Department of Clinical Neuroscience, Institute of Neuroscience and Physiology, Sahlgrenska Academy at the University of Gothenburg, Gothenburg, Sweden
IMED Biotech Unit, Discovery Biology, Discovery Sciences, AstraZeneca, Gothenburg, Sweden

My Andersson
Department of Clinical Sciences, Epilepsy Centre, Lund University, Lund, Sweden

Hana Hall
Department of Biochemistry, Purdue University, West Lafayette, IN 47907, USA

Jingqun Ma
Department of Biochemistry, Purdue University, West Lafayette, IN 47907, USA
Janelia Research Campus, Ashburn, VA 20147, USA

Sudhanshu Shekhar
Interdisciplinary Life Science (PULSe), Purdue University, West Lafayette, IN 47907, USA

Walter D. Leon-Salas
Purdue Polytechnic Institute, Purdue University, West Lafayette, IN 47907, USA

Vikki M. Weake
Department of Biochemistry, Purdue University, West Lafayette, IN 47907, USA
Purdue University Center for Cancer Research, Purdue University, West Lafayette 47907, USA

Herbert Izo Ninsiima
Department of Physiology, Faculty of Biomedical Sciences, Kampala International University, Western Campus, Ishaka, Uganda

Miriela Betancourt Valladares
Department of Human Physiology, University of Medical Sciences, Camagüey, Cuba

Constant Anatole Pie me
Department of Biochemistry and Physiological Sciences, Faculty of Medicine and Biomedical Sciences, University of Yaounde I, Yaounde, Cameroon

Ngala Elvis Mbiydzenyuy
Department of Physiology, Faculty of Biomedical Sciences, Kampala International University, Western Campus, Ishaka, Uganda
Department of Human Physiology, University of Medical Sciences, Camagüey, Cuba
Department of Biochemistry and Physiological Sciences, Faculty of Medicine and Biomedical Sciences, University of Yaounde I, Yaounde, Cameroon

Wonhye Lee, Phillip Croce, Ryan W. Margolin, Amanda Cammalleri, Kyungho Yoon and Seung-Schik Yoo
Wonhye Lee and Phillip Croce have contributed equally to this work Department of Radiology, Brigham and Women's Hospital, Harvard Medical School, 75 Francis Street, Boston, MA 02115, USA

Hong-Lin Su
Department of Life Sciences, Agriculture Biotechnology Center, National Chung-Hsing University, Taichung, Taiwan

Chien-Yi Chiang and Zong-Han Lu
Department of Neurosurgery, Taichung Veterans General Hospital, 1650 Taiwan Boulevard Sec. 4, 40705 Taichung, Taiwan

Fu-Chou Cheng and Chun-Jung Chen
Department of Medical Research, Taichung Veterans General Hospital, Taichung, Taiwan

Meei-Ling Sheu
Institute of Biomedical Sciences, National Chung-Hsing University, Taichung, Taiwan

Jason Sheehan
Department of Neurosurgery, University of Virginia, Charlottesville, VA, USA

Hung-Chuan Pan
Department of Neurosurgery, Taichung Veterans General Hospital, 1650 Taiwan Boulevard Sec. 4, 40705 Taichung, Taiwan
Faculty of Medicine, School of Medicine, National Yang-Ming University, Taipei, Taiwan

Adriana Schatton, Janis Mardink and Constance Scharff
Department of Animal Behavior, Freie Universität Berlin, Takustraße 6, 14195 Berlin, Germany

Gérard Leboulle
Department of Neurobiology, Freie Universität Berlin, Königin-Luise-Straße 28-30, 14195 Berlin, Germany

Julia Agoro
Department of Animal Behavior, Freie Universität Berlin, Takustraße 6, 14195 Berlin, Germany
Department of Neurobiology, Freie Universität Berlin, Königin-Luise-Straße 28-30, 14195 Berlin, Germany

Dmitry A. Sibarov, Ekaterina E. Poguzhelskaya and Sergei M. Antonov
Sechenov Institute of Evolutionary Physiology and Biochemistry, Russian Academy of Sciences, pr. Torez 44 Saint-Petersburg, Russia

Morten B. Schou, Ole Kristian Drange, Karoline Krane-Gartiser and Arne E. Vaaler
Department of Mental Health, Norwegian University of Science and Technology (NTNU), Trondheim, Norway
Division of Mental Health Care, St Olavs Hospital HF, avd Østmarka, Trondheim University Hospital, Postboks 3250, Torgarden, 7006 Trondheim, Norway

Sverre Georg Sæther
Department of Mental Health, Norwegian University of Science and Technology (NTNU), Trondheim, Norway
Division of Mental Health Care, St Olavs Hospital HF, Nidaros DPS, Trondheim University Hospital, Postboks 3250, Torgarden, 7006 Trondheim, Norway

Solveig K. Reitan
Department of Mental Health, Norwegian University of Science and Technology (NTNU), Trondheim, Norway
Division of Mental Health Care, Tiller DPS, St Olavs Hospital HF, Trondheim University Hospital, Postboks 3250, Torgarden, 7006 Trondheim, Norway

Daniel Kondziella
Department of Mental Health, Norwegian University of Science and Technology (NTNU), Trondheim, Norway
Neurology Department, Rigshospitalet, Copenhagen University Hospital, Blegdamsvei 9, 2100 København Ø, Denmark

Sidra Khalid, Hussain Ali and Salman Khan
Department of Pharmacy, Faculty of Biological Sciences, Quaid-i-Azam University, Islamabad 45320, Pakistan

Yeong S. Kim
Natural Products Research Institute, College of Pharmacy, Seoul National University, Seoul, South Korea

Muhammad Ammar Zahid
Department of Pharmacy, Faculty of Biological Sciences, Quaid-i-Azam University, Islamabad 45320, Pakistan

Department of Biotechnology, Faculty of Biological Sciences, Quaid-i-Azam University, Islamabad, Pakistan

Index